PLASTIC SURGERY

Editor

JOSEPH G. McCARTHY, M.D.

Lawrence D. Bell Professor of Plastic Surgery and
Director of the Institute of Reconstructive Plastic Surgery
New York University Medical Center
New York, New York

Editors, Hand Surgery Volumes

JAMES W. MAY, JR., M.D.

Director of Plastic Surgery and Hand Surgery Service
Massachusetts General Hospital
Associate Clinical Professor of Surgery
Harvard Medical School
Boston, Massachusetts

J. WILLIAM LITTLER, M.D.

Past Professor of Clinical Surgery
College of Physicians and Surgeons
Columbia University, New York
Senior Attending Surgeon
The St. Luke's–Roosevelt Hospital Center
New York, New York

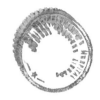

PLASTIC SURGERY

VOLUME 8
THE HAND
Part 2

W.B. SAUNDERS COMPANY
A Division of Harcourt Brace & Company
Philadelphia ※ London ※ Toronto
Montreal ※ Sydney ※ Tokyo

W.B. SAUNDERS COMPANY
A Division of
Harcourt Brace & Company

The Curtis Center
Independence Square West
Philadelphia, PA 19106

Library of Congress Cataloging-in-Publication Data

Plastic surgery.
    Contents: v. 1. General principles—v. 2–3.
The face—v. 4. Cleft lip & palate and craniofacial
anomalies—[etc.]
    1. Surgery, Plastic.   I. McCarthy, Joseph G., 1938–
[DNLM: 1. Surgery, Plastic. WO 600 P7122]

RD118.P536   1990   617′.95   87–9809

ISBN 0–7216–1514–7   (set)

25/7/94

Editor: W. B. Saunders Staff
Designer: W. B. Saunders Staff
Production Manager: Frank Polizzano
Manuscript Editor: David Harvey
Illustration Coordinator: Lisa Lambert
Indexer: Kathleen Garcia
Cover Designer: Ellen Bodner

Volume 1	0–7216–2542–8
Volume 2	0–7216–2543–6
Volume 3	0–7216–2544–4
Volume 4	0–7216–2545–2
Volume 5	0–7216–2546–0
Volume 6	0–7216–2547–9
Volume 7	0–7216–2548–7
Volume 8	0–7216–2549–5
8 Volume Set	0–7216–1514–7

Plastic Surgery

Printed in the United States of America.

Last digit is the print number: 9   8   7   6   5   4   3

Contributors

STEPHAN ARIYAN, M.D.
Professor of Surgery and Chief of Plastic and Reconstructive Surgery, Yale University School of Medicine; Chief of Plastic Surgery, Yale–New Haven Hospital, New Haven; Consultant in Plastic Surgery, Veterans Administration Hospital, West Haven, Connecticut.

PAUL W. BRAND, C.B.E.-M.B.-B.S., F.R.C.S.
Clinical Professor of Orthopaedics and Surgery, Louisiana State University Medical School; Senior Consultant, Gillis W. Long Hansen's Disease Center, Carville, Louisiana.

BENJAMIN E. COHEN, M.D.
Clinical Assistant Professor, Division of Plastic Surgery, Baylor College of Medicine; Academic Chief and Director, Plastic Surgery Residency Program, and Director, Microsurgical Research and Training Laboratory, St. Joseph Hospital, Houston, Texas.

MATTHIAS B. DONELAN, M.D.
Assistant Clinical Professor of Surgery, Harvard Medical School; Chief, Plastic and Reconstructive Surgery, Shriners Burns Institute, Boston; Assistant Surgeon, Massachusetts General Hospital, Boston, Massachusetts.

VINCENT R. HENTZ, M.D.
Associate Professor of Surgery, Stanford University School of Medicine; Chief, Division of Hand and Upper Extremity Surgery, Stanford University Hospital, Palo Alto, California.

LYNN D. KETCHUM, M.D.
Clinical Professor of Surgery, University of Kansas Medical Center, Kansas City; Attending Surgeon, Humana Hospital, Overland Park, Kansas.

J. WILLIAM LITTLER, M.D.
Senior Attending Surgeon, St. Luke's–Roosevelt Hospital Center, New York, New York.

RALPH T. MANKTELOW, M.D.
Professor and Head, Division of Plastic Surgery, University of Toronto Faculty of Medicine; Head of the Division of Plastic Surgery, Toronto General Hospital, Toronto, Ontario, Canada.

IVAN MATEV, M.D.
Professor of Orthopaedic Surgery, The Medical Academy; Head, Department of Upper Extremity Surgery, The Institute of Orthopaedics and Traumatology, Sofia, Bulgaria.

JAMES W. MAY, Jr., M.D.
Chief of Plastic and Reconstructive Surgery and Hand Surgery Service, Department of General Surgery, Massachusetts General Hospital; Associate Clinical Professor, Harvard Medical School, Boston, Massachusetts.

ROBERT M. McFARLANE, M.D.
Professor of Surgery and Head, Division of Plastic Surgery, University of Western Ontario Faculty of Medicine; Head, Division of Plastic Surgery, Victoria Hospital, London, Ontario, Canada.

MARY H. McGRATH, M.D.
Professor of Surgery and Chief, Division of Plastic and Reconstructive Surgery, George Washington University School of Medicine and Health Sciences; Chief of Service, University Hospital; Attending Surgeon, Children's Hospital National Medical Center, Washington, D.C.

ERIK MOBERG, M.D., Ph.D.
Professor Emeritus of Hand Surgery and Orthopaedic Surgery, University of Göteborg Medical School, Göteborg, Sweden.

WAYNE A. MORRISON, M.B., B.S., F.R.A.C.S.
Associate, Department of Surgery, University of Melbourne; Assistant Plastic Surgeon and Deputy

Director, Microsurgery Research Centre, St. Vincent's Hospital, Melbourne; Plastic Surgeon, Repatriation Hospital, Heidelberg, Melbourne; Consultant Plastic Surgeon, Geelong Hospital, Victoria, Australia.

JAMES F. MURRAY, M.D.

Professor Emeritus, Department of Surgery, University of Toronto Faculty of Medicine; Attending Surgeon, Sunnybrook Medical Center, Toronto, Ontario, Canada.

HENRY W. NEALE, M.D.

Professor of Surgery and Director, Division of Plastic, Reconstructive and Hand Surgery, University of Cincinnati College of Medicine; Attending Surgeon, University Hospital, Children's Hospital Medical Center, and Shriners Burns Hospital, Cincinnati, Ohio.

CHARLES L. PUCKETT, M.D.

Professor and Head, Division of Plastic Surgery, University of Missouri–Columbia School of Medicine; Attending Surgeon, University of Missouri–Columbia Hospital and Clinics, Harry S Truman Memorial Veterans Administration Hospital, Boone Hospital Center and Ellis Fischel State Cancer Hospital, Columbia, Missouri.

ROGER E. SALISBURY, M.D.

Professor of Surgery and Chief of Plastic and Reconstructive Surgery, New York Medical College; Director, Burn Center, Westchester Medical Center, Valhalla; Consultant, Plastic and Reconstructive Surgery, Castle Point Veterans Administration Hospital and Glythedale Children's Hospital; Chief of Plastic and Reconstructive Surgery, Metropolitan Hospital Center, New York, New York.

RICHARD J. SMITH, M.D. (deceased)

Clinical Professor of Orthopaedic Surgery, Harvard Medical School, Boston; Director of Hand Surgical Service, Department of Orthopaedic Surgery, Massachusetts General Hospital, Boston, Massachusetts.

JOSEPH UPTON, M.D.

Assistant Professor of Surgery, Harvard Medical School; Active Staff, Division of Plastic Surgery, Department of Surgery, Beth Israel Hospital and Children's Hospital, Boston, Massachusetts.

E. F. SHAW WILGIS, M.D.

Associate Professor of Plastic Surgery and of Orthopaedic Surgery, Johns Hopkins University School of Medicine; Chief, Division of Hand Surgery, Union Memorial Hospital, Baltimore, Maryland.

EDUARDO A. ZANCOLLI, M.D.

Professor of Orthopaedics and Traumatology, Medical School of Buenos Aires; Chief of Orthopaedic Surgery of the Rehabilitation Center of Buenos Aires, Buenos Aires, Argentina.

Preface

Where does a book begin? Initially, I think of a warm September afternoon in a hotel in Madrid when I first organized an outline of the chapters while waiting for an international surgery meeting to begin. However, a scientific book is only an extension of earlier publications. This text is descended from *Reconstructive Plastic Surgery*, edited in 1964 by my predecessor John Marquis Converse, and reedited in 1977. I had been Assistant Editor of the latter. Many of the ideas and principles, if not the exact words, that were integral to the teaching and writing of Dr. Converse live on in the present volumes. *Reconstructive Plastic Surgery* in turn was derived from his earlier collaboration with V. H. Kazanjian, *The Surgical Treament of Facial Injuries*, published in 1949, 1959, and 1974.

Earlier textbooks by Nélaton and Ombrédanne (1904), Davis (1919), Gillies (1920), and Fomon (1939) had played a germinal role in the development of modern plastic surgery. However, even these books represented only a continuum of publications extending back over the centuries to Tagliacozzi and Sushruta. Indeed, there are also the many surgeons who never published but who by their teachings contributed greatly to the body of knowledge that is represented in the present publication. Their concepts, too, have found their way into the plastic surgery literature for the edification of another generation of students.

My own career has been greatly influenced by my teachers, and their spirit has remained an integral part of my personal and professional life. This heritage of the plastic surgeon–teacher represents the spirit of this book.

The title defines the subject—*Plastic Surgery*. Adjectives such as *reconstructive* or *esthetic* are misleading and redundant and represent artificial divisions of this surgical specialty. The parents of the infant undergoing cleft lip repair are more interested in the *esthetic* aspects of the procedure, which traditionally has been regarded as *reconstructive*. The contemporary face lift, long perceived as an *esthetic* operation, represents a surgical reconstruction of the multiple layers of the soft tissues of the face. Plastic surgery, a term first popularized by Zeis in 1838, is preferred.

With the deliberate exception of parts of Chapters 1 and 35, originally written by Dr. Converse and revised through subsequent editions of various books, few paragraphs in these volumes remain unchanged from the 1977 edition. Many of the authors, however, have used material from the previous editions. Line drawings prepared for these editions by Daisy Stillwell have been reproduced again where appropriate. With the death of Ms. Stillwell, I was fortunate to recruit yet another outstanding medical artist, Craig Luce, to draw hundreds of new illustrations to reflect the continuing developments in this specialty.

The purpose of this book is to define the specialty of plastic surgery. To accomplish this goal, contributions have been sought from the acknowledged leaders of this discipline in all of its ramifications. The clinical applications of plastic surgery, practiced over the whole of the human anatomy, range from skin grafting to the management of uncommon craniofacial clefts, to replantation of the lower extremity. Its practice varies from uncomplicated procedures to sophisticated multistage reconstructions that ally the plastic surgeon with other specialists. The chapters that follow vary in the same way from the short and direct to the lengthy and complex. More than any other, this type of surgery strives for the restoration or improvement of form as well as the restoration of function. The teaching of plastic surgery thus lends itself to illustration. The contributors to this book have been encouraged to use drawings and photographs liberally as an enhancement of the principles and techniques described in the text. Special attention has been given to the sizing and placement of more than 5000 illustrations submitted in accordance with this plan. The contributors and publisher have also made every effort to acknowledge and cite the work of other authors. In a text of this magnitude any omission, while understandable, is regrettable.

In Volume 1 will be found discussions of the essential principles basic to all plastic surgery: wound healing, circulation of the skin, microneurovascular repairs, skin expansion, and grafting of tendons, nerves, and bone, as well as their associated methods of repair. This is the largest of the volumes and testifies to the broadening scope of the field. Much of what is now fundamental to the training of a plastic surgeon was only imagined a generation ago.

After the discussion of general principles in Volume 1, the organization of the text is by anatomic regions. Volumes 2 and 3 are devoted to the face; here, as throughout the book, each chapter draws upon the expertise of acknowledged master surgeons particularly experienced in the subjects on which they have written.

Clefts of the lip and palate as well as severe craniofacial anomalies make up Volume 4. In addition to plastic surgery, these chapters incorporate contributions from the allied fields of embryology, craniofacial growth and development, orthodontics, prosthodontics, speech pathology, and neurosurgery.

Volume 5 covers tumors of the skin and head and neck and Volume 6 the trunk, lower extremity, and genitourinary system. Of particular note, the text details recent advances in reconstruction that involve newly developed flaps of ingenious design and considerable sophistication.

The application of plastic surgical principles and techniques of the upper extremity are discussed in Volumes 7 and 8 under the editorship of Drs. James W. May, Jr., and J. William Littler. The latter, one of the most esteemed and influential hand surgeons of the modern era, edited the upper extremity section in 1964 and 1977. He has been joined in this edition by Dr. May, who is qualified in both hand surgery and microsurgical reconstruction. Both, who are my personal friends, brought their usual enthusiasm, experience, and equanimity to bear on this project. Because surgery of the upper extremity is practiced so extensively, ample space has been afforded for the comprehensive description of the reconstructive procedures specifically designed for the restoration of injured parts. Much of the current progress in plastic surgery of the upper extremity has been made possible by the gradual perfection of microvascular techniques, and these newer developments have been incorporated into the text.

Continuing change, the hallmark of all medical and surgical practice, dictates the need for a reference book such as this and makes its accomplishment a challenging task for everyone involved. With the writing of these words the lengthy process of revising, updating, and improving is ended. The book is committed to the press with the promise that it is both complete and current, in the belief that readers will find it an invaluable resource, and with the hope that it makes a contribution to the body of plastic surgery knowledge and to the education of tomorrow's plastic surgeon.

JOSEPH G. McCARTHY, M.D.

Contents

Paul W. Brand

Tendon Transfer Reconstruction for Radial, Ulnar, Median, and Combination Paralyses: Principles and Techniques

PRINCIPLES

Timing of Tendon Surgery

Time waits for no man. Tissues constantly change and adapt to current patterns of position and stress. The subconscious mind reacts to injury by a restless search for ways to compensate for the disaster. Instincts for survival range over all the options, and react with undue emotion in directions of hope or despair out of all proportion to what would seem a reasonable or sober judgment. All these factors have some effect on the success or failure of reconstructive surgery, and most should encourage us to do what needs to be done as early as possible, so that the patient's own creative efforts may be based on the new pattern of muscle balance, rather than on a situation that will have to be changed again.

The following are some of the factors that should be considered when planning the timing of tendon transfer operations.

Tissue Adaptation

Normal connective tissues and normal skin are constantly responsive to the patterns of mechanical stress imposed on them. Skin is loose at joints to allow normal motion. This loose, excess skin becomes absorbed if motion no longer occurs, as in paralysis. If normal motion is restored by recovery of muscles, the tissues gradually lengthen again. However, if the motion is to be restored by a transferred muscle that lies in a wounded bed, the pattern of scar around the tendon may be determined by the limitation of the reduced joint motion. The muscle may then be unable to overcome the drag of both joint stiffness and tendon scar adhesion.

For this reason, tendon transfers should be done as early as possible. If they have to be delayed for any reason, a program of passive range of motion exercises must be instituted to maintain tissue slack. If joints are already limited in passive range when first seen, any surgery must be delayed until exercises, massage, and splinting have restored the range of motion. This is particularly important if the perpendicular distance between the skin or fascia and the axis of the joint is great enough to result in a strong leverage of restraint. An example of this is the dorsal skin and fascia of the thumb web, which may become contracted after median palsy and is then an overwhelming obstacle to the restoration of pronation and abduction.

Tissue Homeostasis. It is very unwise to perform tendon transfer and tendon grafting procedures while there is any inflammatory state in the tissues through which the tendon must pass. If the wound that caused the nerve injury also involved the local tissues where the tendon must pass, it is better to postpone any elective surgery until the tissues are cool and mobile and without any inflammatory edema.

Psychologic State of Patient

A large part of the success of any muscle balance operation depends on the active cooperation of the patient. A hand injury is a very personal thing. It often involves a person's whole self-image and may induce fear, anger, and despair, or there may be a sort of denial of its reality and significance. After a whole series of rather turbulent mental and psychologic adjustments, the patient finally is able to consider rational and constructive alternatives for the future of his limb, and for its significance to his life and work. It is absolutely vital that the physician and other members of the rehabilitation team keep in touch with the patient and choose the right

moment to begin a discussion of the prospects, and the right moment to intervene with a surgical plan.

Once the patient gets into the hands of a lawyer who works on a contingency fee system, the prospects for recovery are very much reduced. At once it becomes clear to the patient that his best chance for substantial financial compensation, whether from employer or insurance company, is for his residual disability to be severe. The lawyer only has to begin talking in terms of the astronomical figures commonly quoted at the start of a compensation suit, and the patient begins to see his disability as a potential advantage. The subconscious mental conflict makes it very difficult for a patient to put any enthusiasm into the pre- and postoperative discipline that is essential to success.

The reason for the existence of the so-called "ambulance chasing lawyers" is that they know the value of getting their word in first. They want their client to think about money before they begin to admit that they are feeling better. If the physician gets to see the patient first, it is important to establish some basic attitude and goal for recovery. This hand is going to recover; it is going to be a useful hand; he can be proud of it and will be independent. The physician will work with the patient to get reasonable compensation for his injury (perhaps recommend a lawyer who works for an honest fee system), but his real security is his own recovered hands.

The reason the subject of compensation is discussed under the heading of "timing" is that the longer reconstructive surgery is delayed, and the more a patient is forced to remain idle, waiting for nerve regeneration, the more discouraged he becomes. Enforced idleness begets acceptance of idleness, and finally resentment at the prospect of work. It is easy for a surgeon to say "it will take a year for this repaired nerve to grow down to the muscles of the hand, so come back in a year and we will see if you need a tendon transfer." The patient who comes back a year later is a different person, and is less likely to succeed than he would have been a year earlier. Then again there is a real sense in which he may have lost a year of his life. What is a year worth? In some cases it is worth submitting to an operation that is intended only to restore good activity to a hand for a year, after which the old muscles might take over again if they recover. As we discuss various nerve paralyses, we shall point out that in some situations this policy is reasonable, where no real harm is done by an early transfer, even if the nerve should fully recover later. In weighing the value of such advice, let us recognize that the imponderable factors of hope, dignity, and self-esteem are at least as significant as the ponderable factors of grip strength and range of motion of joints.

Recovery of Nerves

This factor is last on this list in relation to timing because it is the one most commonly used to determine the timing of transfers. Obviously one needs to know whether a muscle is going to remain paralyzed before deciding whether to replace it, and the safest way to know is to wait until recovery actually takes place, or fails to take place when it should have. The trouble is that there are no precise rules about how long to wait, so that if a muscle is not recovering the physician may wait half as long again as the calculated time "just to make sure." In the case of a high ulnar nerve injury, this may mean a two year wait to be sure the intrinsic muscles will not recover.

To avoid unnecessary delays, some assumptions are in order. It is known that recovery is more likely in children and less likely in the elderly. It is known that recovery is most likely following a clean cut, and least likely following a contaminated laceration with loss of length and scarring and infection. Recovery is most likely following a fascicular repair by an experienced surgeon and least likely under emergency conditions by unspecialized surgeons. Muscle reinnervation is most likely when the injury is just proximal to the muscle because the motor fasciculae in the nerve are almost pure motor, and least likely when the injury is far proximal where the axons to any one muscle are widely distributed through the whole nerve. For example, repair of an ulnar nerve injury in the upper arm is likely to result in recovery of the affected forearm muscles, but very unlikely to give significant recovery to the intrinsic muscles of the hand, even after careful repair (Gaul, 1982).

If each of these factors is listed and given a weight for prognosis, there will be some patients in whom it is apparent that good recovery is so unlikely that early or immediate transfer of tendons is justifiable. In addition to this, a careful evaluation of nerve recovery, as by quantitative Tinel's sign (Omer, 1983), should be made at intervals, so that a failure of nerve recovery may be recognized early and corrected promptly, or else compensated for by muscle balance surgery without further waste of time.

Balance of Muscle Strength

Bunnell (1948) used to call tendon transfers "muscle balance operations." This brings out an important principle: we cannot add new strength to a hand after some muscles have become paralyzed; all we can do is to rearrange what is left so that *balance* is restored. Radial palsy removes about one-third of the summated tension capability of all muscles below the elbow. Therefore, we should not aim to restore the original extensor power of the wrist or fingers by tendon transfer, but perhaps two-thirds of each. In doing so, it would be reasonable to reduce by about one-third the strength of the activities that remained unparalyzed.

In order to plan a new muscle balance for the hand, after injury or disease, we should be able to calculate the effects of the loss of muscles and the probable effects of transferring others. We should also have some idea of the extent to which a muscle can change its mechanical characteristics after transfer to match the requirements of its new situation.

There are only two major variables that define the active capability of any muscle, and one variable to define its passive reaction to stress. The active variables are tension capability and excursion capability. The passive variable is the viscoelastic response to stretch and recoil. Most previous attempts to grade muscle "strength" have not distinguished among these three, and as a result wrong advice has been given about tendon transfers. Most of us were brought up to grade muscle strength on a scale of 1 to 5, where 5 was normal strength and 1 was just an ineffective twitch. We were further told that after a tendon was transferred it would ordinarily function at about one grade lower than it had in its original situation.

This has to be wrong. When a tendon is transferred, there is no reason for any change in any of its basic active characteristics. It has the same cross sectional area, and its fibers are the same length. It has the same number and quality of sarcomeres. Its blood supply is the same and its nerve supply has not been touched. Why should it be weaker? The answer is that it does not become weaker: it simply has a greater amount of passive drag to overcome before its tension capability can be fully transmitted to the joints where it is inserted. That drag is due mostly to the scar tissue surrounding the tendon and muscle in its new pathway. Once that fact is realized, it becomes obvious that a minor transfer involving the relocation of only the distal centimeter or two of tendon "weakens" a muscle much less than a major change of direction where a tendon and muscle has to be widely freed up and has to negotiate curves and angles, and therefore has to stretch a lot of scar before it can move.

ISOLATED MUSCLE FIBER

When a muscle fiber is considered as an isolated unit, a length-tension curve may be drawn that defines its capability. This curve demonstrates mechanical features that have been well described by Elftman (1966) (Fig. 114–1). When the muscle fiber is in the limb and in equilibrium with all other muscles, it rests more or less midway between its position of full contraction and its position of full passive stretch. In this state it is capable of its maximal contractile force. The tension capability is reduced as it shortens, becoming zero before it reaches one-half its resting length. When the fiber is lengthened its tension capability is also reduced, and it becomes near zero at about 50 per cent longer than its resting length. Thus, the resting length of any muscle fiber is about the same as the length of its maximal possible contraction

from full stretch to full active shortening. This is a useful relationship to remember, since the fiber length can be seen in any fresh cadaver dissection or at any operation when part of a muscle is exposed. If any one fiber of a muscle is traced carefully from its origin to its insertion on tendon, and if the limb is in a neutral position, the length of that fiber is the length through which it might contract under optimal conditions.

Blix (1891, 1893, 1894) extended the basic curve of a muscle fiber to include the length-tension curve of passive stretch and recoil of the muscle and its connective tissue (Fig. 114–2). The dotted line curve on the diagram represents the tension that is put into a muscle fiber when it is passively pulled out and lengthened. At any point, if the passive stretch is discontinued and if the muscle is stimulated to contract at the same time, the two curves, active and passive, may be added together, and the resultant curve shows the summated tension that pulls on the tendon. At full stretch, most of that high tension is simply passive recoil. Near full contraction the active muscle is on its own, with no help from passive recoil.

MUSCLES IN PAIRS

The contracting muscle fiber is not only without help from passive tension when it is short, but it is also hindered by passive tension. When Blix was drawing his curve he included the tension of the muscle he was studying, but he neglected to include the tensions in the opposing muscle with which the primary muscle is inescapably bound. This is ungrateful in that the tension available to augment the contraction of the stretched muscle has been put into it by the muscle on the other side of the limb that

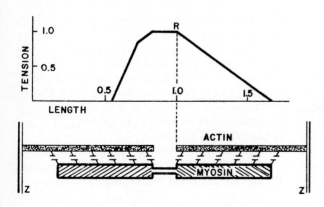

Figure 114–1. *Above,* Length-tension diagram of a single sarcomere unit. R = Physiologic resting length. *Below,* Diagram of sarcomere showing a pair of actin and myosin filaments between a pair of Z-plates.

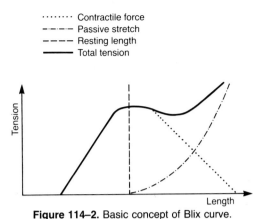

········ Contractile force
—·—·— Passive stretch
— — — Resting length
——— Total tension

Figure 114–2. Basic concept of Blix curve.

stretches it. It is also unrealistic because not only does the primary muscle benefit by its opposite muscle, but it also unavoidably has to return the favor by putting tension into its helper when the tables are turned. At this point, we had better call the muscles A and B and observe the diagram that dramatizes their interaction. Muscles can only contract. They have no ability to lengthen without help. When B contracts, it lengthens A. In doing so it uses some of its own energy and transfers it to A, so that A receives potential energy that it can expend later, to augment its own contraction from the stretched position. As muscle A shortens further, the roles are reversed and A has to use some of its own energy, in order to stretch muscle B. This limits the tension output of A for effective work. Thus the old Blix curve gives an incomplete idea of the length-tension behavior of a fiber.

The author has proposed a new diagram (Brand, 1985) that includes the two major elements of the Blix curve and adds a third element, which is the passive tension of an opposing muscle that must be stretched when the first muscle contracts (Fig. 114–3). When these three elements are added to give the true output of a muscle fiber, it is obvious that a muscle not only is able to generate tension more effectively in the stretched position because of passive stretch, but is able to generate tension *less* effectively in the contracted position because of the need to stretch its partner. The final composite diagram gives a more nearly square curve, with a shorter excursion, through which there is a more sustained tension.

The more one studies the reciprocal assistance that muscles constantly give to each

other, the less appropriate it seems to speak of "opposing muscle": they are partners. As in a dance, one retreats while the other advances in harmony, and either one is lost without the other (Fig. 114–4). This is a reminder that in cases of very severe paralysis, when the few remaining muscles have to be carefully distributed to the most essential functions of the hand, all muscle allocations must be considered in pairs. An isolated muscle is just a twitching lump of flesh until its loyal opposition challenges it to usefulness by putting it on the stretch.

MECHANICAL QUALITIES OF INDIVIDUAL MUSCLES

It is easy to be deceived about the mechanical qualities of a muscle by looking only at its gross appearance. Muscles such as the extensor carpi radialis brevis (ECRB) and the flexor carpi ulnaris (FCU) both look fusiform and seem to be about the same bulk, yet the former has 50 per cent longer fibers while the latter is capable of 50 per cent more tension (Table 114–1) (Brand, Beach, and Thompson, 1981). The author has prepared tables of all muscles below the elbow and has recorded figures for each one, giving tension capability and potential excursion as well as total mass in proportion to all the other muscles. These figures are approximations based on averages from a number of cadaver arms. The graph of these numbers in Figure 114–5 (Brand, Beach, and Thompson, 1981) provides a useful way of comparing the potential performance of various muscles that may be used for transfer. At surgery a quick way to judge muscle cross sectional area (or tension capability) is to observe tendon diameter. Elliott and Crawford (1965a,b) have shown that the cross sectional area of tendons is not exactly proportional to the cross sectional area of the muscle fibers whose tension they transmit, but they are a useful guide. Thus, an inherently weak muscle always has a slender tendon. This applies only to the state of the muscle in health. A recently paralyzed muscle retains a thick tendon for a long time after its muscle fibers have wasted away.

Changes After Transfer

In deciding which muscle to use as transfer, a surgeon may wonder whether a muscle with

Text continued on page 4932

Length—Tension Curve

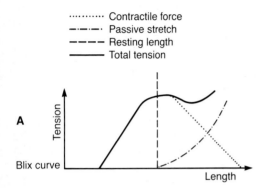

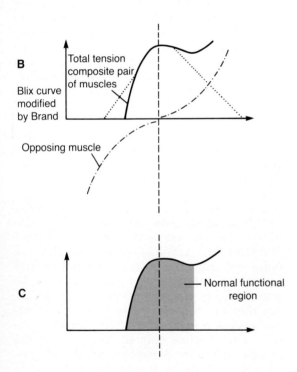

Figure 114–3. *A,* Blix curve, integrating the active contraction and elastic recoil. *B,* Brand curve integrating the above with the elastic curve of the opposing muscle subtracted from the active output of the primary muscle. *C,* Final approximate shape of muscle curve in situ in intact limb. (Note: The curve is more nearly square in shape compared with the isolated sarcomere in Figure 114–1. Also note the excursion is shorter than the potential excursion as judged from Figure 114–1.)

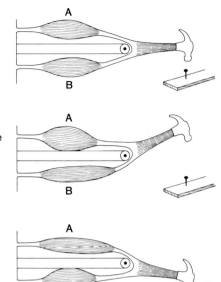

Figure 114–4. When the hammer strikes, it is using both the active contraction of *B* plus the elastic recoil in *B* that has been put into it by *A*.

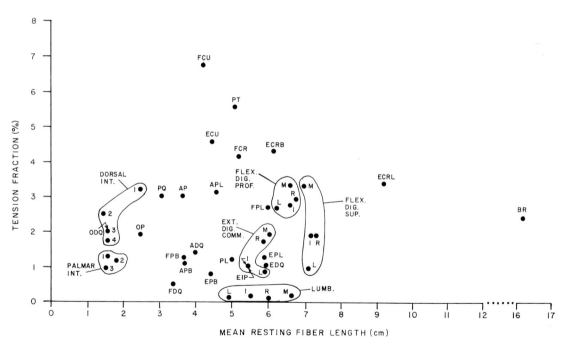

Figure 114–5. Using values from Table 114–1, this diagram shows the relationship between fiber length and tension producing capability. Muscle groups of similar function are circled together for clarity. ADQ = abductor digiti quinti; AP = adductor pollicis; APB = abductor pollicis brevis; APL = abductor pollicis longus; BR = brachioradialis; Dorsal Int. = dorsal interosseous (first, second, third, fourth); ECRB = extensor carpi radialis brevis; ECRL = extensor carpi radialis longus; ECU = extensor carpi ulnaris; Ext. Dig. Comm. = extensor digiti communis (index, middle, ring, little); EDQ = extensor digiti quinti; EIP = extensor indicis proprius; EPB = extensor pollicis brevis; EPL = extensor pollicis longus; FCR = flexor carpi radialis; FCU = flexor carpi ulnaris; Flex. Dig. Prof. = flexor digitorum profundus; FDQ = flexor digitorum quadratus; Flex. Dig. Sup. = flexor digitorum superficialis; FPB = flexor pollicis brevis; FPL = flexor pollicis longus; L = lumbricals (index, middle, ring, little); ODQ = opponens digiti quinti; OP = opponens pollicis; Palmar. Int. = palmar interosseous (first, second, third); PL = palmaris longus; PQ = pronator quadratus; PT = pronator teres.

Table 114–1. Alphabetical Reference List of Normal-Expected Values for Fiber Lengths, Mass Fractions, and Tension Fractions in Adult Males and Females

Muscle	Resting Fiber Length (cm) Mean*	Mass Fraction (%) Mean*	Mass Fraction (%) S.D.*	Tension Fraction (%) Mean*	Muscle	Resting Fiber Length (cm) Mean*	Mass Fraction (%) Mean*	Mass Fraction (%) S.D.*	Tension Fraction (%) Mean*
ADQ	4.0	1.1	0.23	1.4	FCU	4.2	5.6	0.66	6.7
AP	3.6	2.1	0.40	3.0	FDP				
APB	3.7	0.8	0.18	1.1	Index finger	6.6	3.5	0.76	2.7
APL	4.6	2.8	0.34	3.1	Middle finger	6.6	4.4	0.94	3.4
BR	16.1	7.7	2.0	2.4	Ring finger	6.8	4.1	1.1	3.0
Shortest fibers	10.9				Little finger	6.2	3.4	0.93	2.8
Longest fibers	21.3				FDS				
First DI					Index finger	7.2	2.9	0.64	2.0
First metacarpal origin	3.1	0.8	0.25	1.3	Middle finger	7.0	4.7	1.1	3.4
					Ring finger	7.3	3.0	0.84	2.0
Second metacarpal origin	1.6	0.6	0.11	1.9	Little finger	7.0	1.3	0.81	0.9
					FDQ	3.4	0.3	0.10	0.4
Total first DI	2.5	1.4	0.29	3.2	FPB	3.6	0.9	0.22	1.3
Second DI	1.4	0.7	0.17	2.5	FPL	5.9	3.2	0.42	2.7
Third DI	1.5	0.60	0.19	2.0	Lumbrical				
Fourth DI	1.5	0.50	0.13	1.7	Index finger	5.5	0.2	0.08	0.2
ECRB	6.1	5.1	1.3	4.2	Middle finger	6.6	0.2	0.06	0.2
ECRL	9.3	6.5	0.77	3.5	Ring finger	6.0	0.1	0.06	0.1
Shortest fibers	6.3				Little finger	4.9	0.1	0.05	0.1
Longest fibers	12.3				ODQ	1.5†	0.6	0.20	2.0
ECU	4.5	4.0	0.52	4.5	OP	2.4†	0.9	0.26	1.9
EDC					PI				
Index finger	5.5	1.1	0.20	1.0	First	1.5	0.4	0.12	1.3
Middle finger	6.0	2.2	0.51	1.9	Second	1.7	0.4	0.11	1.2
Ring finger	5.8	2.0	0.35	1.7	Third	1.5	0.3	0.08	1.0
Little finger	5.9	1.0	0.41	0.90	PL	5.0	1.2	0.34	1.2
EDQ	5.9	1.2	0.35	1.0	PQ	3.0†	1.8	0.32	3.0
EIP	5.5	1.1	0.36	1.0	PT	5.1	5.6	1.24	5.5
EPB	4.3	0.70	0.32	0.8	Superficial fibers	6.5			
EPL	5.7	1.5	0.48	1.3	Deep fibers	3.7			
FCR	5.2	4.2	0.87	4.1	Supinator	2.7†	3.8	0.95	7.1

*Data from 15 hands determined the mean and standard deviation of the mass fraction for each muscle. Mass and fiber length measurements from the last five of these hands were used to calculate tension fractions.

Figures for mass (or volume) of muscles are calculated as percentages of the total mass (or volume) of all muscles below the elbow. Figures for tension fraction also are percentages of the total of all muscles below the elbow.

†The fibers of these four muscles cross the joint axis with wide variation of fiber length. The figures quoted here for the mean fiber length of these four muscles are more visual estimates than mathematical averages. The mass fraction is accurate, but the tension fraction for these four muscles is only as true as the fiber length. Mean fiber lengths are included for the shortest and longest fibers of BR, ECRL, and PT because of the large range of fiber lengths. Values are included for the two segments of the first DI as well as total values. The data were not normalized for skeletal size differences.

From Brand, P. W., Beach, R. B., and Thompson, D. E.: Relative tension and potential excursion of muscles in the forearm and hand. J. Hand Surg., 6:209, 1981.

Table 114–2. Normal Values Abstracted From Table 114–1 and Listed in Order of Magnitude for Mean Fiber Lengths, Mass Fractions, and Tension Fractions for Adults

Mean Resting Fiber Length (cm)		Mass Fraction (%)		Tension Fraction (%)	
BR	16.1	BR	7.7	Supinator*	7.1
ECRL	9.3	ECRL	6.5	FCU	6.7
FDS (ring finger)	7.3	FCU	5.6	PT*	5.5
FDS (index finger)	7.2	PT	5.6	ECU	4.5
FDS (little finger)	7.0	ECRB	5.1	ECRB	4.2
FDS (middle finger)	7.0	FDS (middle finger)	4.7	FCR	4.1
FDP (ring finger)	6.8	FDP (middle finger)	4.4	ECRL	3.5
FDP (index finger)	6.6	FCR	4.2	FDP (middle finger)	3.4
FDP (middle finger)	6.6	FDP (ring finger)	4.1	FDS (middle finger)	3.4
Lumbrical (middle finger)	6.6	ECU	4.0	First DI	3.2
FDP (little finger)	6.2	Supinator	3.8	APL	3.1
ECRB	6.1	FDP (index finger)	3.5	AP	3.0
EDC (middle finger)	6.0	FDP (little finger)	3.4	FDP (ring finger)	3.0
Lumbrical (ring finger)	6.0	FPL	3.2	PQ*	3.0
EDC (little finger)	5.9	FDS (ring finger)	3.0	FDP (little finger)	2.8
EDQ	5.9	FDS (index finger)	2.9	FDP (index finger)	2.7
FPL	5.9	APL	2.8	FPL	2.7
EDC (ring finger)	5.8	EDC (middle finger)	2.2	Second DI	2.5
EPL	5.7	AP	2.1	BR	2.4
EDC (index finger)	5.5	EDC (ring finger)	2.0	Third DI	2.0
EIP	5.5	PQ	1.8	FDS (index finger)	2.0
Lumbrical (index finger)	5.5	EPL	1.5	FDS (ring finger)	2.0
FCR	5.2	First DI	1.4	ODQ*	2.0
PT	5.1	FDS (little finger)	1.3	EDC (middle finger)	1.9
PL	5.0	EDQ	1.2	OP*	1.9
Lumbrical (little finger)	4.9	PL	1.2	Fourth DI	1.7
APL	4.6	ADQ	1.1	EDC (ring finger)	1.7
ECU	4.5	EDC (index finger)	1.1	ADQ	1.4
EPB	4.3	EIP	1.1	EPL	1.3
FCU	4.2	EDC (little finger)	1.0	FPB	1.3
ADQ	4.0	OP	0.9	First PI	1.3
APB	3.7	FPB	0.9	Second PI	1.2
AP	3.6	APB	0.9	PL	1.2
FPB	3.6	Second DI	0.7	APB	1.1
FDQ	3.4	EPB	0.7	EDC (index finger)	1.0
PQ	3.0	Third DI	0.6	EDQ	1.0
Supinator	2.7	ODQ	0.6	EIP	1.0
First DI	2.5	Fourth DI	0.5	Third PI	1.0
OP	2.4	First PI	0.4	EDC (little finger)	0.9
Second PI	1.7	Second PI	0.4	FDS (little finger)	0.9
Third DI	1.5	FDQ	0.3	EPB	0.8
Fourth DI	1.5	Third PI	0.3	FDQ	0.4
ODQ	1.5	Lumbrical (index finger)	0.2	Lumbrical (index finger)	0.2
First PI	1.5	Lumbrical (middle finger)	0.2	Lumbrical (middle finger)	0.2
Third PI	1.5	Lumbrical (ring finger)	0.1	Lumbrical (ring finger)	0.1
Second DI	1.4	Lumbrical (little finger)	0.1	Lumbrical (little finger)	0.1

*See † footnote for Table 114–1.

From Brand, P. W., Beach, R. B., and Thompson, D. E.: Relative tension and potential excursion of muscles in the forearm and hand. J. Hand Surg., *6*:209, 1981.

inadequate mechanical qualities for its new task may develop improved qualities after a period of use and exercise. The answer is that muscles may improve their strength, or tension capabilities, but not their excursion potential. Regular exercise can increase the bulk and cross sectional area of muscle fibers, but it is doubtful whether more than a 50 per cent increase may be expected, even with a good exercise program. An unduly strong muscle may waste away somewhat and become weaker to match its diminished requirement, but there is danger in transferring a strong muscle to do a job that does not need much strength. If the strong transferred muscle is not synergistic, and contracts out of phase, it may overpower the normal muscle opposite and produce a deformity. The author has seen this when a FCU was used to replace a paralyzed abductor pollicis brevis (APB) and opponens pollicis (OP) in median palsy. The transferred FCU held the thumb in super opposition, and it stayed there.

The length of muscle fibers is *not* determined by the range of motion through which they are actually used. They are changed only in response to a change in their state of tension *at rest*. Thus, fibers that are held in a lengthened position at rest begin to add sarcomeres to each fiber until it is long enough to have a normal resting tension at that length. No amount of active exercise changes a short-fibered muscle to one that has longer fibers; the only way it can be changed is for a surgeon to pull on the tendon at the time of transfer and attach it at higher tension to its new insertion. Then, if it is held with the limb in neutral position, the resting tension of that muscle is high, and it stimulates the adding of length to each fiber until the resting tension is in balance with the other muscles. At this point the muscle is a longer-fibered muscle. This does not mean that it has a longer excursion, because actual excursion depends not only on the length of the muscle fiber, but also on the passive range of joint motion and on the limiting connective tissue. In the case of a transferred tendon, this is liable to be the dominant factor.

Matching of Tendon Excursions

The potential excursion of a muscle has already been defined as being proportional to, and perhaps equal to, the resting length of its fibers. However, the actual excursion of a given muscle in situ is limited by the range required of it, by the full range of motion of the joints that it crosses, and also by the elastic restraint of the connective tissue that invests it in that situation. The term "required excursion" is therefore used to designate the tendon movement that might be required of a tendon by the full movement of the joints it controls. The term "available excursion" (Freehafer, Peckham, and Keith, 1979) is also used as a measure of what is actually found at surgery when a tendon has been cut and pulled out to full stretch and then stimulated to full contraction. The relationship between the fiber length and the excursion at joints has been discussed in the German literature (Weber and Weber, 1836; Fick, 1850, 1904–11; Jansen, 1917) at some length, and the wide variance of opinion suggests that the conditions of measurement have not been defined. The author's experience is that the "available excursion" is usually responsive to the actual use to which the joints and muscles have been subjected. In older subjects this may often be very much shorter than the "potential excursion." The "required excursion" of the muscle in situ is about the same as the "available excursion" if the tendon crosses only one joint. In the case of tendons that cross several joints, it may be that one joint usually flexes while the others extend, and vice versa. If the habit pattern of use is always the same, it is the author's impression that the connective tissue closes in around the range of motion that is actually used, so that the full "potential excursion" is never used. If such a tendon is divided and tested at surgery, it will probably be found to have very limited excursion.

Terminology for Excursion

In view of the variety of ways in which the excursion of a tendon may be measured, the author suggests retaining as a standard the "potential excursion," because it is related to basic anatomy and does not change during adult life. However, this may be very different from the actual "available excursion" of the tendon the surgeon wishes to use. There is no known way to predict this with any accuracy except in the case of single-joint muscles, where it may be calculated from the range of motion of the joint and the known moment arm at the joint. It is suggested that surgeons should try to predict, and then to measure excursion at surgery (see Table 114–1). Figure 114–6 gives the approximate moment arm of every tendon at the wrist. It is known that when a joint moves through 60 degrees (actually 57.29) (Fig. 114–7), all tendons that cross that joint move through an excursion roughly equal to their moment arm at the joint. It may be calculated from the measured range of motion of every affected joint just how much excursion is required of a given tendon to move through its whole range; this is the "required excursion." At operation, after division of the tendon, and

before it is freed up, it may be pulled distally by a stitch through the end of the tendon that is to be discarded. If the operation is being done under local anesthesia, the patient may now be asked to contract the muscle. If there is general anesthesia, the muscle may be stimulated by a fine flexible electrode. The excursion from the stretched position to the contracted position is the "available excursion."

Finally, after surgery and early rehabilitation, the function of the transferred tendon may be evaluated by summating its calculated excursion at each joint, to see if its predicted range comes up to expectations.

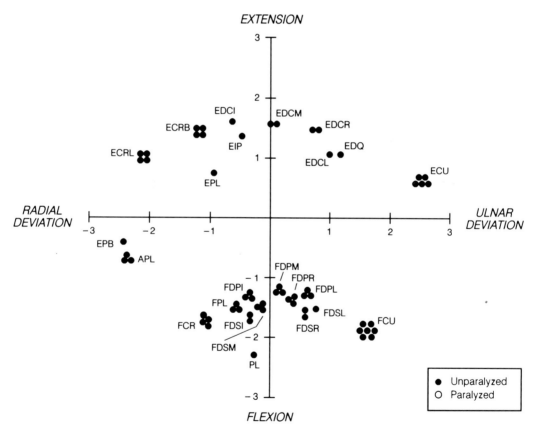

Figure 114–6. This is not an anatomic diagram; it is a simplified mechanical statement of the capability of each muscle to affect the wrist joint. The positions of the tendons in relation to the axes of flexion-extension and of ulnar-radial deviation represent their moment arms at the wrist. The number of dots in each cluster is an indication of the tension capability of that muscle-tendon unit, rounded off to the nearest whole number. APL = abductor pollicis longus; ECRB = extensor carpi radialis brevis; ECRL = extensor carpi radialis longus; ECU = extensor carpi ulnaris; EDCI = extensor digitorum communis (index); EDCL = extensor digitorum communis (little); EDCM = extensor digitorum communis (middle); EDCR = extensor digitorum communis (ring); EDQ = extensor digiti quinti; EIP = extensor indicis proprius; EPB = extensor pollicis brevis; EPL = extensor pollicis longus; FCR = flexor carpi radialis; FCU = flexor carpi ulnaris; FDPI = flexor digitorum profundus (index); FDPL = flexor digitorum profundus (little); FDPM = flexor digitorum profundus (middle); FDPR = flexor digitorum profundus (ring); FDSL = flexor digitorum superficialis (little); FDSI = flexor digitorum superficialis (index); FDSM = flexor digitorum superficialis (middle); FDSR = flexor digitorum superficialis (ring); FPL = flexor pollicis longus; PL = palmaris longus.

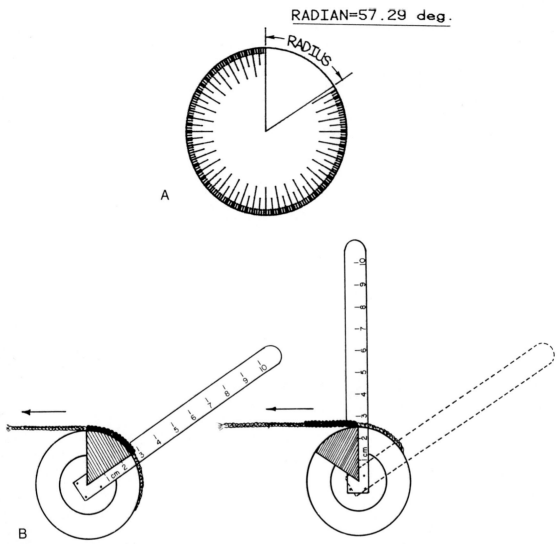

Figure 114–7. *A*, A radian. The length of a radius, measured on the circumference, is joined to the center by two radii. *B*, The way in which the lengthwise movement of a tendon may be used to measure the moment arm of a joint. If the joint (or wheel) moves 57.29 degrees, the length of rope that runs off the pulley must be equal to its moment arm at the joint (i.e., the radius of the pulley).

This may appear tedious, but it is only by using numbers and by checking presumptions that progress is made.

MULTIPLE JOINTS IN PARALLEL

When many muscles are paralyzed it is sometimes a good plan to use one transferred muscle to share more than one task through a number of insertions. A good example is in high ulnar-median palsy when a single wrist extensor tendon may be transferred to power several flexor profundus tendons. This is fine, provided it is recognized that every insertion must move together, or none will move. There are functional implications and the patient must understand that he will be unable, for example, to flex one finger without all fingers becoming flexed. It also means that if one insertion is prevented from moving, as by stiffness, none will be able to move. A severely stiff finger should never be included with mobile fingers in a common transfer.

Another implication of multiple insertions in parallel is that every insertion of one muscle must move exactly the same distance at the same time. If a motor tendon is split between two insertions and if one insertion has a larger leverage or moment arm than the other, the joint served by the larger moment arm will move through a smaller range of motion than the other, since large moment arms mean more power but less motion. If both tendon slips are attached to the same joint (as when two wrist extensors are activated by the pronator teres in radial palsy), the one with the smaller moment arm will transmit the force while the one with the larger moment arm will become slack (Fig. 114–8).

MULTIPLE JOINTS IN SERIES

If one tendon is made to cross more than one joint in series (one after the other), the problem is quite different. The stiffness of one joint does not hinder the action of the tendon at the others; in fact it helps them, by freeing up extra excursion. The problem is that there is no way the muscle can exert selective tension at different joints. The joints are affected in proportion to the leverage or moment arm of that tendon at each joint. There can be individual effect at different joints only by having other muscles oppose or else augment the tendon at one or another joint. A single tendon crossing several joints can produce coordinated motion at all the joints only if the moment arms are in proportion to the local resistance and if there is no external force to work against. For example, a finger or thumb can be fully flexed by a single tendon if the tendon is in a sheath that holds it to the existing pulley system (Fig. 114–9*A*). If external force is applied to the end of the digit (Fig. 114–9*B*), as from a firm pinch action between fingertip and thumbtip, the moment arms of the external force are

much larger at the proximal joints than at the distal ones because the moment arms of the external force are measured along the length of the finger, while those of the tendon are part of the thickness of the finger. The digit will not be under control (Brand, 1985). This is illustrated in the thumb by the hyperextension of the metacarpophalangeal joint and the hyperflexion of the tip (Froment's sign) (Fig. 114–10).

Changing Excursions and Moment Arms

It is sometimes possible to change the pathway of a tendon in such a way that its effect at a joint is modified. Pulley advancement has been used to give flexor tendons greater moment arm at the metacarpophalangeal joint, to compensate for paralysis of the intrinsic muscles. This is not recommended because it is most effective when the joint is flexed, so that the tendon bowstrings. It is least effective when the joint is straight, which is when extra flexion moment is needed.

By making a tendon cross from the palmar to the dorsal side of the limb, or vice versa, it is sometimes possible to reduce or increase the excursion needed for a distal action. For example, if a wrist extensor is to be used in place of the intrinsic muscles in a hand, there are two obvious alternatives. If the ECRB is extended by grafts across the dorsum of the wrist and through the intermetacarpal spaces to cross the metacarpophalangeal joints on the palmar side, it remains as a wrist extensor while it flexes the metacarpophalangeal joints, and extends the interphalangeal joints.

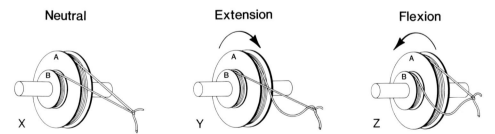

Neutral	Extension	Flexion

Figure 114–8. Two wheels of different diameters, fixed to each other and moving around the same axis, simulate a joint crossed by two tendons, where one tendon is closer to the axis than the other. For example, the rope on wheel *A* could be extensor carpi radialis brevis (ECRB), while that on wheel *B* is the extensor carpi radialis longus (ECRL), closer to the axis of extension-flexion. In *X* the two tendons are joined to each other to share a common motor. In *Y* the motor pulls; the tendon with the big moment arm becomes slack while the tendon nearer to the axis does the work. In *Z* the wrist flexes, and now the ECRL becomes loose and the ECRB does the work. This demonstrates the foolishness of using one muscle to move two insertions if they have different moment arms.

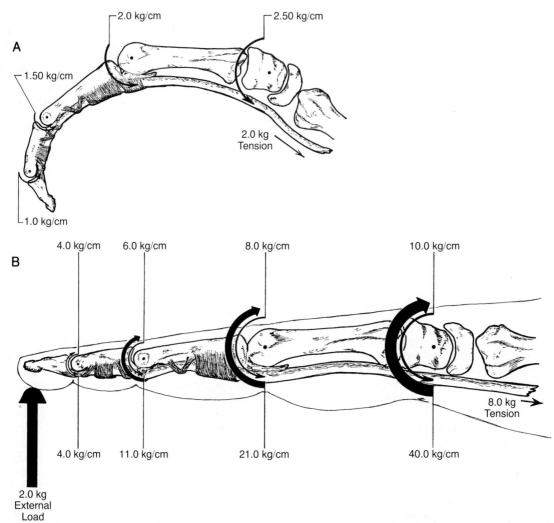

Figure 114–9. *A,* Based on moment arms of the flexor profundus of the distal interphalangeal (DIP) joint 0.5 cm, the proximal interphalangeal (PIP) 0.75 cm, the metacarpophalangeal (MP) 1.0 cm, and at tendon tenson of 2 kg, the actual flexion torque at each joint is shown by an arrow and figures above. *B,* A diagram based on the same moment arms for the profundus, but now with an external force of 2.0 kg at the fingertip, pushing the finger toward extension. There is a tension of 8.0 kg in the tendon to hold the DIP joint in equilibrium; the other joints are seen to be out of balance. The external force has a moment arm of 2.0 cm at the DIP joint, 5.5 cm at the PIP joint, 10.5 cm at the MP joint, and 20 cm at the wrist. The figures for flexor torque (from the tendon) are printed above the joint and that for extensor torque (from external force) are printed below. Equilibrium is impossible without the addition of other muscles at each proximal joint.

These three actions commonly occur together, and the ECRB needs to have enough excursion for them all. This might be 1.5 cm for 60 degrees of wrist extension, plus 1.5 cm for metacarpophalangeal flexion, plus 0.5 cm for interphalangeal extension, totaling 3.5 cm. If the tendon, extensor carpi radialis longus (ECRL) this time, is taken round to the front of the forearm, it becomes a wrist flexor. If it passes deep to the finger flexors in the carpal tunnel, it has only about 1.0 cm flexion moment arm for the wrist. Since hand synergism still calls for wrist extension with finger flexion, the ECRL will be lengthened at the wrist about 1.0 cm for 60 degrees extension while it is shortened at the metacarpophalangeal joints 1.5 cm, and at the interphalangeal joints 0.5 cm. This means that a typical move into the position of intrinsic action with 60 degrees of wrist extension may be accomplished with 1.0 cm excursion of the ECRL. It could almost be accomplished with a tenodesis and no muscle, as suggested by Riordan (1953), but that would have the disadvantage

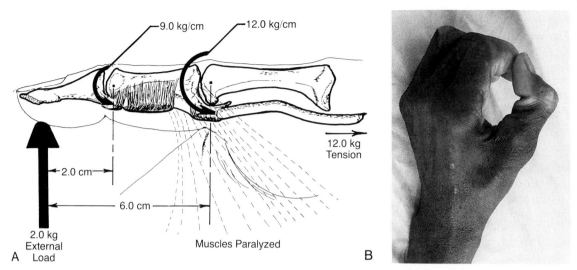

Figure 114–10. *A,* When 2 kg force is applied at the tip of the thumb, at right angles to its length, pushing it into extension, it exerts about three times as much torque at the metacarpophalangeal (MP) joint as at the interphalangeal (IP) joint. The long flexor tendon, which has less than twice the torque at the MP joint than at the IP joint, cannot hold the MP joint in balance without the help of the intrinsic muscles (adductor pollicis). In ulnar palsy, the flexor pollicis longus (FPL) can hold the MP joint in balance against 2 kg force only by providing excessive flexor torque at the IP joint. This results in IP flexion (Froment's sign), which can be corrected only by an extra flexor for the MP joint or by fusion of one of the joints (the MP). *B,* Froment's sign.

that every wrist extension would be accompanied by intrinsic action. It cannot be switched off.

Those who use the FCU for finger extension in radial palsy make similar assumptions. They assume that the patient will want to extend his wrist every time he flexes his fingers. Therefore, the very short-fibered FCU can be an effective finger extensor, but only if the wrist is flexed. It can allow wrist flexion, but only if the fingers are extended. This is acceptable only if better alternatives are not available; usually they are available (see under Radial Nerve Paralysis).

Management of Passive Soft Tissue Resistance

Tendon transfers fail more often from the effects of adhesions than from any other cause. It might be better to leave a hand unbalanced from nerve damage than to transfer a tendon that then becomes adherent. Not only does the transferred tendon fail to do its new job, but it is also lost from its original function, and it inactivates the muscles that oppose its new function, since those muscles cannot contract without the mobility of their partner. Very little is written about this problem, and it is difficult to learn about it, even

from one's mistakes, because there is no easy way to quantify stiffness or to follow the process of mobilization with really repeatable measurements.

The very word "adhesions" does not cover the problem fully, for there are aspects of postoperative stiffness that are unrelated or only indirectly related to adhesions. The author prefers to use the term "drag" to cover all soft tissue resistance to active movement. Ways can then be devised to measure total resistance and plot it against total active moment or torque. Once we begin to use repeatable measurements, we shall be in a position to identify techniques that promote mobility and factors that oppose it.

It has already been shown how muscle tension may be plotted against fiber length in Elftman's curve (see Fig. 114–1). Figure 114–2 showed how, in the Blix curve, the passive elastic recoil of a muscle in situ may be plotted on the same graph, and summated to reveal how they work together in the contraction of a stretched muscle. It was then shown how the need to stretch the opposing muscle required work to be done that diminished the ability of the primary muscle to contract at the short end of its length-tension curve. Thus, the output of an intact muscle in its own bed is determined by a dynamic balance between active and passive forces that can be represented on the length-tension curves of a pair of opposing muscles and shown to *augment* and to *diminish* each other.

When a muscle tendon unit is transferred, it is necessary to add a new factor to that curve and integrate it into the total pattern. That new factor is the scar that surrounds the muscle and tendon in its new bed after transfer, and resists movement in any direction.

Yamada (1970) has collected mechanical data about many different tissues (Fig. 114–11). Some have had tension applied to them while their changing length has been measured and recorded as length-tension curves. From a broad spectrum of these curves, it is possible to recognize three major types. Tissues such as fascia, tendon, and ligament are designed to resist lengthening and to transmit tension. They have a rather steep, straight length-tension curve. They may be lengthened a maximum of about 10 per cent with high tension. Others, such as skin and fatty connective tissue, permit up to about 100 per cent lengthening under moderate tension before the curve turns steeply upward, indicating a limit to stretch. A third type of tissue, exemplified by *paratenon*, is specialized to permit extensive free movement. It has a long, low curve where very little tension results in considerable length-

ening before the curve finally turns up into a terminal steeper section.

Scar tissue composed of undifferentiated collagen tends to have a steep length-tension curve. When a tendon is transferred from a bed in which it is attached to *paratendinous* "gliding" tissue to a new bed in which it lies on raw bone or fascia, the curve of elastic resistance to movement changes from a long, low type of curve to a short, steep one. If the new bed of the transferred tendon is composed of fatty connective tissue with no raw bone or cut fascia, the new curve will be intermediate in profile, because although the scar may not stretch easily, the fatty tissue that becomes attached to the tendon moves with it and stretches, to give a more compliant profile to the length-tension curve. The curve of the tendon that lies on naked bone and fascia will be very steep and may not change much in subsequent weeks, because scar models slowly. The length-tension curve of the tendon lying only on fat changes much faster and begins to look more like a paratenon curve if the patient keeps it stimulated by frequent movement. This is because normal fatty connective tissue is much more responsive and remodels under stress, even though the scar that binds it to the tendon changes little or not at all.

The composite functional curve of a trans-

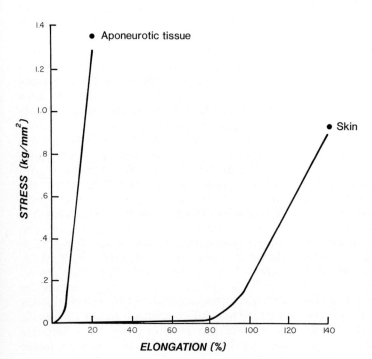

Figure 114–11. Length-tension curves of two different soft tissues. Tendons and ligaments behave like aponeurotic tissue.

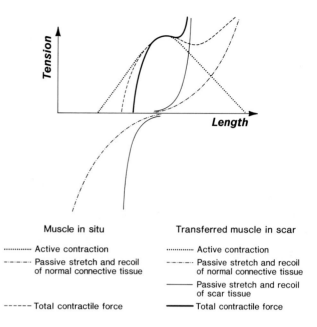

Figure 114–12. Theoretical length-tension diagram of a muscle fiber as part of a muscle that has been transferred into a bed where it is restricted by scar tissue adhesions. Note that the muscle still retains its previous active and elastic qualities, but is not able to use them because it is held close to its resting length by scar. Below the baseline are passive forces that resist shortening of muscle.

ferred muscle (Fig. 114–12) shows that the peak tension is not very different from that of the same muscle before it was moved. However, the range through which it can exercise that tension is grossly shortened. It is this shortening of range that makes the muscle less effective, and has led surgeons in the past to claim that a muscle is "weaker" by one grade after transfer. The shortened range can be gradually lengthened again, but it takes time and discipline to do so, and the success of the process depends a great deal on the quality of the tissues that have become attached to the muscle-tendon unit.

In view of the importance of the factor of *drag* in tendon transfers, it is suggested that surgeons and therapists should make a habit of trying to measure the changing profile of this passive restraint during rehabilitation. They should try to relate it to surgical technique and to different programs of exercise or splinting after surgery.

It is not possible to measure length or tension of individual tissues without opening up the hand again. However, it is possible to obtain a very repeatable gross measurement of total drag by applying measured torque to a joint that is crossed by the tendon, and recording the changes of angle that occur with each successive change of torque. This gives a torque-angle curve that may be repeated at intervals to follow the gradual freeing-up of the tissues that restrain tendon

and joint movement (Brand, 1985). The author uses a standardized method based on an unchanging lever arm for the torque and the application of a series of standard forces on the digit, while measuring the angle of the joint at each change of torque. The tension force may be applied at right angles to the limb segment through a loop of string at the joint crease beyond the joint being measured (Fig. 114–13). A succession of tensions are applied through a calibrated spring, while the joint angles are measured for each tension. The torque is the *ordinate* of the graph, while the joint angles are on the *abscissa*.

To evaluate the drag due to the tendon transfer separately from the factor of joint stiffness, the proximal joints (e.g., the wrist) should be held stable first in a position that relaxes the tendon and then in a position that results in the distal joint being limited by tendon tightness within its own free range of motion. The difference between the two torque-angle curves demonstrates the restriction due to tendon adhesions and drag.

Surgical Techniques to Minimize Drag

It is a principle of tendon transfers that the tendon should run as straight a course as possible from its origin to its new insertion. However, there should not be any unneces-

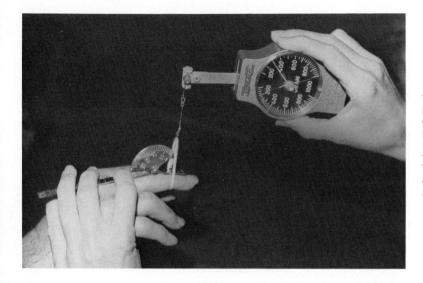

Figure 114–13. Measuring the torque angle of a proximal interphalangeal (PIP) joint. The force gauge measures the tension applied at the distal interphalangeal (DIP) joint crease to provide extension torque at the PIP joint. The goniometer measures the angle at 300 gm force at the lever arm from the joint to joint/crease.

sary freeing-up of the muscle or tendon, because this creates scar. Freeing-up at surgery results in binding-down later and is only justified if definite lateral attachments are present (as in the brachioradialis) or if a marked change of direction is involved.

Whenever possible, the route of the tendon should not be dissected at all. It should be tunneled with a round-nosed tunneling instrument, designed to allow the jaws to be opened without opening the shaft (Fig. 114–14). The thickest part of the tunneler should be near the tip, so that the surgeon can be sensitive to each tissue as it is first being traversed. Careful tunneling ensures that the tendon pathway is lined with loose areolar tissue from end to end.

In those parts of the path that have to be dissected open, no bone or fibrous septum should be cut or scratched. If this is unavoidable, there should be an attempt to cover the raw surface with a flap of fat or loose connective tissue.

The tendon itself should never be scratched or bruised or held by forceps except at the end that is to be discarded. When it is to be pulled out through a proximal incision, before rerouting, the instrument used should be large and smoothly rounded, like a large uterine dilator; never one with edges. No real force should be used. It is far better to make an additional small incision to find out why a tendon does not come easily than to pull harder and risk even minimal bruising of the tendon or tearing at the musculotendinous junction. The most intractable adhesions often occur at the site of suture lines between a tendon and a graft or other tendon. Meticulous care must be taken to have all tendon edges accurately apposed. No cut end of ten-

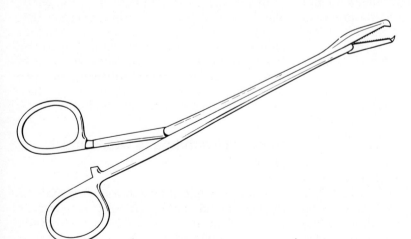

Figure 114–14. Tendon tunneling forceps (Andersen). When the jaws are closed, the nose is smooth rounded. The viper-shaped head places the thickest part of the tunneling forceps just behind the nose.

don should be left exposed in the wound. When possible it is good to have the suture of the tendon to the tendon graft completed before the composite tendon is tunneled, so that the junction itself may come to lie in an intact, unwounded part of the pathway.

Tendons should never be left to dry while the new pathway is being prepared; especially they should not be allowed to lie on bare skin. All incisions must be made first; then, all necessary dissections should be completed; finally, the tendon may be withdrawn proximally and *immediately* placed or tunneled into its new bed. If delay is necessary, the tendon must be wrapped in moist gauze and any exposed parts kept wet by dribbled saline.

Since adhesions are inevitable, the surgeon should plan for them to occur in an optimal position. Adhesions form in the position where the tendon lies during healing, postoperatively. Their elastic recoil always assists movement toward that position, and resists movement away from it. In most cases the hand should be positioned so that the limb and digits are near the position toward which the new transfer is planned to move them. This means that the main movement of the transfer will be helped by its adhesions. It also means that the task of lengthening the adhesions falls on the unoperated opposing muscle rather than on the transferred muscle, which will feel unsure of itself for quite a while after transfer. The tendon need not be at its full terminal position, however, since there is advantage in having adhesions move both ways. A 2 mm lengthening of an adhesion allows 4 mm of extra tendon motion if it is pulled both distally and proximally, but only 2 mm if its attachment is at the extreme end of its trajectory.

Points of Technique. In transferring one motor tendon to move two or more distal tendons, as in reactivating finger extensors, it is important to look carefully at the inevitable distally open V-junctions (or Y-junctions). If such junctions are made and the hand is then immobilized with the junction lying in the most proximal position of its normal range of movement, there is a danger of an absolute block to movement caused by any structure that lies between the two legs forming the "V." This is like the predicament of a downhill skier who allows the two limbs of his own "V" to go one on each side of a tree in his path. He comes to a halt, not

gradually but suddenly and finally. The surgeon must make sure there is no septum or scar between the two tendon limbs in the range of excursion of the tendon. This would happen if a single motor were attached to the tendon of the extensor pollicis longus and also to the extensor indicis proprius or extensor digitorum communis to the index finger. The tendon junction might be made just proximal to the retinaculum, with the digits extended. The septum between the compartments of the retinaculum would impinge in the crotch of the tendon junction and prevent finger flexion.

SUGGESTED PATTERNS FOR SPECIFIC NERVE INJURIES

Radial Nerve Paralysis

The radial nerve is wholly responsible for wrist extension. It also controls the extension of the metacarpophalangeal joints of the fingers and thumb, and it stabilizes the base of the thumb in extension for effective pinch. The only one of these that is essential for every basic hand function is wrist extension; the hand is useless without it. If quick recovery is to be expected, as when the injury to the nerve is distal and clean-cut, the patient should be fitted with a cock-up splint for the wrist and encouraged to use his hand freely. The splint must be worn day and night to avoid shortening of muscles on the flexor side. If the recovery of the nerve is in doubt or is expected to take several months, it is worth considering a transfer of the pronator teres (PT) to the ECRB, leaving the latter in continuity. This can be done immediately so that the patient can use his hand freely while awaiting the recovery of all the muscles. If they do recover, there is often no need to undo the transfer, since the pronator continues to pronate with its new attachment.

In planning definitive transfers, it is worth looking at the diagram of moment arms around the wrist (Fig. 114–15). This shows that no active muscle remains dorsal to the axis of flexion-extension after radial palsy. It also shows that the most effective radial and ulnar deviators are gone. Thus, if a transfer for wrist extension should be eccentric in relation to the deviation axis, the remaining muscles may not be able to compensate for it.

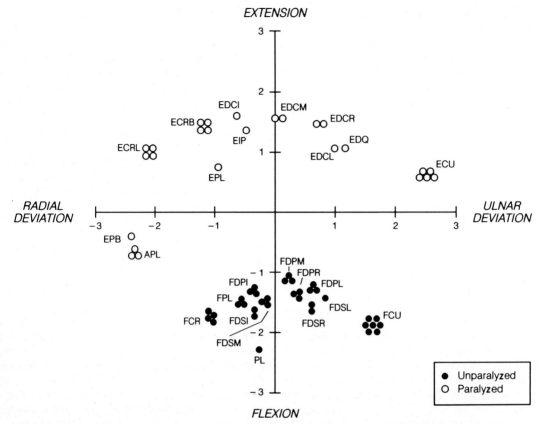

Figure 114–15. Radial palsy: effect at the wrist. In this diagram each tendon that crosses the wrist is represented by a group of circles, each of which denotes 1.0 unit on our scale of relative tension (see Table 114–1). We have used the nearest whole number. Each tendon lies in its mechanical relationship to the axes of flexion-extension and of radial and ulnar deviation. The black circles are normal muscles and the white circles are paralyzed muscles. (See Fig. 114–6 legend for abbreviations.)

WRIST EXTENSION

In the normal wrist the three dedicated extensors have a total relative tension capability of about 13 on the scale used by Brand (1981) the ECU having the highest, but with the smallest moment arm. Their total relative moment is also about 13, the ECRB being the highest because it has the largest moment arm. Since the total tension capability of all muscles crossing the wrist is reduced by about 45 per cent in radial palsy, a good final balance should aim at all functions being about three-fifths of normal. An ideal tendon transfer for wrist extension should provide a relative moment of about 8 (three-fifths of 13). Several different muscles have been used in the past.

The flexor carpi ulnaris (FCU) was used by Weitz (1916). This muscle can provide plenty of tension, but is out of phase.

The flexor carpi radialis (FCR) was used by Henry (1916). This gives acceptable tension and excursion. It is out of phase.

The flexor digitorum superficialis (FDS) was used by Biesalski and Mayer (1916). This muscle is in good synergistic phase, but is preferred by some for finger extension, where it is out of phase but avoids adhesions because it has a long tendon and needs no proximal suture.

The pronator teres (PT) was used by McMurray (1919). This is preferred by most surgeons today. It has a relative tension of about 5½ and provides about 8 units of moment when attached to the ECRB insertion.

PRONATOR TERES AS A WRIST EXTENSOR

This is an ideal muscle so far as tension is concerned. It is also easy to reeducate and it does not have to change direction, so it needs minimal dissection and develops few adhesions. It also continues its original function after transfer, since it does not alter its relationship to the axis of pronation and supination. So it is perfect? Not quite! The PT has a number of different muscle fiber lengths, because it is one of the few forearm muscles whose fleshy fibers cross the axis of its action. Thus, the superficial fibers that are farther from the pronation-supination axis are longer than the deep fibers. All the fibers need the same amount of *extra* excursion in relation to their new action at the wrist joint. This is only a small *percentage* more excursion than is available from the superficial fibers, but is a much larger *percentage* of what is available from the shorter deep fibers. This may limit the range of wrist flexion during supination, and of wrist extension during pronation. Overall, however, the PT makes an excellent substitute for the wrist extensors.

There are various ways to insert the pronator for wrist extension. If it were to be inserted into the ECRL, it would be a weak wrist extensor because the moment arm of the ECRL for extension is short. Also, the wrist would be in uncontrolled radial deviation, because the ECRL has a very large moment arm for that.

If the pronator is inserted into the tendon of the ECRB, it will have an effective moment for wrist extension, but some difficulty in achieving the full range of extension-flexion because of the shortness of some deep pronator muscle fibers. This is acceptable, but it also has the problem of uncontrolled radial deviation, though less severely than the ECRL insertion. The author uses a yoke or bridle insertion to avoid this problem. The pronator is attached to the ECRB tendon, then the ECRL tendon is detached from its insertion and withdrawn through the proximal incision. Tunneling forceps are then introduced through a small incision over the base of the fourth metacarpal bone, and passed under the extensor retinaculum and subcutaneously to the proximal incision. The end of the ECRL tendon is there grasped and pulled through and attached to ligamentous fibers at the base of the fourth metacarpal. Finally, the ECRL and ECRB tendons are matched for tension proximally, with the wrist in neutral deviation, and are then attached to each other at the junction with the pronator. Thus, the ECRL becomes a tendon graft in situ, to compensate for the radial deviating moment of the ECRB. We have found that the attachment to the base of the fourth metacarpal has the same moment arm for wrist extension as the ECRB, and matches its radial deviating moment by an equal one on the ulnar side (Fig. 114–16).

A few details of technique are important at the junction of the pronator with the ECRB.

The first concerns the length of the tendon of the pronator, which is adequate for attachment to the tendon of ECRL, but is a little short to reach the shorter tendon of the more useful ECRB. The tendon of the pronator is short and flat. It winds spirally around the radius, blending with the periosteum. It should not be divided where it reaches the bone, but should be lifted off the bone by a blunt elevator, and divided further distally where it is a blend of periosteum and tendon. This gives an extra 1 or 1.5 cm of length of tendon. It also leaves a bed of raw bone that readily becomes attached to anything that lies on it. To prevent reattachment of the pronator to the bone, the tendon should be pulled back and then passed superficially to the brachioradialis without changing direction. If it still does not reach the tendon of the ECRB, a few muscle fibers of the latter may be detached to expose raw tendon. The pronator tendon should lie, raw surface down, on the ECRB tendon and be sutured into place at relaxed tension to the proximally pulled ECRB, with the wrist extended 45 degrees. Then, the edges of the ECRB may be lifted and brought across the pronator to meet each other so that they tube the tendon and cover the anastomosis. This ensures a minimum of adhesions and very little change of direction.

If a yoke insertion is planned, the pronator tendon should first be attached to the ECRB as in Figure 114–17A. Then, after rerouting the tendon of the ECRL and attaching it distally to the fourth metacarpal base, the tendon of the ECRL should be tested for matched tension with the ECRB. Finally the ECRL tendon is laid over the pronator tendon junction and the edges of the ECRL and the ECRB are attached to each other, creating a sandwich of ECRL-pronator-ECRB. This avoids the need to tube the ECRB, as in Figure 114–17B.

THUMB EXTENSION

Since the thumb with radial palsy has all its intrinsic muscles, it is enough to replace the extensor pollicis longus (EPL) motor, and

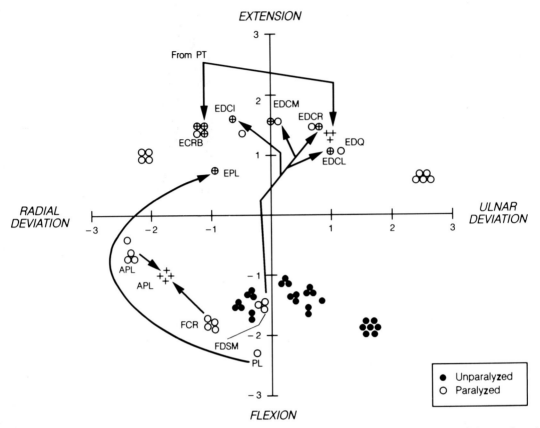

Figure 114–16. Our own preferred pattern of transfer for radial palsy. Note: When normal muscle ● is transferred to the site of the paralyzed muscle ○, the symbol ⊕ indicates activation of the paralyzed tendon, while the original tendon becomes ○. (See Fig. 114–6 legend for abbreviations.)

neglect the brevis. The ideal transfer for this is the palmaris longus (PL) when it is present (Pennell, 1919). The EPL is divided at its musculotendinous junction and the tendon is withdrawn distally just proximal to the meta-

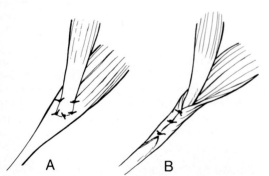

Figure 114–17. *A,* The tendon of the pronator teres lies flat on the tendon of the extensor carpi and radialis brevis (ECRB) and is sutured in place. *B,* The edges of the ECRB tendon are lifted and sutured side to side across the pronator where the two tendons are sutured.

carpophalangeal joint of the thumb. It is tunneled subcutaneously to overlie the tendon of the abductor pollicis longus (APL). The PL is divided at its insertion and withdrawn about 10 cm proximally, from which point it is tunneled subcutaneously to meet the tendon of the EPL. The two tendons are sutured end to end, or with a short interlace. The incision through which they are sutured may be used also in the replacement of the APL. If there is no PL, it is probably best to use one of the flexor superficialis tendons, as part of the operation to provide finger extension.

EXTENSION OF METACARPAL OF THUMB

This function, performed by the abductor pollicis longus (better called by its old name extensor ossis metacarpi pollicis) is important though sometimes forgotten. It holds the metacarpal out and widens the web space, forming the basis of a "circle" pinch. Without an APL the thumb metacarpal will collapse inward under the pull of the adductor. The adductor is so strong, and has such a large moment arm at the carpometacarpal joint of the thumb, that it takes a strong muscle to hold the metacarpal out against it, so that the adductor can be effective at the metacarpophalangeal joint. It is no use transferring a weak muscle to replace the APL. The APL is also a flexor and radial deviator of the wrist, at which it has a much larger moment arm than at the thumb. Thus, if a strong ulnar deviator remains to the wrist (the FCU), the APL tendon could be tenodesed to the radius, and would be activated by contracting the FCU. This is not to be recommended in cases of simple radial palsy, since it renders the FCU captive to thumb abduction, destroying its independence for control of wrist deviation and flexion.

The best replacement for the APL is the FCR (see Fig. 114–16). These two muscles are of comparable strength (APL 3.1, FCR 4.1) and tendon diameter. Both are wrist flexors, both are radial deviators of the wrist, and the shift of the FCR can be accomplished with minimal dissection. The APL tendon must be cut in the sheath, about 4 cm proximal to its insertion, withdrawn at the base of the thumb, directed forward, and sutured end to end to the FCR. Each tendon is redirected 1 or 2 cm toward the other. In this way the final effect on the wrist is a blend of the two, and the effect on the thumb is to add a little true abduction to the normal extension effect of the APL at the carpometacarpal joint.

FINGER EXTENSION

There is no consensus yet about the best way to manage paralysis of the finger extensors. The author has used many of the suggested methods and offers the following comments on his experience.

The classic operation of Jones (1916) was to transfer the FCU around the ulnar border of the forearm and attach it to all finger extensors (Fig. 114–18). Some surgeons have excised some of the lower muscle fibers of the FCU to avoid creating a bulge at the border of the forearm. This operation works. It does the job. The FCU is the strongest forearm muscle to cross the wrist and is well able to provide the needed tension.

There are two problems that together make one reluctant to use this transfer today. The first is that the muscle fibers of the FCU are only about 4 cm long. This is just long enough to control the flexion and ulnar deviation of the wrist, but not long enough to allow a full range of finger extension as well. If the tendon is made to cross the wrist dorsally toward the middle line, it uses less excursion for deviation; it then can cover 120 degrees of wrist motion using perhaps 3.5 cm of excursion, but is still short 1.5 cm for 90 degrees of finger metacarpophalangeal motion. The result is that the patient is able to extend the fingers fully or extend and flex the wrist fully, but not both together. This may not be very important, because people usually flex the wrist a little when extending their fingers, and vice versa. So perhaps it is acceptable. The second problem, a more serious one, is that the FCU is important in its own position as an ulnar deviator. A large number of common actions, like hammering, swinging an ax, and chopping vegetables on the kitchen table, all need ulnar stabilization or ulnar activation of the wrist. If the FCU can be left where it is, the patient will be grateful.

The FCR has been used for finger extension (Murphy, 1914). The author has done this many times, taking the tendon around the radius and attaching it to all the finger extensors (Fig. 114–19); actually attaching it directly to the extensors of the middle and ring fingers, then attaching the tendon of the index to the middle, and the little finger to the ring on the back of the hand. It has worked very well, the only problem being the scar of all the tendon junctures in the region of the extensor retinaculum. It has taken a while to mobilize them all. The fibers of the FCR are longer than those of the FCU and therefore more suitable for crossing more than one joint. The FCR is missed from its own place less than the FCU; it also has a smaller muscle bulk distally, so it makes less of a bulge on transfer.

The FDS tendons to the middle and/or ring fingers have been recommended as motors for the finger extensors by Boyes (1960) and Goldner and Kelly (1958). The tendons are taken through the forearm, through a window in the interosseous membrane, on either side of the flexor tendon mass. The tendons are long enough to obviate any need for a suture proximal to the retinaculum, and there is less problem of adhesions. The fibers of the FDS muscles are amply long enough to allow full

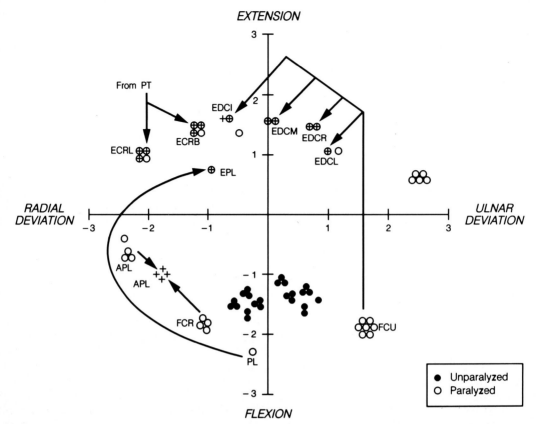

Figure 114–18. The common pattern of tendon transfer for radial palsy. The author does not recommend this. Note the overwhelming radial side dominance. Note: When normal muscle ● is transferred to the site of the paralyzed muscle ○, the symbol ⊕ indicates activation of paralyzed tendon, while the original tendon becomes ○. (See Fig. 114–6 legend for abbreviations.)

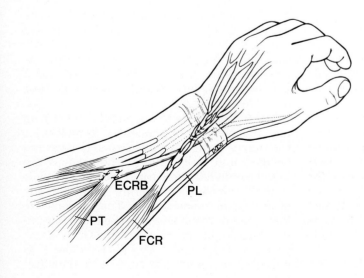

Figure 114–19. One pattern of tendon transfer for radial palsy: pronator teres to tendon of extensor carpi radialis brevis; flexor carpi radialis to extensor digitorum; palmaris longus to extensor pollicis longus.

and independent motion of wrist and fingers. The only problem is one of synergism. More recently the author has used this operation in all but elderly patients. The FDS is easy to reeducate, and is probably the muscle of choice for finger extension in radial palsy.

If there is a palmaris longus available to extend the thumb, the FDS to the middle finger may be used for the extension of all four fingers. If there is no palmaris, two FDS tendons may be used, from the middle and ring fingers, one for extending the three ulnar fingers, and one for the thumb and index finger. Alternatively, and preferably, the stronger FDS to the middle finger may be used for extending four fingers, and the ring finger FDS for the EPL. It is a good thing to keep the thumb independent. (See under *Points of technique* concerning the danger of activating multiple tendons with one common motor.)

Ulnar Nerve Paralysis

TIMING

In high (above elbow) ulnar nerve injury the best results from fascicular nerve suture may restore motor power to the forearm muscles, and protective sensation to the hand, but it is very unlikely to restore significant control to the intrinsic muscles of the hand. Since it may take up to two years to be sure that no recovery is going to take place in the intrinsic muscles, this gives ample time for the development of joint contractures, and habit patterns that make it very difficult to restore balance, full range of motion, and effective use to the hand afterward.

Clawing of fingers and thumb are both progressive deformities. Normal metacarpophalangeal joints are restrained from hyperextension by skin and palmar plates and fascia. Once the intrinsic muscles have become paralyzed, all the palmar soft tissues begin to be lengthened by persistent imbalance of muscles. If the muscular imbalance is corrected early, all the soft tissues retain their normal relationships, and the prognosis for normal use is much better.

Thus, the author recommends early tendon transfers for intrinsic palsy following high division of the ulnar nerve. In low level injury, where the axons are already grouped to divide into superficial (sensory) and deep (motor) branches, there is a likelihood of recovery of the intrinsic muscles and it may be worth waiting. High forearm nerve injury is treated as above elbow if the injury has involved sepsis, crush, or loss of length or if the patient is old. If the injury is clean-cut and has been repaired by an expert, and if the patient is a child, the author may treat it as a low injury, and wait before transferring tendons.

PARALYSIS OF ULNAR-SUPPLIED FOREARM MUSCLES

The loss of the FCU and the ulnar part of the FDP does not result in deformity, but is a serious loss for a manual worker (Fig. 114–20). The whole hand and wrist feels weaker and grip strength is reduced in two ways. The first is the total grip strength, as measured by a dynamometer. The second is the active dynamic control of instruments held in the hand. In most manual activity it is less important to squeeze the instrument hard than it is to wield it or turn it in an effective way. This latter most often involves a radial-ulnar turn or swing. The use of a hammer, ax, broom, sword, club, or table knife requires a broad hand that selectively transfers force from the radial to the ulnar side as the object is moved. In using a fishing pole, the index and middle fingers take the strain in pulling the rod back, but the ring and little fingers work with the thumb to make the cast, by forming an effective torque couple (Fig. 114–21).

In high ulnar palsy this manipulative strength is very grossly diminished. The whole ulnar side of the torque couple, usually powered by the FCU and the FDS and FDP of the ring and little fingers, is left with only the FDS to the ring and little fingers. Since the FDS to the little finger is always small (often almost vestigial); the manual worker and the sportsman feel severely handicapped. Many hand surgeons think of ulnar palsy as a problem mainly of the intrinsic muscles, and attribute the patient's sense of weakness to intrinsic palsy alone. Failure to restore strength to an ulnar-paralyzed hand is blamed on the use of a weak or ineffective transfer for intrinsic muscle palsy. This is false reasoning. The function of intrinsic replacement is to restore balance to the chain of digital joints and to assist in providing flexion torque to the metacarpophalangeal joints. Patients should be told that this will not restore full strength to the hand. If strength and dexterity are of major impor-

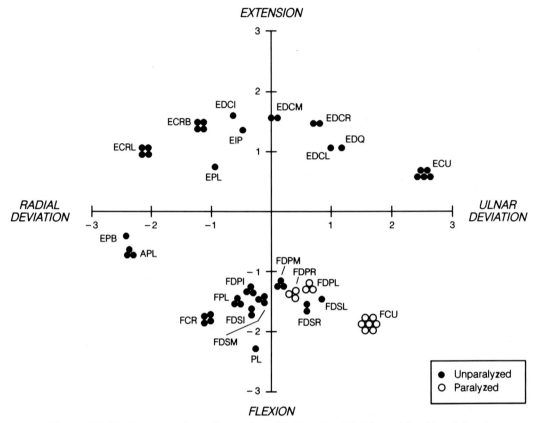

Figure 114–20. Ulnar nerve loss: effect at the wrist. (See Fig. 114–6 legend for abbreviations.)

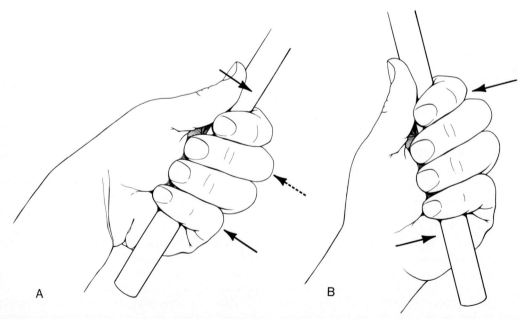

Figure 114–21. *A,* The torque couple used in casting with a fishing pole is provided by the thumb in one direction, and the ring and little fingers in the other. The torque couple becomes much narrower if the little finger is so weak that the middle finger becomes the effective flexor *(dashed arrow). B,* The torque couple used to withdraw a fishing pole (with fish) is powered by the index and middle fingers in one direction, and the heel of the palm in the other.

tance, an attempt should be made to broaden grip strength across the hand and balance the wrist as well.

The simplest way to broaden grip strength is to ensure that the little and ring fingers share the flexor profundus strength of the middle finger, supplied by the median nerve. This may not be necessary in cases where the ring and little fingers already move strongly with the middle finger owing to existing cross connections between the profundus tendons. If it is possible for the surgeon to passively open the little finger while the patient tries to hold his fist clenched, it may be beneficial to operate and attach the middle, ring, and little finger profundus tendons to each other, side to side, proximal to the wrist. At the same operation there may be advantage in moving the FCR to the FCU, since the APL provides flexor moment on the radial side of the wrist. None of this should be considered until after the final status of nerve repair has been achieved, the operation for intrinsic replacement has been performed, and the hand has been tried out in normal activity.

DISTAL EFFECT OF ULNAR PALSY

In contrast to this proximal muscle weakness, the distal results of ulnar nerve loss should be evaluated early, and some sort of corrected balance should be achieved before many months have passed.

In all cases in which tendon transfer has to be postponed, hyperextension of the metacarpophalangeal joints should be prevented, in the interval, by constant wearing of a metacarpophalangeal extension block splint set at about 20 degrees short of full extension (Fig. 114–22).

CHOICE OF METHOD

Two Fingers or Four? After complete ulnar palsy, it often appears that only the ring and little fingers are affected, and even these may not be severely clawed. This is because the palmar soft tissues are tight enough to hold the metacarpophalangeal joints short of hyperextension, allowing the long extensors to extend the interphalangeal joints. Also, the lumbrical muscles to the index and middle fingers, supplied by the median nerve, may hold the metacarpophalangeal joints of those fingers in a straight position even though all the interossei are

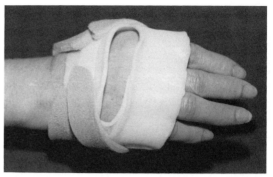

Figure 114–22. A metacorpophalangeal block extender.

paralyzed. As months and years pass, all the palmar tissues become stretched at the metacarpophalangeal level, resulting in progressive clawing of the ring and little fingers, and in the removal of support from the other fingers to an extent that may leave the lumbricals inadequate to work without interosseous support. The author suggests restoring muscle balance to all four fingers in most cases (Brandsma and Watson, 1982). A finger need not be included for surgical correction, if the patient can hold the fingers straight at the interphalangeal joints while holding the metacarpophalangeal joints flexed (without external support), and maintain the position against a backward push on the proximal segment by the examiner. A finger should also be omitted from the tendon transfer if the proximal interphalangeal joint remains stiff in marked flexion, even after therapy. A single stiff finger will prevent a common tendon from being effective for the mobile fingers. In such cases, proximal interphalangeal arthrodesis may be suitable for the omitted finger.

The Motor. To replace the whole power of the paralyzed intrinsic muscles, one would need to use a major muscle, such as a FDS, for each finger. Such a multiple transfer would not only deplete other important actions, but would tend to twist the finger if it were attached to only one side. The use of eight slips of tendon, supplying both sides of all four fingers, using four FDS muscles, was advised at one time by Bunnell (1948). However the addition of so much torque at the metacarpophalangeal joint in a finger that has lost the prime flexor of its proximal interphalangeal joint results in an imbalance that may lead to a swan-neck deformity as a late complication.

The palmaris longus, extended by free grafts through the carpal tunnel, is the motor of choice for mobile hands that are operated on *early*, before metacarpophalangeal hyperextension has time to develop and become a habit. Its early use is easy to justify even if recovery of the intrinsic muscles should occur later, since so little is lost in donor function.

For hands that are operated on after claw deformity is established, a stronger muscle may be needed for correction. A wrist extensor may be used, extended by four free-grafts. The extensor carpi radialis longus (ECRL), withdrawn in midforearm and tunneled around the radial side of the forearm to the palmar side, makes a good transfer and is easy to reeducate. It uses almost no excursion when the fingers flex at the metacarpophalangeal joint while the wrist extends.

Pathway Through Carpal Tunnel. Whatever motor is used, if it approaches the fingers from the volar side of the forearm, the tendon grafts have to pass through the carpal tunnel. This worries many hand surgeons who are aware of the carpal tunnel syndrome and who fear that the addition of grafts may cause compression of the median nerve. This is a pity, because the fear robs them of the best tendon pathway into the hand. The author has used it in more than 2000 cases and his trainees in many thousands more without median nerve problems. Although most of these patients had leprosy and many had already lost their median nerves from that disease, many more had median nerves that were enlarged on account of the disease and would thus be more than usually subject to damage from carpal tunnel compression. The incidence of median nerve complications in such patients after tendon transfers through the carpal tunnel proved to be no more than when other pathways were used (Brandsma and Brand, 1985).

The carpal tunnel is an excellent pathway for tendon grafts if the following points of technique are carefully followed:

1. The junction of motor tendon with grafts should be kept proximal to the carpal tunnel and distal to the transverse forearm incision through which the suture is made. Therefore, the forearm incision should be at least 5 cm proximal to the wrist crease.

2. A longitudinal rerouting incision is made in the proximal one-third of the palm along a line that runs from the palmaris tendon to the middle–ring finger space. This incision may be about 3 cm long and is as proximal as possible, back to the distal edge of the transverse carpal ligament. The skin is incised, the palmar fascia is split along its fibers, and the palmar fat is pushed bluntly aside, taking care to avoid damage to palmar arch blood vessels. The floor of this wound is the skeletal plane of metacarpal bases and ligaments. All longitudinal palmar fibrous septa should be distal to the center of this incision.

3. Lateral incisions are made at the base of each finger, exposing the lateral bands on the radial side of each digit except that it is on the ulnar side of the index finger (to keep fingers side by side rather than constantly abducted). The lateral bands are seen and further exposed as they pass into the palm on the volar side of the intermetacarpal ligament and into the lumbrical canal.

4. Tendon graft material, either the plantaris tendon folded into two and split lengthwise to make four strands, or a 12 mm wide strip of fascia lata split into four strands distally, is now attached to the motor tendon that is projecting from the anterior forearm incision.

5. A tendon tunneling forceps, preferably of the Andersen design (see Fig. 114–14), is inserted into the palmar incision where it passes straight back until the rounded nose is rubbing over skeletal structures. These are easily felt as rough and rigid. The nose of the forceps is passed proximally, deep to all structures, through the carpal tunnel. If, by mistake, the instrument is not on the floor of the tunnel, it will be in among the tendons, and this will pull the fingers into flexion. If this happens, the instrument is withdrawn a little and passed strictly on the floor. As soon as the nose of the tunneler is through the canal, the hand is extended and somewhat radially deviated while the tunneler is advanced. This brings the nose of the tunneler to the ulnar side of the muscles and tendons proximal to the wrist, and it quickly and easily appears to the ulnar side of palmaris, in the incision, where it picks up the ends of all four tendon grafts and pulls them into the palmar incision. A nylon thread should be passed loosely around the motor tendon before it disappears so that at the end of the operation it can be pulled to simulate the effect of the motor on the fingers.

6. The grafts are laid back on a wet sponge while the tunneler is inserted into each finger

incision in turn. The nose of the tunneler follows the lateral band across the volar side of the intermetacarpal ligament (this must be identified by feel) and on through the lumbrical canal, to appear in the palmar rerouting incision, where it picks up one strand of graft and pulls it back into the finger.

7. When all grafts are in position, all are pulled distally together to make sure that no septum is in a position to block distal motion (see distal "V," p. 4941). The hand is then positioned with the wrist 30 degrees flexed, the metacarpophalangeal joint 80 degrees flexed, and the interphalangeal joints extended. It is convenient to have a strip of aluminum already bent into shape to hold the hand in this position while all four grafts are stitched into place on the lateral band under equal tension (Fritschi, 1971). For mobile hands and early cases this tension may be almost zero, in this posture. For older cases with established habit, it may be that higher tension should be used. The little finger is sutured last and at an extra 7 mm of tension, because of the mobility of its metacarpal.

8. In the postoperative dressings and cast, the wrist is straight, the metacarpophalangeal joints fully flexed, and the interphalangeal joints fully extended. A plaster of Paris slab may be used on the volar side, without padding, and a plaster bandage, only two or three layers thick, *loosely* applied and rubbed into every contour of the fingers, so that the position of each joint is controlled. This eggshell cast may be reinforced after 24 hours, but the dorsal layers should remain thin enough to be cut with bandage or plaster scissors, because a saw is dangerous over knuckles without padding.

9. There is no standard postoperative therapy for claw hand correction. After the first week or two of exercises the therapist should evaluate progress. If the patient finds it easy to extend the metacarpophalangeal joints, and if there is any tendency for clawing, it may be best to keep light cylinder casts holding each digit in full interphalangeal extension between exercise sessions. If, on the other hand, the patient experiences difficulty getting the metacarpophalangeal joints extended, and if there is limitation of passive metacarpophalangeal extension of more than about 30 degrees, the therapy needs to be reversed, and the patient needs to be encouraged to extend the metacarpophalangeal

joints and perhaps have a flat hand splint at night. This tightness is less common than looseness of the grafts, but when it occurs it needs attention.

Other Motors. The ECRB may be used as a transfer. It must be withdrawn 4 inches above the wrist, then attached to four grafts and tunneled back *through its own sheath* and on through the interosseous spaces between the metacarpals. This transfer needs more reeducation because the ECRB needs to contract without actually extending the wrist, so that the tendon may be effective distally. This is difficult to learn. Failure to do so results in the tendon grafts becoming adherent in the intermetacarpal space, producing a tenodesis effect at the metacarpophalangeal joint in the position at which it has rested postoperatively. However, with good postoperative training, this is an effective motor.

A single flexor superficialis tendon (ring or middle finger), split into four tails, makes a good intrinsic replacement. (See details of tendon detachment on p. 4954.) It sometimes results in a swan-neck deformity in the digit that has been deprived of its FDS especially if the tendon slip is inserted into the lateral band of the same digit. Another problem is that the stump of the FDS, left behind in the sheath, sometimes becomes attached to the wound in the sheath through which it was divided, proximal to the proximal interphalangeal joint. In such cases a flexion contracture of the latter joint develops and may become progressively more severe. If such a proximal interphalangeal flexor tenodesis is observed early, it may be corrected by serial casting of the finger into extension. If it is already months old, the tenodesis has to be excised surgically, followed by cylinder casting for weeks or even months to prevent a recurrent contracture from scar. A third problem occurs occasionally when a superficialis tendon is removed from a finger that already has a paralyzed profundus, leaving a very weak finger.

The use of the extensor indicis and extensor digiti quinti (Fowler's—Riordan, 1953) is an acceptable procedure for intrinsic replacement. The author has modified this operation somewhat, as follows: the extensor indicis proprius (EIP) is divided at the metacarpophalangeal joint, and split lengthwise. Both slips are taken through the second interosseous space, to be attached to the lateral bands on adjacent sides of the index and middle fingers. The extensor digiti quinti (EDQ) is taken through the third interosseous space to avoid the reversal of the metacarpal arch that occurs strongly when the fourth space is used. One slip of the tendon goes to the radial lateral band on the ring finger, and the other is tunneled across the palmar side of the distal part of the fourth metacarpal to the lateral band on the little finger. A slip of tendon usually needs to be taken from the extensor digitorum of the ring finger and transferred to the extensor stump of the little finger, since the tendon slip from the EDC to the little finger is rarely adequate when the EDQ is removed.

The Insertion. No matter what motor is used, the final approach of the tendon or tendon graft to each finger must be on the palmar side of the intermetacarpal ligament, and the insertion should usually be to the lateral band on the radial side of the finger, except that the ulnar lateral band of the index finger is used to keep the fingers side to side. In the case of pianists or typists who may need to abduct the index finger, an extra muscle may be used to insert into the tendon of the first dorsal interosseous (Fig. 114–23).

Many hands with ulnar paralysis exhibit Wartenberg's sign, a chronic abduction of the little finger, which is a problem because it catches onto things and makes it difficult for a patient to put his hand into his pocket.

This is not always corrected by multiple tendon graft transfer, but usually is prevented by making sure that the tunneler enters the palm in a direction that sends it down in the ring finger compartment. The crossover must be so far distal that the vertical palmar septa are not violated. In the case of Fowler's operation, where the tendon comes from the dorsum, the slip to the little finger must enter through the third interosseous space, and cross the front of the neck of the metacarpal of the ring finger.

Brooks (1975) advised inserting tendon transferred for intrinsic paralysis into the A2 pulley rather than into the lateral band of each finger. This has the advantage of being central, avoiding the rotational effect of a one-sided transfer, but the author finds that a more natural sequence of finger closure occurs if the lateral bands are restored to their normal function by the transfer rather than having to depend entirely on the long extensors to straighten the interphalangeal joints.

Capsulodesis (Zancolli, 1957), bone block (Howard, 1948), or tenodesis (Riordan, 1953) have been recommended for correction of claw hand in ulnar palsy. They all correct the clawing, but they do it by preventing hyperextension of the metacarpophalangeal joint, thus allowing the long extensors to become effective at the proximal interphalangeal joint.

The real defect in intrinsic paralysis, however, is not the obvious deformity of clawing, but the functional disability during the flexion of the fingers, by which the distal joints flex ahead of the metacarpophalangeal joints, curling the fingers into a fist before they have been able to reach out and grasp an object. This feature is also responsible for the fact that the fingertips (often without sensation) take all the stress of grasp, rather than the whole palmar surface sharing the stress, as it does when the sequence of closure is normal (Fig. 114–24).

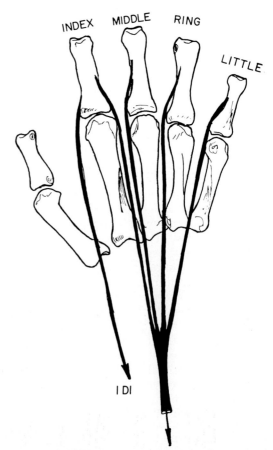

Figure 114–23. For correction of ulnar paralysis a single motor may be used for the radial side of the middle, ring, and little fingers and the ulnar side of the index finger. A separate motor may be used for the radial side of the index finger if necessary. 1DI = first dorsal interosseous.

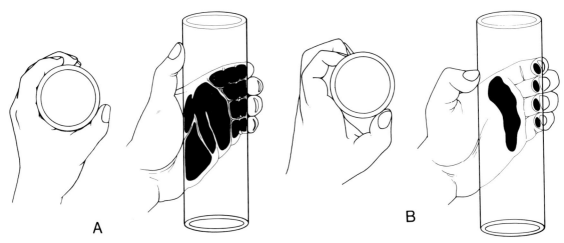

Figure 114–24. *A,* A normal hand grasping a cylinder; the area of skin contact is marked in black. *B,* A claw hand grasping a cylinder; the area of contact is so small that pressure becomes high and damage is common.

Therefore, static methods of correction are to be chosen only when ulnar palsy is part of a much more extensive paralysis, reducing the availability of suitable motors. In such a case the best static correction is a tenodesis crossing the wrist as well as the metacarpophalangeal joints (Riordan, 1953; Tsuge, 1967), allowing some active metacarpophalangeal flexion linked to wrist movement.

ULNAR NERVE PALSY AFFECTING THUMB

Low median nerve palsy prevents proper *positioning* of the thumb, but low ulnar palsy removes the *power* to pinch. Surgeons almost always operate for restoring position, but often neglect the power factor. To the working man or woman a strong pinch is very important, especially in the dominant hand.

Sometimes the median nerve supplies the flexor pollicis brevis and part of the adductor pollicis. In such cases an adequate pinch may be possible in ulnar palsy without any surgical intervention. If a patient with ulnar palsy is able to pinch *strongly* without either hyperextension of the thumb metacarpophalangeal joint or hyperflexion of the interphalangeal joint, there is no need for surgery on the thumb.

In some cases an ulnar-paralyzed thumb may appear to be strong because it rests back in the sling of the thumb web and allows the index finger to pinch down onto the ulnar border of the thumb. This puts stress on the ulnar collateral ligament at the metacarpophalangeal joint. If sensation is normal, strong pinch will result in discomfort in the ligament, causing inhibition of strength and preservation of the ligament. In the case of sensory loss, the pinch is used without inhibition. The ligament becomes stretched and the thumb suffers progressive deformity until it becomes grossly abducted at the metacarpophalangeal joint (like a "gamekeeper thumb").

If the pinch is weak, following ulnar palsy, the surgeon should determine whether the weakness is from the thumb or the fingers. This is done by supporting first one and then the other with the surgeon's own hands and comparing the output on a pinchmeter. If the thumb is weak, it should be strengthened by a replacement for the adductor pollicis. Since the adductor plus short flexor muscle group is strong (3.0 + 1.3 = 4.3),* it is no use replacing it with a weak muscle such as the often used EIP (1.0). The FDS from the middle finger (3.4) may be rerouted, using a split in the palmar fascia near the thenar crease as a pulley.

The exact position of this pulley is important. It should be about halfway between the wrist crease and the crease at the base of the middle finger, and should lie about 0.5 cm to the ulnar side of the thenar crease. It must not be further to the ulnar side, or the tendon will bowstring across the thenar crease and create a painful ridge. It must not be further radialward or it will miss the important strands of palmar fascia that hold it in place.

The distal attachment should be to the

---

*The numbers for muscle tension in this chapter refer to percentages of total muscle tension of all muscles below the elbow (see Tables 114–1, 114–2).

extensor tendon halfway between the metacarpophalangeal and interphalangeal joints, with the interphalangeal joint held extended (Fig. 114–25).

The next incision is across the middle of the proximal segment of the middle finger; care should be taken not to injure the digital vessels or nerves. The incision is deepened bluntly to expose the flexor sheath. The distal edge of the A2 pulley is seen, but not divided. The flimsy sheath distal to the pulley is entered. At that point there appear to be four tendon slips, side by side. The two central ones are profundus (check by flexing the distal joint). The slips on each side (curving to the underside distally) are flexor superficialis. These are picked up and divided and marked by a black stitch, left long for retrieval if needed. The ends are pulled into the wound (flexing the wrist) and the vinculae divided, also the crossconnection between the two slips.

Next the tendon is pulled while the surgeon defines its position in the palm by palpation at the level of the main transverse palmar crease. A 1.5 cm incision is made just to the ulnar side of the thenar crease, and proximal to the transverse crease.

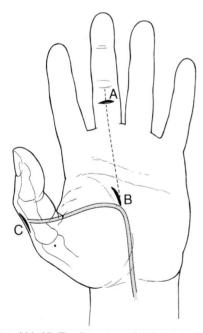

Figure 114–25. The flexor superficialis tendon is divided in the finger through incision A. It is withdrawn through B, leaving a few fibers of palmar fascia intact at the radial edge of the incision. The tendon is then tunneled subcutaneously to the back of the middle of the proximal phalanx to be attached to the extensor tendon (C).

The incision must not divide the palmar fascia, which is split bluntly. The tendon is identified and pulled out in the palm. A pair of straight tunneling forceps is passed from the back of the thumb subcutaneously to the palmar incision. Resistance will be felt at Cleland's ligaments. Approaching the thenar crease, the nose of the tunneler must be strictly subcutaneous, right up against the skin, so that it may appear in the palmar wound between the skin and palmar fascia. Here the end of the tendon is grasped and pulled back to and out of the thumb incision, where it is laced into the split extensor pollicis tendon. The interphalangeal joint of the thumb must be fully extended and the extensor tendon pulled proximally while the tendon transfer is attached. The tension may be zero if tested with the thumb adducted, or 2.0 cm beyond zero in abduction.

While the thumb is immobilized in its postoperative dressings and cast, it should be held in the opposed position, but held out in abduction, keeping the transfer and web a little on the stretch. This is because the transfer has a large moment arm for the carpometacarpal joint and would be difficult to stretch out if it became contracted.

Another motor for thumb adduction is the ECRB (Smith, 1983). The tendon is divided near its insertion and withdrawn proximal to its sheath (about 10 cm up the forearm) where a free graft is attached to it. The extended tendon is taken back through the same sheath and onward to a point about 2 to 3 cm proximal to the metacarpal heads over the second interosseous space. It is brought out here through a small incision. Now a straight tunneler is used, directed from the back of the thumb, straight back through a palpably soft area of the second intermetacarpal space to the incision on the dorsum of the hand, where the tendon graft is picked up and pulled through.

Any transfer to compensate for the adductor and short flexor muscles should approach the middle of the dorsal aspect of the proximal phalanx from a point halfway up the palm at the thenar crease. This gives it a 1.5 cm moment arm for flexion at the metacarpophalangeal joint and about 4.0 cm at the carpometacarpal joint. This gives a good balance for the control of both joints against opposed distal external force.

An alternative to tendon transfer is to arthrodese the metacarpophalangeal joint of the thumb in about 15 degrees flexion. This allows the flexor pollicis longus (FPL) to control the interphalangeal joint, and allows the two arthrodesed bones of the thumb to rest back in the dermofascial sling of the thumb web while the fingers flex down at their metacarpophalangeal joints to meet the thumb. In such a case the FPL, with only 1.5 cm of moment arm at the carpometacarpal joint, will never be able to flex the whole thumb against resistance. The arthrodesis is unsuitable if the web is very wide. It also will not enable a strong key pinch to be used (Brand, 1985) since in key pinch it is the thumb that has to do all the moving. All the fingers need is stability.

Median Nerve Paralysis

PARALYSIS OF DISTAL MUSCLES

The loss of the median-supplied lumbrical muscles can be compensated for by increased activity of the ulnar-supplied interosseous muscles. In cases where part of the flexor-adductor group of intrinsic muscles to the thumb may be median-supplied and therefore paralyzed, it is usually possible to obtain adequate pinch function by what remains. Thus, the only serious imbalance in low median palsy is from the loss of the abductor brevis and opponens pollicis. These two muscles are the only ones that can abduct and oppose the thumb to the fingers. This loss is serious and a replacement must be provided.

Many different motors have been used for the median-paralyzed thumb. Bunnell (1948) said that the motor should approach from the direction of the pisiform bone and the insertion may be to the tendon of the abductor pollicis brevis (APB).

A standard tendon transfer involves division of the flexor superficialis in the ring finger, withdrawal in the distal forearm, making a pulley from a strand of the tendon of the flexor carpi ulnaris just proximal to the pisiform bone, and then tunneling the finger tendon across the thenar eminence toward the axis of the metacarpophalangeal joint of the thumb. This gives a good angle of approach to the thumb, and is satisfactory. We would now prefer to use a window in the roof of the carpal tunnel as a pulley (Fig. 114–26) (Snow and Fink, 1971).

The transferred tendon may be either attached to the tendon of the APB or taken to

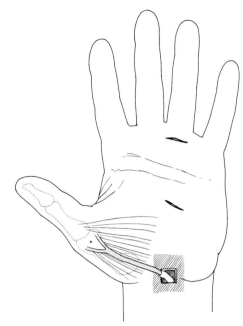

Figure 114–26. Diagram showing the use of the opening in the roof of the carpal tunnel as a pulley for the flexor superficialis tendon (with sheath) for opposition of the thumb.

the dorsum, to the tendon of the extensor pollicis longus (EPL).

The abductor pollicis longus (APL) is not an abductor but an extensor of the metacarpal of the thumb; nevertheless, some patients with hypermobile hands develop a trick movement in which they flex the wrist fully, thus bringing the APL tendon in front of the axis for thumb abduction. Once the thumb is locked in abduction, they can bring the wrist back to neutral without losing the pinch position. Inspired by this observation, the author treated some cases by moving the APL forward to make it a true abductor (Edgerton and Brand, 1965). It works, but the muscle is not really long enough and does not have enough excursion to allow full freedom for thumb abduction with full wrist mobility. This procedure is not recommended now except in cases of extensive paralysis and lack of motors.

Because the active ulnar-supplied adductor is also a supinator of the thumb, there is a tendency for the thumb to adopt a posture of full external rotation after median palsy. This is reinforced by the action of the EPL, which is also an external rotator of the thumb. The thumb lies beside the palm with its pulp facing forward. This is a bad position that results in shortening of the dorsal skin and fascia of the web, as well as shortening of the adductor muscle fibers. These changes are difficult to reverse at the time of late tendon transfer. Therefore, it is very important to keep the thumb abducted and pronated continuously while waiting for the right time to transfer a tendon.

In the case of a high median nerve injury, it is good to restore opposition early even when recovery is expected for forearm muscles. In such cases a method should be chosen that will cause minimal loss due to transferred donor function. The transfer of the extensor indicis proprius (EIP) in a spiral around the ulnar side of the wrist makes a good choice in such a case. The patient can use the thumb opposed to the ring and little fingers while awaiting recovery of the other finger flexors.

It is a common mistake to think that a replacement for low median palsy should run in the same direction as one for low median and ulnar palsy. Figure 114–27A shows the whole fan of intrinsic muscles of the thumb.

It shows by an arrow marked ABD the general direction of the median-supplied muscles and by ADD the direction of the ulnar-supplied muscles. If both are paralyzed and if only one tendon transfer is to be used, that tendon should lie *between* the two arrows, in one of the directions shown in Figure 114–27B, perhaps toward the pisiform bone. For simple median palsy, however, with good ulnar intrinsics, a transfer that approaches from the middle of the wrist crease will result in a good overall balance.

It is on this basis that Camitz (1929) used the palmaris longus tendon in continuity with a long strand of palmar fascia that serves as a tendon graft when it is moved across to lie parallel to the radial fibers of the abductor brevis. This also is a good operation to use when early transfer is to be done in a case in which final recovery of the nerve and muscle is still possible.

Another good replacement for paralyzed thenar muscles is the hypothenar abductor digiti quinti (Littler and Cooley, 1963). This is a whole muscle transfer and has the ad-

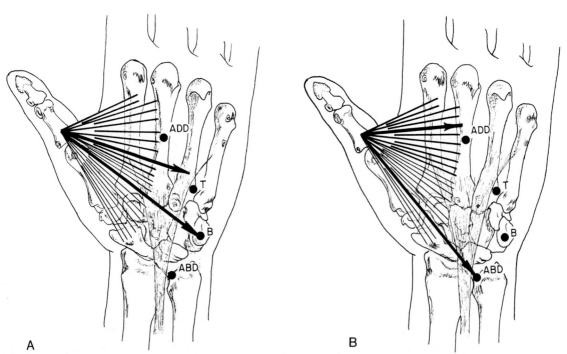

A   B

Figure 114–27. *A,* This fan of muscles represents the APB (abductor pollicis brevis), FPB (flexor pollicis brevis), and AP (adductor pollicis). The heavy lines represent fibers that are usually ulnar supplied, and the lighter lines are median supplied. The long arrow to B is the direction Bunnell (1948) suggested for a single replacement tendon for low ulnar-median palsy. The shorter arrow to T is the direction for a single tendon transfer for the same, as suggested by Thompson (1942). *B,* The same diagram with two separate tendons used together for rebalancing after low ulnar-median palsy, one to replace the adductor-flexor group (ADD) and the other the abductor group of fibers (ABD).

vantage that the muscle mass is bulky enough to restore some of the shape of the thenar mass. The details of the transfer should be carefully studied to avoid the danger of damage to the motor nerve or to the blood supply.

PARALYSIS OF FOREARM MUSCLES IN HIGH MEDIAN NERVE INJURY

Since the prognosis is good for recovery of the forearm muscles after repair of a clean division of the median nerve in the upper arm, and since the waiting period is not very long, there is no real justification for tendon transfers until the pattern of recovery or lack of it has become apparent (Fig. 114–28).

Finger and Thumb Flexion. The middle finger may flex quite well after high median palsy, by its linkage with the ulnar-supplied profundus muscles. If not, this linkage may be enhanced by firm suture of the tendons of the flexor digitorum profundus of the middle and ring fingers side to side in the distal forearm, with carefully matched tension.

The tendon of the extensor carpi radialis longus is a convenient and synergistic transfer for finger flexion. It may be divided distally, withdrawn proximally, and tunneled around the radial side of the forearm to be tapped into the side of the flexor profundus tendon of the index finger, or of the index and middle fingers. It may be used for the index finger and for the flexor pollicis longus (FPL) together, provided the two are matched for tension and for the excursion necessary for pinch. It is usually better to keep the thumb separate and bring the extensor carpi ulnaris (ECU) across from the ulnar side to power its flexion.

The choice of operation in high median palsy must be based on the prognosis for restoration of sensation; on whether it is a dominant hand; and on the age and occupation of the patient. If median sensation is not likely to return, it is not worth trying to restore pulp to pulp pinch between thumb and index finger: it will not be used. Even with partial sensation, the patient usually prefers to use the other hand for precision pinch.

Key pinch, however, is more likely to be

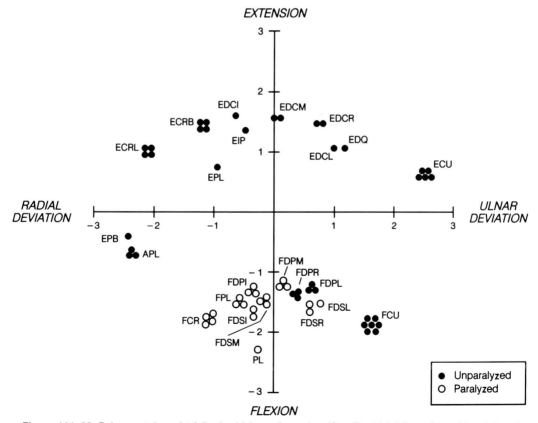

Figure 114–28. Balance at the wrist following high median palsy. (See Fig. 114–6 legend for abbreviations.)

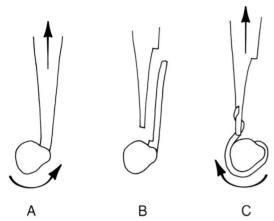

Figure 114–29. *A,* The tendon of biceps insertion on the radius—supinator. *B,* Z division of the tendon—lengthening. (N.B.: Use *long* Z-plasty.) *C,* The distal stump of the tendon passed around the radius to reverse the rotational effects of the biceps on the radius, making it into a pronator (Zancolli).

used because it is broad and secure, and also because the thumb usually pinches against some of the dorsal skin of the proximal part of the index finger where there is normal sensation. For key pinch it is essential that the thumb flexor be independent of the index finger flexor. In fact, key pinch can be accomplished without a long flexor if the interphalangeal joint of the thumb is arthrodesed.

Pronation is lost in high median palsy and needs to be restored. One way to do this is to use the ECU, which may leave its fibrous sheath just below midforearm and then angle across to the distal radial palmar side. It may be extended by means of a graft to the thumb metacarpal, thus serving as an opponens-abductor of the thumb as well as a pronator and wrist flexor. Either one of these actions may be individualized if the other actions are opposed and prevented by contraction of a specific antagonist (supinator, wrist extensor, extensor pollicis longus).

This is a good example of how a single muscle may serve two or three functions *in series* independently, by having selective antagonists at each. This cannot be done when the actions are in parallel, because apparently selective antagonists oppose all actions or none (see p. 4926).

Since it is difficult to restore strong pronation, it is better to weaken supination for fear of having a supine posture for the hand (good only for beggars!). This is accomplished by moving the tendon of the biceps, using the

method of Zancolli (1979) (Fig. 114–29) to reverse the rotation of the radius caused by the biceps.

COMBINED MEDIAN AND ULNER PALSY (WRIST AND LOW FOREARM LEVEL)

The treatment of ulnar-median nerve loss to the fingers is much the same as for the ulnar nerve only, but the problems of the thumb are different. The thumb in low ulnar median palsy is very weak indeed: the FPL is all it has on the flexor-adductor side.

Figure 114–30 shows how the intrinsic muscles converge like a fan toward the base of the middle phalanx. All the strongest of these, and those with the largest moment arms, are the ulnar-supplied adductor–short flexor group. The median-supplied group not only is of lesser cross sectional area (3.0 versus 4.3) but works with a much smaller

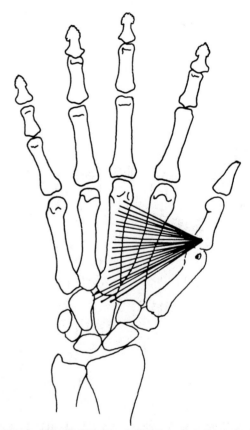

Figure 114–30. The fan of adductor–short flexor muscle fibers. Note the rather constant moment arm at the metacarpophalangeal joint, while at the carpometacarpal joint the distal fibers may have more than double the moment arm of the proximal fibers.

moment arm at the carpometacarpal joint. This contrast also affects their function, since the ulnar group needs power for pinch, while the median group needs only enough for holding position.

In Figure 114–27A the two arrows show the direction taken by the tendons most often advised for transfer in pure ulnar palsy and pure median palsy. In Figure 114–27B two arrows represent two of the directions often advised if only one tendon transfer is to be used to compensate for both palsies. The more proximal arrow is used by those who follow Bunnell's (1948) original suggestion, pulling toward the pisiform bone. The more distal is that suggested by Thompson (1942), who used the ulnar border of the proximal palmar fascia as a pulley. The first favors wide abduction and no adduction, resulting in a weak pinch. The second favors a stronger pinch, at the expense of some abduction.

The author considers pinch to be so important that it is often worth transferring two muscles for the thumb in low ulnar-median palsy, one for abduction (as described for median palsy) and one for adduction (as described for ulnar palsy). In most cases in which a good surgeon has transferred a single good tendon (i.e., without a free graft) using a good muscle (e.g., the flexor superficialis of the ring finger) through a good pulley (Thompson's [1942] palmar fascia or Snow and Fink's [1971] carpal tunnel roof) and with a good insertion (double insertion of Brand [White, 1960]), the result has been good. The pinch may not be very strong, but the patient usually finds it acceptable. However, there is no latitude for error when a single tendon transfer is used. That is why the word "good" keeps recurring in this paragraph and in the next.

A good surgeon will be sure to check that the dorsal skin and fascia of the web is just right. "Just right" is vital here, because not only must the dorsal web be wide enough to allow abduction and *full opposition* or pronation of the thumb, but it *must not be wider than that.*

In simple median palsy the ulnar-supplied adductors take care of the action of pinch. In ulnar-median palsy there is no adductor or short flexor. After only a single tendon "opponens" transfer, there is no muscle that can really adduct the metacarpal against resistance. The FPL has too small a moment arm at the carpometacarpal joint to do this, so the

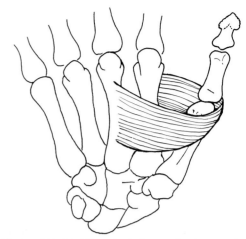

Figure 114–31. When intrinsic muscles are paralyzed, the thumb metacarpal leans back in the passive support of the skin and fascia of the web, leaving the flexor pollicis longus free to control distal joints.

only way to have a strong pinch is for the *fingers* to do the flexing, toward the thumb that rests back in the web (Fig. 114–31).

At one time the author used to do a rather enthusiastic web-plasty to make sure of a wide opening for grasp and pinch. Some thumbs became so widely abducted that where the pinch occurred between the index fingertip and the proximal part of the thumb pulp, the fingers could not reach the tip of the thumb (Brand, 1959).

The author's original web-plasty for the thumb involved a big dorsal flap that was allowed to slide forward with the thumb, supplemented by a Z-plasty of the free edge of the web. This left a crescent-shaped gap over the second metacarpal for a free whole-thickness skin graft.

Today most cases that need a web-plasty get only the sliding flap. The Z-plasty is not used very often, and then it is small, because it lengthens the palmar side of the web, which usually should not be lengthened (Fig. 114–32). This is because it is recognized that, as soon as the thumb is opposed by significant force, the carpometacarpal joint retreats into extension until it is brought to rest by the web. Only the metacarpophalangeal and interphalangeal joints can be flexed by the FPL against resistance (see Fig. 114–31).

Thus, in low ulnar-median palsy single tendon transfers may be used to control only the metacarpophalangeal and interphalangeal joints, leaving the carpometacarpal joint to the passive support of the web. If the

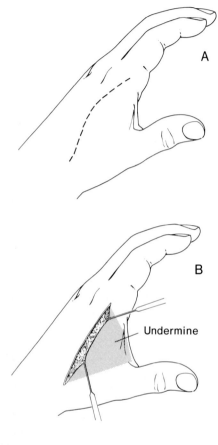

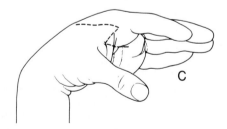

Figure 114–32. *A,* Dorsal web–plasty. An incision is made over the full length of the second metacarpal bone, from a point on the radial side of the metacarpophalangeal joint of the index finger and curving to the dorsal aspect of the bone, and carried proximally almost to the wrist joint. *B,* Undermining. The incision is deepened to the areolar plane in which the skin moves freely over the deeper tissues. The radial flap is reflected and freed back as far as the thumb, dissecting into the free edge of the thumb web and down to the tissue over the carpometacarpal joint of the thumb. While an assistant pulls the thumb into abduction and full opposition, the surgeon divides the dorsal fascia and any tight bands that seem to hinder full opposition. Usually it is not necessary to divide paralyzed muscles. *C,* Z-plasty. At this stage, if the web is still inadequate, a small Z-plasty may be added, using the free edge of the web for its central limb and the distal end of the original incision for its dorsal limb, with an incision down the palmar side of the web as the ventral limb. The Z-plasty should rarely be used, because a very deep web cleft is ugly, and an unduly wide web weakens the pinch in cases of ulnar and median palsy where a web normally acts as a passive check to replace the adductor muscles that are paralyzed.

carpometacarpal joint is to come under control on the flexor-adductor side, it will require an additional muscle, or else the FPL must be rerouted to give it a much greater moment arm (Brand, 1985).

If only a single tendon transfer is to be used, the FPL still will not be able to hold both the metacarpophalangeal and interphalangeal joints when strong pinch is attempted. Therefore, the single tendon transfer should help to *stabilize* the metacarpophalangeal joint, not mobilize it. No one tendon can have two separate actions that can be used in series independently unless there are other effective muscles that can counteract one action or the other. Thus, the FPL must be a prime interphalangeal flexor, and the metacarpophalangeal joint may be fused, or be stabilized so that it need not move during ordinary pinch or grasp. The new tendon should be routed from a pulley in the carpal tunnel roof (Snow and Fink, 1971), and toward the flexion-extension axis of the metacarpophalangeal joint (marked on the skin). The tendon is then brought out through an incision just 2 cm before it reaches the axis and split into two strands. One-half of the tendon is tunneled dorsally across the neck and head of the metacarpal, to be attached to the ulnar side of the base of the phalanx or to the tendon of the paralyzed adductor pollicis at that point. This makes that tendon slip an extensor and an adductor of the metacarpophalangeal joint. The second half of the tendon is tunneled (while the metacarpophalangeal joint is flexed) in front of the axis of the metacarpophalangeal joint and onward to become attached to the extensor tendon of the thumb in the distal half of the proximal phalanx. This tendon slip is now a *flexor* and an abductor of the metacarpophalangeal joint. Thus, one tendon, after transfer, comes to lie on both sides of the metacarpophalangeal joint. Flexor, extensor, abductor, adductor—the tendon slips oppose each other around the joint, tending to restore the neutral position after any thrust in any direction. By fixing the flexor abductor tendon slip last, and using about 4 mm extra tension, one may leave the metacarpophalangeal joint just a little flexed and abducted when the main stem of the tendon is pulled. It will resist further movement in any direction (Fig. 114–33) (White, 1960). Because it holds the metacarpophalangeal joint a little flexed (10 to 15 degrees), the extensor longus will be able to

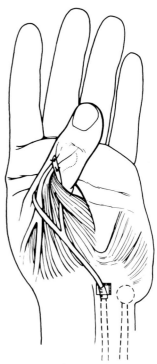

Figure 114–33. Brand transfer to restore opposition. A newer modification in which a different pulley is used is described in the text.

extend the interphalangeal joint to prevent clawing (it corrects the tip flexion of Froment's sign).

If, after the best care, the thumb develops any progressive deformity at the metacarpophalangeal joint, it may be best to operate again and fuse the metacarpophalangeal joint, rather than try to compensate for the deformity by another tendon transfer.

High Ulnar and High Median Palsy

This very disabling condition should not be treated by tendon transfers until it has been determined that recovery after nerve suture is unlikely to occur. There are so few muscles remaining that it would be a mistake to use even one for a task that might later prove to have been unnecessary.

Since any restored grasp or pinch is going to be weak, a single wrist extensor easily provides adequate stabilization of the wrist. The extensor carpi radialis brevis is always the muscle of choice for this, being the most effective wrist extensor, though not the strongest wrist-extending muscle (see Table 114–1). The muscles most commonly used for transfer are the extensor carpi radialis longus (ECRL), the extensor carpi ulnaris (ECU), and the brachioradialis (BR). The BR must be freed from the aponeurotic sheets of fibers that form part of its insertion right up to midforearm. The BR is one muscle that does better if it is transferred through a tunnel of its own, right away from its old bed, because if it is moved only a little there is a likelihood of reattachment to its old extensive insertions. The function of the BR distally is improved if its origin is stripped from the supracondylar ridge of the humerus and reattached a little further down toward the epicondyle, taking care not to stretch or damage the neurovascular bundles that enter the muscle from its deep surface near the proximal end. By moving the origin even a little toward the axis of the elbow, much less excursion is required of the muscle for elbow joint motion. This allows the muscle fibers to have a larger excursion that can be used distally. A good use for this muscle would be to substitute for the intrinsic muscles in the hand. One of the flexor superficialis tendons may be used as a tendon graft in situ. The BR is withdrawn proximally and tunneled forward to be attached to the proximal end of the tendon of the flexor digitorum superficialis (FDS) (middle finger) in the forearm. The distal end of the same FDS tendon is divided in the finger, withdrawn in the proximal palm, and split into four. Each slip is then tunneled to a finger and attached to a lateral band, to flex the metacarpophalangeal joint of each finger and extend the interphalangeal joints.

The ECRL may be attached to each of the profundus tendons in the forearm, and the ECU may be used for the flexor pollicis longus (FPL).

Since the whole palmar surface of the hand is probably insensitive in these cases, it is very unlikely that the hand will be used for any kind of precision pinch, especially if the other hand is normal (contrast tetraplegia cases in which both hands are involved). Therefore, it may be best to aim for a simple grasp action, to assist the other hand that will be dominant.*

---

*Alternatively, one may attempt to restore an area of sensibility, as Omer and associates (1970) have done by removing all the bones of the index finger ray and also its palmar soft tissues, so that its dorsal sensitive surface may be folded over a chosen area of palm.

If it is determined that the thumb is to be used for pinch as well as grasp, the FPL will not be strong enough, even though opposing a weakened hand. It may be best to use the FPL tendon as a graft in situ by detaching it from its muscle and delivering it into the palm. It may then be grasped by a curved tunneler, which enters the palm around the muscles taking origin from the hook of the hamate, and picks up the FPL from behind the profundus tendons. Next the ECU or other motor may be attached to the proximal end of the FPL tendon.

In this new pathway the FPL has at least a 3 cm moment arm at the carpometacarpal joint and may be given a 2 cm moment arm at the metacarpophalangeal joint by advancing the tendon sheath a little. With its original moment arm of 1 cm or less at the interphalangeal joint the rerouted FPL should have a strong balanced action on the whole thumb (Fig. 114–34).

Abduction and opposition of the thumb can be taken care of by rerouting the tendon of the extensor indicis proprius around the ulnar aspect of the wrist. After these transfers the patient should be allowed time for reeducation and must be encouraged to use the hand. After a while, if some imbalance is noted, there are still other muscles that may be used in response to the patient's own sense

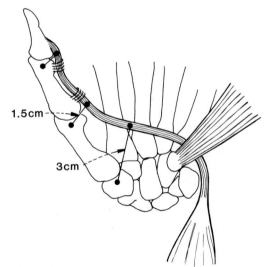

Figure 114–34. A suggested pathway for the flexor pollicis longus tendon when it is to be used as the only motor on the flexor side of the thumb for key pinch. The tendon pulls from the hook of the hamate, behind the long flexors, giving a 3 cm moment arm for flexion at the carpometacarpal joint. The tendon may then be tenodesed to the radius, if the only motor is a wrist extensor.

of need. One of these is the extensor digitorum communis muscle to the middle finger, which is quite distinct. It is proximal in the forearm and has a long tendon that is suitable for rerouting. The only problem is that distally on the back of the hand it has to be dissected free from junctura, which have to be reattached to other slips of extensor tendon (as from the ring finger) that can be moved across to extend the middle finger.

Radial and Ulnar Palsy

This severe paralysis has some good features. There is sensation in the area of pinch, and there are intact long flexors for pinch and for a narrow grasp between thumb and three fingers. (The FDS to the little finger is too weak to produce effective grasp.) In most cases it is best to concentrate only on these two features and aim for a pulp to pulp pinch by fusing the metacarpophalangeal joint of the thumb (except where the median nerve supplies sufficient FPB function).

The wrist drop is treated by the pronator teres as in simple radial palsy, finger extension by transfer of the FDS from the middle finger, and thumb extension by the palmaris longus. Abductor pollicis longus paralysis is not treated, but is not so necessary when the adductors are gone and the metacarpophalangeal joint is fused.

The grasp may be broadened by doing a side to side suture of the middle, ring, and little finger profundus tendons in the distal forearm. Clawing may be corrected by fusing the interphalangeal joints of the fingers or by some form of capsulodesis and/or tenodesis at the metacarpophalangeal joint (Zancolli, 1957; Riordan, 1959).

High Median and Radial

This extremely deprived hand still has most of its intrinsic muscles intact. It may have lost sensation to all but the two ulnar fingers. This kind of hand either should have a free muscle transplant (such as the gracilis) by microneurovascular anastomosis, to power extension of the wrist, or it should have wrist fusion. In the former case, tenodesis of the finger and thumb flexors will allow the power of the transplanted wrist extensor to give finger flexion and pinch. In the latter case,

the aim of surgery should be to develop prehension between the thumb and the ring and little fingers.

After wrist fusion the FCU may be transferred to serve as extensor to all digits, including the thumb. Now the part of the adductor pollicis that goes to the ulnar side dorsal expansion of the thumb may be transferred to the radial side of the thumb, to pull on the tendon of the APB (De Vecchi, 1961). This will not easily reach unless the full length of both tendons is preserved, especially the abductor. Alternatively, a free graft may be used. Now, with the interphalangeal joint of the thumb fused, it gives a strong and effective prehension against the ring and little fingers. The middle finger may be included with the ring and little fingers by side to side suture of the tendons in the forearm.

Considering the severity of the total muscle loss, this type of hand may be surprisingly useful. The tendency toward supination of the forearm may be dealt with by adjustment of the insertion of the biceps tendon, using the Zancolli (1979) technique. Although the *action* of supination is more useful than pronation, the position of supination is bad if it is unopposed.

Partial Brachial Plexus Injury and Other Severe Paralyses

Since tetraplegia and cerebral palsy are dealt with elsewhere, there follows a brief discussion on severe peripheral paralysis in general, including leprosy and muscular dystrophies.

TIME

Time is a most important factor, in relation to the whole life and the hopes and fears of the patient. It is important to be absolutely frank and open about the prospects for recovery of function, and to encourage the patient to struggle with the alternatives and make all the major decisions. One patient had advancing muscular dystrophy affecting both hands, and had already lost all the intrinsic muscles and much of the forearm strength. Some surgeons had discouraged operative intervention because of the poor long-term prognosis. The subsequent tendon transfers for replacement of the function of the intrinsic muscles of both hands have delighted him and continued to prove useful. His whole life was improved, and his new attitude may even have helped to provoke the remission in the disease itself. Leprosy patients often have progressive paralysis for a time, even while the mycobacteria are being brought under control by medical therapy. However, this should not discourage the surgeon who wants to restore balance to the hand; the pattern and sequence of paralysis in leprosy are known (Brand, 1952), and it is safe to use muscles supplied by the radial and high median nerves to compensate for high ulnar and low median paralysis. In poliomyelitis the disease is not progressive, but it used to be the custom to wait two years before advising tendon transfers, because muscles have been known to show recovery for that length of time. It is now known that although recovery may continue for two years, a severely paralyzed muscle will never become really useful if it does not *start* to recover within six months. If an early evaluation of voluntary muscle contraction is made at three months and again at six months, any muscle that is severely paralyzed at three months and has shown no significant sign of recovery at six months may be regarded as lost. It may finally have some minimal recovery but it will never be good enough for real function. Therefore, the surgeon may plan to carry out key tendon transfers within the first year after polio, even at six months, thus avoiding the development of contractures, and also avoiding some of the depression and apathy that make final rehabilitation a problem.

No matter what the cause of paralysis, surgeons must restrain themselves from being too optimistic in trying to restore a wide range of function with only a few muscles. It is better to aim for one good reliable movement that results in one type of prehension. To do this, it is often wise to reserve the strongest muscle as a wrist extensor, and then aim to restore grasp or a key pinch by tenodesis or by a second muscle-tendon unit. It is usually better to use two muscles for each movement, one muscle opposing the other, rather than use each muscle for a different movement, in the hope that gravity will be enough to balance the hand. No muscle can produce a really satisfactory action without another to reciprocate by moving in the opposite direction to open that which is to be closed. Let a severely damaged or paralyzed hand do one thing *well*, rather than two things inadequately.

REFERENCES

Biesalski, K., and Mayer, L.: Die Physiologische Sehnenverpflanzung. Berlin, Julius Springer, 1916.

Blix, M.: Die Länge und die Spannung des Muskels. Skand. Arch. Physiol., 3:295, 1891.

Blix, M.: Die Länge und die Spannung des Muskels. Skand. Arch. Physiol., 4:399, 1893.

Blix, M.: Die Länge und die Spannung des Muskels. Skand. Arch. Physiol., 5:149, 1894.

Boyes, J. H.: Tendon transfers for radial palsy. Bull. Hosp. Joint Dis., 15:97, 1960.

Brand, P. W.: Reconstruction of the hand in leprosy. Ann. R. Coll. Surg., 11:350, 1952.

Brand, P. W.: Deformity in leprosy. *In* Cochrane, R. G. (Ed.): Leprosy in Theory and Practice. Bristol, England, John Wright & Sons, 1959, pp. 265–319.

Brand, P. W.: Tendon transfers in the forearm. *In* Flynn, J. E. (Ed.): Hand Surgery. Baltimore, Williams & Wilkins Company, 1975, pp. 189–200.

Brand, P. W.: Paralysis of the intrinsic muscles of the hand. *In* Rob, C., and Smith, R. (Eds.): Operative Surgery. London, Butterworth, 1977, pp. 238–257.

Brand, P. W.: *In* Clinical Mechanics of the Hand. St. Louis, C. V. Mosby Company, 1985.

Brand, P. W., Beach, R. B., and D. E. Thompson: Relative tension and potential excursion of muscles in the forearm and hand. J. Hand Surg., 6:209, 1981.

Brandsma, J. W., and Brand, P. W.: Median nerve function after tendon transfer for ulnar paralysis. J. Hand Surg., 10B:30, 1985.

Brandsma, J. W., and Watson, J. M.: Clawfinger correction: results of extensor-flexor many-tailed operation. Hand, 14:307, 1982.

Brooks, A. L.: A new intrinsic tendon transfer for the paralytic hand. Proceedings. J. Bone Joint Surg., 57A:730, 1975.

Bunnell, S.: In Surgery of the Hand. 2nd Ed. Philadelphia, J. B. Lippincott Company, 1948, pp. 486, 513.

Camitz, H.: Über die Behandlung der Oppositionslähmung. Acta Chir. Scand., 65:77, 1921.

DeVecchi, J.: Oposicion del pulgar fisiopatologia: una nueva operacion—transplante del adductor. Bol. Soc. Cir. Del., Uruguay, 32:423, 1961.

Edgerton, M. T., and Brand, P. W.: Restoration of abduction and adduction to the unstable thumb in median and ulnar paralysis. Plast. Reconstr. Surg., 36:150, 1965.

Elftman, H.: Biomechanics of muscle. J. Bone Joint Surg., 48A:363, 1966.

Elliott, D. H., and Crawford, G. N. C.: The thickness and collagen content of tendon relative to the strength and cross-sectional area of muscle. Proc. R. Soc. Biol., 162:137, 1965a.

Elliott, D. H., and Crawford, G. N. C.: The thickness and collagen content of tendon relative to the cross-sectional area of muscle during growth. Proc. R. Soc. Biol., 162:198, 1965b.

Fick, A.: Statische Betrachtung der Muskulature des Oberschenkels. Z. Rationelle Med., 9:94, 1850.

Fick, R.: Handbuch der Anatomie und Mechanik der Gelenke unter Berücksichtigung der bewegenden Muskeln, 1904–11. Vol. 3. Specielle Gelenk und Muskelmechanik, Jena, 1911, Verlag von Gustav Fischer.

Freehafer, A. A., Peckham, P. H., and Keith, M. W.: Determination of muscle-tendon unit properties during tendon transfer. J. Hand Surg., 4:331, 1979.

Fritschi, E. P.: Reconstructive Surgery in Leprosy. Bristol, England, John Wright & Sons, 1971.

Gaul, J. S.: Intrinsic motor recovery–a long-term study of ulnar nerve repair. J. Hand Surg., 7:502, 1982.

Goldner, J. L., and Kelly, J. M.: Radial nerve injuries. South. Med. J., 51:873, 1958.

Henry, A. K.: A case of tendon transplantation for wrist-drop. Lancet, 1:1218, 1916.

Howard, L. D.: *In* Bunnell, S. (Ed.): Surgery of the Hand. 2nd Ed. Philadelphia, J. B. Lippincott Company, 1948, p. 491.

Jansen, M.: Ueber die Länge der Muskelbundel und ihre Bedeutung für die Entstehung der spastischen Kontrakturen. Z. F. Orthopaed. Chir., 36:1, 1917.

Jones, R.: On suture of nerves and alternative methods of treatment by transplantation of tendons. Br. Med. J., 1:641,679, 1916.

Littler, J. W.: Tendon transfers and arthrodeses in combined median and ulnar nerve paralysis. J. Bone Joint Surg., 31A:225, 1949.

Littler, J. W., and Cooley, S. G. E.: Opposition of the thumb and its restoration by abductor digiti quinti transfer. J. Bone Joint Surg., 45A:1389, 1963.

McMurray, T. P.: Discussion of the indications, techniques and results of transplantation in gunshot injuries of nerves. J. Orthop. Surg., 1:125, 1919.

Murphy, J. B.: Tenoplasty: tendon transplantation; tendon substitution; neuroplasty. Surg. Clin. North Am., 3:467, 1914.

Omer, G.: Report of the Committee for evaluation of the clinical results in peripheral nerve injury. J. Hand Surg., 8:754, 1983.

Omer, G. E., Jr., Day, D. J., Ratliff, H., et al.: Neurovascular cutaneous island pedicles for deficient median-nerve sensibility: new technique and results of serial functional tests. J. Bone Joint Surg., 52A:1181, 1970.

Pennell, V.: Tendon transplantation in drop-wrist due to nervous injury. Br. Med. J., 1:704, 1919.

Riordan, D. C.: Tendon transplantations in median-nerve and ulnar-nerve paralysis. J. Bone Joint Surg., 35:312, 1953.

Riordan, D. C.: Surgery of the paralytic hand. *In* Reynolds, F. C. (Ed.): American Academy of Orthopaedic Surgeons Instructional Course Lectures, Vol. 16. St. Louis, C. V. Mosby Company, 1959, pp. 79–90.

Smith, R. J.: Extensor carpi radialis brevis tendon transfer for thumb adduction: a study of power pinch. J. Hand Surg., 8:4, 1983.

Snow, J. W., and Fink, G. H.: Use of a transverse carpal ligament window for the pulley in tendon transfers for median nerve palsy. Plast. Reconst. Surg., 48:238, 1971.

Thompson, T. C.: A modified operation for opponens paralysis. J. Bone Joint Surg., 24:623, 1942.

Tsuge, K.: Tendon transfers in median and ulnar nerve paralysis. Hiroshima J. Med. Sci., 16:29, 1967.

Weber, W., and Weber, E.: Mechanik der menschlichen Gehwerkzeuge. Gottingen, Dieterich, 1836.

Weitz, H.: Zur Behandlung der Radialislahmung. Dtsch. Med. Woch., 42:1351, 1916.

White, W. L.: Restoration of function and balance of the wrist and hand by tendon transfers. Surg. Clin. North Am., 40:427, 1960.

Yamada, H.: *In* Evans, F. G. (Ed.): Strength of Biological Materials. Baltimore, Williams & Wilkins Company, 1970.

Zancolli, E. A.: Claw-hand caused by paralysis of the intrinsic muscles: a simple surgical procedure for its correction. J. Bone Joint Surg., 39A:1076, 1957.

Zancolli, E. A.: Structural and Dynamic Bases of Hand Surgery. Functional Restoration of the Upper Limbs in Traumatic Quadriplegia. 2nd Ed. Philadelphia, J. B. Lippincott Company, 1979, p. 236.

Functioning Muscle Transfer for Reconstruction of the Hand

Functioning muscle transfer is the surgical transfer of a skeletal muscle from one site to another by microneurovascular techniques. This procedure is particularly useful to provide finger flexion or extension when flexor or extensor muscles have been lost from the forearm. It should not be used when simpler techniques of tendon transfer are available and are likely to provide a satisfactory result.

The transferred muscle is reinnervated by suturing an undamaged motor nerve from the forearm to the muscle's motor nerve. Circulation is maintained by standard microvascular techniques, anastomosing the muscle's artery and vein to a suitable artery and vein in the forearm. The origin of the muscle is fixed to the proximal forearm fascia and medial or lateral epicondyle, and the insertion to the finger flexor or extensor tendons.

The procedure is complex. Good functional results depend on careful patient selection, use of an appropriate muscle, precise surgical techniques, and a vigorous postoperative therapy program.

HISTORY

Tamai and associates (1970) reported successful microneurovascular muscle transfer in the dog. Their histologic and electromyographic studies indicated that the muscle survived and underwent satisfactory reinnervation, and provided a stimulus to clinical applications. The author studied a patient in Shanghai (1976) who had had a portion of the pectoralis major transferred to the forearm in 1973 by surgeons at the Sixth People's Hospital. This patient had good muscle bulk and contraction in the muscle, which provided a good range of finger flexion and grip strength. Subsequently, the author and others have used microneurovascular muscle transfer in a number of sites, including the forearm for replacement of finger flexion and extension, the upper arm for replacement of the biceps, the shoulder for deltoid reconstruction, and the lower leg for correction of footdrop deformity (1978, 1984).

APPLIED MUSCLE PHYSIOLOGY

The main function of skeletal muscle is to produce a controlled force. The force can be exerted while the muscle is shortening in the performance of work (concentric contraction), or while it is static or lengthening (eccentric

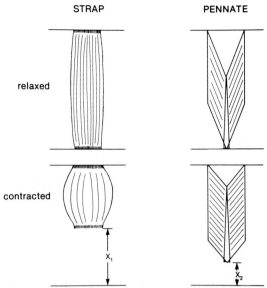

STRAP   PENNATE

relaxed

contracted

X_1

X_2

Figure 115–1. Schematic representation of contraction in a strap and pennate muscle. Note the marked difference in muscle excursions X_1 and X_2 with 50 per cent shortening of the muscle fibers in each muscle.

1 to 40 mm in length. Each cellular unit is composed of many myofibrils lying parallel and enclosed in sarcolemma. Each myofibril is composed of a hexagonal geometric arrangement of thin actin and thick myosin fibers lying adjacent to each other.

Gross muscle fiber configuration is either strap or pennate (Fig. 115–1) or a combination of the two. In a strap muscle, the orientation of the muscle fibers is parallel to the long axis of the muscle. These muscles have a potential range of excursion directly proportional to the overall muscle length. The maximal force of muscle contraction varies with the cross sectional area of the muscle fibers. The maximal tension developed experimentally on tetanic stimulation in mammals is 4 kg/cm² (Carlson and Wilkie, 1974). The maximal potential force of contraction of a strap muscle can be crudely estimated by measuring the cross sectional area of the entire muscle. However, in a pennate muscle, which has much shorter muscle fiber units, the range of contraction of the entire muscle is proportional to the length of these short muscle fibers rather than the overall length of the muscle. For example, if the muscle fiber length in the pennate rectus femoris

contraction), to provide a controlled resistance.

Each muscle is made up of many individual muscle fibers, each of which is a cellular unit

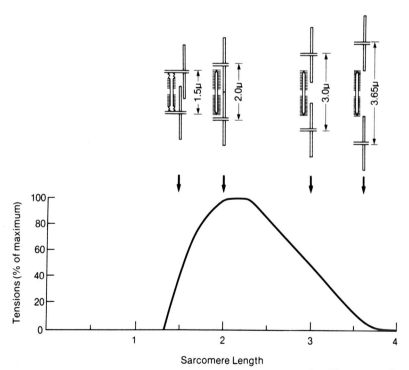

Figure 115–2. Length-tension curve of a single muscle fiber undergoing contraction. The stages of overlap of the thick myosin and thin actin fibers in a sarcomere are shown above the appropriate points on the curve.

muscle is 6 cm, the overall muscle contraction capability is approximately 50 per cent of this, or 3 cm, while the overall muscle length may be 30 cm. However, the aggregate cross sectional area of these pennate muscle fiber units is considerably larger than in a comparable-sized strap muscle, and the muscle is correspondingly more powerful in its force of contraction.

Length-Tension Relationship

When stimulated, a single muscle fiber freed of its connective tissue produces a length-tension curve as shown in Figure 115–2. Muscle contraction consists of a dynamic process of sliding adjacent thick and thin fibers together into an overlap (crossbridging). At maximal extension, there is little overlap, and muscle contraction is weak. As the extent of overlap increases, the strength of the muscle's contractile force increases until there is complete overlap. At the peak of the length-tension curve, there is a total overlap of the actin and myosin fibers. With further contraction there is crumpling of the myosin fibers, less area of overlap, and correspondingly less force of contraction.

The force of contraction of a muscle depends on the number of individual muscle fibers that respond and the length of the muscle at which it is required to contract. The contraction of each muscle fiber is an "all or none" phenomenon. With weak muscle contraction, only a few muscle fibers are functioning; with a strong contraction, most of the fibers respond.

When a noncontracting whole muscle is stretched beyond a certain point, it requires a progressive increase in stretching force. This elasticity within the muscle is produced by the connective tissue network that surrounds the muscle fibers (Fig. 115–3B). Although this elastic component may not be entirely separate and independent of the contractile component, it is generally assumed in estimating an active length-tension curve that these two components can be added to provide the length-tension curve for a functioning muscle unit (Fig. 115–3C). Thus, the extent of connective tissue within the muscle plays a part in determining the useful length of muscle contraction, and the forces generated during contraction from the extended position.

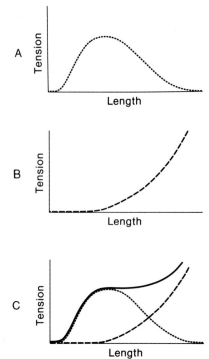

Figure 115–3. *A*, Length-tension curve of a single muscle fiber during contraction. *B*, Length-tension curve of a resting whole muscle being passively stretched. *C*, The total tension developed by a whole muscle under tetanic stimulation (solid line) is the sum of the force produced by active contraction and passive stretching. This curve of total tension varies considerably, depending on the muscle length at which passive stretching begins to produce tension.

The potential range of muscle excursion is finite, depending on the capacity for the actin and myosin fibers to slide apart and together. In a single fiber of a frog's striated muscle, the total range of contraction is 65 per cent of its fully stretched length (Gordon, Huxley, and Julian, 1966). However, this fully stretched fiber length is limited in an intact muscle by the connective tissue network that surrounds each muscle and limits extension.

The author's experience with relatively crude measuring techniques applied to in vivo muscle testing in the human gracilis muscle has demonstrated a shortening of 12 to 16 cm, measured from the physiologic fully extended resting muscle length (Fig. 115–4). The gracilis, which is mostly a strap muscle with a pennate configuration at the distal end, has an average muscle fiber length with a range of 16 to 30 cm. On the basis of these clinical tests and the single muscle fiber testing of Gordon, Huxley, and Julian (1966), it seems reasonable to assume that the useful

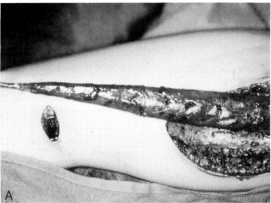 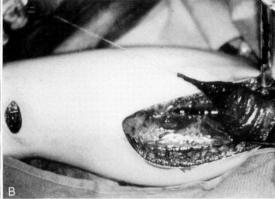

Figure 115–4. *A,* Gracilis muscle dissected free except for origin and neurovascular structures. *B,* Following tetanic nerve stimulation the muscle contracted to 40 per cent of its maximal extended length.

range of powerful muscle excursion of a gracilis muscle, and probably most strap muscles, is at least 40 per cent of the fully extended fiber length.

MUSCLE SELECTION

Many different muscles have been used for functioning muscle microneurovascular transfer. With added experience, additional muscles will probably become popular. The muscles that have been used in the forearm are the gracilis, the latissimus dorsi, the tensor fascia lata, the rectus femoris, and one head of the gastrocnemius. The most commonly used muscle has been the gracilis.

Anatomic Fit

The muscle must have a suitable length to fit the defect, reaching from the intended origin to the tendons for insertion. Usually a tendon of adequate length is needed on the distal end of the muscle to suture to the flexor or extensor tendons.

The location of the neurovascular structures of the muscle must fit those in the recipient area. The distance of the nerve anastomosis from the muscle's neuromuscular hilum should be minimized in order to decrease the duration of muscle deinnervation. The location of the vascular pedicle on the muscle must be in a suitable location for anastomoses to the vessels in the arm. However, the pedicle can be lengthened with vein grafts, as is done in other free tissue transfers.

Mathes and Nahai classified the external vascular anatomy of skeletal muscle into five groups. The type of muscle suitable for free tissue transfer is one that has either a single or a dominant vascular pedicle that is capable of supplying the entire muscle.

Dynamic Suitability

The dynamic requirements of a muscle selected for free transfer are that it have adequate strength and an adequate range of motion to provide the desired function. When the finger long flexors are being replaced, the range of excursion should be 6 to 7 cm to provide full finger flexion in all wrist positions. It is likely that the muscle will be positioned in the arm with slightly different tension than in its original site, and that there will be a proportional loss of useful range of contraction. For this reason, a muscle should be selected that has a range of motion normally greater than that required in the transplanted location. Strap muscles, such as the gracilis, pectoralis major, and latissimus dorsi, have a more than adequate range of contraction to provide full finger flexion throughout all positions of the wrist. Since the strength of a muscle is proportional to the cross sectional area of all muscle fibers, the bulk of a strap muscle is directly proportional to its strength. This relation does not apply to pennate muscles, whose strength is proportional to the aggregate cross sectional area of all the muscle fibers. The pectoralis major and the latissimus have an anatomic disadvantage as there is no tendon for insertion at the muscle origin and the fan-shaped muscle fibers are shorter on the superior margin.

INDICATIONS

This operation is useful for patients who have sustained a major loss of forearm musculature and are unable to flex or extend their fingers. The most common cause of muscle loss is direct traumatic injury to the forearm; other causes are secondary to Volkmann's ischemic paralysis, major electrical burns, and traumatic loss related to amputation and replantation. Occasionally, muscle loss caused by gas gangrene or muscle resection for tumor is suitable for microneurovascular muscle transfer.

The typical patient is one who has lost all flexor musculature and has had sufficient damage to the extensor musculature to preclude extensor carpi radialis transfer. If the extensor muscles are undamaged, a tendon transfer using the extensor carpi radialis brevis is usually the most suitable procedure because of its simplicity and expected good functional results, with early return of function. This typical patient should have the median and ulnar nerves relatively undamaged, providing good sensibility and intrinsic function to the hand. There should be an adequate mechanism for finger and thumb extension, and wrist stabilization. There must be good passive finger joint motion and an intact flexor tendon system in the fingers and palm. In an injured arm, with these functional mechanisms present, the addition of a free muscle transfer can provide useful finger function and can create a very functional hand.

As in most types of hand surgery following complex injuries, the personality, work requirements, and motivation of the patient are important in determining the suitability for operation and the expected patient satisfaction. As the time required for muscle reinnervation and the return of useful muscle strength is lengthy, the patient must be well motivated to pursue a prolonged course of postoperative resisted exercises, which will be necessary before useful function is obtained.

PREOPERATIVE PLANNING

To determine whether a free muscle transfer is feasible, all structures that will be involved in the transfer must be evaluated. The expected location of the flexor tendon stumps in the forearm and wrist can usually be determined from the physical examination or from previous knowledge of the injury. Arterial vasculature in an injured forearm is often difficult to assess with a physical examination. Doppler flow studies and angiography are usually required to determine the location and suitability of an artery for end to end or end to side anastomoses. Usually, veins can be found either as venae comitantes or as superficial veins in the forearm.

The sine qua non for a successful muscle transfer is the availability of an undamaged motor nerve that can be used to reinnervate the transplanted muscle. In the forearm, the anterior interosseous nerve is the preferred one as it is a pure motor nerve and lies in a deep position that is often undamaged despite severe trauma to the more superficial muscle layers. Other suitable nerves are the motor branches of the median and ulnar, which supply the profundus and superficialis musculature. However, it may be difficult to distinguish these from motor branches to the wrist flexors, which do not provide appropriate reinnervation. If the presence of an undamaged motor nerve cannot be predicted from the physical examination and history, a nerve exploration should be made before the anticipated muscle transfer. Histologic examination of the nerve at the intended site of nerve repair will establish the suitability of the nerve for reinnervating the transferred muscle. Neuropathologic frozen section assessment at the time of muscle transfer may also provide information about the integrity of the axons in the nerve that is to be used for reinnervation.

Good skin flap coverage must be available over the distal half of the forearm to facilitate gliding of the distal end of the muscle and the tendon repair site. This may require previous application of a flap, forearm skin tissue expansion, or a myocutaneous muscle transfer. The last-named has not proved entirely satisfactory as it usually provides a very bulky coverage for the forearm.

To select an appropriate muscle, a pattern of the desired muscle is taken from the forearm. The anticipated position of each recipient structure—artery, vein, nerve, tendons, and skin defect—is marked on the forearm. This allows a pattern to be outlined on the forearm indicating the desired location of the muscle's motor nerve, vascular pedicle, ten-

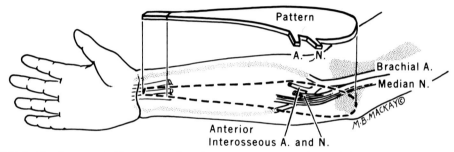

Figure 115–5. After the expected location of all tendons, motor nerves, and vessels is marked on the forearm, a pattern of the desired muscle is created.

dons, and skin cover. A pattern is taken from this outline and can be used to select the most appropriate muscle (Fig. 115–5).

OPERATIVE TECHNIQUE

A two-team approach is useful to allow simultaneous forearm and muscle preparation to minimize operative time. For a more detailed description of the technique, the reader is referred elsewhere (Manktelow, 1986).

Preparation of Forearm

The site of forearm incision should be selected with care, not only to allow adequate exposure of all structures but also to create suitable skin flaps to cover the distal half of the muscle and muscle tendon junction.

Vessels, tendons, and nerve are then prepared for the transfer. A meticulous dissection is required in a badly scarred arm, otherwise these structures can easily be damaged. Dissection from proximal to distal, beginning in an undamaged area, provides a safe exposure for the desired vessels and nerve. If an end to end arterial anastomosis is planned, the artery should be divided and the adequacy of spurt of blood evaluated. If there is not a forceful spurt, it is likely that there is proximal obstruction, or that the artery has been damaged and is in spasm. If this artery is used for anastomoses, thrombosis may occur. The preferred site for a vessel anastomosis is proximal to the zone of injury, where the chance of spasm is diminished. A suitable anastomosis to vessels that are in the zone of injury is an end to side anastomosis, since this technique prevents

vessel retraction and spasm. Fortunately, spasm is not as much of a problem as in the lower leg.

Selection of a suitable motor nerve requires a detailed knowledge of the anatomy of the median and ulnar nerve branches. Although the anatomy is often confused because of previous injury, remnants of functioning muscle often remain in the forearm. Their location and the use of a nerve stimulator may help to identify functioning motor nerves. When a nerve has been selected, it should be examined under magnification to establish whether there is a reasonable fascicular pattern. If intraneural fibrosis is present, the nerve should be trimmed proximally until an undamaged area of nerve is identified.

Suitable tissue for insertion of the muscle origin is prepared. For a flexor muscle transfer, the medial epicondyle and fascia of the common flexor origin is the usual site for the muscle's origin. For an extensor muscle transfer, the lateral epicondyle and common extensor fascia is used. After identification of the flexor or extensor tendons in the wrist, their gliding capability should be assessed by traction on their ends. If the gliding is inadequate, a limited tenolysis may be done. Although some adhesions reform, the postoperative therapy program significantly limits their formation.

Preparation of Gracilis Muscle

The gracilis is the muscle most commonly used for transfer to the forearm. It is completely expendable, leaves an acceptable donor site scar, and has a good anatomic fit for the forearm. The functional capabilities are good, providing a full range of finger excursion and a grip strength of up to 50 per cent of normal.

The gracilis is a broad strap muscle that takes its origin from the body of the pubis and its inferior ramus and adjacent ramus of the ischium. The muscle lies just posterior to the adductor longus and sartorius muscles and immediately deep to the superficial fascia. Muscle fiber length averages 24 cm in the adult. The tendon is long and well defined, lies just anterior to the semitendinosus, and terminates in the shaft of the tibia, just below the tibial tubercle. The muscle fibers attach to the tendon of insertion sequentially, with the anterior fibers inserted most distally. There is a single motor nerve that enters the muscle 6 to 12 cm from its origin and consists of two to six fascicles. There are at least two, and sometimes more, vascular pedicles. The dominant pedicle lies 8 to 12 cm from the muscle's origin. The artery is 1.5 to 2 mm in diameter and at least 6 cm in length. There are two venae comitantes that are slightly larger than the artery. Rarely, the dominant pedicle is a double pedicle, which may create a problem for microvascular anastomoses. The author has used this muscle as a free tissue transfer, both as a functioning and a nonfunctioning muscle, in 90 cases. Many of these involved a small segment of muscle. However, 26 involved free transfer of the entire muscle. Occasionally, with single pedicle repair, the most distal few centimeters of muscle fibers may not perfuse well. These distal fibers are then excised and the cut ends reinserted into the tendon. The functional integrity of the muscle remains intact.

When the gracilis is used as a myocutaneous transfer, the most reliable portion of the cutaneous flap is over the proximal 15 cm of muscle. The distal portion of the muscle does not reliably support a cutaneous flap. However, this distal area is the area in which flap coverage is usually required to provide coverage for the distal muscle tendon junction. The bulk of the cutaneous portion of the transfer has been a moderate disadvantage. Usually, a skin graft on the proximal half of the muscle is preferred as it provides a smooth contour to the forearm and does not limit muscle movement when placed on the proximal muscle belly.

The technique of gracilis preparation is straightforward when the anatomy is well understood (Manktelow, 1986). Elevation of the adductor longus with right-angled retractors allows preparation of the pedicle and adequate exposure for division of side branches.

After the muscle has been completely separated from the leg and left attached to its vascular pedicle, its circulation should be observed. Color, contractility, and epimysial bleeding are adequate signs of muscle viability.

Muscle Transfer

When the forearm is completely prepared, the muscle is separated from the thigh and attached to the forearm. The muscle is positioned so that the motor nerve suture can be placed as close as possible to the neuromuscular hilum, and the vascular pedicle is in a suitable position for anastomosis to the recipient vessels. After a preliminary tacking of the muscle to the forearm, the vessel anastomoses should be done first in order to minimize the ischemia time.

There are five important technical considerations in muscle transfer: revascularization, reinnervation, balanced tendon adjustment, positioning of the muscle at optimal tension, and adequate flap coverage.

Revascularization. Although ischemia time should be minimized, it is unlikely that ischemic damage will occur unless there are operative complications. An ischemia time of two to three hours does not provide ischemic damage to the muscle, as demonstrated in the experimental work of Kuzon and associates (1984). However, the muscle should easily be revascularized in less time than this. Technically perfect anastomoses are necessary, since the ischemic insult that occurs with thrombosis and revision of a thrombosed anastomoses is very undesirable in a functioning muscle transfer. The muscle will be observed to become pink and bleed from the perimysium promptly upon completion of the anastomoses. Any distal musculature that is nonviable should be removed.

While the muscle's origin is held fixed, the insertion is stretched toward the hand and relaxed to simulate extension and flexion movements of the muscle. The movements of the pedicle are observed relative to the intended site of anastomosis on the arm, in order to ensure that with excursion of muscle contraction and relaxation, the anastomosis will be undamaged.

Reinnervation. The nerve repair can usually be placed 2 to 3 cm from the muscle's neuromuscular hilum. As the gracilis motor nerve contains at least 60 per cent fatty connective tissue (Fig. 115–6), a fascicular repair should be made so that fascicles in both nerve ends are accurately approximated. A technically perfect nerve repair should be the surgeon's goal.

Balanced Tendon Fixation. Following revascularization and nerve repair, the muscle's origin is fixed to the medial or lateral epicondyle and the distal attachment to the tendons is planned. If the muscle is being used to produce finger flexion, a balanced grip is required with all fingers flexing in unison. The four profundus tendons are sewn side to side to each other in a balanced position, with each digit slightly more flexed than the adjacent radial digit. When the gracilis tendon is inserted into the group of profundus tendons, mass flexion is produced with the fingers in a balanced grip position.

If the flexor pollicis longus is to be motored with the same muscle transfer as the fingers, it should be sewn to the finger flexors in a position that has some slack so that the fingers start to form a fist before the thumb moves. This brings the thumb to rest on the radial side of the index finger in the position of key pinch. If the flexor pollicis longus is too tight, the thumb is brought into the palm before the fingers, preventing pinch and grip functions.

Muscle Positioning for Optimal Tension. The flexor tendons are sutured to the gracilis muscle at a tension that produces maximal grip strength and a full range of finger motion. In order to accomplish this, a marking system is used to establish the functional length of the muscle. Before removal

of the muscle from its normal site, it is placed at its maximal physiologic stretch by abducting and externally rotating the thigh and extending the knee. Suture markers are then placed along the surface of the muscle at 5 cm intervals (Fig. 115–7A). After the muscle has been placed in the forearm and revascularized, and the origin fixed, the muscle tendon is stretched distally until the distance between each of the markers is once again 5 cm. The fingers and wrist are placed in a fully extended position, and the location of the flexor tendon stumps on the gracilis tendon is noted and marked. The wrist and fingers are then brought back into flexion, and the profundus and gracilis tendons are sutured together at the location marked (Fig. 115–7B,C). An interweaving tendon sutured technique is used. This procedure ensures that with gracilis muscle relaxation, full finger extension is possible. Since the muscle has a useful range of contraction greater than that required for finger flexion, full finger flexion is produced by muscle contraction. The muscle functions within the most powerful range of its length-tension curve, providing its optimal grip capability. The surgeon should not be concerned about the adequacy of blood flow in a muscle that is under mild tension after transfer, as muscles are normally under modest tension at rest and their perfusion is unaffected. With the wrist and fingers semiflexed, the muscle is under moderate tension, which is insufficient to affect circulation or tendon repair during the first few weeks after transfer.

Flap Coverage. The proximal muscle is usually covered with a split-thickness skin graft unless there is adequate forearm skin to cover the muscle without tension. In the distal forearm, good flap coverage must be

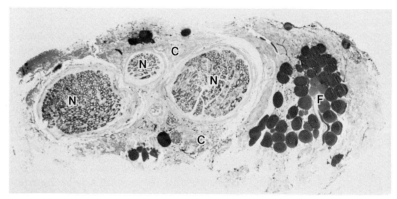

Figure 115–6. Cross section of gracilis motor nerve. *N* = nerve fascicle; *C* = connective tissue; *F* = fat.

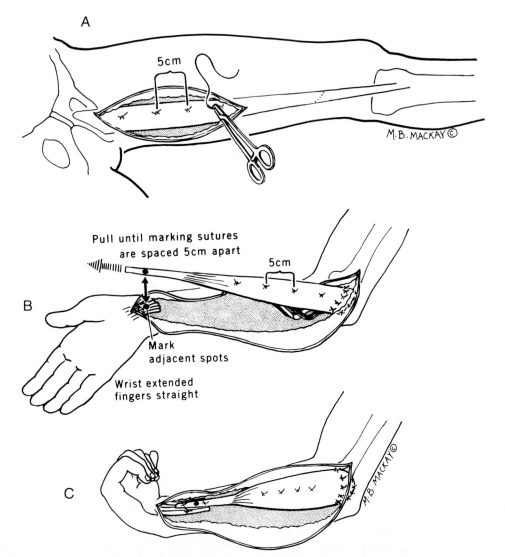

Figure 115–7. *A,* While the gracilis is still in the thigh, it is stretched to its normal maximal length by abducting the thigh and extending the knee. Suture markers are placed on the surface of the muscle at 5 cm intervals. *B,* Following microneurovascular repair and proximal fixation, the muscle is stretched toward the fingers until the suture markers are 5 cm apart. The wrist and fingers are held extended, and adjacent spots are marked on the gracilis and flexor digitorum profundus tendons. *C,* Minimal tension on the tendon repair is accomplished by wrist and finger flexion.

planned before the muscle transfer. If the distal half of the muscle is not covered by a flap or normal forearm skin, good tendon and muscle gliding cannot be expected. If a secondary tenolysis proves necessary, it will be impossible if the distal forearm is not covered by a flap.

POSTOPERATIVE CARE

The anesthetist promotes successful revascularization by maintaining a good peripheral perfusion throughout the duration of the procedure. In the postoperative period, it is important that peripheral perfusion be maintained by adequate intravenous intake and maintenance of body temperature. Antiplatelet agents are unnecessary. Muscles usually have a relatively high volume of blood flow at least twice that of a cutaneous flap, and anastomosis thrombosis is uncommon. If a thrombosis occurs after the patient has left the operating room, the muscle may need to be replaced by another muscle rather than have the anastomosis revised. The duration of the ischemic insult and the effect on function are likely to be uncertain and probably deleterious.

The wrist and fingers are splinted in moderate flexion for three weeks after surgery, followed by a program of passive stretching of the wrist and fingers. Within a few weeks or months a full range of wrist extension and finger extension will be obtained. These early passive extension exercises develop gliding mechanisms between the muscle tendon unit and surrounding tissues, which will be required when active contraction occurs following reinnervation. These gliding mechanisms will not develop if the muscle was not inserted with sufficient tension so that the elastic component of muscle shortening is unable to flex the fingers. Two to four months postoperatively the first clinical signs of reinnervation occur. With reinnervation, a gradually increasing range of muscle contraction and finger excursion is produced. When a full range of excursion has occurred, and there is the beginning of some muscle strength, the patient is placed on a program of resisted exercises and activities of daily living. The best results occur in patients who are well motivated and accept their exercise program with the seriousness of an athlete engaged in a muscle building program. This exercise program should be continued for a further year until grip strength has reached a plateau.

RESULTS

A successful muscle free tissue transfer is one that provides full finger flexion with a powerful grip. The author reviewed the first 12 muscle transfers to the forearm (Manktelow, Zuker, and McKee, 1984). Eleven of these survived completely and one survived partially. Ten out of 12 were successful in providing a useful range of motion and adequate grip for the patient's functional activities. Nine provided full finger flexion from the fully extended position when the wrist was held in neutral. Five of these nine also provided a full range of finger flexion when the wrist was held in the fully flexed or fully extended position. Of the five cases available for measurement of grip strength, four were in adults, who had a grip strength of from 18 to 60 lb with the Jaymar dynamometer. The maximal grip strength in two of the patients was 50 per cent of that in their normal arms.

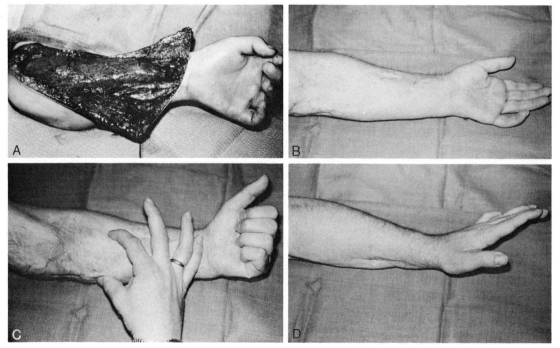

Figure 115–8. Muscle transfer to the left forearm. *A,* A 32 year old man sustained a severe forearm injury with loss of all flexor musculature. The forearm is seen after gracilis muscle transfer. *B,* One year after transfer. *C,* The gracilis can be palpated between the examiner's thumb and index finger when the patient makes a fist. *D,* With muscle relaxation, full finger extension is present.

Table 115–1. Guidelines for Muscle Transfer to the Forearm

Muscle Selection
1. Suitable neurovascular anatomy
2. Adequate strength and range of excursion
3. Suitable anatomy to fit defect—length, location of neurovascular bundle, and tendon availability
4. Ability to be removed without leaving significant functional deficit

Patient Selection
1. Available undamaged motor nerve, artery, and vein at site of muscle transplantation
2. Adequate skin cover for distal half of muscle
3. Supple joints and gliding tendons
4. Good hand sensibility
5. Good patient motivation

One of these patients had a gracilis muscle transfer and one a pectoralis major. All muscles were under precise and spontaneous voluntary control. Some of the patients did heavy farm and construction labor and did not notice any undue muscle fatigue. In most cases, the muscle returned to its pretransfer bulk as evaluated by clinical examination.

CONCLUSION

The most important factors in a successful free muscle transfer are proper patient and muscle selection, careful preoperative planning, and a fastidious surgical technique. For useful muscle function, an undamaged recipient motor nerve must be available for muscle reinnervation.

REFERENCES

Carlson, F. D., and Wilkie, D. R.: Muscle Physiology. Englewood Cliffs, NJ, Prentice-Hall, 1974.

Gordon, A. M., Huxley, A. F., and Julian, F. J.: The variation in isometric tension with sarcomere length in vertebrate muscle fibres. J. Physiol., *184*:170, 1966.

Kuzon, W. M., Fish, J. S., Pynn, B. R., and McKee, N. H.: Determinants of contractile function in free muscle transfers. Surg. Forum, *35*:610, 1984.

Manktelow, R. T.: Microvascular Reconstruction. Heidelberg, Springer Verlag, 1986, Chaps. 6, 19.

Manktelow, R. T., and McKee, N. H.: Free muscle transplantation to provide active finger flexion. J. Hand Surg., *3*:416, 1978.

Manktelow, R. T., Zuker, R. M., and McKee, N. H.: Functional free muscle transplantation. J. Hand Surg., *9A*:32, 1984.

Mathes, S. J., and Nahai, F.: Classification of the vascular anatomy of muscles: experimental and clinical correlation. Plast. Reconstr. Surg., *67*:177, 1981.

Shanghai Sixth People's Hospital: Functioning free muscle transplantation. Chin. Med. J., *2*:47, 1976.

Tamai, S., Komatsu, S., Sakamoto, H., et al.: Free muscle transplants in dogs with microsurgical neurovascular anastomoses. Plast. Reconstr. Surg., *46*:219, 1970.

Surgery for the Spastic, Stroke, and Tetraplegic Hand

The spastic hand, the stroke hand, and the tetraplegic hand, in addition to the total brachial plexus lesion and a few other more rare upper limb disorders, have some important features in common that distinguish them from other cases in everyday hand surgery. Usually the most functional basic parameters, especially kinesthesia, are retained in more simple cases, and so it is necessary to localize and restore only one or a few problems. The defects can easily be "listed" and corrected by separate procedures. The loss is limited and the aim usually is a result close to normality.

In spastic, stroke, or tetraplegic patients, the problem is totally different: the loss is close to subtotal, and any restoration to normality is out of the question. In these severely handicapped patients, some function can be constructed, not always *re*constructed, from the small amount of functional tissues that

exist. The task is not made easier by the fact that what remains may look like a normal, complete hand. In other cases the aim has to be only a cosmetic improvement.

From other points of view there are also enormous differences between the groups mentioned above. In the stroke patient one hand is often normal, whereas in tetraplegia this is not the case. Often mental defects dominate in the spastic child. The young and active tetraplegia victim has his life totally changed without warning in a split second. He never gives up the dream that one day a miracle will restore normal function. Even if his sound judgment is telling him that this is impossible, wishful thinking may prevail, and so he refuses the hope of improvement through surgery, to keep his anatomy intact for the miracle. This is just one of the psychologic problems he may face.

Table 116–1 describes the degrees of proprioception, kinesthetic control, balance, motion, and power seen in normal polio, tetraplegia, and spastic stroke patients. Many reconstructive attempts have failed because of insufficient evaluation of its importance, especially at a time when it was thought that the experience gained from the totally different polio surgery for poliomyelitis could be applied to these patients.

Thus, for the kind of surgery discussed in this chapter, a new concept was necessary. Special personal experience has to be built up, and so it is necessary either to enter the field with enough interest, time, and cases, or to stay outside. The surgeon cannot just perform the operations, but must examine, evaluate, and follow up. If not only cosmetic improvement but also real function is the aim, the patients need much postoperative education and guidance.

Table 116–1. Loss of Function

	Normal	Polio	Tetraplegia	Spastic Hand in Cerebral Palsy and Stroke
Reliable ligaments	45	45	3?	Great variations, often better than in tetraplegia
Muscles for motion and transfer	37	Often 4–8	In the majority 1- 2- 3	Few, if any
Adequate central control of left motor action	Normal	Normal	In most cases sufficient, loss often local	More often than not greatly reduced or absent
Tactile gnosis and proprioception	Normal	Normal	In most cases greatly reduced or absent	Only exceptionally sufficient

LEARNING, KINESTHESIA, AND SENSIBILITY

After surgery the great majority of these patients have to learn to use arms and hands that have been without proper function for a long time. They may have to cope with the still more difficult task to *learn* to use totally new constructions, which were not required before.

Every action (we all function in terms of complicated actions, not in single motor impulses) is an answer to *afferent* impulses, a "feedback" to them. This makes it necessary to distinguish between two kinds of afferents with distinctly different targets and purposes. One group relates to our conscious level, good for making conscious *decisions* and also for *learning*. The other group of impulses relates to our "computer" level and is good for executing the ordered actions with *skill* and *speed*. However, the latter group of afferents are, as Granit (1955) says, "private to the muscles"; they cannot be used directly for learning. When only those related to the computer level are present, patients cannot learn to use new surgical constructions. For those they need the afferent impulses at conscious level, for rehabilitation purposes. Rehabilitation means simply to create a program, using the conscious level, on the computer level system. The presence of the correct afferents must be evaluated preoperatively, as without such a program the surgical result will be a failure.

The next step, therefore, is to find out about these afferents. A prominent physiologist has estimated the number of afferents from a hand in action as roughly 5 million per second, and the ones outgoing to muscles as slightly fewer. The source of the impulses ingoing to conscious level is the next problem. Some of them come from vision, from the balance system, or from hearing. But most must come from the limb itself. In earlier days they were thought to originate from the joints, later they were said to stem from the Golgi apparatus in the tendons and from the muscle spindles. Today (Moberg, 1983b) it has been shown that the cutaneous receptors are the totally dominating ones. Their presence or absence can be evaluated by testing the cutaneous sensibility.

Unfortunately, this testing is currently in a chaotic situation. Almost every new manual has its own points of view, and the practical handling is still worse. Too often it is handed over to helpers with insufficient knowledge and training, as noted by the author in several countries. Seddon (1975) said in the last edition of his final book: "If . . . the recording of sensory recovery can be better defined and generally adopted, it will be a great step forward." The difficult problem of examining sensory function (Moberg and associates, 1984), which must be made different for different purposes, cannot be taken up here. Many test methods produce figures without any correlation to function. In the author's opinion, only the two-point discrimination test, performed correctly with the same degree of attention to detail as a microsurgical procedure, with a very small instrument and adequate bracing done in such a way as to evaluate the presence or absence of tactile gnosis, is of value. The plastic ridge method and the as yet unpublished drum test (Marsh) are inadequate for this purpose, although they measure the correct factors.

Used correctly, the two-point discrimination test evaluates more than the tactile gnosis. It also reveals the presence or absence of proprioception. This test causes a small deformation of the skin surface. Just the same happens when a finger joint is moving—a cutaneous deformation. In flexion there will be tension and elongation of the dorsal skin, and compression volarly; in extension, the inverse. The cutaneous afferents will report these deformations to the central system, which will transform the message to proprioception. Therefore, it is logical that the same test and the same limit, about 10 mm, can be used for tactile gnosis as well as for proprioception. Both factors can be determined segment by segment in the hand, and the result can be given in figures. We can give up the difficult and inaccurate wiggling up and down of digits in the hand.

With a two-point discrimination, accordingly, of at least 10 mm in the thumb pulp, the patient has tactile gnosis good enough to feel that he has an object in the thumb grip and some idea of what it is like. At the same time the test shows that he can control movement to a useful degree and apply the right power (have some proprioception) without help of vision. Without such a quality of cutaneous sensibility, all this is impossible.

For the elbow and shoulder, however, the situation is different (Fig. 116–1).

Muscles

Very little of the necessary detailed information about muscles can be gained during the surgical procedure. As in tetraplegia, it may be necessary to test the extensor carpi

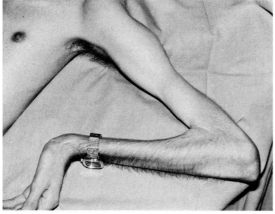

Figure 116–1. This young tetraplegic patient has good elbow flexors and extension through gravity. Unless he can see the arm, however, he is totally unaware of its position. Position sense is lost owing to absence of cutanous afferents of adequate quality. Contrary to the situation in the digits, at this level the two-point discrimination test cannot measure proprioception.

radialis brevis muscle openly, as it is impossible previously to distinguish its pull from that of the longus. Often, however, muscles that have been paralyzed for many years look totally normal in size and color owing to their continuing contact with the anterior horn cells. Although the testing of extremity sensibility is possible, albeit difficult, this may not be so for the muscles, especially in brain lesions. True, there are normal muscles and others with normal, but weakened, power, and for these the scheme of the British Research Council (BRC) is useful. This is contrary to the same scale for sensibility, which now is useless and never had a scientific base. The muscle grade M3 (which means that the muscle can lift the arm against gravity) is the limit for useful function. However, in the hand the part has little weight, so that action only against gravity does not mean useful function. In the wrist and fingers, therefore, Grade 3 must represent the minimum for practical use, otherwise the scale will be distorted.

There is so much more to consider in muscle function than power, however. Especially when one is dealing with the so-called spastic arm, not power but quality is the dominating problem. Here we lack terms as well as suitable tests. We have muscles with only a slightly reduced speed of action, still under voluntary control. Other muscles may have varying degrees of slow muscular contraction and coordination such that a cogwheel action occurs during muscle contraction. Thus, there exists an entire spectrum of defects of voluntary control up to totally athetotic action without any such control. Creeping slow actions occur. Most of these variations, more or less combined (for which the term "overflow" is used) occur when the signals, owing to the lesion in the central nervous system, do not reach parts of the controlling inhibitions. In daily work the term "spastic" is often used for most of what is described, including all variations. When the term spastic is used in such a different way, however, it must always be remembered that paralysis of antagonists and various degrees of dystonia may be a common part of the overall picture. All participating muscle groups must be analyzed.

In the absence of good tests, one can observe or learn from relatives whether real spontaneous, voluntary, and useful actions are performed. One can try to let the patient perform movements with maximal speed. First of all,

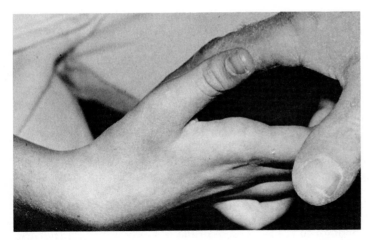

Figure 116–2. A 15 year old girl who had a cerebral lesion at age 11 years. In the totally closed right hand, no voluntary extension was seen. Blocking was performed with local anesthesia of the ulnar nerve at elbow level and of the long flexor muscle group in the forearm. The result is shown in the picture. Weak but voluntarily active extensors now give useful fuction and will gain more power if the abnormal flexor group is weakened, not totally eliminated. This function was masked by the powerful flexors. She is now able to bring the hand into a normal handshaking position. Such tests should be repeated; they give valuable information when surgery is planned.

blocking procedures of nerves or, when this is not possible, individual muscles reveal a great deal. Blocking can also indicate to both surgeon and patient the likely result of planned surgery (Fig. 116–2). Electromyography sometimes is useful, but several experienced authors (Goldner and Ferlic, 1966; Waters, Wilson, and Hecker, 1984) are not very positive about its use. Another fact to remember is that the actions are performed with many muscles together, which individually may be affected quite differently. Just as in tetraplegia, the extensor carpi radialis longus may be found to be very good but the brevis to be weak; neighboring muscles may be affected in different ways. One of the author's patients had "spasticity" in the arm, which by anesthetic blocking could be localized to the brachialis and brachioradialis, keeping the elbow in grave flexion. These two unnecessary muscles were denervated, with an almost normal arm function as the result.

Normal results can be obtained only from the transfer of normal muscles. A dystonic muscle with some voluntary control can be used for a static power, but must never be left without an antagonist, otherwise unhappy new hyperpositions can occur. The more abnormal a muscle is, the more caution must be taken in surgery. Even with very abnormal function, however, a muscle can be weakened or (rarely) eliminated, in order to obtain better balance.

Cooperation

In all surgery the cooperation of the patient (and of the rest of the team) is absolutely necessary. One can only slowly, through close contact with patients, gain the necessary knowledge about their problems and their very often unspoken wishes. Without sufficient cooperation, good results are impossible. Without a very thorough examination (usually repeated several times), performed by the surgeon himself, an adequate evaluation is not possible. Observations by helpers in the team are most useful but surgery should never be based on records, prepared by someone else, no matter how well qualified. For follow-up treatment after surgery, qualified helpers are urgently needed. Even preoperatively positions, contractures, and so on often must be changed with the help of physiotherapy and occupational therapy, and here the hand therapist is needed. In very severe cases one must use a brace shop, which can manufacture corrective splints according to the instructions of the surgeon. The surgeon himself must build up sufficient experience to take charge of every detail of the follow-up procedure. A change of hand therapist during the treatment of a given patient often means disaster. One should learn first from the simpler cases, in which the outcome is predictable. An unhappy result almost always becomes known to a large group of patients and can easily prejudice promising work. On the other hand, a reputation built on a few successful results can reassure new patients while not encouraging unrealistic expectations.

THE SPASTIC HAND AND THE STROKE HAND

This derangement in the shape of palsy, dystonia, and spasticity from central lesions occurs in two large groups; children, and older patients in the form of stroke sequelae. It occurs less frequently in the age groups in between, and then often as a result of trauma, but it often easier to give some help than in the young and the elderly. Surgical rehabilitation is here even less well established than for tetraplegic patients. The percentage of patients who can obtain some little help is also much lower: some authors quote a figure of 20 per cent; others give a much lower figure. Often it is difficult to learn from the literature which kind of groups different authors are dealing with, and not too many centers have entered the field. The number of people getting this help now must be very low. Personal experience means everything, and it is no wonder that different reports often seem contradictory in details. However, it is also clear that this is a field where surgery can give very valuable help. In some cases functional improvement is sought; in others, hygienic or cosmetic improvement is the goal. When function can be improved, it almost always relates to simple opening and closing actions in thumb and finger grips; it almost never involves anything approaching normality.

Examination is already handled in general terms. The value of preoperative electromyography is controversial. Hoffer (1978) and Waters, Wilson, and Hecker (1984) have found it valuable, and Zancolli (1979) employs it, but Goldner (1984) and Treanor (1969b) are in doubt as to its usefulness.

All experts agree upon strict individual indications necessary preoperatively. Hoffer (1978) mentions four factors: cognition, sensibility, placement, and control of muscles. If all four are satisfactory, there is no need for treatment. If three are missing, hygiene perhaps can be improved by surgery; if two are missing, a cosmetic problem might be improved; with only one negative factor, a functional result may be possible. Zancolli (1979) lists three groups, depending on the quality of active finger extension. A patient who is able to extend the fingers with the wrist in neutral extension belongs to Group 1, and good functional improvement can be achieved. Group 2 patients have finger extension only with the wrist flexed, and for these improvement is possible, but less satisfactory. Group 3 patients cannot extend the fingers even with maximally flexed wrist, and for these the results are very poor.

Remnant elementary functions should never be destroyed by reconstructive work.

With children Zancolli (1979) prefers to operate when they are 6 years of age. In younger children, cooperation is lacking; in older patients, the muscles tend to be fibrous.

In stroke cases the situation should have passed the stage of spontaneous recovery before surgery can be planned.

Treanor (1969a) very clearly describes his indications for surgical help as follows:

1. Proprioception should be 75 per cent spared.

2. There should be some volitional finger extension.

3. There should be no rigidity in the triceps.

4. Adequate shoulder stabilization should be present.

5. Patients should understand the limitations of the procedure.

Similar differences occur regarding the surgical procedure itself. Goldner (1984), like Swanson (1975), prefers general anesthesia and a bloodless field. Treanor (1969a), in stroke patients, has found it much easier to get the right tension in transfers if these are performed under local anesthesia. Some authors like to accomplish much at one sitting. Goldner prefers to attempt only a little, in order to check the results. As the goal is better balance, and the less obvious weakness usually improves when the overflow and stronger pull in the flexors are overcome, the main and first step is to weaken the overpowerful flexors.

The Wrist

Denervation is rarely used for the forearm muscles, where lengthening procedures dominate, performed through incisions in the forearm (Fig. 116–3). If more is required, the flexor superficialis tendons can be incised just above the wrist and permitted to slide up to the midpalmar level. In cases where more is required, both the superficialis and the profundus flexor groups can be divided at different levels, and the distal end of the superficialis sutured as a group to the proximal end of the profundus tendons.

The same effect can be obtained by a total flexor group slide from the elbow level (Braun, Moony, and Nickel, 1970). This must include extensive surgery to the fascial septa, combined with good drainage. It is not nec-

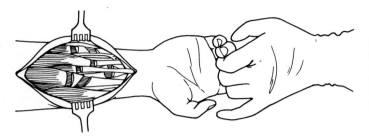

Figure 116–3. Fractional lengthening of the forearm flexors with transverse cuts through the tendinous parts. The fingers are extended by the surgeon to get the desired amount of elongation. (Modified from Walters, R. L.: Upper extremity surgery in stroke patients. Clin. Orthop., *131*:30, 1978.)

essary to obtain full supination, as most useful hand action takes place in slight pronation. This flexor slide is recommended by Zancolli (1979). Other surgeons have found it difficult to control the exact amount of length obtained by this procedure, and prefer other methods.

It is good to measure the necessary elongation; only half the amount necessary to obtain full extension is usually the best. Goldner's (1984) rule is that 0.5 mm for every degree of contracture is the right amount. It is very important that the flexors do not get too weak.

The often forgotten flexor carpi ulnaris muscle can, if necessary, be used as a transfer to the extensor carpi radialis tendon, the Green procedure. Rarely it can also be used for finger extension. However, overaction with hyperextension of the metacarpophalangeal joints and some hyperflexion of the wrist can give rise to unhappy patients.

The Thumb

Usually the thumb is in a position in the palm that from all points of view is very disturbing. A release of the adductor is possible and can be performed either along the third metacarpal (Fig. 116–4) or at the adductor insertion. If the insertion is taken down the muscle can be reinserted at the first metacarpal. Sometimes it is necessary also to release the first dorsal interosseous muscle, and some cases also require release of some long muscles. Reinforcement of the abductor may be useful, when possible.

The Digits

Derangements of the fingers in the form of fixed positions in flexion as well as extension, or in the swan-neck deformity, are not uncommon. Here different procedures on a

stabilization basis can be used, e.g., in the proximal interphalangeal joints in hyperextension deformity. For this, the superficialis tenodesis procedure can be carried out (Fig. 116–5). The thumb, which is poorly controlled by muscles, must often be simplified with the help of joint fusions. Preoperative tests with longitudinally inserted, easily removed K-wires are useful.

Another problem is the hand with very strong intrinsic contractures, which from all points of view, not least the hygienic one, needs a solution. This is one of the rare instances in this surgery when neurotomy can be helpful. After trials with blocking, resection of the ulnar motor branch with postoperative splinting can be most beneficial.

For the hand to which no function can be given, it is almost always a plus for the patient to get rid of exaggerated wrist flexion, maximal forearm pronation, and overadduction of the thumb. In some cases a dorsal tenodesis can provide a solution (Fig. 116–6); even a wrist arthrodesis is sometimes useful. The author has regretted occasions when he has let the patient go without suggesting this procedure, later performed by a wiser colleague. Before final fusion is performed even here the test with a temporary fusion performed with a few 2 mm Steinmann pins through the joint is useful.

Follow-up after surgery (e.g., to supervise the necessary immobilization in plaster) is very important. Sometimes there are no complications; other times it is a most challenging problem for the surgeon, and much psychologic therapy is involved. The hand therapist can be of very great help in such cases.

Results

The whole field is one in which the results are hard to predict and also to evaluate.

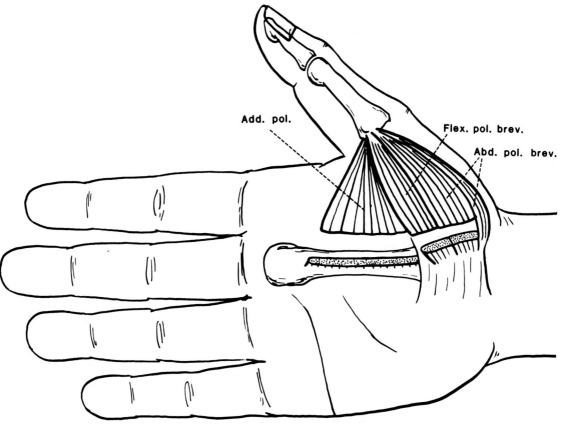

Figure 116–4. Release of an adducted, spastic thumb. (Modified from Swanson, A. B.: Surgery of the hand in cerebral palsy. *In* Flynn, J. E.: Hand Surgery. 2nd Ed. Baltimore, Williams & Wilkins Company, 1975.)

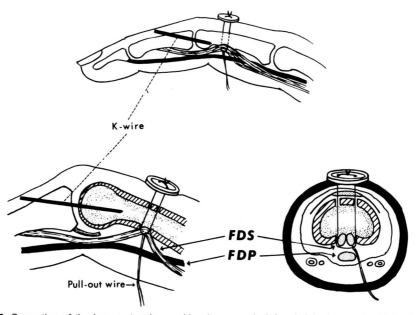

Figure 116–5. Correction of the hyperextension position (swan-neck deformity) in the proximal interphalangeal finger joint in the spastic hand. The superficialis tendon is fixed as tenodesis to the proximal phalanx, with a pull-out wire sutured through bur holes. A raw bone surface must be prepared. The joint is temporarily fixed in 20 to 40 degrees of flexion with a K-wire. FDS = flexor digitorum superficialis; FDP = flexor digitorum profundus. (Modified from Swanson, A. B.: Surgery of the hand in cerebral palsy. *In* Flynn, J. E.: Hand Surgery. 2nd Ed. Baltimore, Williams & Wilkins Company, 1975.)

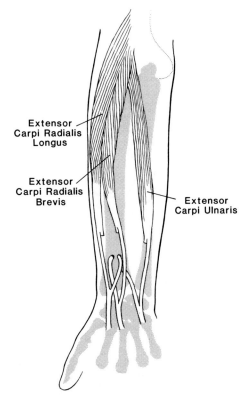

Extensor
Carpi Radialis
Longus

Extensor
Carpi Radialis
Brevis

Extensor
Carpi Ulnaris

Figure 116–6. Wrist extensor tenodesis with the use of half of the tendons of the extensor carpi radialis longus and brevis and the extensor carpi ulnaris fixed to the radius. Remaining parts of the tendons are left in position. (Modified from Waters, R. L.: Upper extremity surgery in stroke patients. Clin. Orthorp., *131*:30, 1978.)

Swanson (1975) produced a scheme for classification of the results, divided into excellent, good, fair, and poor categories.

Treanor (1969a) has provided statistics evaluating the outcome by surgery for the hand in stroke (Table 116–2). He defines failure as the situation in which one of three people involved, "the physiatrist, the surgeon, or the patient, felt that the result had not justified the expense and the attendant period of convalescence." Complications were markedly reduced with added experience.

Table 116–2. Results of Surgery in 341 Stroke Patients—Upper Extremity

Dyskinesia	Success	Failure
Median flexed hand	112	68
Ulnar flexed hand	45	11
Delayed extension	17	5
Remote foci of spasticity	54	29

Data from Treanor, W. J.: The role of physical medicine treatment in stroke rehabilitation. Clin. Orthop., *63*:14, 1969.

The results obtained by the Treanor group were in respect of the lower limb, where the problems are so much easier, on a much better level. Even in this group more emphasis was placed on paresis than on spasticity, and also experience led to increased use of local anesthesia, facilitating better balance between the motors.

Conclusions

This brief survey underlines the fact that only extensive personal experience can lead the work in this difficult field. One must start with the best cases and advance slowly. The percentage of cases to be operated upon will be low. The surgical methods can by no means be said to have reached a stage where "methods of choice" are available, but this is undoubtedly a field in which important help can be given.

TETRAPLEGIA

The terms tetraplegia and quadriplegia are synonymous, meaning paralysis of both arms and legs. In far too many centers of the world there still is no surgical help available for these usually young and active victims of a totally unforeseen accident, and a negative attitude too often prevails. Some unhappy cases from earlier surgical trials are remembered as examples. Even in very recent publications the possibilities of surgical rehabilitation are not mentioned at all. Such an attitude today is clearly out of date. This rehabilitative surgery is now well established, and the principles are much more generally accepted than are those for the spastic hand. Extensive series from Argentina, Finland, France, Scotland, Sweden, and the United States have shown that the risks of such surgery are acceptable, and the results generally can be foreseen. The last 15 years have shown a rapid advancement in the field (Freehafer, Voonham, and Allen, 1974; Moberg, 1975, 1978, 1983; House, Gwathmey, and Lundsgaard, 1976; De-Benedetti, 1979; Hentz and Keoshian, 1979; Zancolli, 1979; Smith, 1981; Hentz, Brown, and Keoshian, 1983; Lamb and Chan, 1983; McDowell, 1983). Progress has been aided by the two "small group international conferences" on the topic, held in 1978 at Edinburgh and in 1984 at Hyères in France (McDowell, Moberg, and Smith, 1979).

Today it is found that 70 to 80 per cent of tetraplegic patients can obtain some improvement in arm and hand function through surgery, depending on how much sensory and motor function remains (see Table 116–1), how many other basic functions are likely to be affected by such surgery, and whether they are psychologically suitable candidates. Even for patients with no useful muscles below elbow level, such help is not out of the question.

In previous years, when only training methods and orthoses were available, the old classification based upon spinal cord level (C_5, C_6, etc.) was sufficient. Nowadays the loss of function must be defined much more clearly. An international classification for this purpose has been worked out, based, as the first step, on remaining afferents: ocular only = O, cutaneous = Cu, and so on, the number of muscles of Grade 4 (BRC-scale) remaining below elbow level (i.e., the brachioradialis being the first of them). Each arm has its own classification. The triceps is also evaluated. An extremity with active extension against gravity of the elbow, a patient with good vision, a thumb pulp with a two-point discrimination of at least 10 mm, a brachioradialis, wrist extension, and pronator function of at least Grade 4 is classified Tr. +, OCu 3. There are other classifications, but they are very complicated and frequently require a "key" every time they are to be used. The need for separate sensory and motor classification is illustrated in Figure 116–7, demonstrating that sensory and motor function can show quite different levels *in the same arm*. In many cases the clinical differences between both arms require different indications for surgery.

In different countries there are remarkable differences between the functional losses reported. Many more higher lesions are seen in Scandinavia and the United States, a higher percentage of lower lesions in Argentina, and Scotland and Australia somewhere in between. These differences are probably due to different survival rates for the worst cases, but also are related to the number of people seeking surgical help.

The correct time to start surgical rehabilitation is usually about one year after the accident or a few months earlier. Earlier than this, so many other problems dominate and the patients are rarely psychologically prepared to discuss what can be offered. Their

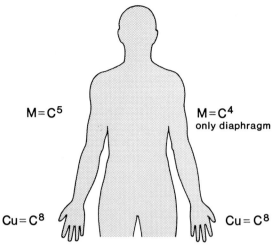

Figure 116–7. An extreme example of differences between sensory and motor loss in the same arm. More than every second tetraplegic case has differences between both arms and between sensibility and motor functions in the same arm of a magnitude that makes C-level classification too inexact for the surgeon. M = muscle; Cu = sensibility; C = cervical cord level.

long-term aim is centered upon being normal again, and no other suggestion is likely to be of interest. Often one meets the opinion that after a couple of years tetraplegic patients have accepted their situation to such a degree, that they are no longer interested in possible improvements. This is totally wrong. In some areas, when a few patients have had surgery, those with older lesions are most interested to ask what can be done for them. In the author's series there were happy results from patients operated on even more than 20 years after the accident.

Spasticity is an important arm-hand problem in only a limited number of cases. On occasion, spasticity may even be useful. One of the author's patients, with no other hand grip, could voluntarily start spastic action in the legs, bring it over to the arm, and so for a few seconds get a hand grip strong enough to lift a heavy lamp. It took him about half an hour to "load up" this again. Spasticity is usually a minus, and, as described earlier, such muscles do not work well as transfers. Sometimes the spasticity is localized to a few muscles that are not necessary, in which case it is possible to eliminate these by denervation. Of course, this must all be tested by several blocking procedures. Unfortunately, no strict rules exist about dealing with spasticity under these circumstances.

To examine or evaluate patients for surgery, they must be in a wheelchair, never in bed. Upper limb surgical rehabilitation depends on the patient's full attention and should not be performed at the same time as any other surgical procedure, for example, for pressure sores or urinary problems. Too much should not be attempted at the same time. For example, trials to restore elbow extension function on both sides at the same time has led to unhappy results. A hand should not be operated on after an elbow procedure before the patient is able to flex the elbow again to 90 degrees.

In several early cases where sensibility was absent and thus the patient had only vision to assist in hand function and hand placement, bilateral hand surgery was performed. It was found postoperatively that in spite of the presence of bilateral grip motor function, only the leading hand was used by the patients, the other not at all. Only in one exceptional single case did the patient have use of good grip in both hands. Therefore, it is wise to perform a grip procedure in just the leading hand in cases led only by vision, and to tell the patient that it is not likely that he will use a similar grip in the other hand. If, however, the vision can lead one hand, and tactile gnosis is good enough in the other, it may be worthwhile to perform grip-establishing surgery on both hands. One should always start with the leading or best hand. The attitude often found in patients that they will "risk" the nonleading hand "for a trial" must be strongly resisted by the surgeon as unrealistic. It will have unhappy results.

In old cases often the first step to accomplish is to take out contractures and train muscle groups, which often can be improved in power half a step, e.g., from Grade 3.5 to the important Grade 4, making them useful for a transfer. In all this work and also in the postoperative training and splinting, the specially trained hand therapist plays a great role. So much is special in this field and in personal contact and cooperation between patient and therapist. A change of therapist during the treatment is very undesirable and should be avoided, especially therapy for the elbow extensor, where a lack of continuity can mean disaster.

The surgeon's role is to tell the patient what can be achieved and what is not possible. He must also try to evaluate the patient's understanding and the amount of active co-operation he can count on. The patient must want the surgery and make his own decision.

Elbow Extension

In earlier days one often met from colleagues the feeling that if the patient could not regain elbow extension power enough to lift themselves, the procedure was useless. This was in no way the view of the patients, for whom control was everything, power much less important. Elbow extension (even Grade 2 or 3) provides better and more useful range of motion. This degree of activity is useful for kitchen work, eating in bed, writing without assistance from the other hand, and also the ability to get rid of shoulder contractures. Experience led to another important discovery. The brachioradialis muscle, an elbow flexor, is also often one of the few forearm muscles with power preserved. This muscle does not easily take over other functions, when used as a transfer; for this it must have a good antagonist, which must be an elbow extensor. Without it, it will be a weak and unreliable motor for the new purpose. Therefore, if the brachioradialis is intended as a transfer for work at the wrist or the hand (exception: as a pronator it is good without an antagonist), the elbow extensor reconstruction should be made first. Another reason is that when useful hand reconstruction already has given the patient a good hand grip, a secondary elbow extensor operation takes this advantage away from him for quite a time, during which the hand is idle. Active elbow extension is a great plus, even when nothing can be done to improve hand function, and should be considered in many high extremity cases.

One way to get an active elbow extensor (Fig. 116–8) is to use the posterior part of the deltoid, which with separate innervation can work independently of the anterior part (Moberg, 1975). It is accomplished by tendon grafts joined with the triceps tendon.

Unfortunately, the procedure I have used, now in 60 cases, requires long-term rehabilitation if the elbow flexion is to be restored without losing some of the extension power. One modification (Castro-Sierra and Lopez-Pita, 1983) involves the use of a reflected central strip of the triceps aponeurosis up to the end of the deltoid. The angle point of the tendinous reflection is reinforced by a Dacron

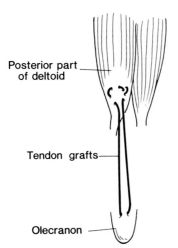

Posterior part
of deltoid

Tendon grafts

Olecranon

Figure 116–8. Procedure to provide active elbow extension. The posterior part of the deltoid is transferred to the triceps aponeurosis (not to the olecranon), extending it with free tendon grafts.

sheath to help production of fibrous tissue. Another graft, the tibialis anterior tendon, is used by Freehafer and associates (personal communication), and shorter follow-up treatment is also reported by them. The author's extensive trials with the first-mentioned modification has not produced the desired results. One of the difficulties is to find the right kind of Dacron. Trials are continuing with the second modification. Zancolli (1979) often uses transfer of the biceps tendon to the triceps to obtain elbow extension.

Hand-Gripping Function

If the elbow extension problem can be met with a more or less standard solution, this is by no means possible with the hand, for which very different degrees of loss require a thoroughly planned approach. Often it is an advantage for the patient with severe deficiencies to achieve two different degrees of function with the two hands under reconstruction. This is advantageous because it allows certain functional purposes for one hand and a different degree of functional purposes for the other hand. This must be thoroughly discussed in detail with the patient before reconstructive surgery is undertaken. Patients often have quite individual points of view. The basic rule, when, as usual, little is available, is to collect all resources in one single action. If the small resources are divided up, the result will be too weak for practical purposes. The wrist extension factor is the key. When the extensors are too weak, they can often be reinforced by the brachioradialis transfer (see above). Wrist flexion for opening of the grip, if no flexors exist, must be obtained by gravity. Wrist fusion should never be performed in order to obtain more muscles for transfer.

The first aim is the key grip, which is obtained by a flexor pollicis longus tenodesis. This must usually be supported by simplification of the thumb through joint arthrodeses. Three different ways to obtain a key grip are shown in Figures 116–9, 116–10, and 116–11.

If more is available, e.g., if each of the two radial wrist extensors are strong enough to handle the wrist extension alone, the longus can be used for finger flexion, transferred to the profundi tendons. To learn whether this is the situation, the extensor brevis must be tested in open surgery. If it can pull 5 kg, the transfer of the longus is possible. If not, such

Figure 116–9. Basic steps in the procedure to provide key grip. *(a),* The brachioradialis is used as a wrist extensor. *(b), (d),* The flexor pollicis longus is tenodesed to the volar surface of the radius, and the annular ligament at the metacarpophalangeal joint is resected to permit the tendon to bowstring and increase the strength of the key grip. *(c),* The thumb interphalangeal joint is arthrodesed with a 2 mm K-wire (a Steinmann pin) to prevent flexion (Froment's sign) and to maintain broad contact surfaces. (A 1.5 mm K-wire is too weak and would break.) The ends must be blunt, otherwise the pin will come out. Sometimes the flexion of the metacarpophalangeal joint must be diminished by a dorsal tenodesis. This is the author's original method to obtain a key grip, but now in many cases the one shown in Figure 116–10 has been found better and even less complicated.

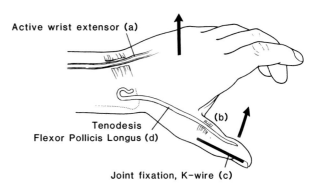

Active wrist extensor (a)

Tenodesis
Flexor Pollicis Longus (d)

(b)

Joint fixation, K-wire (c)

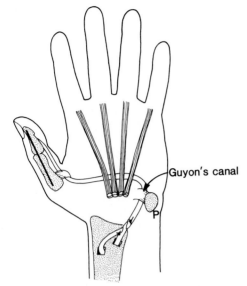

Figure 116–10. The Brand-Moberg transpalmar way to obtain a key grip, using the flexor pollicis longus tenodesis. This tendon is dissected free from the muscle as high up as possible in the forearm; taken out through a small incision close to the thumb metacarpophalangeal joint; brought in again under flexors, nerves, and vessels to an incision just 1 cm distal and radial to the pisiform bone *(P)*; and taken through Guyon's canal and again under tendons, nerves, and vessels to the radius. Here it is anchored as a sling through holes in the cortex. The distal thumb joint is arthodesed with a buried 2 mm Steinmann pin.

a transfer can easily be disastrous for the hand.

Dorsal tenodesis can provide finger extension, but if not the natural tenodesis effect is sufficient. In order to open the grip, a brachioradialis transfer to the finger extensors is possible in some cases.

To obtain useful and different left and right hand function, it is sometimes good to use an active thumb flexor. Again, a good brachioradialis can be transferred to the flexor pollicis longus tendon (Lamb and Chan, 1983), but the power is usually not as effective as with the tenodesis solution. The brachioradialis muscle can also be used under various conditions as a transfer for other purposes, e.g., as a thumb abductor. The opposition function is often mentioned in tetraplegia hand work, but the result actually is much more the key grip than opposition. True opposition has such a small digital contact surface. It is therefore of little use for tetraplegic patients, who do not want to pick up needles and small nuts; their main problems are the handling of clothing, tools for eating, and so forth.

If more motor function is available, the next step can be to provide a strong adductor for the thumb. In the small minority in whom still more is retained, it may be good to use transfers instead of tenodeses. In hands in which sensibility is close to normal, reconstructive work can follow the principles of everyday hand surgery and tendon transfer (see Chap. 114).

The Future

The field of research is now making very rapid progress, with new and detailed solutions being found. A new way to construct a key grip with the use of the supination effect of the biceps, even when no active forearm muscles are left, has been worked out by Brummer (personal communication). It seems also possible that the experiments with implanted electric stimulators (Freehafer, Voonham, and Allen, 1974) may be of help to the higher lesions, perhaps in combination

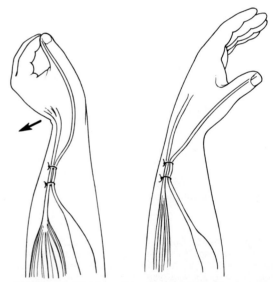

Figure 116–11. Zancolli has several interesting ways to obtain key grip, which differ, depending on the presence of wrist extensors and their power. The *first* stage includes (1) a fusion of the carpometacarpal joint of the thumb in 45 degrees of antepulsion and 30 degrees of abduction, (2) a transfer of the brachioradialis to the tendons of the finger and thumb extensors, and (3) a volar stabilization of the metacarpophalangeal joints of the fingers with a modified Zancolli "lasso" technique. This illustraton shows the *second* stage, which uses a short laterolateral fusion of the flexor pollicis longus tendon to the extensor carpi radialis brevis tendon. If the latter muscle is strong enough to handle wrist extension alone, the longus is of course used for finger flexion.

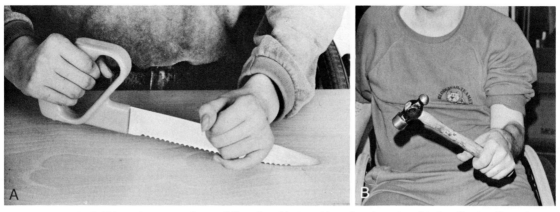

Figure 116–12. *A,* This patient wanted especially to be able to cut bread and meat and to handle utensils such as a frying pan. A transpalmar key grip was performed and a transfer added of the extensor carpi radialis longus to the profundi flexors, which proved sufficient for the desired functions. The hand was classified before surgery as OCu2, indicating some tactile gnosis and wrist extensors of force four, but totally lacking active thumb and finger motion. *B,* In the same way, a similar hand could be given enough power to handle a hammer. The left side was by far the better.

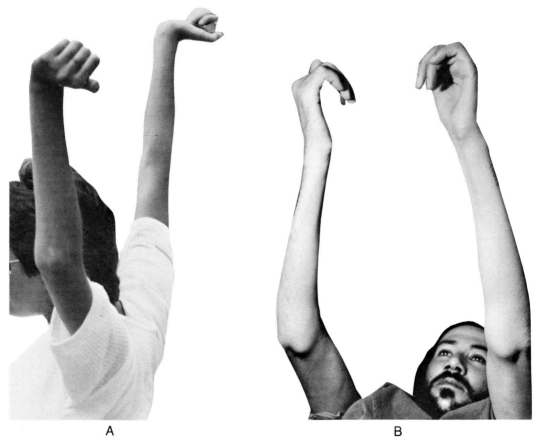

A   B

Figure 116–13. *A,* This patient had no elbow extension but wanted especially to be able to swim. On both sides the deltoid was transferred to the triceps tendon, making possible not only swimming but also other new activities. *B,* Elbow extension obtained by a transfer on both sides of the biceps to the triceps. (Reproduced by permission from Dr. E. Zancolli, Buenos Aires.)

with surgery. Finally, it must be emphasized, that patients with very little left are the ones who need the most help. Some results of current surgical practices are shown in Figures 116–12 and 116–13.

REFERENCES

Braun, R. M., Moony, V., and Nickel, V. L.: Flexor-origin release for pronation-flexion deformity of the forearm and hand in stroke patients. An evaluation of early results in eighteen patients. J. Bone Joint Surg., *52A*:907, 1970.

Brummer, H.: Personal communication.

Castro-Sierra, A., and Lopez-Pita, A.: A new surgical technique to correct triceps paralysis. Hand, *15*:42, 1983.

DeBenedetti, M.: Restoration of elbow extension power in the tetraplegic patient using the Moberg technique. J. Hand Surg., *4*:86, 1979.

Freehafer, A. A.: Determination of muscle-tendon unit properties during tendon transfer. J. Hand Surg., *4*:331, 1979.

Freehafer, A. A., Voonham, E., and Allen, V.: Tendon transfers to improve grasp after injuries of the cervical spinal cord. J. Bone Joint Surg., *56A*:951, 1974.

Goldner, J. L.: The upper extremity in cerebral palsy. *In* Samilson, R. (Ed.): Orthopaedic Aspects of Cerebral Palsy. Philadelphia, J. B. Lippincott Company, 1975.

Goldner, J. L.: Upper extremity reconstruction in cerebral palsy. *In* Hunter, J. M., Schneider, L. H., and Mackin, E. J. (Eds.): Tendon Surgery in the Hand. St. Louis, C. V. Mosby Company, 1987.

Goldner, J. L., and Ferlic, D. C.: Sensory status of the hand as related to reconstructive surgery of the upper extremity. Clin. Orthop., *46*:87, 1966.

Granit, R.: Receptors and Sensory Perception. New Haven, Yale University Press, 1955.

Granit, R.: The functional role of the muscle spindles: facts and hypotheses. Brain, *98*:531, 1975.

Hentz, V. R., Brown, M., and Keoshian, L. A.: Upper limb reconstruction in quadriplegia: functional assessment and proposed treatment modifications. J. Hand Surg., *8*:119, 1983.

Hentz, V. R., and Keoshian, L. A.: Changing perspectives in surgical hand rehabilitation in quadriplegic patients. Plast. Reconstr. Surg., *54*:509, 1979.

Hoffer, M. M.: The upper extremity in cerebral palsy. *In* Fredericks, S., and Brody, G. S. (Eds.): Symposium on the neurologic aspects of plastic surgery. St. Louis, C. V. Mosby Company, 1978.

House, J. H., Gwathmey, F. W., and Lundsgaard, D. K.: Restoration of strong grasp and lateral pinch in tetraplegia due to spinal cord injury. J. Hand Surg., *1*:152, 1976.

Lamb, D. W., and Chan, K. M.: Surgical reconstruction of the upper limb in traumatic tetraplegia. A review of 41 patients. J. Bone Joint Surg., *65B*:291, 1983.

Marsh, D.: Personal communication.

Marsh, D. R.: Use of a wheel aestesiometer for testing sensibility in the hand. J. Hand Surg., *11B*:182, 1986.

McDowell, C. L.: Tetraplegia. *In* Green, D. P. (Ed.): Operative Hand Surgery. Vol. 2. New York, Churchill Livingstone, 1983, p. 1109.

McDowell, C. L., Moberg, E., and Smith, A. G.: International conference on surgical rehabilitation of the upper limb in tetraplegia. J. Hand Surg., *4*:387, 1979.

Moberg, E.: Criticism and study of methods for examining sensibility in the hand. Neurology, *12*:8, 1962.

Moberg, E.: Surgical treatment for absent single-hand grip and elbow extension in quadriplegia. J. Bone Joint Surg., *57A*:196, 1975.

Moberg, E.: Reconstructive surgery in tetraplegia, stroke and cerebral palsy: some basic concepts in physiology and neurology. J. Hand Surg., *1*:29, 1976.

Moberg, E.: The Upper Limb in Tetraplegia: A New Approach to Surgical Rehabilitation. Stuttgart, Thieme, 1978.

Moberg, E.: Upper limb surgical rehabilitation in tetraplegia. *In* McCollister Evarts, C. (Ed.): Surgery of the Musculoskeletal System. New York, Churchill Livingstone, 1983a.

Moberg, E.: The role of cutaneous afferents in position sense, kinaesthesia, and motor function of the hand. Brain, *106*:1, 1983b.

Moberg, E., Hagert, C. -G., Nordenskiöld, U., Traneus, M., and Svens, B.: Splinting in Hand Therapy. New York, Thieme-Stratton, 1984.

Perry, J., and Waters, R. L.: Surgery. *In* American Academy of Orthopaedic Surgeons: Instructional Course Lectures 24. St. Louis, C. V. Mosby Company, 1975.

Seddon, H.: Surgical Disorders of the Peripheral Nerves. 2nd Ed. Edinburgh, Churchill Livingstone, 1975.

Smith, A. G.: Early complications of key grip hand surgery for quadriplegia. Paraplegia, *19*:123, 1981.

Swanson, A. B.: Surgery of the hand in cerebral palsy. *In* Flynn, J. E. (Ed.): Hand Surgery. 2nd Ed. Baltimore, Williams & Wilkins Company, 1975.

Treanor, W. J.: The role of physical medicine treatment in stroke rehabilitation. Clin. Orthop., *63*:14, 1969a.

Treanor, W. J.: The hemiplegic posture and its correction. Clin. Orthop., *63*:113, 1969b.

Waters, R. L., Wilson, J. D., and Hecker, R. S.: Rehabilitation of the upper extremity after stroke. *In* Hunter, J. M., Schneider, L. H., Mackin, E. J., and Callahan, A. D. (Eds.): Rehabilitation of the Hand. St. Louis, C. V. Mosby Company, 1984.

Zancolli, E. A.: Structural and Dynamic Bases of Hand Surgery. 2nd Ed. Philadelphia, J. B. Lippincott Company, 1979.

E. F. Shaw Wilgis

Ischemic Conditions of the Upper Extremity

HISTORICAL PERSPECTIVE

The development of the field of reconstructive vascular surgery has followed an interesting course characterized by bursts of knowledge and advances over several centuries. The earliest recorded examples of vascular reconstruction date to the time of Celsus when hemorrhage, whether accidental or resulting from operative intervention, was dealt with by blood vessel ligation. The first recorded arterial repair was performed on an injured brachial artery by Hallowell in Newcastle-upon-Tyne, England, in 1759. The method was suggested by Lambert, who subsequently described it to Hunter, and was derived from the steel pin approximation used in that day for harelip. This was the first reconstructive surgical operation on the vascular system in which vascular continuity was restored. It was a remarkable feat for that period and one not duplicated for many years. Progress was quite slow thereafter. Most of our modern techniques, including

autographs and homographs, were summarized in the classic works of Carrel and Guthrie. Alexis Carrel was recognized as the true father of experimental vascular surgery. He received the Nobel prize in 1912 for his pioneering contributions to this field. His classic paper on the subject (Carrel, 1907) outlined the essential technical and operative principles necessary for reconstructive surgery of the vascular system. These principles are still being used today, equally applicable to the microvascular reconstructive surgery that is now done routinely. By 1910, over 100 lateral repairs and 46 end to end anastomoses or segmental vein grafts had been performed clinically. In the early years of World War I, German surgeons repaired a few vascular injuries, but the effort did not last. Great delay in treatment was caused by the long evacuation times when horse transport was more common than vehicular transport. Treatment priorities imposed by vast casualty situations caused further delays. The lack of antibiotics and blood banks, and the crude nature of instruments and suture material, further dictated that vascular reconstruction would not be successful.

During the years between the two World Wars, several major advances were made, the benefits of which would not be appreciated for several decades. Heparin was discovered by McLean in 1916, but a suitable preparation was not produced in the laboratory until the middle 1930's. Antibiotics were just being used in the clinical setting and transfusions became a clinical reality. Blood banking soon followed, making transfusions a more feasible solution for treatment of shock. Despite these advances, however, ligation of a transected artery and accompanying vein remained the standard form of treatment throughout World

War II. Only 3 per cent of 2471 arterial injuries were repaired; the rest were ligated to control hemorrhage. The overall amputation rate after major vessel injury was 49 per cent.

The Korean war produced a very different experience. Rapid evacuation, ample blood replacement, heparin, antibiotics and new vascular instruments combined with the availability of trained surgeons to change the management of vascular injuries from amputation to reconstruction. Of the 304 major repairs carried out, the amputation rate was reduced by 13 per cent. The experience in Vietnam was similar. In 1000 patients from the Vietnam Vascular Registry, Rich, Baugh, and Hughes (1970) reported a 13 per cent amputation rate. Stimulated by the repair of vascular wounds in the war setting, there was a tremendous revival of interest in reconstructive surgery during the 1950's and 1960's in civilian life. Many of the surgeons trained in emergency reconstruction in the battlefield came back to civilian life and proceeded with sophisticated vascular reconstruction. The creation of vessel banks and vascular substitutes (including homographs and prostheses), the development of sophisticated angiographic and noninvasive studies, and the development of artificial suture material, with its corresponding small needle for anastomosis of small vessels, stimulated an explosion of research. These events opened the field for clinical reconstructive vascular surgery. Mutilating vascular surgery, i.e., vessel ligature with acceptance of the ischemic complications, was replaced by reconstructive vascular surgery.

The advancement of microsurgical techniques in the late 1960's and 1970's led to clear-cut thinking concerning the treatment of ischemic conditions within the hand. In addition to the repair of trauma, the reconstruction of occlusive and compressive disorders became commonplace. The indirect approach to ischemic conditions of the hand, with pharmacologic and surgical manipulation of the sympathetic nervous system, has improved the quality of life for many people with vasospastic disorders.

Computer technology and advanced imaging techniques have led to more precise diagnosis and localization of lesions. Noninvasive recordings of pulse flow have made possible dynamic and provocative testing.

EMBRYOLOGIC DEVELOPMENT AND ANATOMY

In the embryo lymphatics, veins, and arteries are all developed as tissue spaces that become confluent and form a connected system of channels. These channels communicate freely among themselves in a plexiform arrangement, and function as conduits for any of these fluid types. During development, these vessel systems are isolated and become separate entities. Persistence of various patterns in the embryonic vascular channels results in lymphangiomas, hemangiomas, and arteriovenous fistulas. The plexus of blood vessels develop on the yolk sac, the body stalk, and the chorion of the embryo. The differentiation in the blood vessels occurs first in the chorionic region, arising from the need for vessels to extract nourishment and oxygen from the internal situation and to distribute them to the tissues of the embryo. Concomitantly, capillary plexus form in several regions, preceding the formation of definitive arterial and venous trunks. Initially the arteries and veins are structurally indistinguishable; their development occurs later as differentiation in the embryo proceeds. What determines this eventual differentiation is not completely known. Presumably, hemodynamic factors as well as the mechanical conditions of the blood flow, including velocity and pressure, are involved. However, the definitive vessels arise through the selection, enlargement, and differentiation of appropriate paths. Those capillary plexus from which the flow has been diverted atrophy.

After the arterial and venous trunks have formed, the paired aortic arches develop. Thus, by the time the embryo is four-weeks old, the primitive vascular system consisting of four pairs of aortic arches is established. The paired precardinal and postcardinal veins drain into the heart, while the dorsal aorta fuses into the descending aorta and the branching of the great vessels begins. At about four weeks the limb buds appear as lateral swellings. The upper limb continues to grow over the next few weeks as it lengthens; and the elbow, wrist, and hand develop. During this time, the embryo enlarges from approximately 7 mm to about 25 mm. As the limb develops, the vascular system within the limb becomes more definitive. The capillary plexus in the limb bud gives rise to an axial vessel system that initiates with a subclavian axillary artery as a sole stem. The brachial artery develops in the upper arm and the interosseous artery branches off from the brachial artery to develop in the forearm. Figure 117–1 illustrates the vascular system as it develops from four weeks to eight weeks. The capillary plexus remaining in the hand develop as the hand is developing. The process continues with the median artery branching off from the brachial artery and annexing the vessels of the hand. Next the ulnar, followed by the radial, arteries arise as brachial branches. These two arteries become the most prominent vessels in the forearm. As they anastomose with the vessels developing in the hand, they bypass the median artery, which (being of no further use) eventually atrophies in most cases. Thus, the development is complete.

The main arterial supply to the forearm and hand is derived from the continuation of the axillary to the brachial artery. At the elbow or just distal to it, the brachial artery divides into the radial and ulnar arteries and the anterior and posterior interosseous arteries. These vessels course through the forearm with the interosseous branches terminating at the wrist. The hand is supplied by the radial and ulnar arteries and is supplemented by the anterior interosseous artery and its posterior branch. The radial and ulnar arteries, with contributions from the other arteries, form the arterial arches of the hand. The variations observed in the formation of the

arches in the digital branches result from differences in size of the five contributing arteries: the radial, the ulnar, the anterior interosseous, the dorsal branch of the anterior interosseous, and the median nerve artery. The retention of the embryonal type with predominance of one of these arteries is responsible for the variations.

The general pattern of the hand's arterial supply consists of two systems for the volar aspect and a single system for the dorsal aspect. The volar supply is arranged into a superficial and a deep group.

Variation in the formation of the arterial supply in the forearm and hand has been studied. There were major variations in the brachial and antebrachial arteries in 18 per cent of 750 extremities studied by McCormack, Cauldwell, and Anson (1953). Generally, the deviations were observed more often on the right than on the left side. The most common deviations were high origin of the radial artery; high origin but usual course of the ulnar artery; and a common trunk formed by the superficial brachial artery for both radial and ulnar arteries. Variations in the arterial arches in the hand have also been studied. McCormack, Cauldwell, and Anson studied the superficial volar arch in 650 specimens. They found a complete arch in 80 per cent and an incomplete arch in the remaining 20 per cent. "Complete" means that the digital circulation can be maintained from the ulnar artery alone. Five types of complete arches were found (Fig. 117–2):

Type I, formed by the superficial palmar

Figure 117–1. Development of the vascular system throughout embryonic weeks 4 to 8. (From Wilgis, E. F. S.: Vascular Injuries and Diseases of the Upper Limb. Boston, Little, Brown & Company, 1983. Copyright 1983, Little, Brown & Company.)

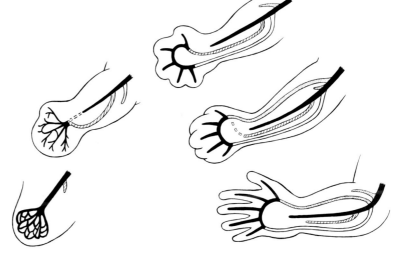

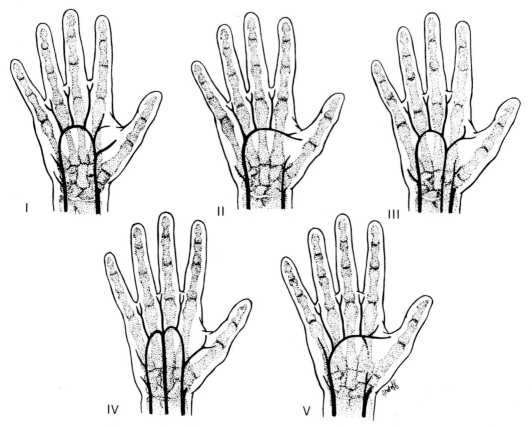

Figure 117–2. Anatomic abnormalities of the superficial arch. (From Wilgis, E. F. S.: Vascular Injuries and Diseases of the Upper Limb. Boston, Little, Brown & Company, 1983. Copyright 1983, Little, Brown & Company.)

branch of the radial artery and the larger ulnar artery (found in 34.5 per cent of the specimens).

Type II, formed by the ulnar artery entirely (found in 37 per cent of specimens).

Type III, formed by the enlarged median artery (found in 3.8 per cent of specimens).

Type IV, formed by the radial, median, and ulnar arteries (found in only 1.2 per cent of specimens).

Type V, formed by the ulnar artery, joined by a large sized vessel from the deep palmar arch and joining the superficial arch at the base of the thenar eminence (found in 4.5 per cent of specimens).

The deep volar arch is less variable than the superficial arch and was complete in 97 per cent of the specimens examined. The authors noted four types of perforating arteries passing from volar vessels through the metacarpal interspaces to anastomose with the dorsal metacarpal arteries and provide the principal arterial supply to the dorsum of the hand. These metacarpal arteries play a significant role in supplying blood to the digits when the common and proper digital arteries have been divided.

Stimulated by the development of hand ischemia in a young patient after the radial artery had been cannulated, Mozersky and associates (1973) studied 70 patients, using noninvasive testing techniques to determine the adequacy of the normal palmar anastomosis of blood vessels. They found that 12 per cent displayed radial dominant circulation and had an incomplete superficial palmar arch. The remaining patients had ulnar dominant circulation, and one-fifth of these had incomplete superficial palmar arches. The dominant circulation was symmetric in all but four of the patients studied. This characteristic of radial or ulnar dominance takes on great significance when the surgeon sees an individual with acute trauma or is planning reconstruction. For instance, a patient with a radial dominant hand circulation with a thrombosed ulnar artery would naturally be a poor candidate for ulnar reconstruction.

Conversely, a patient with ulnar thrombosis and an ulnar dominant circulation desperately needs ulnar artery reconstruction. Thus, the application of dynamic testing for the anatomic variance becomes very important.

CIRCULATION AND ISCHEMIA

In studying the natural course of vascular conditions of the hand—whether traumatic and occlusive, vasospastic or compressive—the most frequent complication is ischemia of varying degrees. Ischemia can be manifested at times of increased need for circulation, such as a very cold exposure or increased demands of the muscle during extreme exercise. This is very mild ischemia, which during the resting state is not manifested at all. As ischemia progresses to more total ischemia, the individual can experience pain, paresthesia, and absence of pulses, indicating a significant deprivation of the tissues of the blood supply. Ultimately more profound ischemia can lead to tissue loss with gangrene. Many times in the natural course of vascular disease, such as gradually occlusive or vasospastic diseases, one sees the ischemia syndrome progress from very mild to marked ischemia with marginal tissue loss. However, in the traumatic occlusive or embolic categories, the ischemia is frequently total, and if not diagnosed and treated appropriately it can lead to massive tissue loss.

When one thinks of the macroscopic circulation system, one should envision the heart as the central pumping system that sends out blood to various sites of the body through a system of channels called arteries. The pressure throughout the system should essentially be constant, as it is the single most important ingredient of the fluid mechanics and is responsible for the constant delivery of the blood to the various sites, which have continually changing demands. It is these changing demands that cause the shunting of blood from one site to another. The whole system is under a complex control regulated through the autonomic nervous system, which changes the diameter of the various channels to supply the flow necessary to the various demand sites. The whole system is under the control of the basic laws of hemodynamics. If the diameter changes and the pressure remains constant, the rate of flow is increased through the more narrow site; if the peripheral resistance increases, the rate of flow is significantly less; and if the peripheral resistance equals the head of pressure, there is no effective flow. A basic understanding of these fluid dynamics is necessary to treat most of the conditions that arise in the vascular system of the upper extremity. With these changing flow patterns, dynamic testing is imperative. The patient should be tested in multiple positions and under various conditions. Stress conditions such as cold and exercise should be employed to study the changes of the pulse during these maneuvers. In the normal state, there are marked changes, and the most critical part of the evaluation is the quality and time it takes the pulse to return to its prestress state. In other words, the only abnormal finding in some conditions may be that the pulse does not return to its prestress state after the stress is induced. This may mimic an obscure clinical situation and can be duplicated with provocative testing.

Vasospastic conditions that can cause hand and upper extremity ischemia are discussed in Chapter 118.

TRAUMA

Although it is not the purview of this section to deal with traumatic injuries, revascularization, and replantation (see Chap. 93), a short review of the reaction of the cellular components of the artery to injury leads to some clinical conclusions.

Arteries are lined by a continuous monolayer of endothelium that is not thrombogenic and serves as a permeability barrier and intermediary between the blood and underlying cells of the vessel wall. Smooth muscle cells in the main reside within the media and are responsible for the structural integrity of the vessel wall as well as vasomotor tone. They exist in a quiescent state, yet in response to various stimuli they are capable of exuberant proliferation. From experiments on injured arteries, it is now known that the endothelial and smooth muscle cells interact with one another both to promote and to inhibit growth, although the factors that affect endothelial and smooth muscle cell population in a normal vessel wall remain obscure.

When an artery is denuded of its endothelium by trauma, both endothelial and smooth muscle cells are stimulated to proliferate. Such extensive injury can be produced by the mere passage of a balloon embolectomy catheter, as has been demonstrated in animal models. The fibroproliferative intimal lesions induced by the injury stimulus resemble the advanced fibrous atherosclerotic plaques found in man. The similarity between human and experimental lesions has led Ross and Glomset (1976) to propose the injury hypothesis of atherosclerosis. This hypothesis states that the fibrous lesions in man are the result of endothelial damage and adherence of platelets to the denuded wall with release of smooth muscle mitogens, and subsequent stimulation of smooth muscle proliferation of the intima. How this injury occurs in man is not clear. Nevertheless, trauma models and the injury hypothesis serve as a useful starting point for an investigation of arterial endothelial smooth muscle interactions.

Immediately after an artery is stripped of its endothelium, platelets adhere to the denuded surface, spreading and degranulating as they coalesce to form a monolayer. This process is most active in the first few hours and stops within 24 hours of an injury. The released platelet granule content, as indicated by platelet factor 4, enters the wall but appears to be cleared within hours. Within 24 hours smooth muscle cells begin to proliferate. What exactly causes this marked burst of proliferative activity of the smooth muscle

cells is not known. Platelet-derived growth factor (PDGF) is secreted with platelet factor in the alpha granule, and is a potent mitogen for vascular smooth muscle cells in vitro. PDGF is probably present in the media bound to matrix, and might in fact account for the initiation of smooth muscle growth. This process is illustrated in Figure 117–3. Within two and four days after surgery, proliferating medial smooth muscle cells begin to migrate through clefts in the internal elastic lamina into the intima. They continue to proliferate for seven to ten days, at which point the proliferation rate rapidly declines. The proliferative activity in the intima and media is reduced to normal by one month except at the surface of the region lacking endothelium. However, the intimal smooth muscle cells under regenerated endothelium resume the quiescent state and do not exhibit the persistent elevated level of proliferative activity. Thus, as healing progresses, the intima is thickened by the accumulation of smooth muscle cells and connected tissue. How the endothelium heals has been the subject of intense investigation. There appears to be an interaction between the endothelial cells and the smooth muscle cells. In essence, the endothelial lining of denuded arteries is restored by migration and proliferation of endothelium from untraumatized sources adjacent to the zone of injury. Most endothelial healing occurs in 14 days, and after that time the endothelial cells appear incapable of any further replication. A natural substance, hepa-

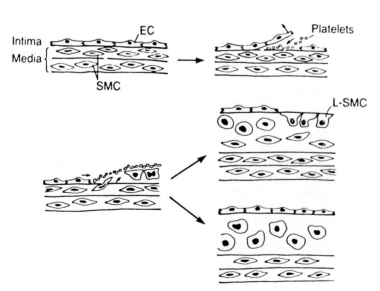

Figure 117–3. Schematic of arterial injury (after Clowes). EC = endothelial cell; SMC = smooth muscle cell.

rin sulfate, is found in vessel walls and is synthesized by endothelium and, to a more limited extent, by smooth muscle cells. There appear to be increased amounts of heparin sulfate in post-traumatic reendothelialized vessel walls, and it may be that heparin or a heparin-like substance may play an active role as an inhibitor of smooth muscle cell growth.

All these observations have some practical importance for vascular surgery. First, in dealing with the traumatic condition, the natural response of the vessel to injury makes it mandatory to remove all of the injured vessel. Endothelium does not bridge a defect greater than 20 mm, and early endothelial coverage of an injured artery may be expected to reduce myointimal thickening, and therefore luminal narrowing. The exact delineation of cellular response to injury within the vessel wall leads clinical surgeons to perform finer vascular technique.

Traumatic injuries in the upper extremity can be either closed or open. Direct blunt trauma sometimes associated with fractures can cause disruption of the vascular system. The most common site of this kind of vascular injury is at the joint level, where there is a looser anatomic arrangement of the vessels to allow for motion than in areas proximal and distal to the joint. Injuries to the clavicle and shoulder region can seriously damage the underlying subclavian and axillary arteries. As the vessels course over the first rib, they can be caught between the clavicle and the first rib and damaged. Venous injuries are also common in this region. At the level of the shoulder, damage to the axillary artery following shoulder dislocation is a devastating complication. The mechanism of injury to the axillary artery is that it is fixed by the circumflex and subscapular arteries, with the tendon of the pectoralis minor muscle acting as a fulcrum over which the artery is bent. The vessel can in fact be transected at this level.

The brachial artery in the region of the elbow is a common complication of fracture dislocation of the elbow and supracondylar fracture of the humerus.

Open injuries to the vascular system in the upper extremity usually are heralded by a large hematoma or profuse bleeding.

Diagnosis of these injuries should include determination of pulses distal to the area of trauma by clinical palpation, use of the Dop-

pler ultrasonic flow detector, and possibly pulse volume recordings. The presence of profuse bleeding in the acutely injured patient is suggestive of a partial arterial laceration. If the vessel is completely severed, the artery goes into spasm and occludes its cut end. An arterial angiogram usually is not needed in treating a sharp laceration with arterial involvement. The normal noninvasive studies indicate arterial damage and this is confirmed during surgery when appropriate repair is made. In the avulsing, tearing type of injury, however, one must be careful that there is not a proximal arterial lesion. In this case, contrast arterial angiogram may yield useful information of a proximal lesion. At surgery, if there is no proximal flow, an operative arterial angiogram should be obtained to clarify the level of injury.

In the acutely injured patient, the physician must be aware of ischemia due to compartmental pressure elevation. Tenseness in the forearm compartment, pain, paresthesias, and pain on extension of the digits indicate increased compartmental pressure. The fascial compartment of increased pressure feels tense. The onset of this condition is often insidious and the results of its not being recognized can be disastrous. Pulses are often present and unaltered. Increased compartmental pressure can be directly measured, as advocated by Whitesides and associates (1975), Mubarak and associates (1978), and others. In the awake, cooperative patient, the symptoms of persistent, progressive pain aggravated by extension of the digits, which passively stretches the ischemic muscle, indicates increased compartmental pressure; objective testing only confirms the diagnosis. However, objective testing is most useful in patients with associated complicating problems, such as coma or systemic diseases, that mask the normal pain responses. Patients on anticoagulation or with bleeding disorders who are poor candidates for surgery should also be tested by the objective technique before they are subjected to extensive fasciotomy; in such patients a fasciotomy could be life-threatening and should not be done without substantial evidence of increased intercompartmental pressure.

Finally, in the patient with an acute injury, once arterial reconstruction has been carried out, all the pulse-detecting maneuvers must be repeated to make sure there is adequate flow in the immediate postoperative state.

COMPRESSION SYNDROMES AND DISORDERS

The neurovascular supply to the upper limb traverses the shoulder area and is confined to narrow rigid anatomic spaces that offer little cross sectional latitude. These structures are subject to the compressive forces of respiration and movement of the shoulder girdle. The subclavian artery emerges from the thoracic cavity behind the sternoclavicular joint and must pass behind the scalenus anterior muscle on its way to the axilla. It ascends across Simpson's fascia, which is a semi–cone-shaped sheet of fascia roofing the cervical pleura, and curves posteriorly as well as outwardly to pass just distal to the scalenus anterior muscle and its tendon before turning slightly forward again as it enters the apex of the axilla. Thus, the artery is angulated in two places over the first rib and behind the tendon of the scalenus anterior muscle. There is a natural tendency for the artery to slide down the slope of the rib, drawing the vessel against the tendon, which acts as a fulcrum over which the vessel must pass. Behind the subclavian artery are the scalenus medius and posterior muscles. As the vessel passes between the scalene, it is compressed by contractions of these muscles. It is interesting to note that this is the only region of the body where a large artery passes through muscle tissue without a fascial sheath.

The three anatomic structures most often associated with vascular compression syndromes in the shoulder and neck region are (1) the cervical rib and its fascial remnants, (2) the rudimentary first thoracic rib, and (3) anomalous insertions or dispositions of the anterior and middle scalene muscles (Fig. 117–4). Less frequent causes of compression include a bifed clavicle, a bony protuberance of the first rib, enlargement of the costal element of the transverse process of the seventh cervical vertebrae, hypertrophied omohyoid muscle, and adventitious fibrous bands. Of all these factors, cervical rib is the most common and the most easily identified.

In 1869, Gruber divided cervical ribs into four groups according to the extent of growth. These vary from ribs of slight degree that reach beyond the transverse process and end freely to complete cervical ribs that possess a true cartilaginous end uniting with the cartilage of the first rib. Cervical ribs are usually

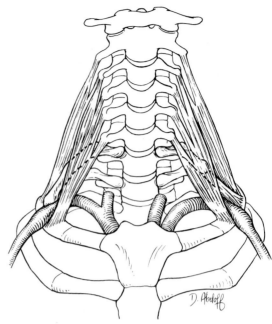

Figure 117–4. Anatomic abnormalities about the shoulder girdle, cervical rib, and fascial strip. (From Wilgis, E. F. S.: Vascular Injuries and Diseases of the Upper Limb. Boston, Little, Brown & Company, 1983. Copyright 1983, Little, Brown & Company.)

incomplete and are united to the normal first thoracic rib by fibrous bands. Their incidence is said to be in 0.5 to 1 per cent of the population, or 5.6 people in 1000. However, symptoms do not arise in every person with a cervical rib, and only when they are correlated with the presence of a cervical rib should attention be drawn to this area. Symptoms occur when the patient attempts to carry heavy objects. Cervical ribs and their fibrous bands cause compression by narrowing the interscalene triangle through which the subclavian artery and nerves pass.

A rudimentary first thoracic rib is one that fails to reach the sternum. Its anterior end is usually attached to the second rib by ligaments. This is a rare condition whose symptoms mimic those of a cervical rib. The third anatomic factor in this region is the formation of the scalene muscles. Occasionally, adventitious ligaments or fibrous bands develop within the scalenus anterior muscle and can cause compression of the subclavian artery.

Costoclavicular compression can occur when the angle between the clavicle and the first rib is narrowed, or when there is an abnormality of the clavicle from fracture or a bony protuberance of the first rib. Figure 117–5 illustrates a patient with an osteochon-

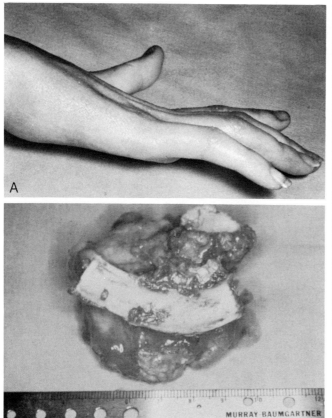

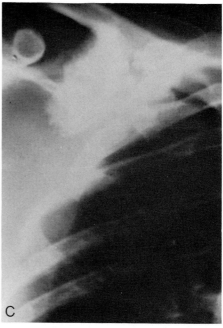

Figure 117–5. A patient with osteochondroma of the first rib, vascular compression, and ulnar nerve palsy. *A,* Illustrating ulnar nerve palsy. *B,* Radiograph of osteochondroma of the first rib. *C,* Pathologic specimen.

droma of the first rib that narrowed the angle between the clavicle and the first rib and compressed the neurovascular structures.

The axillary artery may be compressed when it is tensed and bowed beneath the coracoid process and pectoralis minor tendon during hyperabduction of the arm. When the arm is fully abducted and externally rotated, the head of the humerus moves anteriorly from the glenoid fossa, stretching the axillary artery across the humeral head and compressing it along the undersurface of the pectoralis minor tendon.

Diagnosis of the compression syndrome should be as precise as possible. The symptoms, which may not appear until after age 40, are dependent on the frequency, duration, and degree of compression of the vessels in the lower chords of the brachial plexus. The neurologic symptoms consist of pain segmental in distribution, paresthesias and numbness, and occasionally weakness. The symptoms of arterial compression and insufficiency include coldness, weakness, fatigability of the limb, and pain that frequently cannot be distinguished from that caused by a compressed nerve root. Signs of arterial insufficiency consist of diminution or absence of peripheral pulses, blanching of the hand on elevation, and ulceration and gangrene in advanced stages. In the diagnosis of shoulder girdle compression, the general vascular examination is first elicited. Diagnostic tests and positional maneuvers are then performed with the aid of pulse volume recording. Every effort must be made to localize the general area of compression, be it supraclavicular, retroclavicular, or subclavicular. Radiologic examination of the lower cervical spine will confirm the presence of a cervical rib. Occasionally, further diagnosis by contrast angiography is necessary. This must be performed with the patient in both supine and erect positions. As the contrast medium is injected, the arm is taken through the positional maneuvers in an effort to visualize the obstructing element. With the use of digital subtraction angiography and the venous injection, this diagnosis has been made considerably easier.

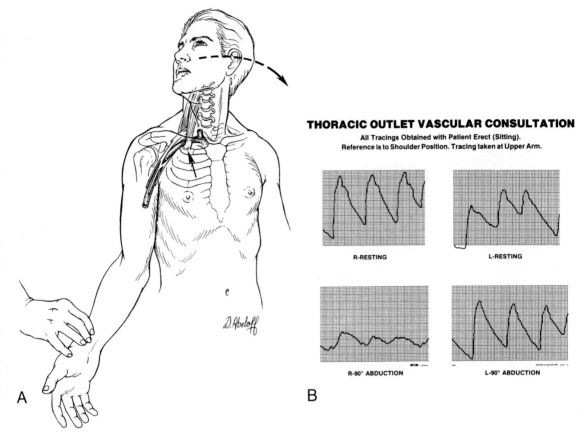

THORACIC OUTLET VASCULAR CONSULTATION

All Tracings Obtained with Patient Erect (Sitting).
Reference is to Shoulder Position. Tracing taken at Upper Arm.

R-RESTING

L-RESTING

R-90° ABDUCTION

L-90° ABDUCTION

A

B

Figure 117–6. *A,* Adson's maneuver. (From Wilgis, E. F. S.: Vascular Injuries and Diseases of the Upper Limb. Boston, Little, Brown & Company, 1983. Copyright 1983, Little, Brown & Company.) *B,* Pulse volume recording showing positional pulse deficit.

There are three positional maneuvers that should be performed in both clinical examination and pulse volume recording, and utilized when performing angiographic studies.

The Adson Maneuver. The patient is instructed to take and hold a deep breath to elevate the rib cage, extend his neck fully, and turn his chin toward the side that is being examined with the arm at his side. The limb is externally rotated with the wrist in a dependent position. The head can also be rotated toward the contralateral side. The observer then looks for any changes in the radial pulse that may be produced by this maneuver. Any resulting decrease in pulse volume, particularly if accompanied by paresthesia, suggests that the upper extremity symptoms described by the patient are caused by abnormal pressure at the intrascalene triangle formed by the borders of the anterior scalene and posterior scalene muscles and the first rib. This can be confirmed by pulse volume recording, as illustrated in Figure 117–6.

The Costoclavicular Maneuver. This is used to detect compression in the costoclavicular interval. The patient assumes an exaggerated military stance with shoulders drawn downward and backward, the arm by his side in a slightly externally rotated position. The maneuver narrows the costoclavicular space between the clavicle and first rib by approximating the clavicle to the first rib, thus tending to compress the structures that lie between them. This maneuver normally causes a dampening of the pulse in many perfectly normal people without symptoms. If this reproduces symptoms, this test indicates that the compression is between the clavicle and the first rib. This can also be confirmed by pulse volume recording (Fig. 117–7) and by contrast angiography. In this series of photographs the exact area of compression is isolated by the provocative test. Therefore,

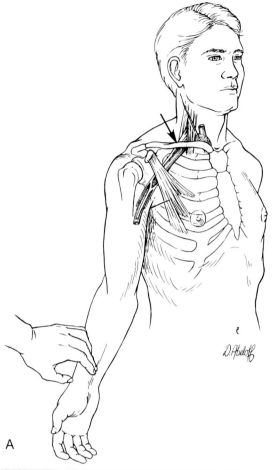

Figure 117–7. *A,* Wright's maneuver. (From Wilgis, E. F. S.: Vascular Injuries and Diseases of the Upper Limb. Boston, Little, Brown & Company, 1983. Copyright 1983, Little, Brown & Company.) *B,* Pulse volume recording showing positional pulse deficit. *C,* Digital subtraction angiogram—normal. *D,* Digital subtraction angiogram—abnormal (during Wright's maneuver).

THORACIC OUTLET
VASCULAR CONSULTATION

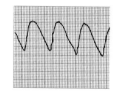

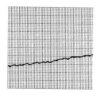

R-90° ABDUCTION
SHOULDERS BRACING;
NEUTRAL HEAD POSITION

L-90° ABDUCTION
SHOULDERS BRACING;
NEUTRAL HEAD POSITION

A

B

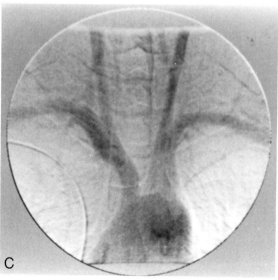

C

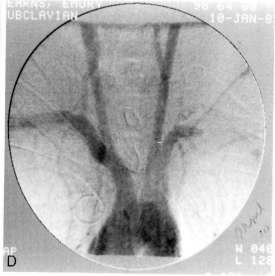

D

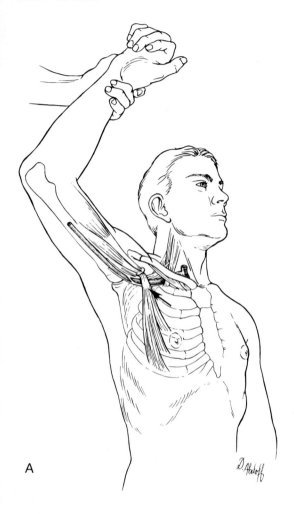

A

Figure 117–8. *A*, Hyperabduction maneuver. (From Wilgis, E. F. S.: Vascular Injuries and Diseases of the Upper Limb. Boston, Little, Brown & Company, 1983. Copyright 1983, Little, Brown & Company.)

one can logically assume that the surgical approach should be to the clavicle or first rib region.

The Hyperabduction Maneuver. In this maneuver the arm undergoes hyperabduction to 180 degrees (Fig. 117–8). When this is done the components of the axillary vessel and the brachial plexus are bent to form 90 degree angles at the junction of the glenoid and humeral head, subjecting the artery and vein to maximal compression against the axillary pulley and the pectoralis minor tendon. This maneuver with corresponding symptoms may indeed indicate that the compression is at this level. Positive studies with pulse volume recordings reproducing the objective pulse diminution and digital subtraction angiography, as in Figure 117–9, would illustrate that the patient might indeed have total occlusion of the axillary artery with the hyperabduction maneuver. Thus, it can be seen that by combining clinical, noninvasive, and invasive testing, the precise area of compression in the shoulder girdle syndrome can be elicited. This provocative testing while the patient is undergoing contrast angiography has made the precise diagnosis of this condition much easier.

There is general agreement that conservative management should be the first approach in managing patients with shoulder girdle compression syndromes. The importance of exercise to improve the posture of the shoulder girdle should be emphasized and the patient should be counseled on how to avoid the extremes of movement that produce the symptoms. Lord and Stone (1956) report that with conservative management, more than 70 per cent of patients show significant relief within four to 12 weeks. For example, patients with hyperabduction syndrome who habitually sleep with arms upraised may be able to adopt another sleeping posture. Some patients may even consider a change in oc-

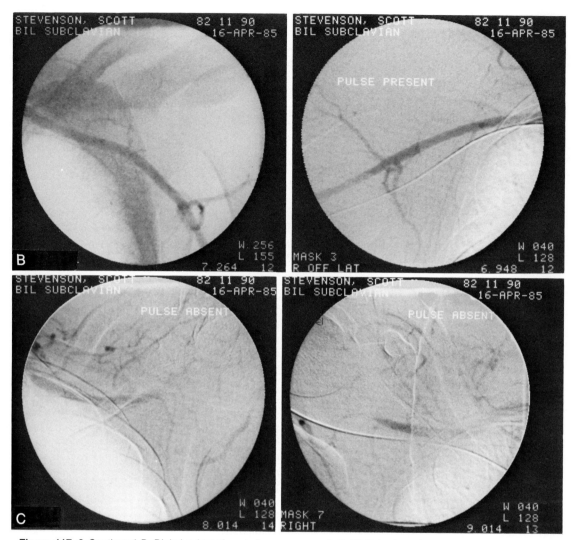

Figure 117–8 *Continued B,* Digital subtraction angiogram—normal. *C,* Digital subtraction angiogram—abnormal, with occlusion of axillary artery during hyperabduction bilaterally.

cupation if this is thought to be an important factor in producing symptoms, e.g., in the case of a waiter who must carry a tray in a hyperabducted position. The most successful patients treated conservatively are those, usually sports enthusiasts, who have suffered an injury to the hand, elbow, or shoulder and who go on to develop an ulnar pattern of use of the arm, subsequently experiencing vascular symptoms of thoracic outlet compression. The appropriate exercises frequently reverse the process in this group of patients. The exercises should be instituted under the direction of a physical therapist and should consist of stretching the muscles and strengthening the weakened muscles, so that the sagging of the shoulder girdle is reversed.

When the patient's symptoms are severe or refractive to conservative treatment, surgery must be considered. If the arterial insufficiency is accompanied by ischemic changes, embolization, or gangrene, surgery should not be delayed. Several surgical approaches have been reported to be successful. Roos (1971) has advocated total first rib resection from the transaxillary approach as the complete treatment for shoulder girdle compression. This in fact does relieve all the areas of possible compression, in that the entire rib is removed along with all of its muscular attachments so that the subclavian artery and brachial plexus are entirely decompressed. However, because surgical exposure is limited, there have been complications with this

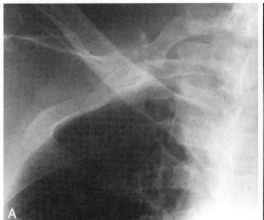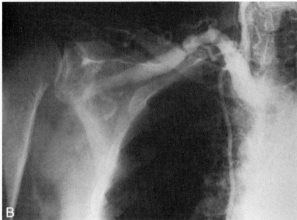

Figure 117–9. *A,* Cervical rib. *B,* Angiogram illustrating almost total occlusion of the subclavian artery. (*B* from Wilgis, E. F. S.: Vascular Injuries and Diseases of the Upper Limb. Boston, Little, Brown & Company, 1983. Copyright 1983, Little, Brown & Company.)

approach, including both nerve and arterial damage. Dale and Lewis (1970) reviewed their personal series of 76 patients treated by this approach, of whom 64 had transaxillary first rib resection. Fifty-five per cent had excellent results, 35 per cent had good results, and 9 per cent were failures. What is more important is that these authors included the results of a national inquiry made of surgeons performing the transaxillary first rib resection. Complete postoperative paralysis due to brachial plexus dysfunction was reported in 102 instances. Twenty-two of these patients did not recover, an additional seven patients experienced partial neurologic deficit, and 30 instances of failure of complete recovery were reported. Patients having first rib resection through the transaxillary approach should be warned of the potential complications of brachial plexus neuritis, neuralgia, or even paralysis. The significant traction and abduction that is necessary for the exposure through this approach may lead to these lesions; therefore, the author recommends careful positioning of the arm if this approach is used, and a discontinuance of the abduction and traction every 20 minutes during the operative procedure.

The supraclavicular approach can be used in patients having primarily compressive lesions in the intrascalene region. The scalenus anterior muscle and its fibrous tissue and/or the cervical rib can be resected and the subclavian artery totally visualized. In the author's opinion, cervical rib should always be removed by the supraclavicular approach.

However, the lower portion of the brachial plexus cannot be well visualized through this access. If the patient does have these symptoms, the author would approach it in a different manner. Also, if the patient has significant arterial disease with occlusion, the subclavian approach is unwise because only a portion of the subclavian artery can be visualized and control is inadequate. Division of the clavicle provides easy access to the entire region with good visualization, but it adds significantly to the procedure, and risks potential nonunion of the clavicle. If, however, the operation is performed because of a malunion of the clavicle, osteotomy and total visualization would be the procedure of choice.

The posterior operation popularized by Clagett and Martinez (Martinez, 1979) is an excellent technique and is recommended in any patient who has scarring from a previous approach by either the transaxial or the supraclavicular route. In the posterior approach, the scapula is detached and rotated superiorly, allowing removal of the first and second ribs by direct visualization. This allows the neurovascular structures to fall away from the first rib and eliminates the chance of a traction lesion. Once the ribs are removed, the neurovascular decompression is complete. In this operation, the rhomboids, a portion of the serratus, and a portion of the latissimus dorsi are divided, allowing the scapula to be elevated. With the patient in a lateral position, the upper rib cage is visualized. The second rib is resected to allow complete exposure to the first rib for its ultimate removal. The patient has only two to three days of postoperative pain, can leave the hospital, and recuperates at the same rate as if the transaxillary approach had been made. The potential brachial plexus injury is less and this approach affords the best visualization. It is recommended for all complicated cases.

If a diagnostician is certain that the patient has axillary artery compression beneath the tendon of the pectoralis minor muscle, sectioning of this tendon through an anterior approach by elevating the pectoralis major muscle yields excellent results.

The group of compression syndromes involving the vascular tree and accompanying nerves represents a complex diagnostic and therapeutic area. Meticulous and precise diagnosis must be carried out because the presenting symptoms are often vague and can be construed as psychosomatic. The consequences of undiagnosed compression with frank arterial thrombosis and ischemia are grave; however, repeated operations on a patient with psychosomatic illness are just as grave. The clinician therefore must be rigorous in his diagnosis, demanding in his conservative treatment, and exacting in his surgery.

OCCLUSIVE DISEASE

Occlusive disease in the upper extremity can produce symptoms because of the chronicity of its nature, with increasing pain, numbness, chronic ulceration, and frank gangrene. The patient with acute occlusive arterial disease presents with severe arterial insufficiency of the hand and fingers, indicating obstruction of flow within one or more arteries. It is characterized by the sudden onset of pain, paresthesia, a "cold" feeling in the extremity, and uniform tissue ischemia. The diagnosis of acute occlusive disease can be suspected when there is an absence of pulse. This can be confirmed by various pulse detection techniques, including the Doppler ultrasonic flow detector and pulse volume recording. A radionuclide angiogram is an excellent test for screening the patient with acute and chronic occlusive disease.

When the symptoms of acute occlusive disease are seen in association with a recent or present cardiac arrhythmia or marked cardiac infarction, arterial embolism must be immediately suspected. In patients with arterial emboli of the upper extremity from a cardiac etiology, approximately two-thirds show atrial fibrillation due to arteriosclerotic heart disease. Embolism from sources other than cardiac arrhythmia or infarction is uncommon, but it becomes an emergency if the embolus originates in a larger, more proximal vessel, such as the subclavian artery in shoulder girdle compression. The embolus breaks off and lodges at the brachial artery bifurcation in the upper arm, and the patient presents with a serious ischemic condition. Angiography, utilizing the digital subtraction venous route, confirms the site of the embolus, and surgical embolectomy should be performed as soon as possible. No effort should be made to delay the operation in order to allow conversion of rhythm, full digitalization, or other medical treatment. Since the site of the embolus in the upper extremity is usually at the bifurcation of the brachial artery, the operation can normally be done under local anesthesia. The brachial artery is exposed and arteriotomy is performed. A Fogarty balloon catheter is passed proximally to remove the embolus from the subclavian artery or from the brachial artery itself, and is then passed distally to extract any peripheral emboli from the small vessels. Afterwards the proximal blood flow should be brisk and the appearance of back-bleeding after removal of the distal embolus indicates that the peripheral circulation is now devoid of further emboli. The arteriotomy should be closed so as not to compromise the lumen of the brachial artery. A vein patch graft can be used if necessary. A normal pulse in the peripheral extremity should be demonstrated and can be confirmed by pulse volume recording in the operative setting. Embolectomy in the upper extremity is an uncomplicated procedure if done at the time of diagnosis and when the clot is still soft.

Arterial thrombosis in the upper extremity may also occur quite suddenly and may mimic embolism. However, the absence of a primary embolic site, the usually irregular distal distribution of necrosis, and a nonuniform picture of tissue ischemia help to differentiate arterial thrombosis from acute embolism. Acute thrombosis of the wrist vessels can be caused by occupational trauma. The two most common causes of surface-induced thrombosis are injury to the normal endothelium and an ulcerating atherosclerotic plaque that attracts platelets to the exposed subendothelial connective tissue. Of course the combination of trauma and atherosclerotic plaquing within one region predisposes it to thrombus formation.

Only rarely does acute thrombosis arise from trauma in a large vessel such as the subclavian, axillary, and brachial arteries. However, thrombosis of the subclavian and axillary vessels does occur when severe persistent compression causes arterial damage, as in the thoracic outlet syndrome (Fig. 117–9). In these patients, a combined upper extremity and thoracic approach is necessary to either bypass or alleviate the thrombotic segment by thrombectomy.

Thrombosis of the ulnar artery at the wrist secondary to blunt trauma was first described by VonRosen in 1934. Further studies have confirmed a relatively high incidence of this problem among laborers. Multiple methods of treatment have been utilized including conservative management, use of vasodilators, local and regional sympathectomy, ligation and excision of the thrombosed segment, and arterial reconstruction. All these methods have some merit, but none has given 100 per cent satisfactory results. Koman and Urbaniak (1981) reviewed 28 cases of ulnar artery thrombosis of the wrist and presented a guide to treatment. Successful management of an artery such as the ulnar artery thrombosed at the wrist depends on an appropriate diagnosis. Examination should include radioisotope scanning techniques and pulse volume recordings to determine whether the thrombosed ulnar artery is dominant. If there is any diminution of flow to the digits normally supplied by the affected vessel, excision of the thrombosed segment and arterial reconstruction should be strongly considered. Once the preoperative pulse volume recordings are done and surgery is deemed necessary, the author routinely performs intraoperative pulse volume recordings, after the patient has been anesthetized by either the regional or general route. The tourniquet is then inflated, the vessel exposed, and the thrombosed segment excised. The tourniquet is then released and repeat pulse volume recording is done. If the circulation to the digit is, in fact, improved and equal to that to the other digits, no further surgery is performed. If, however, the circulation to the ring and little finger or another digit is not equal to that to the other

digits, further reconstruction including vein grafting is done. The most common measurement of circulation used is the digital brachial index, which is the pressure of the digit expressed as a fraction of the brachial pressure. If the digital brachial index in the affected digit studied is below 0.85, further reconstruction should be done. This is illustrated in Figure 117–10. In this patient, interposition vein grafting was done because the circulation was deemed inadequate after excision of the thrombosed segment.

Thrombosis of the smaller vessels, if recognized early, can be treated by thrombectomy and/or excision of the thrombosed segment and replacement with vein graft or direct anastomosis. However, one is rarely given the opportunity to perform this early because diagnosis is usually delayed and the artery has undergone secondary changes with fibrosis.

Diffuse intravascular coagulopathy presenting as ischemia and impending gangrene is an example of acute thrombotic disease at multiple sites. This can be seen in patients with shock, sepsis, or far-advanced malignant conditions. Surgical treatment including thrombectomy is rarely useful; however, Fogarty catheterization of the vessels at the wrist and palm level sometimes can yield positive results. Thrombolitic agents such as streptokinase or urokinase have been used, although they must be monitored carefully and the patient must be checked for any allergic reaction or excessive systemic lytic state.

Moore and Weiland (1979) reported a case of heparin-induced thrombosis of the brachial artery. Thrombocytopenia induced by the heparin occurred several days after the drug was started, and platelet clots formed. The arm in this case needed to be amputated. Coagulopathy can be caused by a number of different pharmacologic agents or intra-arterial injections. Generally, intra-arterial surgery is not beneficial and secondary surgery such as fasciotomy is the only treatment available.

Symptomatic chronic occlusive arterial disease of the upper extremity occurs infrequently. Its diagnosis and treatment present challenging problems. Most of the treatable lesions arise in the large vessels, namely, the subclavian or axillary vessels. With proximal occlusive disease of the subclavian vessels, the patient may exhibit a subclavian steal

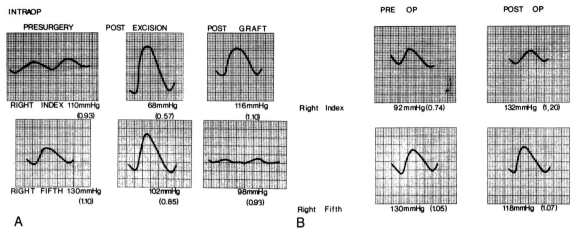

Figure 117-10. A, Pulse volume recording of an ulnar artery thrombosis patient during surgery. B, Pulse volume recording one day later—note the return to a normal digital brachial index.

syndrome in which there is a hemodynamic abnormality that causes blood to flow into the subclavian artery retrograde from the vertebral artery, because the blood pressure in the subclavian artery distal to the occlusion is lower than the vertebral artery pressure. This produces transient vertebrobasilar insufficiency. The classic symptom of this syndrome is dizziness or vertigo on repetitive use of the arm. Intermittent claudication of the upper extremity is seen in patients with obliteration of the subclavian artery distal to the origin of the vertebral artery. This lesion is relatively uncommon, but occasionally appears in patients complaining of tiredness and weakness or claudication of the extremities after use.

It should be emphasized, however, that patients with generalized atherosclerotic occlusive vascular disease who experience the symptoms of obliterative disease of the upper extremity have a systemic problem. Significant lower extremity or coronary occlusive disease could preclude treatment of the upper extremity disorder. The clinician must be cognizant of all the areas that may be involved and not be led into treating just one segment of a generalized disease problem, unless there is a potential loss of limb or tissue.

TUMORS

Although tumors of the hand are covered elsewhere (see Chaps. 133 and 134), special reference to several tumors is made below.

Vascular tumors are not commonly encountered, but when they are, they frequently occur in the hand and upper extremity. Various studies indicate that approximately 14 to 25 per cent of the vascular tumors seen involve the upper extremity. Most vascular tumors can be classified as "congenital" and are usually due to a failure of differentiation of a common embryonic vascular channel, resulting in hemangioma, lymphangioma, and arteriovenous fistula. Malignant change in these tumors is rare, but can be found occasionally. Of the acquired tumors, aneurysms may appear in the hand and may be either true or false. A true aneurysm consists of uniform dilatation of the arterial wall, whereas a false aneurysm is essentially caused by leakage of blood from the arterial wall and the formation of a hematoma that becomes surrounded by fibrous connective tissue to form a false sac. Both these aneurysms are usually traumatic in origin. An arteriovenous fistula can also have a traumatic origin and can present as a vascular tumor. Other tumors, such as glomus tumor, hemangiopericytoma, hemangioendothelioma, and sarcoma, can also arise. Kaposi's sarcoma is extremely rare.

Diagnostic tests should include clinical pulse detection examination of the mass with the Doppler ultrasonic flow detector, radionuclide angiography, venous angiography, and contrast arterial angiography. Digital plethysmography can yield useful information. The mass should be carefully described in the initial evaluation report, since one of the major problems in treating vascular tumors is recurrence. Later examinations must include study of the original tumor site so that if a questionable recurrence arises, the treating surgeon will know whether the current problem is a direct extension of the initial one or a new condition.

Because specific tumors are described elsewhere in this book, only several points deserve mention here. First, when evaluating a vascular tumor, one must be aware of the role the tumor plays in the hemodynamic assessment. The examining physician must be cognizant of whether the tumor itself is shunting the blood away from distal phalanges causing ischemia, or whether ligation and removal of the tumor will, in fact, cause peripheral ischemia and perhaps tissue loss. Therefore, in the overall assessment, one must occlude the inflow site in the preoperative state and assess the effect on distal circulation, as one would do in surgery. This is particularly true in treating arteriovenous fistulas and hemangiomas, which is quite clearly demonstrated in Figure 117–11. There is a vascular tumor arising on the radial side of the wrist that appears to be a traumatic arteriovenous fistula. A review of the digital brachial indices and digital pressure studies shows that the digital pressure in the little finger is not recordable as is the digital brachial index. The index finger shows a marked reduction in both the perfusion pressure and the digital brachial index. When the fistula is occluded by occlusion of the radial artery, the indices in both the index and little fingers improve dramatically. However, when occluding the ulnar artery, both the index and little fingers show no demonstrable perfusion pressure. Essentially, these data lead to the inevitable conclusion that there is an arteriovenous fistula between the radial artery and the accompanying vein, which is, in fact, stealing blood from the available ulnar system, so that there is relative ischemia in both the index and little fingers. When occluding the radial artery and thereby the arteriovenous fistula, the ulnar system is allowed to perfuse the digits in a more normal fashion, with subsequent improvement in the digital brachial indices. Furthermore, when one occludes the ulnar system, all flow to the index and little finger is stopped, proving that this is a vascular

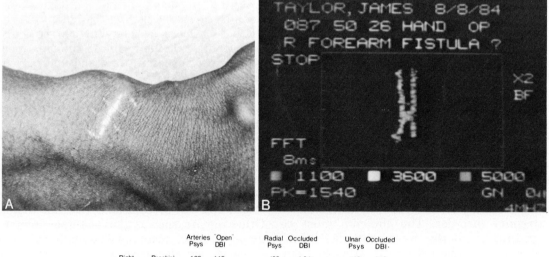

		Arteries "Open" Psys	DBI	Radial Occluded Psys	DBI	Ulnar Occluded Psys	DBI
Right	Brachial	120	1.18	108	1.04	118	1.13
	Radial	104	1.02			116	1.12
	Ulnar	98	0.96	110	1.06		
	Index	50	0.49	80	0.77	0	0
	Fifth	0	0	52	0.50	0	0
Left	Brachial	102 used for DBI		104		104	

C

Figure 117–11. *A,* A traumatic arteriovenous malformation at the wrist level. *B,* Doppler visualization of an arteriovenous malformation. *C,* Digital brachial index studies of an arteriovenous malformation, illustrating the "steal" effect.

tumor producing a steal phenomenon and causing digital ischemia.

The stealing of blood from the peripheral digits caused the ischemia to the peripheral digits and was the presenting complaint of this particular patient. At operation the fistula was closed, reproducing the relatively normal digital brachial index to the index finger and an improved digital brachial index pressure recording to the little finger. At follow-up some nine months later, this too had returned essentially to normal. The important point is that this dynamic provocative noninvasive testing yielded the information to enable an intelligent surgical decision to be made for this particular patient. This kind of testing can also be applied to other vascular tumors such as aneurysms. The author advocates noninvasive testing with pulse volume recording preoperatively, during surgery, and in the postoperative period when dealing with tumors.

Malignant blood vessel tumors are extremely rare. They consist of hemangioendotheliomas, hemangiosarcomas, and hemangioperiocytomas. Radical surgery is the treatment of choice for all these tumors.

One tumor now becoming more frequent in incidence is Kaposi's sarcoma, first described by Kaposi in 1872. It is essentially a malignant degeneration of the reticuloendothelial system and is characterized by a lesion that frequently begins in the skin of the hands or feet. The initial lesion is usually a pinhead-sized, flat nodule of reddish or bluish-red color. The lesion seems to coalesce and form larger plaques. Occasionally, wide surgical excision of the early solitary tumor may yield gratifying results, but aggressive treatment consists of controlled radiation in small doses. A poor five-year survival rate has been reported by McCarthy and Pack (1950). There is now significant evidence linking multiple-lesion Kaposi's sarcoma and acquired immune deficiency syndrome (AIDS). The combination of Kaposi's sarcoma and AIDS is usually fatal within several months. The case illustrated in Figure 117–12 shows a Kaposi's

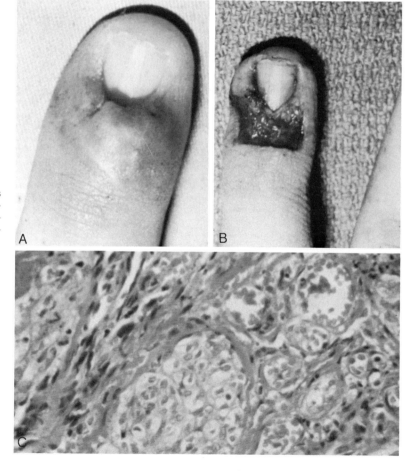

Figure 117–12. *A,* Kaposi's sarcoma in the paronychial region. *B,* After excision. *C,* A histologic section of Kaposi's sarcoma.

sarcoma lesion in the paronychial region. This was initially unrecognized and treated as a paronychia until excisional biopsy showed the true lesion. It is estimated that over 200,000 cases of AIDS exist in the United States today, so Kaposi's sarcoma will become more frequent. If the physician is faced with one of these devastating lesions, diagnosis should be made by pathologic biopsy and the patient should be referred to an AIDS center for treatment.

REFERENCES

Adson, A. W.: Surgical treatment for symptoms produced by cervical ribs and the scalenus anticus muscle. Surg. Gynecol. Obstet., *85*:687, 1947.

Allen, E. V., and Brown, G. E.: Raynaud's disease: a critical review of minimal requisites for diagnosis. Am. J. Med. Sci., *183*:187, 1932.

Arey, L. B.: Developmental Anatomy. 7th Ed. Philadelphia, W. B. Saunders Company, 1974.

Baird, R. J., and Lajos, T. Z.: Embolism in the arm. Ann. Surg., *160*:905, 1964.

Bardeen, C. R., and Lewis, W. H.: Development of limbs, body wall and back in man. Am. J. Anat., *1*:1, 1901.

Barker, N. W., and Hines, F. H., Jr.: Arterial occlusion in the hands and fingers associated with repeated occupational trauma. Mayo Clin Proc., *19*:345, 1944.

Beyer, J. A., and Wright, I. S.: Hyperabduction syndrome with special reference to its relationship to Raynaud's syndrome. Circulation, *4*:161, 1951.

Carrel, A.: The surgery of blood vessels. Bull. Johns Hopkins Hosp., *18*:18, 1907.

Clowes, A. W.: Arterial endothelial–smooth muscle cell interactions. *In* Bergan, J., and Yao, J. (Eds.): Evaluation and Treatment of Upper and Lower Extremity Circulatory Disorders. Florida, Grune & Stratton, 1984, p. 25.

Coleman, S. S., and Anson, B. J.: Arterial patterns in the hand based on a study of 650 specimens. Surg. Gynecol. Obstet., *113*:409, 1961.

Cranley, J. J.: Vascular Surgery. Vol. 2. Hagerstown, Harper & Row, 1975.

Curtis, R. M.: Congenital arteriovenous fistulae of the hand. J. Bone Joint Surg., *35A*:917, 1953.

Dale, W. A.: Occlusive arterial lesions of the wrist and hand. J. Tenn. Med. Assoc., *57*:402, 1964.

Dale, W. A., and Lewis, M. R.: Management of ischemia of the hand and fingers. Surgery, *67*:62, 1970.

Darling, R. D., Raines, J. K., Brener, B. J., and Austin, W. G.: Quantitative segmental pulse volume recorder: a clinical tool. Surgery, *72*:873, 1972.

DeBakey, M. E., and Simeone, F. A.: Battle injuries of the arteries in World War II: an analysis of 2471 cases. Ann. Surg., *123*:534, 1946.

Edwards, W. S., and Lyons, C.: Traumatic arterial spasm and thrombosis. Ann. Surg., *140*:318, 1954.

Egloff, D. V., Mifsud, R. P., and Verdan, C.: Superselective digital sympathectomy in Raynaud's phenomenon. Hand, *15*:110, 1982.

Fisher, C. M.: New vascular syndrome "subclavian steal." N. Engl. J. Med., *265*:912, 1961.

Gross, W. S., Flanigan, P., Kraft, R. O., et al.: Chronic upper extremity arterial insufficiency: etiology, manifestations and operative management. Arch. Surg., *113*:419, 1978.

Gruber, W.: Über die Halsrippen des Menschen mit Vergleichand Anatomischen Bermerkunger. Mem. Acad. Imp. D. Sc., St. Petersburg, 1869.

Inui, F. K., Shannon, J., and Howard, J. M.: Arterial injuries in the Korean conflict: experiences with 111 consecutive injuries. Surgery, *37*:850, 1955.

Koman, L. A., Nunley, J. A., Urbaniak, J. R., and Wilkinson, R. H.: Upper extremity radionuclide imaging. J. Hand Surg., *7*:412, 1982.

Koman, L. A., and Urbaniak, J. R.: Ulnar artery insufficiency—a guide to treatment. Proc. Am. Soc. Surg. Hand. J. Hand Surg., *6*:16, 1981.

Lord, J. W., Jr., and Stone, P. W.: Pectoralis minor tenotomy and anterior scalenectomy with special reference to the hyperabduction syndrome and "effort thrombosis" of the subclavian vein. Circulation, *13*:537, 1956.

Martinez, N. S.: Posterior first rib resection for total thoracic outlet syndrome decompression. Contemp. Surg., *15*:13, 1979.

Matsen, F. A., Mayo, K. A., Krugmier, R. B., et al.: A model compartmental syndrome in man with particular reference to the quantification of nerve function. J. Bone Joint Surg., *59A*:648, 1977.

Maurer, A. H., Holder, L. E., Espinola, D., Rupani, H., and Wilgis, E. F. S.: Three-phase radionuclide scintigraphy of the hand. Radiology, *146*:761, 1983.

McCarthy, W. D., and Pack, G. T.: Malignant blood vessel tumors: a report of 56 cases of angiosarcoma and Kaposi's sarcoma. Surg. Gynecol. Obstet., *91*:465, 1950.

McCormack, L. J., Cauldwell, E. W., and Anson, B. J.: Brachial and antebrachial arterial patterns. A study of 750 extremities, Surg. Gynecol. Obstet., *96*:43, 1953.

Moore, J. R., and Weiland, A. J.: Heparin-induced thromboembolism. A case report. J. Hand Surg., *4*:382, 1979.

Morgan, R., Riesman, N., and Wilgis, E. F. S.: Anatomic localization of sympathetic nerves in the hand. J. Hand Surg., *8*:283, 1983.

Mozersky, D. J., Buckley, C. J., Hagood, C. O., Jr., et al.: Ultrasonic evaluation of the palmar circulation—a useful adjunct to radial artery cannulation. Am. J. Surg., *126*:810, 1973.

Mubarak, S. J., Owen, C. A., Hargens, A. R., Garetto, L. P., and Akeson, W. H.: Acute compartment syndromes. Diagnosis and treatment with the aid of the wick catheter. J. Bone Joint Surg., *60A*:1091, 1978.

Peet, B. M., Henricksen, J. D., Anderson, T. P., et al.: Thoracic outlet syndrome: evaluation of a therapeutic exercise program. Proc. Staff Meet. Mayo Clin., *31*:265, 1956.

Pick, J.: The Autonomic Nervous System. Philadelphia, J. B. Lippincott Company, 1970.

Rich, N. M., Baugh, J. H., and Hughes, C. W.: Acute arterial injuries in Vietnam: 1000 cases. J. Trauma, *10*:359, 1970.

Roos, D. B.: Experience with first rib resection for thoracic outlet syndrome. Ann. Surg., *173*:429, 1971.

Rosati, L. M., and Lord, J. W., Jr.: Neurovascular compression syndromes of the upper extremity. Ciba Clin. Symp., *10*:35, 1958.

Ross, R., and Glomset, J. A.: The pathogenesis of atherosclerosis. N. Engl. J. Med., *295*:369, 1976.

Stout, A. P.: Tumors of the soft tissues. *In* Armed Forces Institute of Pathology Atlas of Tumor Pathology, Washington, 1953.

VonRosen, S.: Ein Fall von Thrombose in der Arteria ulnaris nach Einwirkung von Stumpfer gewalt. Acta Chir. Scand., *73*:500, 1934.

Whitesides, T. E., Haney, T. C., Morimoto, K., and Harada, H.: Tissue pressure measurements as a deter-minant for the need of fasciotomy. Clin. Orthop., *113*:43, 1975.

Wilgis, E. F. S.: Vascular Injuries and Diseases of the Upper Limb. Boston, Little, Brown & Company, 1983.

Wilgis, E. F. S., Jezic, D., Stonesifer, G. L., Jr., et al.: The evaluation of small-vessel flow: a study of dynamic non-invasive techniques. J. Bone Joint Surg., *56A*:1199, 1974.

Lynn D. Ketchum

Vasospastic Disorders of the Hand

Many otherwise normal individuals have "cold hands," hands that are cold to touch, especially when stimulated by even modest drops in ambient temperature. Most people can be shown to demonstrate on digital plethysmography marked drop in pulse volume after smoking two cigarettes. These are examples of vasoconstriction (Fig. 118–1).

In this chapter, vasospasm is defined as an intense constriction of an artery sufficient to obstruct blood flow beyond the point of constriction. It is possible for a fingertip to remain pink with as much as an 85 per cent reduction in blood flow. With vasospasm, blanching of the fingertip indicates that there is insufficient or no blood flowing through the digit for that variable period.

Anyone who has seen a patient experiencing Raynaud's phenomenon appreciates that vasospasm is a definite entity. However, such vasospasm is usually a temporary and benign, though recurring, phenomenon; intensive vasospasm in a coronary artery may endanger life and, in the traumatic setting in a limb, is a serious problem that must be

dealt with expeditiously to avoid loss of tissue or even the limb.

ANATOMY

The structure of blood vessels varies according to their location. Central large arteries are rich in collagen and elastin, which supply tensile strength (Pick, 1970; Flatt, 1980). As the vessels course peripherally to terminate in the specialized vascular beds of the extremities, there is a progressive reduction in collagen and elastin, so that smooth muscle provides most of the vascular tone of the arteries supplying the digits.

Vascular smooth muscle undergoes constant asynchronous contractions, the summation of which produces vessel wall tone. Vascular tone of the skin of the hands appears to be largely a function of neuroregulation via the activity of sympathetic vasoconstrictive nerves. Vasodilatory innervation of these areas is thought not to exist (Metzler and Silver, 1979).

There are both alpha- and beta-adrenergic receptors in the vascular smooth muscle. Catecholamine stimulates the alpha receptors, whereas vasodilatory polypeptides such as bradykinin stimulate beta receptors. Prostaglandins may be both vasopressors and vasodilators (Strong and Bohr, 1967).

The amount of nicotine absorbed from the smoking of two cigarettes has been shown to decrease blood flow to the skin of the feet by 40 per cent and to increase peripheral resistance by 100 per cent.

Physical agents may affect vascular smooth muscle. Digital response to cold is both a central, sympathetically mediated phenomenon and a local vascular phenomenon. A cold

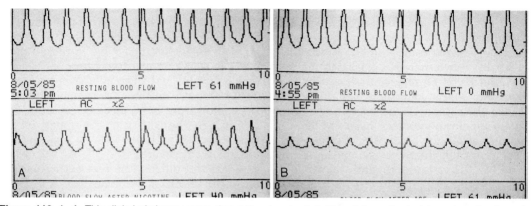

Figure 118–1. *A,* This digital plethysmogram shows the drop in digital blood flow after just two cigarettes have been smoked. Because of the increase in resistance, there was an increase in digital blood pressure. *B,* This digital plethysmograph shows a decrease in blood flow after a digit was immersed in ice for four minutes. There was a concomitant drop in blood pressure to the finger.

stimulus of the opposite extremity or the lowering of the core temperature produces digital vasoconstriction, which is abolished by sympathectomy. However, the vasculature of a digit whose sympathetic innervation has been interrupted also responds with vasoconstriction to direct application of cold (Fig. 118–2).

In Raynaud's phenomenon, intense vasoconstriction is usually brought about by exposure to cold; a moderate drop in temperature, e.g., to 60° F, can precipitate an attack (McGrath and Penny, 1974; Porter and associates, 1975). Central stimulation of the sympathetic nervous system as a result of anxiety can also be the cause. Because of vasospasm, the finger or fingers blanch from almost total lack of blood flow; with the ingress of some blood but with insufficient pressure for the blood to be pumped back into the venous circulation, deoxygenated blood pools, giving the fingers a blue color. Finally, the third phase or reactive hyperemia occurs and the fingers become red (Fig. 118–3).

The entire system complex can also be initiated by connective tissue diseases (e.g., scleroderma, lupus erythematosus, rheumatoid arthritis), occlusive arterial diseases including peripheral arteriosclerosis, certain neurologic diseases including carpal tunnel syndrome, blood disorders, chemical intoxication, and trauma. This group of symptoms, however vague, has come to be referred to as "Raynaud's phenomenon." If a specific cause has not been identified and the symptoms persist for two years (and is bilateral with

Figure 118–2. *A,* This depicts the digital Allen test used to assess the degree of vasospasm. Both digital arteries are compressed and the blood is milked out of the finger. *B* shows the radial digital artery being released and blood flowing back into the finger, the ulnar side remaining blanched. The time that it takes for the blood to come back into the finger after release of the digital artery gives a quantitative component that helps to assess the amount of vasospasm.

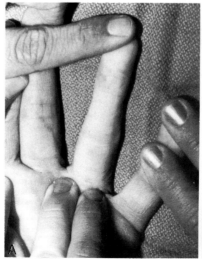
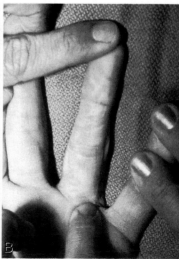

minimal gangrene), the entity is usually referred to as Raynaud's disease; however, the differentiation between Raynaud's phenomenon and disease is confusing and conflicting. It is felt by many that this classification and categorization is clumsy and should be discarded. All these conditions should be referred to as vasospastic disorders.

The peripheral vascular beds, which are most susceptible to vasospastic disorders, are subject to a high degree of sympathetic regulation but also possess capabilities for local regulation and response to circulating vasoactive substances.

What we have discussed so far are two mechanisms of vasoconstriction. First, an effect on the smooth muscle in the media of the small vessels produced by humoral factors such as ischemia or catecholamines, and second, stimulation of the sympathetic nervous system, again acting on the smooth muscle of the media from pain, anxiety, or cold.

Through the course of the upper extremities, the sympathetic nerves innervate the vessels from several sources. At the level of the brachial plexus, the cervicothoracic sympathetic trunk is not the sole supplier of sympathetic nerves to the upper extremity.

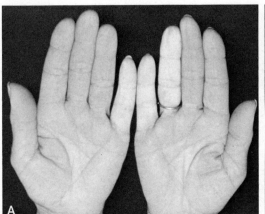
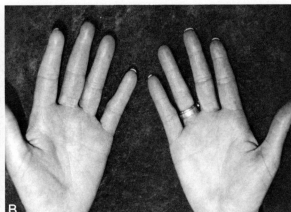

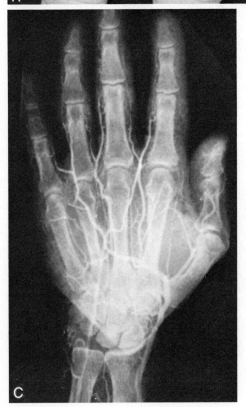

Figure 118–3. *A,* The phases of vasoconstriction with blanching of the fingers from cold exposure in a patient who experiences periodic Raynaud's phenomenon. In just a few minutes, unoxygenated blood pools in the fingers from lack of sufficient pressure to move the blood back into the systemic circulation, and so the second phase of cyanosis is seen. This is followed by the phase of hyperemia (not shown) in which the fingertips are red. *C,* the arteriogram of a patient with vasospasm of the common digital artery to the little finger.

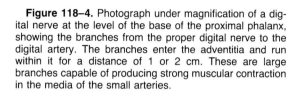

Figure 118–4. Photograph under magnification of a digital nerve at the level of the base of the proximal phalanx, showing the branches from the proper digital nerve to the digital artery. The branches enter the adventitia and run within it for a distance of 1 or 2 cm. These are large branches capable of producing strong muscular contraction in the media of the small arteries.

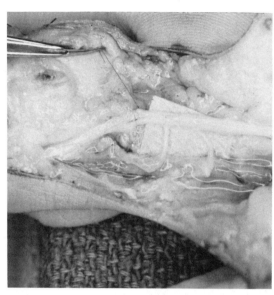

It is also supplied by the vertebral nerve, the sinuvertebral nerve, the carotid plexus, and the nerve of Kuntz (Woollard and Phillips, 1932; Kaplan, 1965; Pick, 1970). Intermediary sympathetic ganglia, placed in spinal nerve roots or rami communicantes, bypass the sympathetic trunk. These pathways, especially the intermediary ganglia, are often untouched during sympathectomy and later play an important role in residual sympathetic activity.

Pick dissected out the large number of possible routes of nerve supply to the vascular tree of the hand. The distal third of the radial artery is innervated by one filament of the superficial branch of the radial nerve and by eight additional twigs from the lateral cutaneous nerve of the forearm. The distal third of the ulnar artery receives three direct branches from the ulnar nerve and a branch from the medial cutaneous nerve of the forearm (Pick, 1970).

Within the hand, the superficial palmar arterial arch receives nearly a dozen branches from the common digital nerves arising from the median and ulnar nerves. The deep palmar arch receives two branches. The deep palmar arch receives two branches from the deep branch of the ulnar nerve and one from the median nerve. The digital arteries themselves are said to receive from three to 12 twigs (Fig. 118–4) (Wilgis, 1981).

Mitchell has shown in electron microscopic studies that the sympathetic fibers ramify in the adventitial layer of the vessels (Flatt, 1980).

Interruption of the sympathetic fibers in the hand produces a significant and lasting vasodilatation and a six- to tenfold increase in blood flow to the digits (Morgan, 1985). Nevertheless, the smooth muscle of the vessel media is still susceptible to humoral factors such as catecholamines and ischemia, even in the sympathectomized state.

MECHANISMS OF VASOSPASM

Because of its impact on death from myocardial infarction, much of the experimental work on vasospasm has been done on coronary arteries. Spasm in these vessels occurs most frequently from midnight to early morning and least often in the afternoon because of the circadian variation of the tone of the coronary arteries (Zuberbuhler and Bohr, 1965; Yasue and associates, 1979).

Coronary spasm is caused by a strong contraction of coronary smooth muscle cells that is triggered by an increase of intracellular calcium ions (Bohr, 1963; Fleckenstein, 1977; Karaki, Kubota, and Urakowa, 1979); calcium antagonists such as diltiazem, nifedipine, and verapamil, which block the entry of calcium ions into coronary vascular smooth muscle cells and dilate large coronary arteries, prevent coronary spasm (Fleckenstein and associates, 1976). Alpha-adrenergic stimulation increases intracellular calcium ions by using calcium from intra- and extracellular sources and causes contraction of vascular smooth muscle.

Hydrogen ions compete with calcium ions; anything that increases hydrogen ion concentration tends to prevent arterial spasm. Hydrogen ions are produced by metabolism and increase after exercise during the day when metabolism increases; the reverse is true at night. Hyperventilation, which decreases hydrogen ions, can stimulate smooth muscle contraction (Yasue, 1980).

Calcium channel blockers are now being used to treat Raynaud's disease as well as coronary artery vasospasm.

Severe arterial spasm leading to gangrene of the extremities and coronary artery spasm can be produced by ergot poisoning (Ricci and associates, 1978). The alkaloid ergotamine, used for relief of migraine headache and as an oxytocic in obstetrics, can produce intense peripheral vasoconstriction that lasts for days. It probably exerts its action through alpha-adrenergic stimulation.

Agents that have been used to reverse the arteriospasm from ergot poisoning include anticoagulants, vasodilators, and sympatholytic drugs. There are reported cases in which not only were these drugs ineffective but stellate ganglion blockade and arterial stripping were ineffective, so intense was the vasoconstriction.

Because the extremities were in danger of gangrene in these instances, Shifrin and associates (1980) produced immediate and long-standing relief with mechanical intra-arterial dilatation. They found experimentally that bladder muscle could be caused to contract intensely when bathed in ergotamine and that the contraction could not be reversed with phentolamine, propranolol, or atropine; however, mechanical stretching to a tension of 4 to 5 gm produced muscle relaxation that was sustained even after the tension was released. The analogy is probably valid.

In microvascular surgery, vasospasm can compromise tissue perfusion even though the microsurgical anastomoses remain patent. One of the most potent stimuli for peripheral vasoconstriction is circulating catecholamine (Nikki and associates, 1972; Hjemdahl, Belfrage, and Daleskog, 1979). Human catecholamine levels are markedly elevated by elective or emergency surgery, and increase in response to virtually any type of emotional stress such as pain or anxiety.

Richards, Seaber, and Urbaniak (1985) demonstrated in denervated rat hind limbs that catecholamine in the form of norepinephrine, when injected intra-arterially, induced vasospasm, decreasing blood flow by 78 per cent within five minutes of norepinephrine administration. Flow did not return to normal levels for 30 minutes. Norepinephrine administration in the presence of ischemia decreased flow by 95 per cent with one hour of ischemia before the injection, normal flow occurring only after 90 minutes. The clinical applications are obvious for the individual having an arterial repair and resumption of flow after a variable ischemic period (Strock and Majno, 1969).

One form of vasospasm, traumatic segmental arterial spasm (TSAS), deserves special comment, since it is frequently suspected as being the cause of an ischemic extremity (Samson and Pasternak, 1980).

The term was coined by Montgomery and Ireland (1935), who found that fractures and gunshots accounted for 36 of the 44 cases they reviewed from the world literature. Once universally accepted as a clinical entity, TSAS has passed through a period when it was thought to exist only in the minds of some vascular surgeons; it is currently controversial.

What has been reported in the literature is that injured arteries have a natural predisposition to contract. Kroh described an arterial injury from a gunshot in which the femoral artery was seen "to be contracted to the size of a knitting needle," but while it was being dissected the vessel dilated to normal size (Samson and Pasternak, 1980). From the German literature during World War I, it was noted that many contracted arteries were not damaged; however, adjacent nerves and veins frequently had been severed.

Cohen (1940–41) reviewed 50 reported cases of TSAS spasm in which the diagnosis was confirmed by surgical exploration, and concluded that the condition was more common than the literature suggested. However, surveys of arterial injuries collected from World War II, the Korean war, and the Vietnam conflict indicate a progressive decrease in the incidence of diagnosed TSAS. DeBakey and Simeone (1946) recognized TSAS in 28 of 62 cases of arterial injuries sustained by American Soldiers in World War II. Hughes (1955) found only two reported cases of TSAS in the Korean war. Perry, Thal, and Shires

(1971) noted two instances of arterial spasm among 259 civilian arterial injuries reported from Dallas.

Hardy and Tibbs (1960) felt that TSAS had become a mystique based on imprecise observations, and that for all purposes the entity did not exist. Samson and Pasternak (1980) concluded that TSAS "is a definite entity that can occur in the absence of organic injury but is extremely rare."

Localized segmental arterial constriction has been produced experimentally in response to stretching of an artery. Every hand surgeon has witnessed this phenomenon after the release of a contracted finger, as from a burn. If the finger has been contracted for several months or more, with release and extension of the digit, it is not uncommon for the digital arteries to go into spasm for up to an hour. Usually the spasm spontaneously abates; however, if the digit is still blanched after an hour, return of the digit to a more relaxed state of flexion relieves the spasm in most cases; the digit can then be progressively extended over a period of days. The spasm is a myogenic reaction independent of the autonomic nervous system, usually occurring in medium-sized muscular arteries; it may be localized to a segment of one vessel or may occupy the entire limb. Although usually encountered in the arteries of the extremities, TSAS has been described in the mesenteric vessels after catheterization. Once the stretching mechanism becomes powerful

enough to produce intimal damage, thrombosis of the artery usually follows.

In the experience of Samson and Pasternak (1980), arterial spasm occurs frequently in children and adolescents. Femoral or brachial arteriography in this age group is commonly followed by disappearance of the distal pulses, with full return of distal circulation several hours later (Fig. 118–5). Any open procedures on the arteries in this age group usually allow the surgeon to observe a spastic response of the arteries to direct handling. In such patients, return of palpable pulses may be delayed for several days despite arteriographically proved absence of an obstruction. In adults the occurrence of such spasm is much less frequent.

A commonly observed delay in the appearance of palpable pulses after successful revascularization of the extremities may represent a variant of such a spastic response of the arteries. It certainly is often given the onus for the "no-reflow phenomenon" as termed by May and associates (1978).

Vasoconstriction decreases blood flow, which is undesirable. In addition, edema subsequent to direct injury, prolonged ischemia, or inadequate venous outflow may exert sufficient external hydrostatic pressure to collapse the smaller vessels and obstruct flow. Burton and Yamada (1951) have advanced the concept of critical closing pressure, which implies that if the intravascular pressure falls below the pressures that tend to reduce

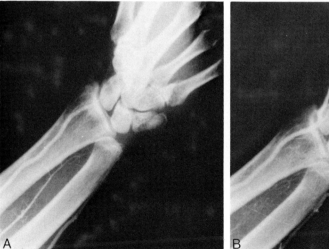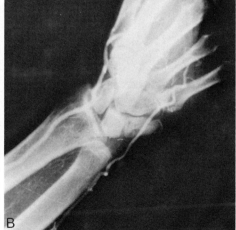

Figure 118–5. *A,* Arteriogram showing spasm of the radial and ulnar arteries in the distal forearm from the injection of a bolus of radiopaque dye. *B,* Release of vasospasm after an intra-arterial injection of isoxsuprine hydrochloride (Vasodilan).

the vessel lumen (autonomous vessel tone, external tissue pressure), small vessels not merely conduct less circulation but may totally collapse with complete cessation of flow. Thus, diminished distal intravascular pressures and reduced flow are detrimental to tissue perfusion and survival. Diminished perfusion initiates a cycle wherein capillary permeability increases, resulting in greater edema, elevated extravascular tissue pressure, and ultimately further reduction of perfusion.

THE NO-REFLOW PHENOMENON

Extended periods of ischemia secondary to vasospasm, prolonged tourniquet use, or replantation of an amputated digit can result in the obstruction to blood reflow in peripheral tissues. In their studies, May and associates (1978) revealed a definite pattern of change developing with increasing periods of ischemia. For example, after 12 hours of ischemia (using the rabbit epigastric island flap model) isolated intravenous aggregates were common and, although the epigastric artery demonstrated vigorous pulsation, no venous filling was visible during 20 minutes of observation. With increasing periods of ischemia, the progressive delay in venous filling after reperfusion suggested an ischemia-related increase in the peripheral resistance to blood flow.

In the study (May and associates, 1978) in which the vessels were denervated, 80 per cent of flaps survived eight hours of warm ischemia, but 100 per cent (15 flaps) died after 12 hours of warm ischemia. These authors showed that as flap ischemia time was prolonged from one to 12 hours, sludge and thrombosis were noted increasingly in the microcirculation; furthermore, with increasing ischemia there was an increase in leakage of fluorescein from the vessels and a decrease in the extent of vascular perfusion.

Zdeblick, Shaffer, and Field (1985) performed quantitative testing of the incidence of irreversible no-reflow at various controlled ischemia times. They studied replanted rat hind limbs with warm ischemia times of two, three, four, and five hours, including operating time. They measured the time elapsed from removal of the arterial clamp to venous filling; looked for venous microthrombi in the femoral vein; and measured the pH of the gastrocnemius muscle continuously for one hour. After four hours of warm ischemia, 50 per cent of the limbs became necrotic.

A consistent pattern of irreversible no-reflow was found. Microscopically, initial arterial and venous flow was brisk in all limbs. In those that eventually progressed to necrosis, large numbers of venous microthrombi were noted at three to five minutes. Flow then became noticeably sluggish. The time to venous filling ranged from two to 45 seconds in the limb survival group and five to 20 seconds in the necrosis group; i.e., there was no significant difference. Flow meter measurement showed an 18 to 20 per cent increase after replantation in the survival group, compared with a 41 to 46 per cent decrease in the necrotic group, which was significant.

Muscle pH decreased to an average of 6.57 during ischemia. Further decrease to 6.52 occurred in the first five minutes after clamp removal. The pH in the survival group then increased to an average of 7.08 in one hour, while the no-reflow limbs rose to 6.82; this difference was significant. Regarding venous microthrombi, no limbs survived when aggregate assessment was $4+$ to $5+$. All limbs survived when 0 to $2+$ aggregates were noted.

Perfusion of the isolated extremity with numerous solutions before surgery has not been found to increase survival and may in fact be deleterious to the limb.

Concerning the theory of swollen endothelial cells causing no-reflow, the lack of correlation of limb survival with the time to venous filling does not support the idea of a static obstruction (Leaf, 1973). If the cellular edema occurred during the ischemic interval, obstruction should be present immediately upon clamp removal. Thus, if cellular swelling occurs, it does so after revascularization.

The findings of May and associates (1978) showed that with denervation of the limb some arteriovenous shunting occurred but was not the cause of no-reflow, since in legs that eventually failed, flow decreased markedly both in the pedicle and at the tissue level.

The pH of skeletal muscle closely follows that of intra-arterial pH and has been found to be a reliable indication of peripheral blood flow. In this study, the rate of increase of pH when flow was restored correlated with limb survival rather than absolute pH. Rising pH corresponded to lactate washout and increased flow.

The most reliable observation in predicting limb failure was the number of red blood cell aggregates found intravenously after replantation. Although the exposure to subintimal collagen in the vessel wall may lead to increased thrombogenicity after ischemia, the observation of free-floating aggregates may also suggest a regional defect in the ability to lyse microthrombi. Puckett and associates (1985) showed that an impaired fibrinolytic system existed after prolonged ischemia in a rat groin flap.

May and associates theorize that microthrombi form and are unable to be lysed, which leads to aggregates of red blood cells and platelets. If the insult is moderate, the phenomenon is reversible; with prolonged ischemia, the microthrombi coalesce and the defect is irreversible. Venous thrombosis follows, which eventually results in tissue necrosis.

TREATMENT

The treatment of vasospastic conditions may be separated into that for acute and that for chronic phenomena. The therapeutic approach to acute vasospastic conditions may be divided further into pharmacologic and surgical approaches, in which various agents are used to counteract the effect of humoral factors on muscular layers of the arterial wall, and surgical approaches directed at interrupting the sympathetic innervation of that muscle layer or at physical dilatation of the spastic lumen.

Pharmacologic

Reserpine. Low dose intra-arterial reserpine has been used in a variety of conditions to relieve acute vasospasm localized to an extremity.

Hurst, Evans, and Brown (1982), using human volunteers in whom vasoconstriction was produced in one extremity by cold stress, established a dose-response curve for intra-arterial reserpine. The average temperature difference in the cold stressed and control extremities was 8° C, which occurred in two hours. There was a dramatic increase in the height of the pulse wave following reserpine injection after cold stimulation; however, there was no change in systemic or digital blood pressure in any individual. The effects lasted a minimum of 48 hours, and in some individuals up until the 15th day, with a marked clinical difference between the two arms in most subjects for at least 96 hours.

Reserpine is a *Rauwolfia* alkaloid that produces its effect by interfering with the granular storage mechanism in sympathetic nerve endings (Porter and Reiney, 1975; Serafin, Puckett, and McCarty, 1976; Nobin and associates, 1978). The granules play an important part in norepinephrine synthesis, storage, and reuptake following sympathetic nerve discharge. They also provide protection from intraneuronal inactivation by monoamine oxidase. Reserpine appears to exert a direct toxic effect on the intraneuronal norepinephrine-containing vesicles. It acts as a long-acting blocking agent of intracellular amine storage function. Only minute amounts of reserpine are required, since the active reserpine is highly bound. After a single intra-arterial dose, arterial segments showed diminished norepinephrine content within 30 minutes. Maximal reduction in arterial wall catecholamine content was shown by Porter and Reiney (1975) to occur two weeks after injection, with recovery complete by four weeks. Intramuscular injections of the same dose produce no effect on vessel wall catecholamines.

Another effect of reserpine is its effect on platelets (Hurst, Evans, and Brown, 1982). Blood surrounding a vessel produces vasoconstriction as a result of vasoactive amines that are released from platelets. Reserpine inhibits storage of these vasoactive amines in platelets, decreasing the vasospastic effect of extravasated blood.

Hurst, Evans, and Brown found that in adults the maximal effect with a single intra-arterial injection with a minimum of side effects (symptoms of a cold for 24 hours) was 1.25 mg.

Phentolamine (Regitine). Richards, Seaber, and Urbaniak (1985) found that in situations of vascular ischemia compounded by increased levels of catecholamines, pretreatment of the extremity with ipsilateral, proximal, intra-arterial injection of phentolamine caused a marked increase in blood flow. To a lesser extent, this increased blood flow also happened after ischemic treatment with phentolamine.

Denervated tissue perfusion is regulated by the intrinsic activity of vascular smooth muscle, which responds in turn to blood-borne substances and local metabolites.

In general, local metabolic factors including increased lactate, decreased oxygen tension, increased carbon dioxide tension, increased potassium, and local hyperosmolality are potent stimuli for vasodilatation (Hjemdahl, Belfrage, and Daleskog, 1979).

The study of Richards, Seaber, and Urbaniak (1985) suggests that vascular smooth muscle in ischemic tissue may be hypersensitive to the vasoconstrictive effects of catecholamines even in the face of increased concentrations of the metabolic factors mentioned above. The effect of vessel occlusion by itself was primarily responsible for the increase in vasospasm, since local metabolic changes, if anything, would tend to produce vasodilatation. In these authors' model, which was the denervated rat hind limb, the presence of ischemia or a temporary vessel occlusion, as commonly encountered in replantation and free tissue transfer, increased the vasospasm induced by norepinephrine. Pharmacologic treatment with phentolamine was effective in blocking vasospasm induced by norepinephrine and prevented the establishment of a low flow state. When phentolamine was given after the induction of chemical vasospasm, blood flow improved within five minutes.

Phentolamine is an alpha-adrenergic blocking agent, part of a group of drugs that includes phenoxybenzamine (Myers and Cherry, 1968) and tolazoline. These agents make the alpha-adrenergic receptors unresponsive to either direct adrenergic neural stimulation or the effect of blood-borne agents such as norepinephrine.

Phentolamine does cause gastrointestinal stimulation, which may result in abdominal discomfort, nausea, and vomiting. It also may cause tachycardia and hypotension. The intravenous dose of phentolamine is 5 mg for adults and 1 mg for children (the intra-arterial dose for humans has yet to be established).

Topical Agents. Numerous topical agents have been used to dilate vessels constricted from ischemia and manipulation in microvascular surgery. Local anesthetic agents such as procaine and lidocaine, nonspecific smooth muscle relaxants such as papaverine, and even simple salts such as magnesium sulfate have been used as first-aid measures when vessel constriction has been encountered.

These agents have been found to be effective on occasion, but their action is unpredictable in terms of length and amount of effectiveness; they are usually ineffective in situations of intense vasoconstriction.

Surgical

Surgical stripping of the adventitia of arteries to interrupt the innervation to the smooth muscle of the vascular media has been tried in situations of acute vasospasm following trauma or during microsurgery. However, this technique is often ineffective because of the vasoconstrictive effect on the smooth muscle by humoral factors, including catecholamines encountered in ischemic conditions that are not affected by the sympathetic nervous system.

Because of the myogenic nature of the spasm, as may be seen in TSAS or following ergot poisoning or intense postischemic vasoconstriction, treatment should not be directed toward the autonomic nervous system. Not until the nature of the lesion has been ascertained, intimal damage with or without thrombosis has been ruled out, and pharmacologic treatment has been found to be ineffective should the vessel constriction be treated by physical dilatation. A closed technique may be tried first in which a heparinized saline solution is injected under pressure between occluding vascular clamps. Finally, an arteriotomy may be required and the vessel dilated with a Fogarty catheter.

The principle of mechanical dilatation is based on the observation of Bard (1941), who noticed that a vessel in a state of tonic contraction may respond with reflex dilatation when mechanical dilatation is attempted.

If spasm is not relieved by any of the means suggested, the affected arterial segment should be resected and replaced by an appropriate graft.

CHRONIC OR RECURRING VASOSPASM

Cold Avoidance. Since exposure to cold can precipitate an episode of vasospasm, the use of insulation when a person is handling cold objects or is out in cold weather is important, as is physical hand warming (Folkow and associates, 1963).

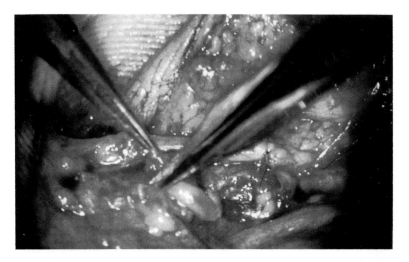

Figure 118–6. Technique of digital sympathectomy. Using an operating microscope and instruments, the surgeon incises the adventitia as shown here, dissects it circumferentially for a distance of 1.5 to 2 cm, and excises it.

Thermal Biofeedback. This technique employs voluntary control over automatically, reflexly regulated body functions such as circulation (Surwit, 1973). The patient monitors the effect of his voluntary control over the temperature of the digits. He hears or sees physiologic changes that he produces through voluntary control, and through repeated efforts is able to reinforce and augment this control, which can be as much as a 4° to 5° C rise in temperature with each biofeedback session. The drawback to biofeedback is that the improvement is transitory, and only 70 per cent of patients in one series tested could sustain an improvement; nevertheless, since Raynaud's phenomenon can be caused by stress and anxiety, this is one modality that can help in stress management.

Pharmacologic. The effects of nicotine are so dramatic in its reduction of blood flow to the digits that abstinence from nicotine is the single most important pharmacologic treatment.

As mentioned previously, calcium channel blockers such as diltiazem, nifedipine, and verapamil have been used successfully to treat coronary artery spasm and now have been found to be effective in the treatment of Raynaud's phenomenon (Fleckenstein and associates, 1976). The initial dose of diltiazem is 30 mg orally q.i.d., with a progressive increase to an optimal dose of 180 to 240 mg a day.

Phenoxybenzamine, an alpha-adrenergic blocking agent, has been used in a dosage of 10 mg three to four times a day and has been effective in some patients, as have tolazoline and isoxsuprine (Myers and Cherry, 1968).

Intra-arterial reserpine injections into the brachial or radial artery have improved symptoms for periods ranging from several weeks to several months (Abboud and associates, 1967).

Surgical Treatment. Digital sympathectomy as first advocated by Flatt (1980) has been found to produce a sustained increase in blood flow and thereby to be an effective treatment of nonhealing digital ulcers in Raynaud's disease. As Flatt has pointed out, the more distal the sympathectomy is performed, the more likely is there to be an effective denervation of the sympathetics to the digital vessels. This is a microsurgical technique that involves adventitial stripping of the digital vessels for a distance of 1 to 2 cm (Fig. 118–6). For multiple digits, the procedure is usually done at the level of the common digital vessels; if only one digit is involved, the adventitial stripping can be done at the level of the proximal phalanx.

In a series of 18 digits in ten patients, there was no recurrence of symptoms in 17 digits; pain was relieved almost immediately and ulcers healed in about two weeks (Wilgis, 1983).

REFERENCES

Abboud, F. M., Eckstein, J. W., Lawrence, M. S., et al.: Preliminary observations on the use of intra-arterial reserpine in Raynaud's phenomenon. Circulation (Suppl. 2), *36*:49, 1967.

Bard, P. H.: Macleod's Physiology in Modern Medicine. St. Louis, C. V. Mosby Company, 1941.

Bohr, D. F.: Vascular smooth muscle: dual effect of calcium. Science, *139*:597, 1963.

Burton, A. C., and Yamada, S.: Relation between blood pressure and flow in the human forearm. J. Appl. Physiol., 4:329, 1951.

Cohen, S. M.: Traumatic arterial spasm. Guy's Hosp. Rep., 90:201, 1940–41.

DeBakey, M. E., and Simeone, F. A.: Battle injuries of the arteries in World War II: an analysis of 2471 cases. Ann. Surg., 123:534, 1946.

Flatt, A. E.: Digital artery sympathectomy. J. Hand Surg., 5:550, 1980.

Fleckenstein, A.: Specific pharmacology of calcium in myocardium, cardiac pacemakers, and vascular smooth muscle. Annu. Rev. Pharmacol. Toxicol., 17:149, 1977.

Fleckenstein, A., Nakayama, K., Fleckenstein-Grun, G., and Byon, Y. K.: Interactions of H ions, Ca-antagonistic drugs and cardiac glycosides with excitation-contraction coupling of vascular smooth muscle. In Betz, E. (Ed.): Ionic Actions on Vascular Smooth Muscle. Berlin, Springer-Verlag, 1976.

Folkow, B., Fox, R. H., Krog, J., Olderam, H., and Thoren, O.: Studies on the reactions of the cutaneous vessels to cold exposure. Acta Physiol. Scand., 58:342, 1963.

Hardy, G., and Tibbs, D. J.: Acute ischaemia in limb injuries. Br. Med. J., 1:1001, 1960.

Hjemdahl, P., Belfrage, E., and Daleskog, M.: Vascular and metabolic effects of circulating epinephrine and norepinephrine. J. Clin. Invest., 64:1221, 1979.

Hughes, C. W.: The primary repair of wounds of major arteries: an analysis of experience in Korea in 1953. Ann. Surg., 141:297, 1955.

Hurst, L. N., Evans, H. B., and Brown, D. H.: Vasospasm control by intra-arterial reserpine. Plast. Reconstr. Surg., 70:595, 1982.

Kaplan, E. B.: The blood and nerve supply of the hand. In Functional and Surgical Anatomy of the Hand. Philadelphia, J. B. Lippincott Company, 1965, pp. 143–168.

Karaki, H., Kubota, H., and Urakowa, N.: Mobilization of stored calcium for phasic contraction induced by norepinephrine in rabbit aorta. Eur. J. Pharmacol., 56:237, 1979.

Leaf, A.: Cell swelling. A factor in ischemic tissue injury. Circulation, 48:455, 1973.

May, J. W., Chait, L. A., O'Brien, B. M., and Hurley, J. V.: The no-reflow phenomenon in experimental free flaps. Plast. Reconstr. Surg., 61:256, 1978.

McGrath, M. A., and Penny, R.: The mechanisms of Raynaud's phenomenon (I). Med. J. Aust., 2:328, 1974.

Metzler, M., and Silver, D.: Vasospastic disorders. Postgrad. Med., 65:79, 1979.

Montgomery, A. H., and Ireland, J.: Traumatic segmental arterial spasm. J.A.M.A., 105:1741, 1935.

Morgan, R. F.: Post-sympathectomy thermal changes in a rabbit ear model. Presented at the 40th Annual Meeting of the American Society for Surgery of the Hand, Las Vegas, NV, 1985.

Myers, M. B., and Cherry, G.: Enhancement of survival in devascularized pedicles by the use of phenoxybenzamine. Plast. Reconstr. Surg., 41:254, 1968.

Nikki, P., Takki, S., Tammisto, T., and Jaatela, A.: Effect of operative stress on plasma catecholamine levels. Ann. Clin. Res., 4:146, 1972.

Nobin, B. A., Nielsen, S. L., Eklov, B., and Laasen, N. A.: Reserpine treatment of Raynaud's disease. Ann. Surg., 187:12, 1978.

Perry, M. O., Thal, E. R., and Shires, G. T.: Management of arterial injuries. Ann. Surg., 173:403, 1971.

Pick, J.: The Autonomic Nervous System. Philadelphia, J. B. Lippincott Company, 1970.

Porter, J. M., and Reiney, C. G.: Effect of low dose intra-arterial reserpine on vascular wall norepinephrine content. Ann. Surg., 182:50, 1975.

Porter, J. M., Snider, R. L., Bardana, E. J., et al.: The diagnosis and treatment of Raynaud's phenomenon. Surgery, 77:11, 1975.

Puckett, C. L., Winters, R. R., Geter, R. K., and Goebel, D.: Studies of pathologic vasoconstriction (vasospasm) in microvascular surgery. J. Hand Surg., 10A:343, 1985.

Ricci, D. R., Orlick, A. E., Doherty, P. W., Cipriano, P. R., and Harrison, D. C.: Reduction of coronary blood flow during coronary artery spasm occurring spontaneously and after provocation by ergonovine maleate. Circulation, 57:392, 1978.

Richards, R. R., Seaber, A. V., and Urbaniak, J. R.: Chemically induced vasospasm: the effect of ischemia, vessel occlusion and adrenergic blockage. Plast. Reconstr. Surg., 75:238, 1985.

Samson, R., and Pasternak, B. M.: Traumatic arterial spasm—rarity of nonentity. J. Trauma, 20:607, 1980.

Serafin, D., Puckett, C. L., and McCarty, G.: Successful treatment of acute vascular insufficiency in a hand by intra-arterial fibrinolysin, heparin, and reserpine. Plast. Reconstr. Surg., 58:506, 1976.

Shifrin, E., Perel, A., Olschwang, D., Diamant, Y., and Cotev, S.: Reversal of ergotamine-induced arteriospasm by mechanical intra-arterial dilatation. Lancet, 2:1278, 1980.

Strock, P. E., and Majno, G.: Vascular responses to experimental tourniquet ischemia. Surg. Gynecol. Obstet., 129:309, 1969.

Strong, C. G., and Bohr, D. F.: Effects of several prostaglandins on vascular smooth muscle. In Ramwell, P. W., and Shaw, J. E. (Eds.): Prostaglandin Symposium of the Worcester Foundation for Experimental Biology. New York, Interscience Publishers, 1967.

Surwit, R. S.: Biofeedback: a possible treatment for Raynaud's disease. Semin Psychiatry, 5:483, 1973.

Wilgis, E. F. S.: Evaluation and treatment of chronic digital ischemia. Ann. Surg., 193:693, 1981.

Wilgis, E. F. S.: Vascular Injuries and Diseases of the Upper Extremity. 1st Ed. Boston & Toronto, Little, Brown & Company, 1983.

Woollard, H. H., and Phillips, R.: The distribution of sympathetic fibres in the extremties. J. Anat., 67:13, 1932.

Yasue, H.: Pathophysiology and treatment of coronary arterial spasm. Chest (Suppl.), 78:216, 1980.

Yasue, H., Omote, S., Takizawa, A., Nagao, M., Miwa, K., and Tanaka, S.: Circadian variation of exercise capacity in patients with Prinzmental's variant angina: role of exercise-induced coronary arterial spasm. Circulation, 59:938, 1979.

Zdeblick, T. A., Shaffer, J. W., and Field, G. A.: An ischemia induced model of revascularization failure of replanted limbs. J. Hand Surg., 10A:125, 1985.

Zuberbuhler, R. C., and Bohr, D. F.: Responses of coronary smooth muscle to catecholamines. Circ. Res., 16:431, 1965.

Charles L. Puckett

Lymphedema in the Upper Extremity

Lymphedema is a particularly unpleasant and difficult disease. Fortunately it only occasionally affects the upper extremity. It is worth noting that the condition is presently incurable, frequently poorly understood, and thus often poorly managed by both patient and physician. Lymphedema has failed to capture the imagination or even the attention of most plastic surgeons, and consequently our management of patients with the disease has been haphazard at best. Many physicians have realized that the surgical "solutions" have often proved unpredictable and unreliable, and since conservative management has not been particularly interesting for the surgeon, many have avoided participation in the treatment of lymphedema patients, who are often "starved" for physician attention. The involved plastic surgeon will find them to be quite enthusiastic if he evinces some interest in their care. Indeed, they are often some of his most grateful patients.

PATHOPHYSIOLOGY

Lymphedema basically represents a failure of the lymphatic system to execute its physi-ologic role, which appears to be twofold: (1) the removal of macromolecules from the interstitial space and (2) assistance in the return of interstitial fluid to the venous compartment. Failure of the system occurs when the lymphatic channels are rendered inadequate by virtue of either obstruction or diminished numbers. Although a distinction is made in classifying lymphedemas into primary and secondary types, the fundamental pathologic condition is the same. There is a relative obstruction of lymphatic flow occasioned by either physical obstruction of a normal complement of lymphatics or an inadequate number of normal lymphatics, thus resulting in a bottleneck restricting flow. However, it is interesting that even with severe obstruction, flow never totally stops but continues at a retarded rate inadequate to keep up with the generation of tissue fluid, until tissue pressure is quite elevated (Puckett and associates, 1974).

Classification of Lymphedema

Primary lymphedema is recognized in patients who have a congenital inadequacy of lymphatics manifested by lymphedema occurring earlier in life and without a dramatic precipitating event (Milroy, 1892). *Secondary lymphedema* is generally referred to as *obstructive lymphedema*, the type that manifests itself as a result of some event that causes a significant destruction of existing lymphatics. Postsurgical (postlymphadenectomy) lymphedema and that occurring in filariasis are examples of this type. However, the common denominator with either type of patient is that eventually there are too few lymphatic channels to handle the interstitial fluid that needs to be removed. It is presumed in the primary lymphedema patient that a reduced but marginally competent number of lymphatics are able to handle the fluid load until some relatively minor event results in further destruction of lymphatics (i.e., infection) or greater demand on the system (i.e., menarche). The time of onset of clinical signs in primary lymphedema may simply represent relative degrees of initial lymphatic inadequacy. This concept may aid an understanding of why some patients develop postmastectomy lymphedema of the upper extremity and others do not. If it is presumed that these patients had a reduced but marginally competent complement of lymphatics before surgery, we can envision how ablation could result in relative obstruction. This would also explain why the vast majority of patients do not develop postmastectomy lymphedema.

DIAGNOSIS

Certainly, most patients with lymphedema of the upper extremity represent postlymphadenectomy cases. Although the primary lymphademas occasionally involve the upper extremity (Fig. 119–1), they are much more commonly manifest in the lower extremity, presumably owing to the effect of gravity. When the physician is faced with a swollen arm or hand, a brief differential diagnosis must be considered. However, a history of mastectomy and/or axillary lymphadenectomy and the chronicity of the swelling clearly label the diagnosis in most cases (Figs. 119–2, 119–3). With swelling of briefer duration one must consider venous obstruction, either with acute thrombosis of the axillary and subclavian veins, or obstruction related to tumor, such as with the superior vena cava syndrome. Pancoast's tumor may rarely obstruct venous return sufficiently to cause arm swelling. The typical lymphedema patient has swelling involving the lower portion of the arm, forearm, and hand. A characteristic of lymphedema is often involvement of the digits, whereas in venous obstruction digital swelling usually is not apparent. (Puckett and Silver, 1984). Infection of the extremity, with attendant swelling, must be considered and a primary site of infection sought. The sympathetic dystrophies (Chap. 113) may result in a remarkably swollen hand and forearm. In these cases, the history of a traumatic event for the hand, burning pain, and hyperhidrosis may be directing clues. Certainly, iatrogenic causes of hand and arm swelling must be eliminated; these would include constricting dressings or clothing and factitious etiology such as is suspected in Secrétan's syndrome (Fig. 119–4). However, in the patient with chronic lymphedema of the upper extremity requiring treatment there is almost always an etiology related to lymphatic ablation.

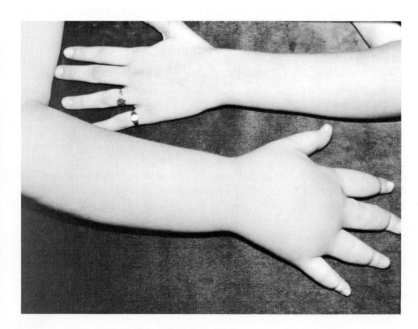

Figure 119–1. A patient with primary lymphedema, lymphedema praecox. Note the involvement of the hand and the swelling of the digits. This seems more characteristic of the primary lymphedemas than it does of the secondary varieties.

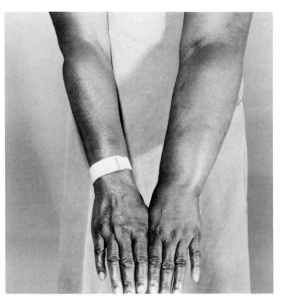

Figure 119–2. Secondary lymphedema of moderate degree after radical mastectomy. There is some involvement of the hand dorsum, but none apparent in the fingers. This patient should be fairly well managed with supportive measures.

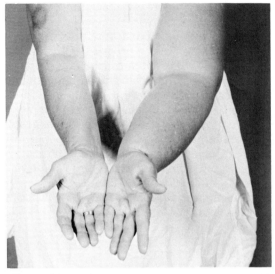

Figure 119–3. A secondary lymphedema patient who has more brawny lymphedema with involvement of the arm and forearm predominantly. She complains of heaviness and easy fatigability of the arm.

The lymphedema patients typically complain of a heavy (leaden) arm and hand. If the dominant extremity is involved they often indicate rapid fatigue as a common problem even when their activities are relatively sedentary. Patients note decreased dexterity and limitation of range of motion of joints. Advanced stages of lymphedema with brawny infiltration of the subcutaneous tissue can result in a nearly useless arm and hand. The elimination of the swelling (by any mechanism) seems to ameliorate virtually all symptoms. Thus, there appears to be no pathology other than the volume and weight problem of excessive fluid retention. These patients are prone to frequent and sometimes severe bouts of lymphangitis-cellulitis. Compromised immunologic capability of the lymphatic system in the involved extremity leads to a retarded clearing of bacterial contamination. A relatively minor skin injury can result in an infection with fever of 103 degrees or more and systemic toxicity.

Lymphangiography is an interesting procedure but actually has very little diagnostic value. With it one can differentiate hyperplastic and hypoplastic forms of lymphedema, but it rarely offers any insight into appropriate therapeutic regimens (Kinmonth, 1952,

Figure 119–4. This chronic factitious ulceration of the hand, present for many years, and the multiple secondary surgeries that have been associated with it have resulted in a chronic brawny edema of the forearm that is indistinguishable from secondary lymphedema. The forearm swelling remained even after complete healing of the hand was achieved.

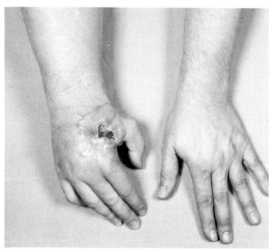

1954). Indeed, some evidence suggests that lymphangiography with Lipiodol dye further damages lymphatics and may actually cause the disease process to progress (O'Brien and associates, 1981). The author has eliminated lymphangiography from his diagnostic armamentarium, although it is still used in his research projects to characterize and document lymphatic status. It has been suggested that the information obtained by the injection of a vital dye such as patent blue (indicating either rapid clearance, stasis, or even dermal backflow) is just as valuable as x-rays with contrast material (Kinmonth, 1952; O'Brien and associates, 1981).

TREATMENT

Medical

The fundamental treatment for lymphedema of the upper extremity is a well-conceived and religiously executed regimen of prophylaxis with prompt attention to change or deterioration in status. Surgery should be considered only when there is failure of control with the medical regimen (Kinmonth, 1972; Casley-Smith, 1976; Puckett and Silver, 1984).

Treatment objectives in the medical management consist of (1) aid in removing the edema fluid, (2) decrease in the generation of edema fluid, and (3) avoidance of infection. Certainly the hallmark measures of care are elevation and elastic support. A harness or sling apparatus to permit efficient elevation at night is most helpful (Fig. 119–5). An arm stocking or sleeve with strong elastic compression (e.g., the Jobst) provides good daytime control and helps lymph egress from the arm (Fig. 119–6). More severe degrees of lymphedema may require an intermittent compression device (e.g., the Jobst) to help "pump" the fluid out of the extremity. These are particularly useful at night during sleep.

Dietary control with avoidance of obesity seems to decrease the fluid load somewhat. Salt restriction may be of some help, and diuretics occasionally, assist in mobilizing recalcitrant fluid.

With regard to avoidance of infection, the first step is meticulously careful hygiene and prompt attention to any minor injuries that could result in a bacterial portal of entry. Any inflammation, fever, or other signs of infection must be carefully evaluated. Par-

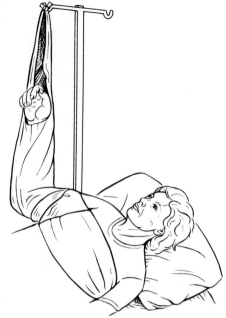

Figure 119–5. The stockinette sling provides nonconstricting elevation of the hand and forearm, and yet allows some movement in bed.

enteral antibiotics are often indicated and local wound measures must be aggressive. Full-blown episodes of lymphangitis-cellulitis require hospitalization and should be considered medical emergencies; these bouts probably result in further lymphatic damage that compounds the lymphedema problem. Therefore, the preservation of existing lymphatics requires vigorous anti-infection efforts.

In the late 1970's, the European literature showed considerable enthusiasm for the benzopyrones as a treatment for lymphedema (Casley-Smith, 1976; Piller, 1976; Clodius and Piller, 1978). Presumably, these compounds have some effect in lymphedema, not on the basis of anticoagulation, but on the breakdown of macromolecular structures to smaller particle size that can, theoretically, more easily get back into the vascular compartment. Clinical trials in the United States have not yet been forthcoming.

Daily attention to and scrupulous observation of these principles satisfactorily control most patients. Warm weather is definitely trying for those attempting to wear an arm stocking, and lapses in regimen are frequent. Observation has shown, however, that fastidious patients generally do well. Careless or less compulsive patients tend to have progressive arm swelling and more frequent bouts of infection.

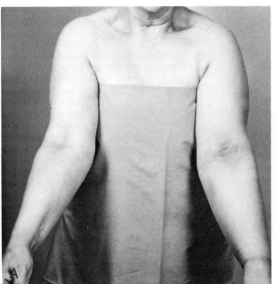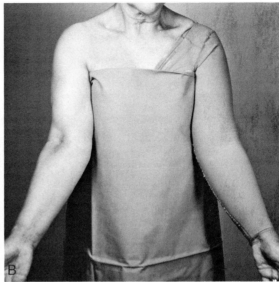

Figure 119–6. *A,* Mild to moderate secondary lymphedema following modified radial mastectomy. *B,* The typical Jobst arm stocking gives compression from the wrist to the shoulder. An elastic glove can be added if involvement of the digits or hand is significant.

Surgical

The surgical treatment for lymphedema has had a long and fickle history. Traditionally, "new" operations for lymphedema have enjoyed enthusiastic endorsement as early results seemed encouraging, but as time passed and this relentless process continued its inevitable progression, failures of therapy became apparent. Eventually the "cure rates" were found to be relatively modest. For those who are routinely involved in the care of lymphedema patients, it is generally accepted that approximately one-third of patients obtain significant long-term benefit from surgery, one-third are ultimately unchanged, and one-third continue a slowly progressive deterioration. As yet, no precise substitution for the lymphatic system or repair of its inadequacy has been consistently accomplished. Ingenious ideas have been offered and some have shown promise. However, in the author's view, at the present none can consistently offer cure. In interpreting the results of surgery, confusion has resulted from the frequent inclusion of subjective criteria in evaluating success. As stated previously, these neglected patients are often so pleased to have an interested physician involved in their care that they indicate improvement when objective findings suggest none, presumably to please their surgeon. Also, intensified medical measures are often a part of postsurgical regimens, and several surgical approaches are occasionally used in the same patient. Consequently, it has not been easy to determine any factual, legitimate surgical improvement.

The approaches to the surgical treatment of lymphedema have generally evolved in one of two directions. Attempts are made either to *ablate the offending tissue,* leaving behind only those tissues served by the presumed competent deep lymphatic system, or to assist or *augment lymph flow* from the involved part.

Ablation. The eponym frequently associated with the ablative procedures for lymphedema of the lower extremity is that of Kondoleon (1912). However, this is something of a misnomer, since Kondoleon's interest was primarily in creating a fascial window to enable communication between the incompetent superficial lymphatics and the "normal" deeper ones. Charles (1912) and Sistrunk (1918) both described resection procedures covered either by skin grafts (Charles) or skin flaps (Sistrunk). Sistrunk actually established the misconception with regard to Kondoleon's name by titling his paper: "further experiences with the Kondoleon operation . . . ." Homans (1936) described a modification using thin skin flaps to cover the resected area, and this procedure has had more application to the upper extremity than the original Charles or Sistrunk operations.

Miller (1977, 1978) described and chronicled his experiences with a modification of Homans' operation, using particularly thin skin flaps to create an esthetically satisfactory end result. This operation has enjoyed good application to upper extremity lymphedema, and it, or some modification of it, is the standard ablative approach used in the arm and forearm. The Charles-type procedure is rarely ever indicated. Miller described the elevation of an anterior and posterior flap from both medial and lateral incisions (Fig. 119–7). These flaps are approximately 1 cm thick, and the lymphedematous subcutaneous tissue remaining is then excised down to muscle fascia. The flaps are trimmed and sutured. (Fluorescein dye may aid in the determination of viability of the skin edges in these rather large random skin flaps, and may obviate some late necrosis.) Suction drains are routinely used.

Good success is reported with this technique from an esthetic and functional standpoint in the upper extremity (Fig. 119–8). However, second and occasionally even third operations are indicated to either maintain correction or obtain the maximal benefit possible.

Augmentation of Lymph Flow. The procedures that have been proposed to augment lymph flow or egress from the lymphedematous extremity have generally fallen into one of three categories: (1) attempts to establish communication between the superficial (compromised) lymphatics and the deep system, (2) the provision of an alternative lymph drainage mechanism, and (3) the construction of direct lymphatic to venous anastomoses.

Establish Communication Between Superficial and Deep Lymphatics. Efforts to improve lymph flow were initiated by Kondoleon (1912). His fascial window to accomplish this was apparently unsuccessful, however, and only the tissue resection portion of his operation has been retained. Thompson (1967, 1970) reported on a unique technique to merge dermal lymphatics with the deep system by burying a dermal flap (Fig. 119–9). The operation is done in a manner not unlike that of Miller. Instead of trimming the flaps and discarding the redundant portion, Thompson described deepithelizing them, the extra length being folded in to establish contact with the deep fascia. (One wonders about the viability of this even longer random skin flap when there is occasionally loss of the abbreviated flaps in Miller's operation.) Thompson reported twice on his procedure and claimed good results in 92 per cent of a series of 79 cases. While Chilvers and Kinmonth (1975) endorsed this operation as their procedure of choice, others were less enthusiastic about its long-term results (Sawhney, 1974). To date, there are no studies that document any communication between these dermal lymphatics and the deep system. Many surgeons have suggested that the beneficial effects of the operation are related to the ablative aspect of this surgery rather than to the creation of new lymphatic pathways.

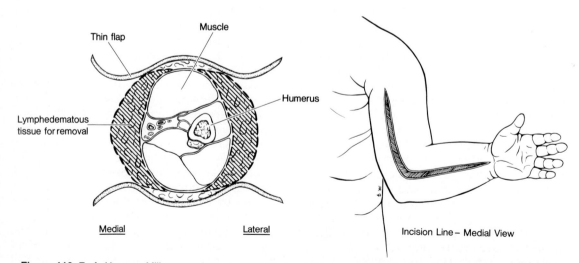

Figure 119–7. *A,* Homans-Miller procedure—a cross sectional diagram at the midarm level to show the thin skin flaps elevated and the lymphedematous tissue *(outlined in dashed lines)* to be resected down to the muscle fascia. *B,* Location of medial incision.

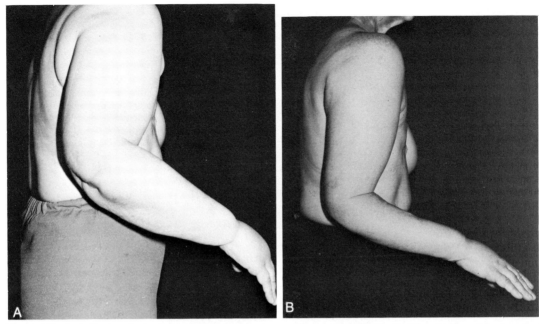

Figure 119–8. *A,* Postmastectomy, secondary lymphedema patient preoperatively. *B,* After ablation of the lymphedematous tissue with replacement of thin skin flaps (Miller). A satisfactory, functional, and esthetic result is apparent. Note that only a medial incision was used here. (Photos courtesy of Dr. Timothy Miller.)

Provide Alternative Lymph Drainage.
The idea of providing alternative methods or avenues of lymph drainage has stimulated the invention of several ingenious procedures. Handley (1908) proposed the wick lymphangioplasty, burying silk threads to augment lymph flow by capillary attraction. Long-term improvement was nonexistent and this procedure was abandoned. It was revived in modified form by Degni (1974a) and by Silver and Puckett (1976). The installation of multistranded Teflon or nylon threads to serve as wicks is a very simple procedure that can easily be done on an outpatient basis with very minimal morbidity (Fig. 119–10). It is easily applied to the patient with upper extremity lymphedema. The procedure does not appear to offer long-term improvement, but there is some short-term reduction in the swelling and it has been proposed as a possible measure to "buy time" in patients in whom a brief palliation might be of benefit.

Goldsmith (1974) proposed the transfer of omental flaps to provide a new resource of lymphatics to aid in drainage of lymphadematous limbs. Like many such procedures, early results gave grounds for optimism. However, follow-up has revealed recurrence or persistence of lymphedema in most of the patients, and omental transfer has been associated with an alarming incidence of serious complications, such as hernias. Furthermore, the procedure would have limited application to the upper extremity.

Lymphatic To Venous Anastomosis.
Since lymph is ultimately returned to the

Figure 119–9. A diagram of the Thompson buried dermal flap procedure. The deepithelization of the flap is usually done with the dermatome, and this flap is then folded in to establish contact with the deep muscle and fascia. A significant reduction (ablation) of the lymphedematous tissue is simultaneously done. Therefore, it is difficult to assign responsibility for improvement to the establishment of new pathways of lymph flow versus the improvement gain by tissue ablation.

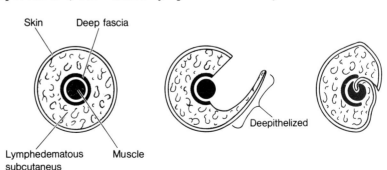

Skin   Deep fascia

Lymphedematous subcutaneus tissue   Muscle

Deepithelized

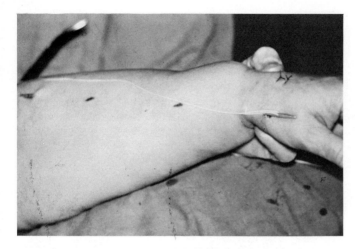

Figure 119–10. A patient at the time of wick lymphangioplasty. A modified knitting needle is inserted subcutaneously, and a multistranded Teflon No. 2 suture is placed from the wrist level, up the arm, and over the shoulder onto the chest. A series of tiny skin incisions allows this placement with minimal surgery.

venous system, it is appropriate to consider surgical mechanisms to facilitate this within the lymphedematous limb. If one can establish and maintain the patency of a lymphatic to venous anastomosis, decompression of the lymphedematous tissue should be achievable. A number of investigators and clinicians have contributed to this concept (Degni, 1974b). Lane and Howard (1963) reported the first direct lymphatic to venous anastomoses in normal dogs. Politowski, Bartkowski, and Dynowski (1969) recommended lympho-nodo-venous anastomoses in which the collecting node for the lymphatics of the lymphedematous limb was sectioned and sutured as a conduit directly to a venotomy (Fig. 119–11). The idea was ingenious, but long-term patency is not believed to have persisted. O'Brien and co-workers (O'Brien and associates, 1977; O'Brien and Shafiroff, 1979; Franklin and O'Brien, 1980) have been the major proponents in the English-speaking literature of direct lymphovenous anastomoses. In several publications, they have reported on 46 patients. However, in more recent years O'Brien has added segmental resection to his lymphovenous anastomosis

procedure, and it is difficult to determine how much permanent improvement is related to that and how much to the functioning lymphovenous anastomoses. Huang and associates, describing 91 patients treated in this manner, reported success in the mild and moderate cases but little or none in the severe cases. There has been no opportunity or mechanism to study these patients in such a manner as to document patency of the anastomoses. The author's experience with lymphovenous anastomoses in an obstructive lymphedema model in dogs suggests that, while patent, the lymphovenous anastomosis has legitimate potential to relieve lymphedema (Fig 119–12) (Puckett and associates, 1980). However, in the author's model, long-term patency was not demonstrated and he remains pessimistic about the potential to maintain patency of such anastomoses. Once adequate decompression of the lymphedema occurs, the pressure differentials are such that venous backflow into the lymphatics would be allowed and could result in thrombotic occlusion. On the other hand, if patency of the anastomoses could be maintained, there should be permanent improvement in

LYMPHO-NODO-VENOUS ANASTAMOSIS

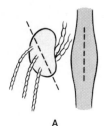
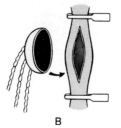
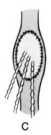

A   B   C

Figure 119–11. Lympho-nodo-venous anastamosis (Politowski) in which the receiving lymph node is sectioned (A), the lymphatic tissue is removed (B), and the node shell is anastomosed to a vein (C).

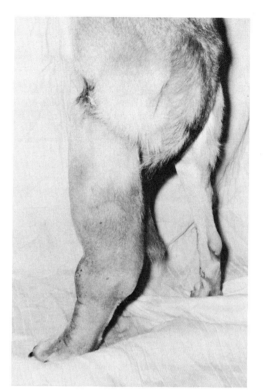

Figure 119–12. A representative animal from our lymphedema dog colony. A series of lymphovenous anastomoses was performed to determine effectiveness and permanency.

the lymphedematous state. The author's personal clinical experience with lymphovenous anastomoses has thus far been unrewarding. However, a survey of several microsurgeons who continue to perform occasional lympho-

venous anastomoses for lymphedema suggests that *some* rather dramatic successes have been produced and that improvement in as many as 50 per cent of these cases has apparently been permanent (Franklin; Shaw).

The procedure is carried out using the operating microscope and standard microsurgical technique. Multiple anastomoses are recommended, in the presumption that some will fail and that fewer ones may be inadequate to decompress the lymphedema. End to end, end to side, and rarely side to side anastomoses all seem appropriate in various locations (Fig. 119–13). Visualization of the lymphatics may be aided by vital dye installation in the finger web spaces.

In summary, the final story on surgery to augment lymph flow is clearly not yet written. This is certainly the most physiologic approach to the problem and many surgeons have been teased by the short-term good results. Investigation must continue in this area to determine the final role of surgery to augment lymph flow. The surgical treatment of lymphedema must for now remain a recourse for assistance in the patient who fails to respond to a conservative medical regimen. Until an operation is discovered that can consistently cure these individuals, surgery must take a secondary role in the treatment.

Since most patients with this problem have undergone radical mastectomy, lymphedema of the upper extremity may significantly decrease. Already fewer cases are seen as con-

LYMPHOVENOUS ANASTAMOSES

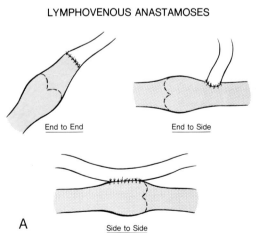

End to End   End to Side   Side to Side

A

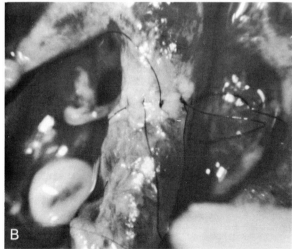

B

Figure 119–13. *A,* Examples of end to end (most common), end to side, and side to side (rare) lymphovenous anastomotic possibilities. Since the direction of flow in either lymphatic or vein is occasionally difficult to determine, end to side and side to side anastomoses are desirable. However, the two structures are rarely in sufficient juxtaposition to allow these options. *B,* A completed end to end lymphovenous anastomosis.

servative operations have evolved. Modified radical mastectomy has currently replaced radical mastectomy, and it is anticipated that with the use of procedures preserving even more tissue, such as tumorectomy or lumpectomy and axillary node "sampling," fewer and fewer problematic lymphedema cases will be created. Other causes of upper extremity lymphedema are sufficiently rare to be curiosities in the United States, and therefore this problem may largely solve itself, at least in the upper extremity.

REFERENCES

Casley-Smith, J. R.: The medical treatment of lymphoedema. Experientia, *32*:825, 1976.

Charles R. H.: Elephantiasis scroti. *In* Latham, A., and English, T. C. (Eds.): A System of Treatment. Vol. 3. London, Churchill, 1912.

Chilvers, A. S., and Kinmonth, J. B.: Operations for lymphoedema of the lower limbs. J. Cardiovasc. Surg. *16*:115, 1975.

Clodius, L., and Piller, N. B.: Conservative therapy for postmastectomy lymphedema. Chir. Plast. *4*:193, 1978.

Degni, M.: New technique of drainage of the subcutaneous tissue of the limbs with nylon net for the treatment of lymphedema. Vasa, *3*:329, 1974a.

Degni, M.: New technique of lymphatic-venous anastomosis (buried type) for the treatment of lymphedema. Vasa, *3*:479, 1974b.

Franklin, J. D.: Personal communication.

Franklin, J. D., and O'Brien, B. McC.: Microlymphatic surgery. *In* Barron, J. N., and Saad, M. N. (Eds.): Operative Plastic and Reconstructive Surgery. London, Churchill Livingstone, 1980, pp. 85–93.

Goldsmith, H. S.: Long-term evaluation of omental transposition for chronic lymphedema. Ann. Surg., *180*:847, 1974.

Handley, W. S.: Lymphangioplasty, a new method for the relief of brawny arm of breast cancer and for similar conditions of lymphatic oedema. Lancet, *1*:783, 1908.

Homans, J.: The treatment of elephantiasis of the legs. N. Engl. J. Med., *215*:1099, 1936.

Huang, G. K., Hu, R. Q., Liu, Z. Z., Shen, Y. L., Lan, T. D., and Pan, G. P.: Microlymphaticovenous anastomosis in the treatment of lower limbs' obstructive lymphedema: analysis of 91 cases. Plast. Reconstr. Surg., *76*:671, 1985.

Kinmonth, J. B: Lymphangiography in man. Clin. Sci. *11*:13, 1952.

Kinmonth, J. B.: Lymphangiography in clinical surgery and particularly in the treatment of lymphoedema. Ann. R. Coll. Surg. (Engl.), *15*:300, 1954.

Kinmonth, J. B.: Conservative treatment of lymphoedema. *In* Kinmonth, J. B. (Ed.): The Lymphatics. Baltimore, Williams & Wilkins Company, 1972, p. 314.

Kondoleon, E.: Die operative Behandlung der elephantiastischen Odeme. Zentralbl. Chir. *39*:1022, 1912.

Laine, J. B., and Howard, J. M.: Experimental lymphatico-venous anastomosis. Surg. Forum, *14*:11, 1963.

Miller, T. A.: A surgical approach to lymphedema. Am. J. Surg., *134*:191, 1977.

Miller, T. A.: Surgical management of lymphedema of the extremity. Ann. Plast. Surg., *1*:184, 1978.

Milroy, W. F.: An undescribed variety of hereditary edema. N.Y. Med. J., *1892*:505, 1892.

O'Brien, B. M., Das, S. K., Franklin, J. D., and Morrison, W. A.: Effect of lymphangiography on lymphedema. Plast. Reconstr. Surg., *68*:922, 1981.

O'Brien, B. M., and Shafiroff, B. B.: Microlymphaticovenous and resectional surgery in obstructive lymphedema. World J. Surg., *3*:3, 1979.

O'Brien, B. M., Sykes, P. J., Threlfall, G. N., and Browning, F. S. C.: Micro-lymphaticovenous anastomoses for obstructive lymphedema. Plast. Reconstr. Surg., *60*:197, 1977.

Piller, N. B.: Drug-induced proteolysis: a correlation with oedema-reducing ability. Br. J. Exp. Pathol. *57*:266, 1976.

Politowski, M., Bartkowski, S., and Dynowski, J.: Treatment of lymphedema of the limbs by lymphatic-venous fistula. Surgery, *66*:639, 1969.

Puckett, C. L., Helfrich, L. R., Carter, R. D., Joyner, W. L., Mishriky, et al.: Studies of lymph flow during experimental obstructive lymphedema. Surg. Forum, *25*:530, 1974.

Puckett, C. L., Jacobs, G. R., Hurvitz, J. S., and Silver, D.: Evaluation of lymphovenous anastomoses in obstructive lymphedema. Plast. Reconstr. Surg., *66*:116, 1980.

Puckett, C. L., and Silver, D.: Complications of Lymphadenectomy and Lymphedema. *In* Greenfield, L. J. (Ed.): Complications in Surgery and Trauma. Philadelphia, J. B. Lippincott Company, 1984, pp. 91–100.

Sawhney, C. P.: Evaluation of Thompson's buried dermal flap operation for lymphoedema of the limbs: a clinical and radioisotopic study. Br. J. Plast. Surg., *27*:278, 1974.

Shaw, W. W.: Personal communication.

Silver, D., and Puckett, C. L.: Lymphangioplasty: a ten year evaluation. Surgery, *80*:748, 1976.

Sistrunk, W. E.: Further experiences with the Kondoleon operation of elephantiasis. J.A.M.A., *71*:800, 1918.

Thompson, N.: The surgical treatment of chronic lymphedema of the extremities. Surg. Clin. North Am., *47*:445, 1967.

Thompson, N.: Buried dermal flap operation for chronic lymphedema of the extremities. Plast. Reconstr. Surg., *45*:541, 1970.

120

Eduardo A. Zancolli, M.D.

Ischemic Contractures

VOLKMANN'S ISCHEMIC CONTRACTURE

Over 100 years ago, Richard von Volkmann (1881) of Halle, Germany, identified ischemia to be the cause of certain post-traumatic contractures. Prior to that time, these contractures were generally attributed to nerve damage. Volkmann believed the reason to be extrinsic pressure imposed by tight bandages on already swollen limbs. Fractures of the distal humerus and their treatment were the chief contributor to the classic contracture. Later, internal pressure and venous obstruction were considered; Murphy (1914) recommended splitting the fascia of the forearm from the elbow distally. After World War I, interest shifted to arterial trauma. Thus, Griffiths in 1940 proposed the etiology of Volkmann's contracture to be arterial injury with reflex spasm of collateral circulation.

We now understand the acute ischemic condition to be a compartment syndrome that may or may not be associated with an initial major arterial injury, and the residual contracture to be the result of the untreated state (Holden, 1975; Hargens and associates, 1978; Mubarak and Carroll, 1979; Louis, 1980; Matsen, Winquist, and Krugmire, 1980; Sarokhan and Eaton, 1983).

PATHOPHYSIOLOGY

The common factor in all cases of Volkmann's ischemia (compartmental syndrome) is an increase in tissue pressure in a closed osteofascial compartment sufficient to cause occlusion of the small vessel circulation. The occlusion quickly leads to muscle and nerve ischemia (Mubarak and associates, 1978; Sarokhan and Eaton, 1983) and finally to muscular contracture and nerve damage (Volkmann's contracture).

Much work has been done on the tolerance of muscle and nerve tissue to ischemia. Nerve ischemia produces altered sensation within 30 minutes, and irreversible loss begins and progresses after 12 hours. Muscle ischemia produces functional changes the first four hours and irreversible changes after four to six hours. Compartment syndromes lasting more than 12 hours usually lead to permanent damage (Sheridan and Matsen, 1956; Matsen, 1975; Hargens and associates, 1981).

Volkmann's contracture may occur in any compartment of the extremities. It is more common in the smaller compartments distal to the elbow and knee. Knowledge of the muscles and nerves in various compartments is important in understanding, diagnosing, and treating the various stages. Like the leg, the forearm contains four compartments; the hand has five, and the foot four (Bonutti and Bell, 1979).

The mechanism of muscular and nerve ischemia represents a traumatic ischemia-edema cycle (Eaton and Green, 1972) that begins with a trauma, usually associated with an initial arterial occlusion (vascular lesion or spasm), and produces progressive intramuscular edema due to increased capillary permeability. This intramuscular pressure, in a closed osteofascial compartment, causes occlusion of the small vessels and necrosis of muscles and nerves.

All patients with swollen, painful extremities and palpably tense compartments should be closely examined and followed. Most compartment syndromes can be diagnosed clinically. Pain in the extremity increases with time or passive stretch of the involved muscles. Progressive loss or change in sensation occurs.

In equivocal cases or those in which the patient is comatose or unable to cooperate, direct tissue pressure levels are measured. The most common methods are those advocated by Whitesides and associates (1975) and by Mubarak and colleagues (1976, 1978).

Normal tissue pressure is zero to 8 mm Hg. It rises with muscle contracture and almost immediately drops with relaxation. A resting compartment pressure of over 30 mm Hg has been shown to cause pain, paresthesias, and interference with capillary circulation.

Tissue ischemia passes through three different stages: *initial* or *acute, evolutionary* or *subacute,* and *established* or *final.*

Initial or Acute Stage (Vascular Crisis)

Ischemia of the muscles and nerves of the forearm is more common in childhood. The compartment syndrome may begin after any injury of the major vessels above the elbow, usually in association with a displaced supracondylar fracture or after a severe and progressive edema or hemorrhage at the forearm. These latter two etiologies occur with crush injuries, burns, forearm or humeral fractures, operative complications, and constrictive bandaging.

Early clinical symptoms and signs are pain, both at the site of trauma and with passive digital extension; severe edema at the volar aspect of the elbow and forearm; hypoesthesia of the volar aspect of the digits; weakness of finger and wrist flexion; flexion contracture of the digits and wrist; and cool and cyanotic forearm and hand. The absence of the radial pulse is an unreliable sign and has far less significance than progressive pain (on finger extension), paresthesia, and forearm swelling (Littler, 1977) because the radial artery passes only superficially through the forearm.

The muscles most commonly affected are those located at the deep volar compartment of the forearm (flexor digitorum profundus and flexor pollicis longus), which are supplied by "end arteries," branches of the ulnar and interosseous arteries in the antecubital fossa. Occasionally, the flexor digitorum superficialis and flexors of the wrist are involved. The nerves most commonly affected are the median and ulnar nerves. The muscles of the dorsal compartment of the forearm can also be involved. In a series of 83 cases of muscular ischemia and contracture at the level of the upper limb, 61.5 per cent were located in the hand muscles (Finochietto's ischemic contracture) and 38.5 per cent in the forearm (Zancolli, 1963). In the latter group 87 per cent of patients presented with classic Volkmann's ischemic contracture of the volar compartment of the forearm, and in 13 per cent the dorsal muscular compartment was also affected.

The goal of treatment during the acute

stage is to reestablish the circulation of the affected muscles and nerves.

In the case of a displaced supracondylar fracture, the following corrective measures should be instituted: (1) remove all constricting bandages and (2) reduce the fracture by gentle manipulation or by Dunlop's traction. These measures will frequently restore the radial pulse and reduce symptoms. The elbow should not be placed in acute flexion for the first few days. Pinning of the fracture may be necessary to maintain position. The limb is not elevated but rather is placed at heart level. Elevation significantly increases anoxia in the face of high intercompartmental pressures (Matsen and associates, 1977).

If these measures do not improve the circulation in 3 to 4 hours and bring relief of symptoms, and intracompartmental pressure is greater than 30 mm Hg, surgery is undertaken. An extensive fasciotomy of the involved compartments is performed to avoid irreversible tissue damage. Both the superficial and deep flexor compartments are opened in an incision from the flexor crease of the elbow distally to the wrist (Fig. 120–1). The lacertus fibrosus is opened to decompress the median nerve and brachial artery. The median and ulnar nerves are released past the muscular arches in the proximal forearm. Individual muscles are palpated, and the epimysium is opened if there is any doubt as to increased pressure in it (Eaton and Green, 1972). If the dorsal and lateral compartments are tight, they are also opened.

About 10 to 15 minutes after the fascia is opened, small vessel bleeding will increase as circulation returns. This bleeding is controlled, and the wound left open.

If a lesion of the brachial artery is present, the damage is located. Lacerations are repaired. Localized narrowing in the artery

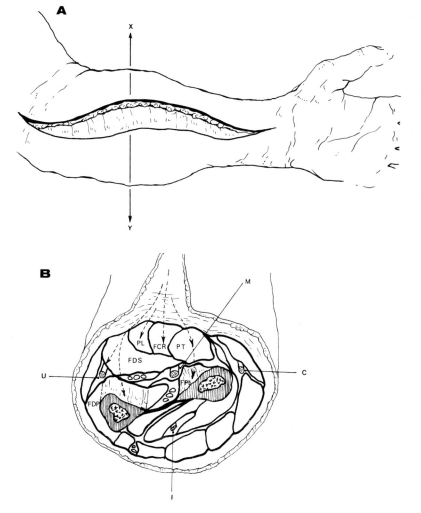

Figure 120–1. *A,* Skin incision at the forearm and elbow to decompress the volar muscles and the brachial artery. *B,* A transverse section at the middle of the forearm (X–Y of part *A*). Decompression of muscles is obtained by division of the antebrachial fascia and the fascial sheath of all the muscles affected. The deep muscles—flexor digitorum profundus and flexor pollicis longus—irrigated by the anterior interosseous artery are particularly decompressed. M = median nerve; U = ulnar nerve; C = cutaneous branch of the radial nerve; I = posterior interosseous nerve; PL = palmaris longus; FCR = flexor carpi radialis; PT = pronator teres; FDS = flexor digitorum superficialis; FDP = flexor digitorum profundus; FLP = flexor pollicis longus.

may be a tearing of the intimal lining, and a clot is frequently palpable. In this case the artery is opened, the clot removed, and flow reestablished by graft or repair. Mechanical spasm may frequently be overcome by injecting a bolus of fluid through the narrow segment from above. Fractures are usually stabilized (Rich, 1978; Holden, 1979).

After fasciotomy and restoration of circulation, an adaptive nonconstrictive, moistened dressing is applied. Delayed skin closure or grafting is done in three to five days.

Evolutionary or Subacute (Paralytic) Stage

This stage has somewhat vague boundaries ranging from one to two days, when muscular and nerve sequelae are present, up to 3 to 6 months (Seddon, 1956), when spontaneous recovery of muscles and nerves ends and established final deformity appears.

The main goals during this period are: (1) re-education of hand movements, (2) prevention of articular stiffness, and (3) release of nerves compressed by retraction of the scar tissue (Leviche, 1938).

Conservative treatment is indicated immediately after the end of the acute period, when the damage to muscles and nerves has been definitive. In the most favorable cases, muscular recovery depends on the recovery of the nerves and regeneration of muscles.

Neurolysis is particularly indicated for the median nerve when spontaneous recovery does not occur. In this situation, excision of the scar tissue and the infarct is performed simultaneously with neurolysis. The nerve must be displaced from within the flexor muscle mass and allowed to lie in the subcutaneous tissue free from any fibrous incarceration (Littler, 1952). The median nerve is usually compressed beneath the pronator teres and the proximal origin of the flexor superficialis muscle. In severe lesions (axonotmesis III and neurotmesis), the nerve should be replaced by nerve grafts. After this procedure perfect tactile gnosis cannot be expected, but in a child the prognosis for a return of useful sensibility is exceptionally favorable (Littler, 1977).

Another indication for early surgery during the evolutionary period is a severe flexion contracture of the digits for which stretching exercises and splinting have been ineffective.

In these cases all fibrotic and ischemic tissues are excised. During the evolutionary period no definitive procedures, such as tendon transfers, should be performed (Seddon, 1956). It is preferable to perform surgery only to prevent complications.

Final Stage (Established Deformity)

Many descriptions of the final deformity stage have been published. Bunnell (1944) classified Volkmann's contracture as *simple* or *severe* according to the characteristics of the deformity at the level of the forearm and hand. Pedemonte (1948) of Uruguay divided the deformity into two types: (1) classic or favorable and (2) useless hand. Merle D'Aubigne and Tran-Ngoc-Ninh (1955) also divided the deformity into two types: (1) without clawhand and (2) with clawhand. Seddon (1956) suggested three groups divided in accordance with the severity of the ischemia: group I, with diffuse ischemia and without infarct, in which spontaneous recovery occurs; group II, with typical muscular infarct and with or without nerve damage; and group III, with diffuse fibrosis and severe paralysis and deformity.

Since 1959 the author has been classifying the established contracture into four types based on the condition of intrinsic hand muscles (Zancolli, 1959, 1965, 1971) (Fig. 120–2). In all four types the wrist is flexed. This classification system has been helpful in determining the surgical program. In type I, the intrinsic muscles are normal; in type II, they are paralyzed; in type III, they are contracted. In type IV there is some combination of the preceding three types.

TYPE I: CONTRACTURE OF THE FOREARM MUSCLES WITH NORMAL INTRINSIC MUSCLES

The wrist and fingers are deformed in flexion, and the forearm is fixed in pronation. The median and ulnar nerves are in good condition. Usually there is no finger joint stiffness.

In some patients, the metacarpophalangeal joints are in hyperextension in spite of normal intrinsic muscles. This imbalance is produced during attempted finger extension, the result of the tenodesic effect of long extensors with retracted finger flexors.

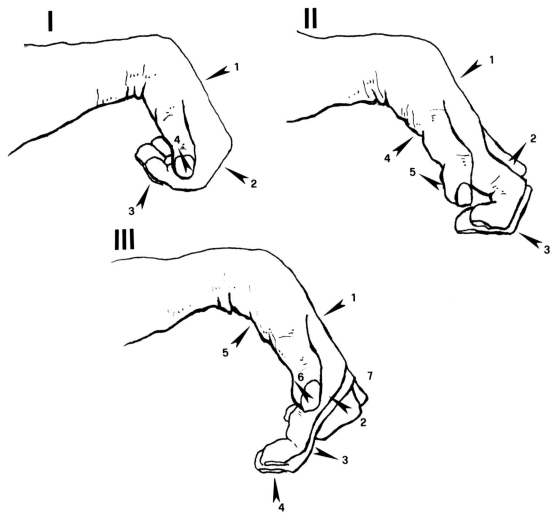

Figure 120–2. Different types of hands in established Volkmann's ischemic contracture. *Type I*: flexion contracture of the wrist *(1)*, fingers *(2)*, *(3)* and thumb *(4)*. Fixed pronation contracture. Nerves are not affected. *Type II*: flexion contracture of the wrist *(1)* and interphalangeal joints *(3)*. Hyperextension of the metacarpophalangeal joints of the fingers *(2)* due to intrinsic clawhand. Opposition paralysis of the thumb *(4)* with flexion contracture of its interphalangeal joint *(5)*. In this case the ulnar and median nerves are affected. *Type III*: flexion contracture of the wrist *(1)* and distal interphalangeal joint of the index and middle fingers *(4)*. The proximal interphalangeal joints of these fingers are in recurvatum *(3)* owing to ischemic contracture of the interosseous muscles. Thenar muscles are paralyzed *(5)* owing to paralysis of the median nerve, and the IP joint of the thumb is in flexion contracture *(6)*. The ring and little fingers have a clawhand deformity *(7)* owing to paralysis of the ulnar nerve (combined type II and III).

TYPE II: CONTRACTURE OF THE FOREARM MUSCLES WITH INTRINSIC MUSCLE PARALYSIS
(intrinsic-minus clawhand with opponens paralysis)

Wrist flexion, fixed pronation of the forearm, and intrinsic paralysis of the hand constitute the common presentation. Frequently, the median or ulnar nerve is involved. Occasionally, the intrinsic clawing is simple, but in the majority of cases it is complicated by finger joint stiffness in a claw position. The extensor mechanism over the middle finger joint may be attenuated. Opponens paralysis of the thumb is usually present.

In general it is preferable to deal with the motor problem of an ulnar nerve clawhand rather than with a severe median nerve lesion, as the latter generally presents difficulty in restoration of adequate sensation.

TYPE III: CONTRACTURE OF THE FOREARM AND INTRINSIC MUSCLES
(intrinsic-plus contractures of
the fingers and thumb)

The interosseous contracture is usually localized in the radial fingers. This type is rare. The wrist is in flexion. The metacarpophalangeal joints are in flexion, the proximal interphalangeal joints in extension, and the distal interphalangeal joints in flexion. The thumb may be adducted into the palm with the metacarpophalangeal joint flexed and the interphalangeal joint extended.

TYPE IV: COMBINED TYPE

Deformities are often a combination, usually of types I and II. Opposition paralysis may occur with normal interosseous and lumbrical muscles or an intrinsic-minus clawhand with a normal thumb. Some fingers may be paralyzed but others have normal or retracted intrinsic muscles. In a type II and III combination deformity, the interosseous contracture usually involves the radial fingers, and the ulnar fingers are in an intrinsic-minus deformity (Fig. 120–2, part III).

SIGNS OF DIFFERENT TYPES OF CONTRACTURE

Specific signs are helpful. In Volkmann's type I, finger extension is obtained by increasing wrist flexion. In type II, the fingers actively extend when the wrist is flexed, and hyperextension of the proximal phalanx is prevented (Bouvier's maneuver). In complicated clawhand, interphalangeal extension is lost owing to stiffness. In type III, proximal interphalangeal flexion increases only after the metacarpophalangeal joints are passively flexed, as in other intrinsic contractures of the fingers. In these cases, passive extension of the proximal phalanx increases hyperextension of the middle joint and flexion of the distal joint.

SURGICAL TREATMENT

Surgical treatment is discussed separately for each type of deformity. Surgical reconstruction is indicated after maximum spontaneous muscle recovery but before definitive articular stiffness of the fingers occurs. Saving passive mobility of the finger joints is of fundamental importance in correcting Volkmann's contracture.

TYPE I (NORMAL INTRINSIC MUSCLES)

This type is most favorable for correction of deformity and restoration of function, because intrinsic muscles and sensation are normal. Surgical correction is directed to the pathology of the forearm. The surgical procedure the author prefers is excision of retracted muscles, lengthening of tendons, and reconstruction by tendon transfers. This method was developed by Parkes (1951) and Seddon (1956). The author advocates excision-reconstruction of the forearm when the following conditions are present: mild or severe retraction of the long flexor muscles; available muscles for transfers; and moderate or no voluntary contraction in the finger flexor muscles after sufficient time for recovery.

The technique consists of "Z" lengthening of the principal flexor tendons of the wrist (flexor carpi radialis and ulnaris) and the flexor pollicis longus (Fig. 120–3). When this last muscle is completely fibrotic or paralyzed, it is sectioned and activated by transfer of the brachioradialis. The palmaris longus is lengthened or sectioned. The flexor digitorum sublimis tendons are excised completely to the distal forearm. The tendons of the flexor digitorum profundus are excised at their musculotendinous junction to avoid retraction of the distal stump of the tendons into the carpal tunnel and to permit their activation by tendon transfers. If the flexor tendons of the fingers are only divided, partial recurrence of the deformity is possible.

After the deformity is corrected, the lengthened wrist flexor tendons are repaired. The extensor carpi radialis longus is transferred to the distal stumps of the flexor digitorum profundus tendons.

This technique may vary according to different pathologic conditions. In some cases, the wrist flexors are not retracted. In severe pronation contractures it is necessary to excise the distal part of the pronator teres muscle. Occasionally, the flexor superficialis muscles are partially retracted with good voluntary contraction. In this situation, their tendons are divided distally, above the wrist, and transferred to reinforce the reconstructed flexor profundus tendons. One of these tendons can be used to activate the flexor pollicis

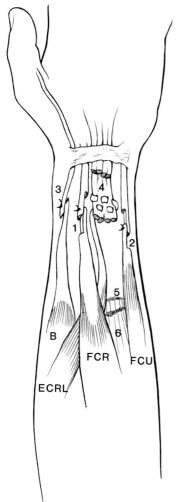

Figure 120–3. Excision-reconstruction procedure to correct contracture of the forearm muscles. The usual technique is as follows: lengthening of the flexor carpi radialis (FCR) and flexor carpi ulnaris (FCU) tendons *(1, 2)*. Tendon transfer of the brachioradialis *(B)* to the flexor pollicis longus tendon *(3)*, and the extensor carpi radialis longus (FCRL) to the distal stumps of the flexor digitorum profundus tendons *(4)*. The fibrotic tendons and muscles of the flexor digitorum superficialis and profundus are excised *(5, 6)*. This is the complete procedure indicated for type I established Volkmann's contracture. In types II and III, other procedures are added to correct intrinsic paralysis or contracture of the hand.

longus tendon. Postoperative re-education is usually simple after excision-reconstruction, because the extensor carpi radialis muscle is a synergist of finger flexion. The brachioradialis is a good candidate for transfer to the flexor pollicis longus.

In general, the author believes that there is little indication for the classic *proximal muscle slide operation,* as it allows for little control of the release and may lead to excessive weakness. It also may affect the blood supply to the flexor muscle bellies. The only indication for this procedure is in the presence of good function of the retracted flexor muscles, but even in this case the author prefers the tendon transfer procedure.

Postoperative re-education, particularly in children, is difficult in the presence of abnormal patterns of finger flexion. One of these patterns is *intrinsic dominance,* which produces metacarpophalangeal flexion and promotes adhesions of the reconstructed long tendons. Another pattern is flexion of the interphalangeal joints by a tenodesic action with the long digital flexors through wrist extension and metacarpophalangeal hyperextension. To break this pattern, a splint is used to maintain the wrist in neutral and the metacarpophalangeal joints in mild flexion, and full excursion of the transferred tendons is encouraged through correct movements.

TYPE II (INTRINSIC MUSCLE PARALYSIS)

For patients with type II deformity, treatment is divided into two surgical stages. During the first stage, the retracted forearm muscles are corrected. As in type I deformity, excision-reconstruction is the operation the author prefers. Postoperatively, finger re-education is encouraged for several months. Splinting is employed to prevent "clawing" of the fingers.

The second stage is reconstruction of the intrinsic muscle paralysis. The method chosen depends on available muscular motors for transfers and the type of deformity at the level of the fingers and thumb.

Clawhand, without significant complications such as definitive joint stiffness or stretched extensor apparatus of the middle joints, is treated like any other intrinsic paralysis by active or passive surgical procedures. The "lasso" operation and metacarpophalangeal capsuloplasty are the author's operations of choice (Zancolli, 1979). If a motor is available—usually the brachioradialis—the indirect "lasso" technique is indicated (Fig. 120–4). The motor is lengthened by adding distal stumps of flexor superficialis or tendon grafts. These are fixed at the A1 pulley of the flexor tendon sheath of each finger. When no motors are available, capsuloplasty with bony fixation is utilized. In clawhand with definitive interphalangeal

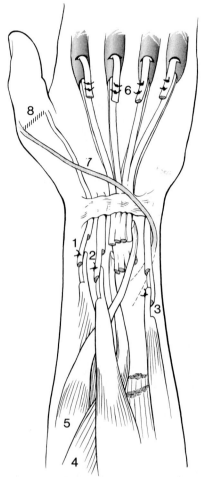

Figure 120–4. Surgical procedure to correct a type II Volkmann's contracture with opposition paralysis and intrinsic clawhand without finger joint stiffness. Lengthening of the flexor pollicis longus (if active) *(1)*, flexor carpi radialis *(2)*, and flexor carpi ulnaris *(3)* tendons. Tendon transfer of extensor carpi radialis to distal stumps of flexor digitorum profundus *(4)*. Tendon transfer of brachioradialis to flexor digitorum superficialis *(5)*. These tendons are fixed to A₁ pulley of each finger *(6)* to correct the clawhand deformity (the "lasso" procedure). Opposition is restored, transferring the extensor indicis propius to the extensor apparatus of the thumb *(7)* and fusing its MP joint *(8)*.

stiffness, joint fusion in functional position is indicated. If the metacarpophalangeal joints are also stiff, a capsulectomy or excision and arthroplasty with flexible implants is performed. This is a very unfavorable situation to correct.

Paralysis of the intrinsic muscles of the thumb is corrected by tendon transfers. The

extensor indicis proprius around the ulnar wrist is an excellent motor to use to regain opposition (Zancolli, 1979). This transfer is combined with fusion of the metacarpophalangeal joint of the thumb. If there is an adduction contracture of the thumb, it must be corrected before or simultaneously with the opponens transfer. The adductor and flexor pollicis brevis muscles are released, and occasionally the dorsal trapeziometacarpal ligament. A thenar web release requiring a major skin flap necessitates a separate procedure.

TYPE III (INTRINSIC MUSCLE CONTRACTURE)

With type III deformity, the contracture of the forearm and the intrinsic muscles must be corrected during the same surgical procedure. It would be impossible to obtain digital function with contracted intrinsic muscles. Forearm excision-reconstruction is performed as previously described.

The technique to release the interosseous muscles depends on the severity of the contracture. In mild cases, the Littler (1977) technique of intrinsic lateral bands and triangular interosseous laminae excision (distal intrinsic release) is indicated; in cases with flexion contracture of the metacarpophalangeal joints, the interosseous tendons are excised at the level of the neck of the metacarpal bones (proximal intrinsic release) (Zancolli, 1979). In severe cases, the retracted interosseous muscles are excised.

Here the thumb is adducted and in antepulsion. All thenar muscles are retracted and must be released. Again, a major skin flap necessitates a separate procedure.

RESTORATION OF SENSATION

To restore sensation, grafts may be needed to bridge defects. With loss of significant length in both median and ulnar nerves, the pedicle nerve graft devised by Strange may be utilized. This two stage procedure uses the ulnar to replace the median nerve in such a way as to preserve neural circulation. This technique can yield enough sensation in the arm and hand to protect them from injury during daily activities.

ISCHEMIC CONTRACTURE OF THE INTRINSIC MUSCLES OF THE HAND

Ischemic contracture of the intrinsic muscles of the hand is the result of ischemia and secondary intrinsic muscular retraction localized at the intrinsic muscles of the intermetacarpal compartments. According to its pathophysiology this muscular contracture could be called intermetacarpal compartment syndrome.

Whether a particular case is in the initial ischemic or the established deformity stage should be clearly determined, because appropriate treatment is different for each stage.

The initial period is characterized by vascular compression and muscular anoxia and necrosis. In the established deformity stage, there is contracture of the interosseous muscles, the deep intrinsic muscles of the thumb, or both.

The usual causes of ischemia of the intrinsic muscles are traumatic, either direct arterial trauma or severe and persisting edema at the intermetacarpal compartments. This section deals with pathophysiology of the intrinsic muscular ischemia and necrosis and the surgical correction of established deformity.

Post-traumatic ischemic contracture of the intrinsic muscles of the hand was initially described by Ricardo Finochietto (1920), director of one of the most important surgical schools of Argentina. He presented his first communication on the subject to the Buenos Aires Surgical Society. This presentation (concerning one clinical case) deals with (1) the ischemic origin of the intrinsic muscular contracture, (2) a clinical description of the deformity, (3) identification of the clinical test to demonstrate the interosseous muscular contracture, and (4) the surgical procedure (excision of the retracted muscles) to correct the deformity. Finochietto named the deformity Volkmann's retraction of the intrinsic muscles of the hand. Before Finochietto's description, the deformity had been variously attributed to a lesion of the spinal cord (Dubrueil, 1870), a traumatic lesion of the ulnar nerve (Polaillon, 1871), hysteria (Charcot, 1887), and irritation of the ulnar nerve (Tinel, 1916).

Twenty-eight years after Finochietto's presentation, Bunnell, Doherty, and Curtis (1948) remarked on the significant incidence of contracture of the intrinsic muscles in the hand of soldiers wounded in World War II. They described the release of the proximal metacarpal attachments of the interosseous muscles to correct the deformity. Littler (1949) described excision of the lateral bands and the fan fibers of the extensor apparatus to correct contracture of the fingers.

More recently, other authors referred to this syndrome (Smith, 1982; Rowland, 1982). Thermal injuries of the upper limb have been considered significant in the necrosis and contracture of the interosseous muscles and hand disfunction (Zancolli, 1961, 1978; Salisbury and McKeel, 1974). Necrosis of the interosseous muscles (second interosseous compartment) after unaccustomed work has been also mentioned as a cause of the intrinsic contracture syndrome (Vogt, 1945; Reid and Travis, 1973).

ETIOLOGY AND CLINICAL EXPERIENCE

The author's clinical experience consists of a series of 63 cases of intrinsic contractures observed over more than 30 years. In this series the ischemia of the intrinsic muscles was caused by crush injuries with or without carpal or metacarpal fractures (7 cases); mild trauma, but with persisting edema of the hand (8 cases); forearm and Colles' fractures, particularly in patients of advanced age (8 cases); thermal injuries involving all or almost all the upper limb (23 cases); tight plaster casts or constricting bandages applied to the upper limb or hand (4 cases); trauma or obstruction of the principal arteries of the upper limb (subclavian, 3 cases; axillary, 1 case; humeral near the elbow, 3 cases); radiotherapy to the hand (for fibrosarcoma, 1 case; for dermatitis, 1 case); collagenous diseases (2 cases); and tetraplegia after spinal cord lesion (2 cases).

This series shows that the main cause of ischemia of the intrinsic muscles of the hand is severe thermal injury of the upper limb and that the principal mechanisms are reduction of the blood supply of the intrinsic muscles and persistent and severe edema of the hand.

In the majority of the author's cases (41),

the deep muscles of the thumb and the interosseous muscles of one or more intermetacarpal spaces were involved. Occasionally (8 cases), the only digit affected was the thumb; these cases were usually of traumatic origin. Interosseous contracture without thumb involvement was present in 14 cases. In one case the only retracted muscle was the abductor digiti quinti (Zancolli, 1978); the little finger was contracted in permanent abduction.

Of all the patients in this series, 81 per cent were males. The youngest was 18 years and the oldest 73 years of age.

PATHOPHYSIOLOGY

The most common cause of intrinsic ischemic contracture is a decrease in blood supply to the hand. According to the author's experience, the blood deficit to the intrinsic muscles can be produced by either of two mechanisms that cause a compartment syndrome:

1. *Direct injury or disease of the principal vessels* of the upper limb. Circulation is reduced but not stopped. Muscle anoxia is the primary factor in the increase in endothelial permeability, which leads to progressive intramuscular edema and further anoxia by arterial and venous compression (Eaton and Green, 1972; Salisbury and McKeel, 1974).

2. *Severe and persistent edema* in the closed and unexpandable intermetacarpal compartments of the hand. The edema, occasionally associated with deep hematomas, causes muscular anoxia, which leads, as in the first mechanism, to secondary intramuscular edema and progressive compression of the small vessels in the intermetacarpal compartments.

Ischemic contracture of the intrinsic muscles of the hand represents an intermetacarpal compartment syndrome. This term can also be applied to a similar condition in the thumb, because the great majority of the cases in the author's experience in which the thumb was also affected involved the muscles located between the first and second metacarpals.

This theory of an ischemia-edema cycle with consequent muscular anoxia and necrosis is favored by the anatomic characteristics of the deep vessels of the hand that perfuse the intermetacarpal muscles.

According to the author's anatomic investigations and clinical observations, there are three closed fascial compartments where the deep intrinsic muscles of the hand and their supplying vessels can be easily compressed by edema and or tense hematomas: the retroadductor space, the first intermetacarpal space, and the second, third, and fourth intermetacarpal spaces (Fig. 120–5).

The *retroadductor space* is limited volarly by the adductor pollicis muscle and its fascia and dorsally by the interosseous fascia that covers the second and first intermetacarpal spaces volarly. The radial part of the deep palmar arch runs through this space.

The *first intermetacarpal space* is limited volarly by the volar interosseous fascia and dorsally by the fascia that connects the extensor tendons of the fingers with the extensors of the thumb (intertendineal fascia of Anson). This space is occupied by the first dorsal interosseous muscle.

The *second, third, and fourth intermetacarpal spaces* are limited volarly by the volar interosseus fascia and dorsally by the dorsal interosseous fascia. The vessels contained in these compartments are branches of the deep palmar arch of the hand.

Study of the *deep palmar arch of the hand and its branches* gives the surgeon a better understanding of the mechanism of intrinsic muscular ischemia previously described. The author's conclusions as to the anatomy of the deep palmar arch and its branches coincide with those of Fracassi (1945).

The radial artery, which basically forms the deep palmar arch, penetrates into the retroadductor space at the angle formed between the two first metacarpals and through a tendinous ring formed by the two heads of the first dorsal interosseous muscle (Fig. 120–6). From this point the artery runs across the bases of the second and third metacarpals and emerges from the retroadductor space through another tendinous ring formed by the transverse and oblique fascicles of the adductor pollicis muscle.

At the retroadductor space, the deep palmar arch (Delorme's oblique part) (Zancolli, 1978) runs volarly to the volar interosseous fascia and yields two groups of branches: the proximal or recurrent branches of the carpus, and the distal or metacarpal branches. The proximal or recurrent branches might be connected with the anterior interosseous artery of the forearm. This anastomosis may compensate the circulation of the hand in cases

Figure 120–5. *A,* Transverse section of the hand at the level of the deep palmar arch. We observe: the midpalmar fascia (MPF), the thenar septum (TS), the hypothenar septum (HS), the volar interosseous fascia (VIF), the dorsal interosseous fascia (DIF), the adductor pollicis muscle (AP), and the deep palmar arch *(DPA)* that runs superficial to the volar interosseous fascia. Three closed fascial compartments are shown: the first intermetacarpal compartment *(1);* the retroadductor compartment *(2)* and the second, third, and fourth intermetacarpal compartments *(3).* Arrows show the dorsal approaches to open the intermetacarpal and retroadductor compartments *(4)* and the palmar approach to evacuate hematomas deep to the flexor tendons of the fingers. This drawing also shows the descending vessels of the deep palmar arch that perfuse the interosseous muscles (volar and dorsal metacarpal arteries) and perforate the deep interosseous fascia of the hand. *B,* Transverse section of the hand at the level of the distal palmar crease. We observe: the pretendinous bands (PB) of the midpalmar fascia; the lumbrical tunnels (LT), and the volar (VIF) and dorsal (DIF) interosseous fascia of the hand. Between these fascia and the metacarpal bones are the intermetacarpal spaces.

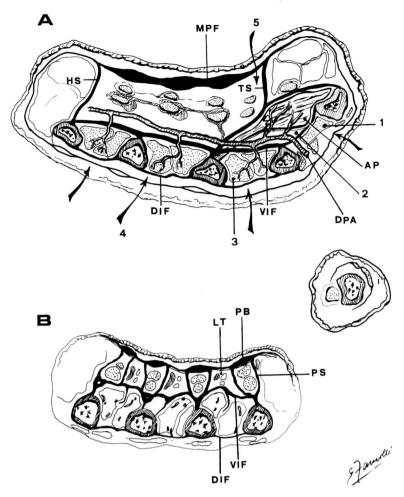

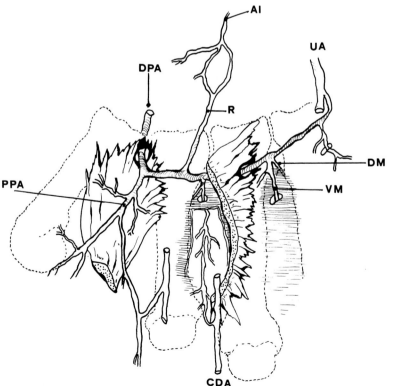

Figure 120–6. Drawing taken from a cadaveric dissection of the deep palmar arch, showing the standard pattern. The deep palmar arch (DPA) runs through the aponeurotic rings formed by the first dorsal interosseous and adductor pollicis muscles. In this dissection, the deep palmar arch gives the following branches: princeps pollicis artery (PPA); recurrent artery (RA), which may anastomose with the anterior interosseous artery (AI), and the branches that perfuse the medial muscles of the thumb and the interosseous muscles of the second intermetacarpal compartment. The metacarpal arteries end at the interosseous muscles and the metacarpal bones. At the distal part of the palm, anastomoses with the common digital arteries (CDA) are seen. The figure shows the volar (VM) and dorsal (DM) metacarpal arteries perforating the volar interosseous fascia.

with combined lesions of the radial and ulnar arteries. The distal or metacarpal arteries may be dorsal or volar.

The volar metacarpal arteries divide into (1) the princeps pollicis artery or first volar metacarpal artery, (2) the volar artery of the radial aspect of the index finger, which may arise in common with the princeps pollicis artery, and (3) the second volar metacarpal artery. The volar metacarpal arteries usually anastomose with the descending branches of the superficial palmar arch and end at the level of the interosseous, adductor pollicis, and flexor pollicis brevis muscles. Other branches end at the level of the metacarpophalangeal joints of the fingers (volar plate and metacarpal metaphysis and epiphysis).

The dorsal metacarpal arteries (called perforating arteries by the classical anatomists) penetrate to the intermetacarpal compartments at their proximal ends after perforating the volar interosseous fascia. Arriving at the dorsal aspect of the hand these vessels perfuse the dorsal interosseous muscles and end at the level of the metacarpal metaphysis (metaphyseal arteries). The second dorsal metacarpal artery may anastomose with the palmar arteries. According to this description, which coincides with that of other investigators (cited by Eaton and Green, 1972), the dorsal metacarpal arteries generally originate from the deep palmar arch and not from the dorsal carpal arch, as described by many of the classical anatomists (cited by Zancolli, 1978).

Ulnar to the retroadductor space, the deep palmar arch gives off the third and fourth volar metacarpal arteries and then connects with the deep volar branch of the ulnar artery, which passes through the hiatus formed by the origins of the abductor and short flexor muscles of the little finger.

On the basis of the previous description, the arteries that supply the intermetacarpal muscles (flexor pollicis brevis, adductor pollicis, and interossei) run in closed fascial compartments (retroadductor and intermetacarpals) and end at the level of the intrinsic muscles and distal end of the metacarpal bones. These two anatomic characteristics permit easy compression of the small vessels when edema or hematomas infiltrate these closed compartments.

This pathophysiology indicates the importance of preventing severe and persisting edema of the hand. Early fasciotomy of the different compartments of the hand is indicated when the surgeon believes that the intrinsic muscles are ischemic.

It is interesting to point out that the lumbrical muscles are not affected by the mechanism of compartment syndrome, because these muscles are not included in the closed fascial spaces. The lumbrical muscles may produce intrinsic-plus deformities by mechanisms other than ischemia.

CLASSIFICATION OF ESTABLISHED INTRINSIC-PLUS DEFORMITY

Deformities may be divided into three groups according to the muscles affected.

Group I: All the interosseous muscles and the medial thenar muscles (flexor pollicis brevis, adductor pollicis, and first dorsal interosseous) are affected. In severe cases (classified as group IV in the author's series) the lateral thenar muscles can be also involved. This group also contains the cases in which the intrinsic contracture is associated with a Volkmann's ischemic contracture of the forearm (2 cases in the author's series). The intrinsic muscles most commonly affected are those perfused by the branches of the volar palmar arch given off at the level of the retroadductor space (medial thenar muscles and interosseous muscles of the index finger and radial aspect of the middle finger.

Group II: The medial thenar muscles or the interosseous muscles are affected, which means that the deformity localizes independently at the thumb or at the fingers.

Group III: Muscular ischemia is localized atypically. Thus, in one of the author's group III cases, the contracture was localized at the abductor digiti quinti, and in another it affected the intrinsic muscles of the middle and ring fingers.

Deformity of the Fingers

The author divides deformities into three types according to the severity of the contracture of the interosseous muscles (Zancolli, 1978) (Table 120–1).

TYPE 1 FINGER DEFORMITY

These cases are characterized by a mild muscular contracture that may be over-

Table 120–1. Classification of Ischemic Contractures of the Intrinsic Muscles of the Hand

Location	Type	Features
Fingers (contracture of the interosseous muscles)	1	Complete finger extension and flexion with inability to place the fingers in "hook" position Delayed flexion of the proximal phalanx Positive intrinsic-plus test
	2	Intrinsic-plus deformity with metacarpophalangeal flexion contracture
	3	Intrinsic-plus deformity with articular stiffness
Thumb	1	Adduction contracture (contracture of the medial thenar muscles)
	2	Adduction and palmar abduction contracture (contracture of medial and lateral thenar muscles)

looked. When intrinsic muscle contracture is mild, the patient can open and close the fingers normally.

Diagnosis of type 1 intrinsic muscle contracture is confirmed by three clinical signs:

1. *Inability to place the affected fingers in a "hook" position.* Normally, to place the fingers in the "hook" position (metacarpophalangeal extension and interphalangeal flexion) it is necessary that the intrinsic tendons—interosseous and lumbricals—shift distally approximately 6 mm. This displacement allows distal shifting of the extensor apparatus, which in turn permits interphalangeal flexion without simultaneous flexion of the metacarpophalangeal joint (Fig. 120–7A). When the

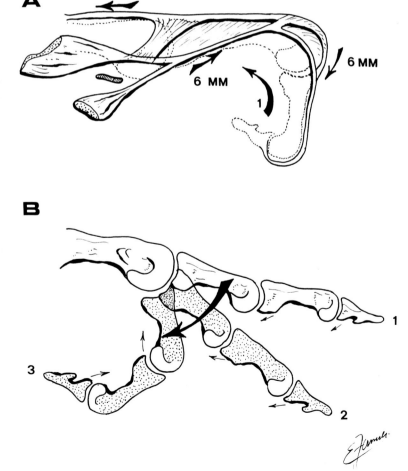

Figure 120–7. *A,* Normally during "hook" flexion the intrinsic tendons glide distally (approximately 6 mm) to allow distal gliding of the extensor apparatus, permitting flexion of the interphalangeal joints. In ischemic intrinsic contracture, "hook" flexion cannot be obtained, because distal gliding of the intrinsic tendons is blocked. *B,* In intrinsic contracture, finger flexion begins by flexion of the metacarpophalangeal joint *(1 to 2).* Flexion of the interphalangeal joints begins after the intrinsic tendons slacken by flexion of the metacarpophalangeal joint *(2 to 3).* The greater the intrinsic contracture, the greater the delay to initiate interphalangeal flexion. In very severe intrinsic contracture, interphalangeal flexion is not produced even after complete metacarpophalangeal flexion.

interosseous muscles are contracted, their tendons cannot be distally displaced and thus it is impossible to flex the interphalangeal joints while the metacarpophalangeal joint remains in complete extension. Owing to this pathophysiology, complete interphalangeal flexion is obtained only if the metacarpophalangeal joint is in flexion. The greater the interosseous contracture, the greater the flexion position of the metacarpophalangeal joint to permit interphalangeal flexion.

2. *Delayed flexion of the proximal phalanx during complete finger flexion (intrinsic-plus type finger flexion)*. This type also depends on the lack of initial distal displacement of the intrinsic tendons when complete finger flexion is attempted. Because of the intrinsic muscle contracture, the patient must first flex the proximal phalanx to permit the initiation of middle and distal joint flexion. This delay of interphalangeal flexion during complete finger flexion produces a rolling rather than simultaneous type of finger flexion (Fig. 120–7B). This rolling flexion differs from that of intrinsic paralysis of the hand. In intrinsic paralysis, finger flexion is initiated at the interphalangeal joints; in intrinsic contracture, finger flexion is initiated at the metacarpophalangeal joint.

3. *A positive intrinsic-plus test*. The intrinsic-plus test was first described by Ricardo Finochietto. The intrinsic-plus test is positive if passive flexion of the interphalangeal joints is blocked when the metacarpophalangeal joint is kept in extension. Interphalangeal flexion is possible when the metacarpophalangeal joint is permitted to flex (Fig. 120–8). The intrinsic-plus test can be masked when intrinsic contracture is combined with interphalangeal stiffness. Under these conditions, the position of the metacarpophalangeal joint will not influence interphalangeal motion. It is important that investigation of the intrinsic-plus test be routine in all clinical examinations, because only through this test can mild interosseous muscle contractures be demonstrated.

TYPE 2 FINGER DEFORMITY

In this type of interosseous contracture, the muscular retraction is greater than in type 1, and therefore, the metacarpophalangeal joint is contracted in flexion. This joint contracture is greater as contracture of the interosseous muscles increases. The interphalangeal joints are in a position of extension. Occasionally the proximal interphalangeal joint is in recurvatum.

The principal functional deficit in type 2 deformity is inability to completely open the hand. Flexion of the interphalangeal joints is more delayed than in type 1 when complete finger flexion is attempted. In these conditions there is a tendency for the proximal interphalangeal joint to be contracted owing to retraction of the collateral ligaments. The intrinsic-plus test is positive.

TYPE 3 FINGER DEFORMITY

This type of intrinsic contracture is complicated by joint stiffness. The principal complication at the metacarpophalangeal joint is retraction of the volar plate and glenoid bundle of the collateral ligaments. The usual complication at the proximal interphalangeal joint depends on the retraction of the collateral ligaments. Occasionally, the affected fingers may show a swan-neck deformity. In this type of deformity, hand function is severely affected. The thumb is usually included in the deformity (Fig. 120–9A).

Deformity of the Thumb

The thumb may have two types of deformities based upon which intrinsic muscles are affected (Table 120–1). The more common deformity depends on the ischemic contracture of the medial thenar muscles (flexor pollicis brevis, adductor pollicis, and first dorsal interosseous muscles). This type of deformity produces a typical adduction contracture of the first metacarpal. The thumb contracts against the radial aspect of the index finger. The first web can be contracted, and also the first intermetacarpal ligament. Passive flexion of the interphalangeal joint is limited when the metacarpophalangeal joint is kept in extension (positive intrinsic-plus test) (Fig. 120–9A).

When the lateral thenar muscles are also affected by ischemia (cases with severe deficit of perfusion) the thumb contracts in adduction and palmar abduction. In these cases the thumb may block flexion of the index and middle fingers (Fig. 120–9B). In these cases the metacarpophalangeal joint is contracted in hyperflexion (intrinsic-plus deformity of the thumb).

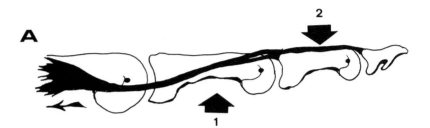

Figure 120–8. Intrinsic-plus test. This test has two parts. *A,* The first part consists of producing passive interphalangeal flexion *(1)* while the metacarpophalangeal joint is held in complete extension *(2). B,* The second part consists of producing passive flexion of all finger joints *(1, 2).* The test is positive when interphalangeal flexion is reduced or totally annulled in the first part and possible in the second part of the maneuver (Finochietto's intrinsic-plus test positive). *C,* In ischemic intrinsic contracture, passive flexion of the interphalangeal joint *(1)* prevents passive extension of the metacarpophalangeal joint *(2).* The angle of flexion contracture of the metacarpophalangeal joint *(3)* increases or decreases according to the severity of the intrinsic contracture.

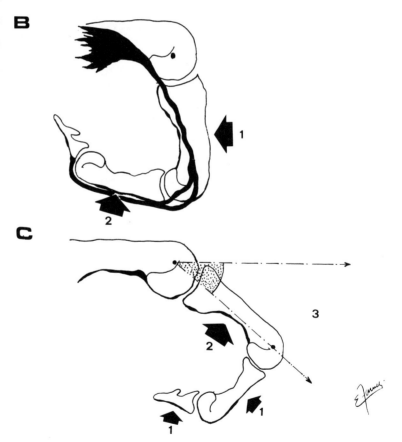

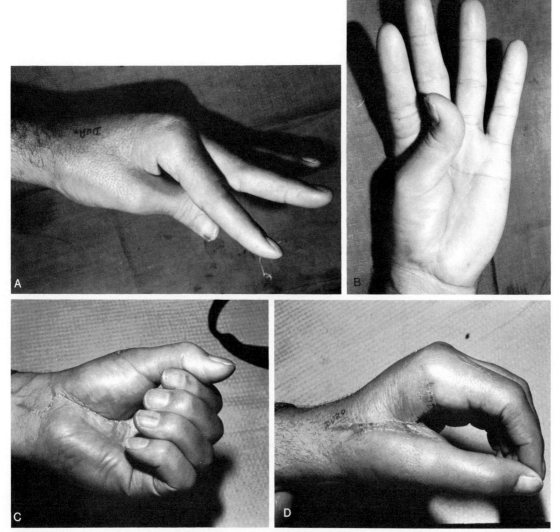

Figure 120–9. *A* and *B,* Severe ischemic intrinsic contracture of all the digits consecutive to thrombosis of the axillary artery. Type 3 interosseous contracture of the fingers and adduction and palmar abduction contracture of the thumb. The surgical program was a complete release of the medial thenar muscles and the interosseus muscles through a transverse palmar approach. A satisfactory result was obtained for grasping *(C)* and pinching *(D).*

SURGICAL CORRECTION

The surgical procedures of preference to correct the established deformity depend on the severity of the muscular retraction and deformity and the localization of the pathology.

Correction of Finger Deformity

The choice of surgical procedure is determined by the severity of the muscular retrac-

tion and the possibility of associated complications.

TYPE 1 FINGER DEFORMITY

This type of deformity is corrected by excision of the intrinsic lateral band and the fan fibers of the dorsal aponeurosis on both sides of each finger affected (Littler technique). This procedure, which represents a distal intrinsic muscle release, has advantages over the isolated excision of the lateral bands because it eliminates the more medial fibers of division of the interosseous tendon, which reach the long extensor tendons in their course over the proximal phalanx. This procedure is performed through a unique longitudinal incision over the proximal dorsal half of the proximal phalanx of each finger (Fig. 120–10A). Damage to metacarpophalangeal dorsal hood fibers must be avoided in order to prevent dislocation of the long digital extensor tendon over the metacarpal head.

Once the intrinsic muscle release has been performed, the interphalangeal joints are flexed passively, very gently, while the proximal phalanx is held extended. Difficulty in passive flexion of the middle joint usually means that the collateral ligaments are retracted. If, under these circumstances, the surgeon were to force interphalangeal passive flexion, an irreversible stretching of the extensor apparatus would be produced, leaving a definitely flexed, painful, semirigid, and swollen middle joint. Other causes of resistance to passive flexion of the middle joint may depend on adherences or retraction of the extensor apparatus over the middle joint.

This technique cannot correct flexion contracture of the proximal joint and therefore must not be used in type 2 or 3 deformity.

During the postoperative period, the hand is immobilized by means of a sufficiently

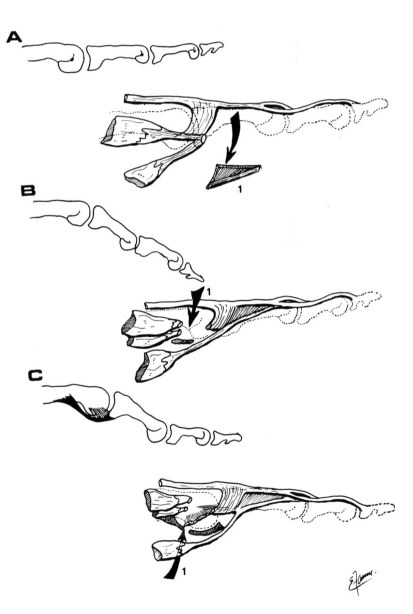

Figure 120–10. Surgical procedures to correct the different types of ischemic interosseous contracture. *A,* Type 1. Release is obtained by excision of the lateral band and fan fibers on both sides of the extensor apparatus *(1). B,* Type 2. Release is performed through separated longitudinal dorsal approaches at the level of the metacarpal necks *(1).* Interosseous tendons are excised. *C,* Type 3. Through a transverse palmar approach (1) release is obtained by excision of the interosseous tendons and release of the volar plate and the glenoid part of the collateral ligament. Capsulotomy of the interphalangeal joint may also be performed.

padded circular plaster cast that keeps the wrist and metacarpophalangeal joints in neutral extension. The interphalangeal joints are left free to allow active flexion-extension exercises during the immediate postoperative period. Active and passive interphalangeal joint flexion must be done to avoid relapse of the deformity. The initial plaster immobilization cast is removed in 10 days, and re-education is started with complete digital movements, with the free hand carrying out the intrinsic-plus maneuver repeatedly to distend the intrinsic tendons. The dynamic splint conceived by Bunnell—metacarpophalangeal extension splint or "reverse knuckle-bender splint"—is very useful during the re-education period, which must continue for several weeks or even months owing to the great and particular tendency of this deformity to recur.

Postoperative re-education is considered to be complete when the patient affirms that on waking up in the morning (1) the hand is the same as it was when going to bed at night or (2) the hand rapidly acquires complete digital movements. The ability to place the operated fingers into "hook" position is evidence of excellent correction.

TYPE 2 FINGER DEFORMITY

Intrinsic muscle contracture is corrected by release of the muscles proximal to the metacarpophalangeal joint (proximal intrinsic muscle release). The interosseous tendons are resected at their musculotendinous junction, at the level of the deep transverse intermetacarpal ligament. Finochietto (1920) employed a similar technique for the case he had the opportunity to treat. Bunnell (1944) insisted on the need to release the intrinsic muscles proximal to metacarpophalangeal joint level when this joint is contracted in flexion.

Proximal intrinsic muscle release is indicated not only to restore the normal rhythm of digital flexion but also to allow complete extension of the proximal phalanx. Correction of flexion contracture of the proximal phalanx is important to allow opening of the hand for grasping functions and also to avoid overpull of the long extensor tendon, which favors recurvatum of the proximal interphalangeal joint.

The procedure is performed through longitudinal incisions on the dorsum of the hand,

at the distal ends of the intermetacarpal spaces. Excision of the interosseous tendons must be complete, with the precaution taken to eliminate all the fibers of the palmar interosseous muscles, which may remain hidden at the depth of the wound (Fig. 120–10B).

If after excision of the interosseous tendons the metacarpophalangeal joint does not passively extend completely, the volar plate is retracted, indicating a type 3 deformity. A palmar approach is needed to obtain correction of the flexion contracture of the joint.

In several series of patients, the author had to combine proximal and distal intrinsic muscle releases. This combination was indicated in cases of interosseous contracture and simultaneous adhesions of the interosseous tendons in their course at metacarpophalangeal level.

TYPE 3 FINGER DEFORMITY

This deformity is a very difficult surgical situation, and the possibility of restoring acceptable digital function varies according to the severity of the case. The most favorable situations are those in which the metacarpophalangeal joints are stiff but the interphalangeal joints are free of periarticular complications.

In type 3 intrinsic muscle contractures, proximal interosseous muscle releases and palmar metacarpophalangeal joint releases should be performed in the same operation through a unique transverse approach at the level of the distal palmar crease (Fig. 120–10C). After dissection of the cutaneous flaps and retraction of the lumbrical tendons and vessels and nerves of the palm, each intermetacarpal compartment is approached. The deep aponeurosis of the palm is opened proximal to the deep transverse intermetacarpal ligament, and the interosseous tendons are exposed and excised. Next, the tunnel of the long digital flexor tendons is opened longitudinally and the tendons are retracted. Through this approach, the metacarpophalangeal volar plate at its middle part and the glenoid fascicle of the collateral ligaments are transversely divided, allowing passive extension of the metacarpophalangeal joint.

Should the middle joint be stiff in extension, it must be either mobilized by excision of its collateral ligaments or, in irreversible cases, fused in the position of function.

In cases with marked circulatory deficit of

the hand, the surgical procedure must be performed with great precaution and always within the limits of the assurance of tissue perfusion.

Correction of Thumb Deformity

The thumb deformity can be corrected in the same procedure in cases of mild contracture in adduction if reconstruction of the first web can be obtained by Z-plasty or local cutaneous flaps. If such reconstruction would demand a distant pedicle flap (abdomen, thorax, or opposite arm), thumb deformity correction must be performed before finger deformity correction. If the thumb and the finger deformities were corrected in the same surgical procedure, immediate postoperative re-education of the fingers will be very difficult because the hand would generally be fixed to a distant pedicle cutaneous flap.

In adduction contractures, the retracted intermetacarpal aponeurosis and the adductor and flexor pollicis brevis muscles must be released. The cutaneous incision in these cases depends on the severity of the skin retraction of the first web. When skin retraction is slight, a Z-plasty is indicated, the branches of which are extended to the dorsal and palmar sides of the first metacarpal compartment. It is important to note that the release of the flexor pollicis brevis muscle is carried out more easily using the palmar branch approach.

When the skin retraction cannot be corrected with a simple Z-plasty, a rotation flap from the dorsum of the hand is indicated. Occasionally it may be necessary also to divide the first intermetacarpal and the dorsal ligaments of the trapeziometacarpal joint or to perform an osteotomy at the base of the first metacarpal to obtain the desired correction.

When cutaneous retraction is extreme, the thumb cleft is released by a dorsal and palmar longitudinal incision that opens the entire intermetacarpal space. A distant pedicle flap may be required to fill the cutaneous defect.

In contractures in adduction and palmar abduction in which all thenar muscles are contracted, the criterion for choice of cutaneous incision is similar to the one used for adduction contractures. The lateral thenar muscles must be included in the release.

REFERENCES

Bonutti, P. M., and Bell, G. R.: Compartment syndrome of the foot. J. Bone Joint Surg., 61B:294, 1979.

Bunnell, S.: Surgery of the Hand. Philadelphia, J. B. Lippincott Company, 1944.

Bunnell S., Doherty, E. W., and Curtis, R. M.: Ischemic contracture, local, in the hand. Plast. Reconstr. Surg., 3:424, 1948.

Charcot, J. M.: Oeuvres completes de J. M. Charcot. Leçons sur les malades du système nerveux. Paris, 1887.

Coleman, S., and Anson, B. J.: Arterial patterns in the hand. Based upon a study of 650 specimens. Surg. Gynecol. Obstet., 113:409, 1961.

Dubrueil, M. A.: D'une espèce connue de contracture siegeant sur les interosseux palmaires. Gazette des Hopitaux, No. 9, p. 33, 1870.

Eaton, R. G., and Green, W. T.: Epimysiotomy and fasciotomy in the treatment of Volkmann's ischemic contracture. Orthop. Clin. North Am., 3:175, 1972.

Finochietto, R.: Retraccion de Volkmann de los musculos intrinsecos de la mano. Bol. Trab. Soc. Cirug. Buenos Aires, 4:31, 1920.

Fracassi, H.: Arterias interoseas de la mano. Prens. Med. Argentina, 1:27, 1945.

Griffiths, D. L.: Volkmann's ischaemic contracture. Br. J. Surg., 28:239, 1940.

Hargens, A. R., Akeson, W. H., Mubarak, S. J., Owen, C. A., Evans, K. L., et al.: Fluid balance with the canine anterolateral compartment and its relationship to compartment syndromes. J. Bone Joint Surg., 60A:499, 1978.

Hargens, A. R., Schmidt, D. A., Evans, K. L., Gonsalves, M. R., Cologne, J. B., et al.: Quantitation of skeletal-muscle necrosis in a model compartment syndrome. J. Bone Joint Surg. 63A:631, 1981.

Harris, C., Jr., and Riordan, D.: Intrinsic contracture in the hand and its surgical treatment. J. Bone Joint Surg., 36A:10, 1954.

Holden, C. E. A.: Compartmental syndromes following trauma. Clin. Orthop., 113:95, 1975.

Holden, C. E. A.: The pathology and prevention of Volkmann's ischaemic contracture. J. Bone Joint Surg., 61B:296, 1979.

Leriche, R.: A propos du mécanisme et de la thérapeutic de la maladie de Volkmann. J. Internat. Chirurg. 3:81, 1938.

Littler, J. W.: Tendon transfers and arthrodeses in combined median and ulnar nerve paralysis. J. Bone Joint Surg., 31A:225, 1949.

Littler, W.: The hand and wrist. In Howorth, M. B. (Ed.): A Textbook of Orthopaedics. Philadelphia, W. B. Saunders Company, 1952.

Littler, W.: The hand and upper extremity. In Converse, J. M. (Ed.) Reconstructive Plastic Surgery. 2nd ed. Philadelphia, W. B. Saunders Company, 1977.

Louis, D. S.: Diagnosis of compartment syndromes of the forearm. J. Hand Surg., 5:296, 1980.

Matsen, F. A.: Compartment syndrome: A unified concept. Clin. Orthop. 113:8, 1975.

Matsen, F. A., Mayo, K. A., Krugmire, R. B., Sheridan, G. W., and Kraft, G. H.: A model compartment syndrome in man with particular reference to the quantification of nerve function. J. Bone Joint Surg., 59A:648, 1977.

Matsen, F. A., Winquist, R. A., and Krugmire, R. B.:

Diagnosis and management of compartment syndromes. J. Bone Joint Surg., *62A*:286, 1980.

Merle D'Aubigne, R., and Tran-Ngoc-Ninh: Syndrome de Volkmann invétéré. Rev. Orthop., *41*:32, 1955.

Mubarak, S. J., Carroll, N. C.: Volkmann's contracture in children: Aetiology and prevention. J. Bone Joint Surg. *61B*:285–293, 1979.

Mubarak, S. J., Hargens, A. R., Owen, C. A., Garetto, L. P., and Akeson, W. H.: The wick catheter technique for measurement of intramuscular pressure. J. Bone Joint Surg., *58A*:1016, 1976.

Mubarak, S. J., Owen, C. A., Hargens, A. R., Garetto, L. P., and Akeson, W. H.: Acute compartment syndromes: Diagnosis and treatment with the aid of the wick catheter. J. Bone Joint Surg., *60A*:1091, 1978.

Murphy, J. B.: Myositis. J.A.M.A., *63*:1249, 1914.

Parkes, A.: The treatment of established Volkmann's contracture by tendon transplantation. J. Bone Joint Surg., *33B*:359, 1951.

Pedemonte, P. V.: Cirugía Plastica de la Mano. Sus deformidades y su tratamiento. Montevideo, Ed. Instituto Traumatológico, 1948.

Polaillon, R.: La contracture des muscles intrinsecos de la main. *In* Dechambre, A. (Directeur): Dictionnaire Encyclopédique des Sciences Médicales. Paris, 1871.

Reid, R. L., and Travis, A. T.: Acute necrosis of the second interosseous compartment of the hand. J. Bone Joint Surg., *55A*, 1973.

Rich, N. M.: Complications of treatment of peripheral vascular injuries of the extremities. *In* Epps, C. H. (Ed.): Complications in Orthopaedic Surgery, Vol. 2. Philadelphia, J. B. Lippincott Company, 1978.

Rowland, S. A.: Fasciotomy. *In* Green, D. P. (Ed.): Operative Hand Surgery. New York, Churchill Livingstone, 1982.

Salisbury, R. E., and McKeel, W.: Ischemic necrosis of the intrinsic muscles of the hand after thermal injuries. J. Bone Joint Surg., *56A*:1974.

Sarokhan, A. J., and Eaton, R. G.: Volkmann's ischemia. J. Hand Surg., *8*:806, 1983.

Seddon, H. J.: Volkmann's contracture: Treatment by excision of the infarct. J. Bone Joint Surg., *38B*:152, 1956.

Sheridan, G. W., and Matsen, F. A.: Fasciotomy in the treatment of the acute compartment syndrome. J. Bone Joint Surg., *58A*:112, 1956.

Smith, R.: Intrinsic contracture. *In* Green, D. P. (Ed.): Operative Hand Surgery. New York, Churchill Livingstone, 1982.

Tinel, J.: Les Blessures de Nerfs. Paris, Ed Masson et Cie, 1916.

Vogt, P. R.: Ischemic muscular necrosis following marching (quoted by Reid and Travis, 1982).

Volkmann, R. von: Die ischemischen Muskellahmungen und Kontrakturen. Centralb. Chirurg., *8*:801, 1881.

Whitesides, T. E., Hanley, T. C., Morimoto, K., and Harada, H.: Tissue pressure measurements as a determinant for the need of fasciotomy. Clin. Orthop., *113*:43, 1975.

Zancolli, E. A.: Clasificacion de las contracturas de Volkmann. Prensa Med. Argentina, *46*:1344, 1959.

Zancolli, E. A.: Cirugia de las secuelas por quemaduras de la mano. Medicina Panamericana. Numero Especial, p. 139, Buenos Aires, 1961.

Zancolli, E. A.: Tendon transfers after ischemic contracture of the forearm. Classification in relation to intrinsic muscle disorders. Am. J. Surg., *109*:356, 1965.

Zancolli, E. A.: Structural and Dynamic Bases of Hand Surgery. 2nd Ed. Philadelphia, J. B. Lippincott Company, 1979.

Robert M. McFarlane

Dupuytren's Disease

Dupuytren's disease is one of the fibroproliferative conditions of unclear etiology and pathogenesis. It is common and has been known to surgeons and treated by them for at least 200 years. Plater (1614) is credited with the first account of the condition, and Cline (1808) and Sir Astley Cooper (both cited by Windsor, 1834) described the contracture of the fingers and suggested treatment by subcutaneous fasciotomy. However, it remained for Dupuytren in 1831 to describe the anatomy, to establish clearly that the disease was located in the palmar fascia, and to suggest treatment by open fasciotomy. In a biography, Barsky (1984) defends the continued association of Dupuytren's name with this condition by stating: "Even if Cline did make the correct observation, the old and perhaps futile question still remains as to where credit is to go: to invention or dissemination. In this case there can be no doubt that the term 'Dupuytren's contracture' is deservedly applied for Dupuytren was first to present a meticulous diagnosis of the condition, to differentiate it with precision from all other types of finger contraction, to observe similar changes in the sole of the foot, to devise a closely reasoned and effective operation, and to make diagnosis and treatment available to the entire surgical world."

Over the years surgeons have failed to understand the disease process. The discovery of the myofibroblast in nodules of Dupuytren's disease by Gabbiani and Majno (1972) has stimulated others to study the more fundamental aspects of this disease. The collagen and supporting matrix produced by the cells has received considerable attention. Because of this interest by many basic disciplines, the etiology and pathogenesis will surely be clarified and treatment will change accordingly.

EPIDEMIOLOGY

Dupuytren's disease has been called a disease of the Celtic race. It is very common in northern Europe and also in countries inhabited by immigrants from northern Europe, notably Australia and the east coast of North

America. The incidence varies, depending on the age and sex of the population (Early, 1962). Mikkelsen (1972) reported an incidence in a Norwegian community of 5.6 per cent of the population over 16 years of age. Hueston (1982a) reported an incidence in Australia of 26 per cent of males and 20 per cent of females over the age of 60. It is said to be rare in the black and Oriental races, but Egawa (1983) examined 3244 Japanese patients between the ages of 20 and 90 and found that 3 per cent of males and 1 per cent of females were affected. He also found an incidence of 11 per cent of males and 4 per cent of females over the age of 60. Dupuytren's disease is not rare in the Oriental but perhaps is uncommon (Chow, Luk, and Kung, 1984). The real difference is that the disease is mainly confined to the palm in the Oriental and does not often cause joint contracture, so that an affected individual is unlikely to be seen by a surgeon.

Mennen and Gräbe (1979) have established that the disease occurs in the black patient who does not possess Caucasian genes. The disease is much less common in southern than in northern Europe. It has been reported in the East Indian, American Indian, and Mexican but must be very uncommon.

Table 121–1 contains some demographic data obtained in a survey (McFarlane, 1985). The preponderance of males in a ratio of 82:16 is consistent in all countries and races, and the female incidence rises with increasing age. The incidence of a positive family history of 27 per cent indicates a strong genetic influence, considering that the history was taken by a surgeon and not a geneticist. Of interest, the incidence in the Japanese patients was only 6 per cent. Both hands are usually involved and this suggests that unilateral disease may be a variant.

ETIOLOGY

Ling (1963) concluded that Dupuytren's disease is genetic in origin and likely due to a single dominant gene. He interviewed 50 patients with Dupuytren's disease, of whom 16 per cent admitted to a positive family history. However, on further investigation 68 per cent of these patients were found to have affected relatives. Ling found, however, that the expression of the gene was less complete in females, and concluded that Dupuytren's is not an etiologically uniform disease. Nyberg and associates (1982) studied Peyronie's disease in three families and concluded that it was autosomal dominant. In these families, 78 per cent of affected individuals had Dupuytren's disease. Seven of eight persons had HLA-B7, which suggests an immunologic influence. Nyberg and associates concluded that Dupuytren's disease and Peyronie's disease are not homogeneous conditions but that contracture of the fingers, penis, plantar fascia, and knuckle pads are pleiotropic effects of the same gene.

Clinically there are phenotypes that are

Table 121–1. Survey of 1227 Patients with Dupuytren's Disease Seen by 108 Surgeons in 12 Countries

Family origin of patients			Sex:	
Northern European:	82%		Male:	82%
Southern European:	2%		Female:	16%
Black African:	1%		Hand dominance	
Japanese and Chinese:	1%		Right:	94%
Polynesian:	0%		Left:	5%
American Indian:	0.2%		Hand involved	
Uncertain:	12%		Right:	23%
			Left:	12%
			Both:	65%
Age at Onset of Disease:	49 yrs (males 49 yrs, females 54 yrs)		Occupation	
Age at Operation:	58 yrs (males 58 yrs, females 62 yrs)		Manual:	45%
Family history of Dupuytren's disease:	27%		Non-manual:	41%
Associated diseases			Other Areas Involved	
None:	62%		Knuckle Pads:	22%
Diabetes:	8%		Feet:	10%
Epilepsy:	2%		Penis:	2%
Alcoholism:	10%			
Trauma:	13%			

different from the common form of Dupuytren's disease, which is bilateral and seen in the male at about 50 years of age. In the female, the disease is usually seen later and is less severe (Matthews, 1979). With unilateral disease the incidence of a positive family history, of associated diseases, and of other areas involved are all less, and also the hand is less severely involved. The disease seen in the diabetic patient is usually confined to the palm, similar to that seen in the Oriental. The thickening of the palmar fascia after injury and immobilization is clinically similar to that seen in Dupuytren's disease and yet is often reversible. Ledderhose (1897) described a similar condition in the plantar fascia.

Hueston (1982a) reported a particularly aggressive form of Dupuytren's disease that appears at an early age (third or fourth decade), is bilateral and extensive, causes severe contracture, is associated with a strong family history, and shows a tendency to recur. He refers to these patients as having a strong Dupuytren's diathesis.

Chromosomes

Bowser-Riley and associates (1975) cultured the fibroblasts of Dupuytren's tissue and found mosaicism in four of six patients. They felt that this was unlikely to indicate a mechanism of inheritance, but rather that the changes were similar to those seen in experimentally induced tumors; thus, chromosomally abnormal cell lines may arise in the development of Dupuytren's disease. In a similar study, Sergovich, Botz, and Mc-Farlane (1983) found mosaicism in nine of 31 fibroblast cultures from the tissue of Dupuytren's disease. Of interest, a trisomy 8 abnormality occurred in five of nine positive cultures. These chromosomal changes are similar to those seen in malignant growth disorders, and suggest a fundamental error in growth regulation and cell division.

Associated Diseases

Dupuytren's disease is seen frequently in association with other diseases. This suggests a common pathological process.

Knuckle Pads, Peyronie's Disease, and Plantar Fibromatosis. These conditions have a similar histologic appearance and are frequently seen with contracture of the hand. For this reason, Hueston (1982b) suggested the term Dupuytren's disease rather than Dupuytren's contracture to indicate a widespread disease process. Knuckle pads are most frequently seen in patients with Dupuytren's disease, and penile fibromatoses the least. Knuckle pads do not cause proximal interphalangeal joint contracture and may occasionally disappear. Peyronie's disease may cause penile contraction on erection, but also may disappear. Plantar fibromatosis does not cause contracture of the toes but often progresses to nodules in the plantar fascia that are many times larger than those seen in the hand.

Diabetes, Epilepsy, Alcoholism, and Trauma. Some publications (Crisp and Heathcote, 1984; Noble, Heathcote, and Cohen, 1984) have clarified the relationship of diabetes mellitus and Dupuytren's disease. Dupuytren's disease is usually mild in the diabetic and therefore (in a diabetic clinic) is detected only by someone who is an expert in examining the hand. The incidence of Dupuytren's disease in the diabetic patient varies with the age of the patient and the duration of diabetes. It is about 30 per cent in patients who have had diabetes for less than five years, and rises to over 80 per cent in patients who have had diabetes longer than 20 years. It is not related to the need for insulin or the control of diabetes (Ravid, Dinai, and Sohar, 1977). As shown in Table 121–1, patients with Dupuytren's disease who are seen by surgeons have an incidence of diabetes similar to that in the normal population for that age group. The common factor between diabetes and Dupuytren's disease is probably a microangiopathy that causes disturbances in the structural macromolecules in the extra cellular matrix and results in inappropriate deposition of connective tissue (Crisp and Heathcote, 1984). The "diabetic hand syndrome" that is similar to carpal tunnel syndrome (Jung and associates, 1971), the "limited joint mobility" seen in the juvenile diabetic (Rosenbloom, 1984) and in Dupuytren's disease, presumably have this common pathology. According to Lawson, Maneschi, and Kohner, (1983), a complex relationship exists among hand abnormalities, retinopathy, age, and duration of diabetes.

There is an increased incidence of epilepsy in patients with Dupuytren's disease. The world incidence of epilepsy is about 0.6 per cent. Table 121–1 shows that the incidence of epilepsy in patients with Dupuytren's disease is 2 per cent. Critchley and associates (1976) found the incidence of Dupuytren's disease in an epileptic colony to be 56 per cent, with a similar incidence in idiopathic and symptomatic epilepsy. These authors felt that Dupuytren's disease is probably a sequela of longterm phenobarbital administration. Interestingly, Fréré, as cited by Critchley, found only one patient with Dupuytren's disease in 134 epileptics at a time before phenobarbital was used.

The relationship of Dupuytren's disease and alcoholism is not established, although reports have shown an increased incidence of Dupuytren's disease in alcoholic patients (Su and Patek, 1970; Sabiston, 1973). In the alcoholic the disease consists primarily of thickening of the palmar aponeurosis without significant contracture, similar to the situation in the diabetic. However, the surgeon occasionally sees an alcoholic patient with extensive disease and severe joint contracture (see Fig. 121–10). If there is an association, the mechanism is unknown. It does not seem to be related to liver function or alcoholic cirrhosis (Pojer, Radivojevic, and Williams, 1972; Houghton and associates, 1983).

It is natural for patients to associate their disease with trauma to the hand. Every hand is subjected to specific episodes of trauma, and many hands to the repetitive trauma of work or play, so that an association with Dupuytren's disease in most instances is coincidental. However, there is evidence that some relationship exists, whether it be microtrauma as suggested by Skoog (1974), Larsen, Takagishi, and Posch, (1960) and Flint (1985), a specific episode (Hueston, 1968), or occupation (Mikkelsen 1978; Bennett 1982). Mikkelsen found a greater incidence of Dupuytren's disease in heavy manual workers, including those who had not sustained a specific injury to the hand. In Table 121–1 the incidence of trauma overall is seen to be 13 per cent. Further analysis revealed that in males the incidence was 13 per cent, in females 5 per cent, in manual workers 16 per cent, and in nonmanual workers 9 per cent. These figures are somewhat supportive of this view. Of more interest is the fact that two-thirds of patients described in Table 121–1 related the onset of Dupuytren's disease to a single episode of trauma. This disease (at least according to the patients) appeared within six months in 23 per cent and after five years in 50 per cent. About one-half of these patients had Dupuytren's disease only in the injured hand. In terms of the relationship with trauma, this is the most interesting group. In this group the disease appeared at an earlier age; was not associated with penile or plantar fibromatosis, diabetes, or epilepsy; and was less extensive. This type of Dupuytren's disease may be another phenotype, if in fact there is any genetic basis for its appearance.

PATHOLOGY

The Fibromatoses

According to Enzinger and Weiss (1983), Dupuytren's *contracture* is one of a group of superficial fibromatoses that also includes knuckle pads, Peyronie's disease, and plantar fibromatosis. Therefore, Dupuytren's *disease* (as defined by Hueston) is the only type of superficial fibromatosis. This is in contrast to the deep or desmoid type of fibromatoses, which are more aggressive and produce larger tumors. The fibromatoses as a group are intermediate between benign fibrous lesions and fibrosarcoma. Interestingly, work by Azzarone and associates (1983) suggests that the nodule of Dupuytren's disease has some features of a benign tumor and in fact is a model of tumor progression in a benign situation. Seemayer and associates (1980) call Dupuytren's disease a quasineoplastic proliferative disorder.

Cells, Collagen, and Ground Substance

The cell of Dupuytren's disease is the fibroblast or some modification of it. Since Majno and associates (1971) described the myofibroblast, others have related the presence of the myofibroblast to the contracting process (Ryan and associates, 1974; Rudolph and associates, 1977; Ariyan, Enriquez, and Krizek, 1978). The fibroblast is found in very early nodules, whereas the myofibroblast is the principal cell seen during the stage of contraction. The fibrocyte is the occasional cell seen in the tendon-like cords of long-standing contracture (Chiu and McFarlane, 1978). Seemayer and associates (1980) suggest that the myofibroblast is a functional modification of the fibroblast. However, all new cells likely arise from the pericyte, which retains its mesenchymal potential in adult life and which is known to be the source of young fibroblasts in the repair process (Ham and Cormack, 1979). Kischer and Speer (1984) favor the origin of the myofibroblast from the pericyte and believe that the initial stimulation to this transformation is hypoxia due to luminal occlusion of the microvasculature. It is important to our understanding of the disease process to know that the myofibroblast is capable of manufacturing collagen and elastin in addition to its contractile properties.

A study of the collagen of Dupuytren's disease has revealed two important findings. First, it is similar to that found in reparative tissue. There are increased amounts of Types III and V and Type I trimer collagen. These changes are similar to those found in granulation tissue, healing wounds, and hypertropic scars (Bailey and associates, 1977; Menzel and associates 1979; Bazin and associates, 1980; Brickley-Parsons and associates, 1981; Ehrlich, Brown, and White, 1982; Hanyu and associates, 1984; Parsons and associates, 1985). Brickley-Parsons states: "The biochemical changes in the collagen of Dupuytren's fascia are not the underlying basis for the gross shortening of the tissue fiber seen. Rather the changes represent the usual changes which occur in rapidly synthesized new collagen during the active stages of repair and healing of connective tissues." Second, the biochemical changes in the palmar fascia are widespread. They are found not only in the obviously diseased fascia but also in apparently normal-appearing fascia (Delbrück, Reimers, and Schönborn, 1981; Hamamoto and associates, 1982; Delbrück and Schröder, 1983; Flint, 1985; Parsons and associates, 1985). Therefore, Dupuytren's disease is multifocal in the fascia of the hand.

Flint, Gillard, and Reilly, (1982) and Slack, Flint, and Thompson, (1982) studied glycosaminoglycans in Dupuytren's disease and found that the concentration of chondroitin sulfate is 11 times greater than normal and the dermatin sulfate four times greater, while the level of hyaluronic acid is normal. These macromolecules play a role in determining the physical and functional characteristics of connective tissue. Flint believes that these biochemical changes are a physiologic adaptation to compressive loading. That is, the glycosaminoglycans are altered as a result of physical forces to which the tissues are subjected, rather than being the cause of the contracture.

Pathogenesis

The pathognomonic lesion of Dupuytren's disease is the nodule. Luck (1959) emphasized that the nodule is the site of the contracting process and also that it is usually multiple (Fig. 121–1). The nodule is frequently seen just proximal or just distal to the distal crease of the palm. There may be multiple nodules in the palmar aponeurosis. Nodules are frequently seen at the base of the little finger in association with the abductor digiti minimi tendon, and at the base of the thumb and in the thumb web. Nodules are also seen in the proximal segment of the finger and at the level of the proximal interphalangeal joint. They are occasionally seen at the level of the distal interphalangeal joint, particularly in the little finger. To understand the pathogenesis of Dupuytren's disease, it must be appreciated that collections of cells of microscopic size or larger are scattered throughout the

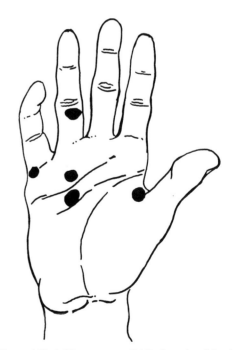

Figure 121–1. The common distribution of nodules in the palm and digits.

diseased tissue in addition to those present in the visible and palpable nodules (Mac-Callum and Hueston, 1962).

There are three stages of Dupuytren's disease: early, active, and advanced. These stages correlate clinically, histologically, and biochemically (Luck, 1959; Chiu and Mc-Farlane, 1978; Meister, Gokel, and Remberger 1979; Gelberman and associates, 1980). Early disease is characterized by thickening and nodularity in the palmar or digital fascia. Histologically the prominent cell is the fibroblast, and biochemically Type III collagen is present (Bailey and associates, 1977). In the stage of active disease, contraction occurs. The first indication of contraction is blanching of the skin of the distal palm on extension of the fingers. The skin then becomes fixed to the underlying fascia, as evidenced by the appearance of grooves and pits. Joint contraction follows. Nodules are large and visibly apparent. Histologically the myofibroblast is seen. Biochemically there are increased amounts of Types III and V collagen and an increase in the glycosaminoglycans. With advanced disease the nodules have disappeared, the joints are contracted severely, and tendon-like cords are both visible and palpable. Histologically the tissue resembles tendon. The few cells that are present are fibrocytes, and the collagen bundles are longitudinally oriented. There is less Type III and more Type I collagen in the cords.

The first sign of contraction is the appearance of a palpable cord proximal to a nodule in the palm or finger. The nodule is cellular as described above but also contains abundant collagen (Legge, Finley, and McFarlane, 1981). Under the electron microscope, frequent myofibroblasts are seen. Histologic examination of the cord reveals fewer cells but nevertheless collections of cells forming small nodules interspersed throughout the collagenous tissue (see Fig. 121–16*E*).

Flint (1985) made interesting observations on the pathogenesis of Dupuytren's disease. He noticed the disappearance of subdermal fat pads in the palm with age, and believes that this is due to progressive fibrotic replacement of the fat. He suggests that, in those races in which Dupuytren's disease is not seen or is infrequent, the fat pads persist into later life. He feels therefore that the initial lesion is damage to the fascia owing to this loss of protection. This leads to thickening of the longitudinal strands of fascia because of the loss of absorption of compression and stress forces provided by the fat pads. He believes that the cellularity and nodule formation is a reparative reaction around damaged longitudinal fibers. This repetitive damage and healing would account for the presence of fibroblasts, the increase in Type III collagen, and the changes in the ground substance. Again, these changes are not specific to Dupuytren's disease but rather to inflammation and repair. What is not explained to date is why this process of repair continues (unnecessarily) until severe joint contracture has occurred.

Mechanism of Contraction

At one time it was thought that collagen contracted or could shrink in vivo, but this is not so. The contraction of the digits in Dupuytren's disease is the result of an active cellular process similar to that of contraction of granulation tissue and scar. The myofibroblasts are known to contain contractile proteins similar to those of smooth muscle in the form of myofibrils. Also, the myofibroblasts have cell to cell and cell to stroma junctions that permit a synchronized contraction process similar to that seen in smooth and cardiac muscle (Fig. 121–2 and see Fig. 121–16*F*) (Gabbiani, Chaponnier, and Huttner, 1978; Salamon and Hamori, 1980). Badalamente, Stern, and Hurst (1983) showed that the contraction of the myofibroblast is driven by the dephosphorylation of adenosine triphosphate. A concept of the mechanism of contraction that involves fibroblasts, myofibro-

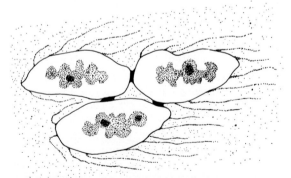

Figure 121–2. The significant features of the myofibroblast pertaining to Dupuytren's disease and contraction. The indented nuclei indicate contraction, cells are attached by intercellular junctions, and the cells are capable of producing collagen.

blasts, and the remodeling of collagen is illustrated in Figure 121–3.

In addition to this biologic explanation, there are biomechanical forces to consider. As the strands of diseased fascia mat together, there is lack of compliance of the fixed mass of tissue (Flint, 1985). McGrouther (1982) showed that in normal fascia the longitudinal, transverse, and vertical fibers of the palmar aponeurosis glide upon each other, but with disease these fibers adhere to each other. As stated by Hunter and Ogdon (1975), "when the disease spreads to join the dermis to aponeurosis, the strains produced in these tissues by normal hand movements act on the Dupuytren's tissue which is remodeled to cope with these stresses." Finally, Brody, Peng, and Lawdel (1981) believe that (once the disease begins) the fascia of Dupuytren's disease thickens in response to compressional and buckling forces caused by finger flexion.

Therefore, the contraction process is cellularly induced and follows the expected pattern of the process of repair. Why it begins and why it continues remains unanswered. However, the biomechanical forces applied to this tissue by the normal movements and functions of the hand may account for the continuation of the process to a severe and fixed contracture.

ANATOMY

In Dupuytren's disease the normal fascia is replaced by diseased tissue. In order to re-move this tissue safely and efficiently, one must know the normal anatomy of the fascia involved and the changes that take place with disease. Stack (1973) and Thomine (1974) studied the developmental anatomy of the fascia of the palm and digits in detail. Mc-Grouther (1982) demonstrated the three-dimensional relationship of the longitudinal transverse and vertical fibers and their relation to disease. McFarlane (1974, 1984) correlated the normal and pathologic anatomy.

Palm

There are only two components of the palmar fascia that become diseased: the pretendinous bands of the palmar aponeurosis and the natatory ligament (Fig. 121–4). The pretendinous bands, when diseased, cause contraction at the metacarpophalangeal (MP) joint, and in fact these bands are the only cause of contraction at this joint in Dupuytren's disease. Luck (1959) suggested that the normal fascia be referred to as bands and the diseased fascia as cords. This is a good way to differentiate the normal (bands) from the diseased (cords).

The natatory ligament is frequently involved in Dupuytren's disease. Beginning on the ulnar side of the hand, it passes from one tendon sheath to the next, supporting the skin of the web space and also sending fibers down either side of the digit (Fig. 121–5). From the radial side of the index finger, the natatory ligament continues in the thumb web to attach to the skin at the proximal

Figure 121–3. A concept of the mechanism of contraction that assumes a contractile role of the myofibroblast, and includes continuous resorption and replacement of collagen during the course of the disease. *A,* Three fibroblasts are shown in the early stage of disease, with surrounding collagen. *B,* These three cells become myofibroblasts, and contract; at the same time, new cells appear. *C,* With contraction of the second generation of cells the original collagen develops a wave form. *D,* With further contraction the original collagen is replaced so that it has a normal appearance, but the mass of tissue is shorter.

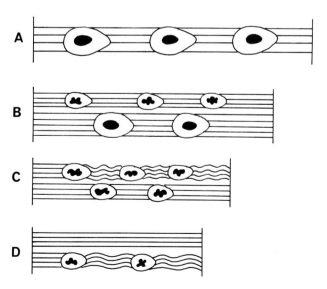

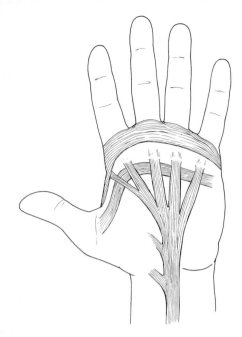

Figure 121–4. The components of the palmar fascia that become diseased. The pretendinous bands of the palmar aponeurosis are variable and often multiple. The band to the index finger frequently terminates on the radial border of the hand, and the band to the thumb is inconsistent. The superficial transverse ligament (transverse fibers of the palmar aponeurosis) is not often diseased in the central palm, but the fibers passing to the base of the thumb are frequently diseased. The natatory ligament is often diseased throughout its entire course, including the thumb web.

Figure 121–5. The detailed anatomy of the fascia of the finger web. The pretendinous bands, in addition to attaching to the skin just distal to the distal crease of the palm, bifurcate on either side of the metacarpophalangeal joint and reach the side of the finger deep to the neurovascular bundle. The fibers of the natatory ligament pass from side to side, attaching to the superficial surface of each flexor tendon sheath. In addition, fibers pass distally on each side of the finger to form the lateral digital sheet. A three-dimensional chiasm consisting of the fibers of the pretendinous band and the natatory ligament is formed, with the neurovascular bundle between these two layers of fibers.

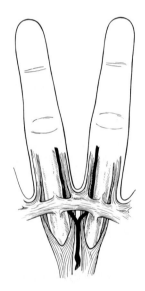

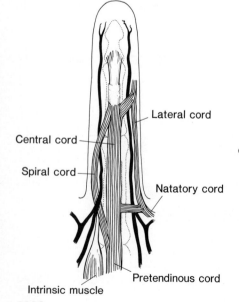

Lateral cord

Central cord

Spiral cord

Natatory cord

Pretendinous cord

Intrinsic muscle

Figure 121–6. The components of normal fascia that become diseased.

crease of the thumb. Contraction of the natatory ligament draws the fingers together, converting the normal U-shaped web to a "V." With severe contracture the skin of the web and adjacent sides of the fingers become macerated and the site of chronic infection. The fibers from the natatory ligament that enter the fingers join the fibers of the lateral digital sheet.

Fingers

Fascial disease in the finger results in contraction at the proximal interphalangeal (PIP) and occasionally at the distal interphalangeal (DIP) joint. The normal fascia that becomes diseased and the cords that result from this change are illustrated in Figures 121–6, 121–7, and 121–8. It is interesting that only the superficial fascia of the finger becomes diseased. Cleland's and Landsmeer's ligaments are not involved, whereas the lateral digital sheet, the superficial volar fascia, and Grayson's ligament become diseased. Knuckle pads originate in the dorsal subcutaneous tissue and are usually located over the dorsum of the proximal interphalangeal joint in the wrinkle ligaments described by Law and McGrouther (1984). Knuckle pads do not restrict proximal interphalangeal flexion. They are often tender and sometimes disappear, (Fig. 121–9) (Lagier and Meinecke, 1975; Hueston, 1984). Occasionally a plaque of diseased tissue is seen over the dorsum of the middle phalanx and in this location it may prevent distal interphalangeal flexion (Fig. 121–10) (Hueston, 1982b).

The central, lateral, and spiral cords terminate in the tendon sheath and adjacent

Figure 121–7. The diseased cords that develop from the normal fascial structures in Figure 121–6. The spiral cord can originate from the pretendinous cord or from an intrinsic muscle.

bone of the middle phalanx just distal to the proximal interphalangeal joint. One or any combination of the three cords can be found in the same patient. The central cord is the most common cause of proximal interphalangeal joint contracture, followed closely by the spiral cord, which is particularly common in the ring and little fingers. In the little finger, the spiral cord also arises from the abductor digiti minimi tendon (Barton, 1984) and is the cause of particularly severe proximal interphalangeal joint contracture. The lateral cord is not often seen alone except on the ulnar side of the little finger. The contracting cord or cords in the finger are almost always

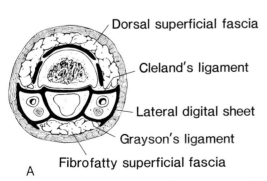

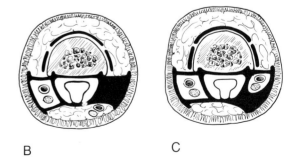

Figure 121–8. Cross sections of the normal and diseased fascia in the finger. *A,* The normal structures. *B,* The displacement of the neurovascular bundle toward the midline by a spiral cord or a lateral cord. *C,* The encasement of the neurovascular bundle by a central cord, which arises from the fibrofatty superficial fascia but usually is directed to one side of the midline of the finger.

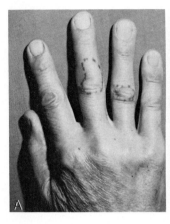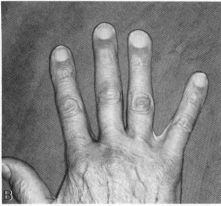

Figure 121–9. The appearance of knuckle pads. *A,* A large knuckle pad over the dorsum of the middle finger and a typical knuckle pad over the dorsum of the proximal interphalangeal joint of the ring finger. *B,* Ten years later, the knuckle pad has disappeared over the dorsum of the middle finger and is much smaller over the dorsum of the ring finger.

on one or the other side. It is unusual to have diseased cords on both sides.

The neurovascular bundle is not displaced or distorted from its course by a pretendinous cord, a central cord, or a lateral cord, although the bundle can be intimately surrounded by diseased fascia. There is always a plane of dissection between the fascia and the neurovascular bundle that can be developed by blunt dissection. However, the spiral

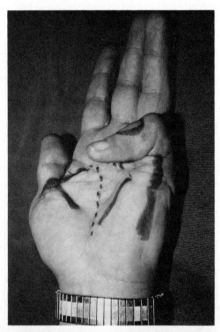

Figure 121–10. Severe contracture of the thumb web and little finger in a 57 year old alcoholic who had similar involvement of the other hand. His disease appeared at the age of 25. He had bilateral plantar fibromatosis and a positive family history. He is unable to flex the distal interphalangeal joint of the little finger because of a deposit of Dupuytren's tissue over the dorsum of the middle phalanx.

cord displaces the neurovascular bundle toward the midline, as illustrated in Figures 121–11 and 121–12. It is important to identify spiral cord contracture early in the operation in order to avoid damage to the neurovascular bundle.

The retrovascular cord of Thomine (1974) may be of the same fascial layer as Cleland's ligaments, but the author of this chapter believes that it is just superficial to Cleland's ligaments, as illustrated in Figure 121–13. It is seen as a longitudinal, cordlike structure originating from the periosteum of the proximal phalanx and passing distally, deep to the neurovascular bundle but superficial to the axis of movement of the proximal interphalangeal joint. The fibers can be traced distally to attach to the side of the distal phalanx. These fibers can develop into a diseased cord that causes contracture at both the proximal and distal interphalangeal joints. If the proximal interphalangeal joint cannot be fully extended after excision of obviously diseased fascia, one should look for the retrovascular cord as the cause of the contracture. This cord is a common cause of persistent or recurrent proximal interphalangeal joint contracture and the cause of contracture at the distal interphalangeal joint.

Thumb and Thumb Web

As described by Tubiana and Defrenne (1976), fascia arrives at the base of the thumb from three directions (see Fig. 121–4). The palmar aponeurosis frequently has a pretendinous band to the thumb, and this band can become diseased in the same way as those to the finger. This results in flexion contracture

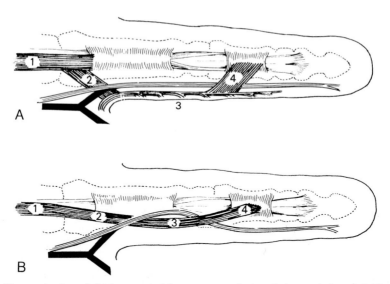

Figure 121–11. The mechanism of displacement of the neurovascular bundle by a spiral cord. *A,* The normal structures that produce the spiral cord in disease—the pretendinous band, the spiral band, the lateral digital sheet, and Grayson's ligament. *B,* As these four structures become diseased, the complex shortens and straightens, and the neurovascular bundle is displaced toward the midline of the finger.

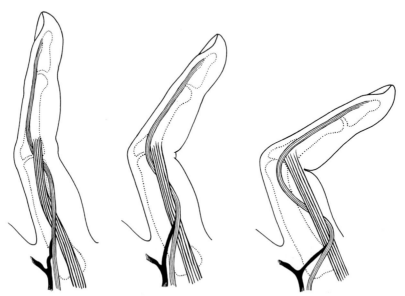

Figure 121–12. With increasing proximal interphalangeal joint contracture, the neurovascular bundle is displaced closer to the midline, and the point of displacement becomes more proximal and more superficial.

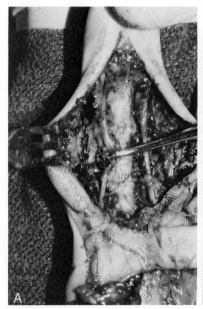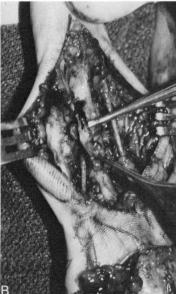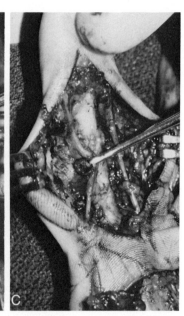

Figure 121–13. A demonstration of the retrovascular cord. *A,* The neurovascular bundle is retracted toward the midline to display the cord. *B,* The cord has been resected. *C,* With the retrovascular cord completely removed, the oblique fibers of Cleland's ligament remain.

at the metacarpophalangeal joint. The natatory ligament continues in the thumb web to attach to the skin at the base of the thumb, and again this portion of the ligament can become diseased, causing an adduction contracture of the thumb. Finally, the fibers of the superficial transverse ligament of the palm (transverse fibers of the palmar aponeurosis) terminate at the base of the thumb. These fibers are frequently diseased in the region of the thumb web and cause an adduction contracture of the thumb. One, two, or all three of these fascial bands can be involved in the same patient. All of them are superficial to the neurovascular bundles, and therefore they do not disturb the course of the bundles to the thumb or index finger. Nevertheless, the fascia can be adherent to these bundles, and care should be taken when removing the diseased fascia to identify the neurovascular bundles.

TREATMENT

Incision or excision of the diseased fascia is the only available therapy to correct joint contracture. Surgical treatment does not cure the disease and in some cases does not even control its progress. Manipulation of the biologic process is needed. Seemayer and associates (1980) suggest that a determined search for the molecular signal(s) of myofibroblast induction be undertaken.

Indications

The indications for treatment depend on the severity of contracture and the joint involved. Patients may complain of a tender nodule in the palm and even insist upon having it removed, but usually tenderness is transient, especially when the nature of the nodule is explained. About 30 degrees of metacarpophalangeal joint contracture becomes a nuisance to the patient simply because the finger gets in the way. This is a good guide to recommending surgery. There is never an urgency to correct a metacarpophalangeal joint contracture. Long-standing and severe contractures are readily corrected. However, it may not be possible to fully correct a proximal interphalangeal joint contracture even when it is of short duration. For this reason, the patient should be advised to have an operation as soon as the contracture appears.

Goals

The surgeon should have realistic goals and should convey these to the patient. The results of treatment at the metacarpophalangeal and proximal interphalangeal joints are very different. Usually the metacarpophalangeal joint contracture is completely corrected and recurrent contracture does not occur. In contrast, proximal interphalangeal joint contracture more often than not is not completely corrected, and on occasion is made worse by surgery. Recurrent contracture typically occurs at the proximal interphalangeal joint. These observations are borne out by the data in Table 121–2.

Types of Surgery

Many surgical techniques have been described but they fall into three categories: fasciotomy, regional fasciectomy, and extensive fasciectomy (Table 121–3).

Fasciotomy. In this procedure the fascia is simply incised. Classically, as performed by Sir Astley Cooper, the fascia is incised subcutaneously. The knife penetrates the skin at a distance from the contracting cord and reaches a position between the cord and the skin. With the finger forced into extension, the cord is incised. This operation is very successful in correcting metacarpophalangeal contracture because only the pretendinous cord need be incised. There is no danger of damaging a neurovascular bundle. It is not as successful in correcting a proximal interphalangeal joint contracture because more than one cord can be involved and all the diseased tissue cannot be divided for fear of dividing a neurovascular bundle (Rowley and associates, 1984).

A more reliable procedure is an open fasciotomy (Watson, 1984). Through a short incision, the cord is exposed and divided under direct vision. This is much preferable in the finger because the neurovascular bundle can be visualized before the cord is incised. Even with complete division of the diseased fascia, the joint may not extend because of foreshortening of the articular structures. The wound is closed by direct suture, Z-plasty, or skin graft.

This operation is usually performed under local anesthesia. The morbidity rate is low and the patient usually gains a maximal range of motion quickly. The only disadvantage is that contracture is likely to recur. Therefore, the operation is reserved for patients who are unable, because of disease or infirmity, to tolerate a more extensive procedure.

Regional Fasciectomy. This term means that only the diseased fascia is removed. In the palm, this involves excision of the diseased pretendinous cords and parts of the natatory ligament. In the finger, only those fascial cords that are obviously diseased are removed. The operation is performed on the assumption that the disease is not likely to extend beyond the fascia that is obviously diseased, and that therefore normal-appearing fascia need not be removed. Even though it is now known that Dupuytren's disease exists in normal-appearing fascia, a regional fasciectomy has proved successful in the palm where this type of surgery is usually performed. A modification of this operation has been described by Gonzalez (1971) in which a segment of disease that is sufficient to correct the joint contracture is excised, and the wound is covered by a full-thickness skin graft.

Extensive Fasciectomy. This term means that as much fascia as possible is removed, both diseased and potentially diseased. In the palm an attempt is made to remove the entire palmar aponeurosis as well as the natatory ligaments. In the finger, the diseased cords and also the normal-appearing bands are excised. McIndoe and Beare (1958) popularized an extensive palmar fasciectomy, but the operation is not often performed today because of the morbidity associated with it. Hematoma was common followed by prolonged swelling and stiffness. McCash (1964) solved the problem of hematoma formation by simply leaving the palmar wound open to heal secondarily. The McCash principle continues to gain support (Noble and Harrison, 1976; Lubahn, Lister, and Wolfe, 1984). In the finger an extensive operation is often performed. More than one fascial cord is frequently found to be contracting the proximal interphalangeal joint, but contracture also often recurs. It seems only logical to remove as much fascia as possible to be assured that the contracture has been corrected and that recurrent contracture is unlikely.

An even more extensive operation is a dermofasciectomy in which the diseased fascia and overlying skin are excised together.

TABLE 121–2. Correction of Flexion Contracture in Each Joint in Each Finger in 1202 Operations 6–18 Months Postoperatively

	Little			Ring			Middle			Index			Thumb		
	N	Pre	Post	N	Pre	Post	N	Pre	Post	N	Pre	Post	N	Pre	Post
MP joint	258	44.1±24.8*	3.2±11.1	251	36.3±20.0	2.5±8.4	126	28.1±16.3	2.3±7.5	27	23.3±15.2	4.6±9.3	16	19.6±11.6	8.8±17.2
Outcome†															
Perfect	84%	42.8±24.1	0	86%	34.3±18.9	0	87%	27.9±15.9	0	78%	21.1±12.2	0	69%	21.5±11.2	0
Improved	13%	54.9±25.3	14.3±11.2	12%	52.5±20.4	15.3±14.0	10%	31.1±20.8	14.8±8.1	11%	45.0±26.0	20.0±10.0	6%	35.0	30.0
Same/worse	3%	31.4±31.5	46.4±35.9	2%	22.0±16.8	29.0±21.3	3%	25.0±17.3	27.5±20.6	11%	16.7±5.8	21.7±2.9	25%	10.4+7.1	27.5±24.0
PIP joint	263	52.9±25.2	27.2±23.0	138	49.5±26.5	16.9±21.0	42	39.6±21.6	20.8±21.5						
Outcome															
Perfect	19%	46.5±23.8	0	45%	41.7±24.1	0	36%	30.3±14.3	0						
Improved	56%	63.2±21.3	28.8±17.4	42%	64.3±22.8	29.0±18.2	43%	50.4±20.7	26.4±13.4						
Same/worse	25%	34.9±22.7	44.9±23.3	13%	28.2±19.8	36.2±22.7	21%	33.7±25.6	44.2±22.1						
DIP joint	52	26.9±17.0	8.8±11.9	23	32.8±28.1	4.0±10.5	6	18.3±16.0	9.2±20.1						
Outcome															
Perfect	56%	20.9±15.2	0	82%	29.5±23.8	0	66%	12.5±5.0	0						
Improved	33%	38.6±15.4	16.6±7.7	9%	87.0±4.2	32.5±17.7	17%	10.0	5.0						
Same/worse	11%	23.0±13.7	29.7±8.9	9%	10.0±7.1	14.0±1.4	17%	50.0	50.0						

*Mean ± Standard Deviation.
†Perfect: Flexion contracture was completely corrected.
Improved: Flexion contrcture was less but not completely corrected.
Same/worse: There was no correction or the flexion contracture was worse.

**Table 121–3. Involvement of Hand and Type of Treatment Provided by
108 Surgeons to 1227 Patients***

Hand involvement				Number of rays involved		
	Palm:	95		None:		6
	Thumb:	25		1:		31
	Index:	13		2:		31
	Middle:	33		More than 2:		33
	Ring:	65				
	Little:	71				

Type of Operation Performed	Palm	Thumb	Index	Middle	Ring	Little
Fasciotomy	9.9	10.6	14.8	10.0	9.1	9.5
Regional fasciectomy	63.1	68.1	44.3	48.7	46.8	35.9
Extensive fasciectomy	27.0	21.3	41.0	41.3	44.1	53.6
Type of incision						
Longitudinal	68.2	84.0	80.3	84.7	87.0	89.6
Transverse	29.4	10.6	14.7	11.3	7.9	5.8
Type of wound closure						
Suture	70.3	85.1	83.6	84.0	86.3	78.1
Leave open	14.6	4.3	0	4.0	1.8	2.5
Free graft or flap	15.0	10.6	11.5	9.3	7.0	17.9
Procedure at PIP joint: 11						

*All figures are percentages.

A skin graft is used to close the wound. Hueston has observed that recurrence rarely follows a full-thickness skin graft. This operation is usually reserved to treat recurrent disease, but has also been recommended for aggressive disease in patients with a strong Dupuytren's diathesis (Hueston, 1982a; Tonkin, Burke, and Varian, 1984).

With long-standing or severe proximal interphalangeal joint contracture, the joint may not extend after an extensive fasciectomy. The surgeon must then decide whether to accept the correction obtained, whether to rely on postoperative splinting and therapy to gain more extension, or whether an arthroplasty is indicated. If the joint is corrected to less than 30 degrees' flexion, it is likely that splinting and therapy can maintain, if not improve, this state so that an arthroplasty is not indicated. A flexion contracture greater than 30 degrees is troublesome, and therefore some type of soft tissue release is indicated. The simplest procedure is to incise the flexor tendon sheath and try to extend the finger passively. Frequently the foreshortening of the tendon sheath is all that need be released. If this procedure is not successful, the attachments of the accessory collateral ligaments to the volar plate can be excised, as recommended by Curtis (1954). This procedure frequently permits full passive extension at the proximal interphalangeal joint. Alternatively the check-rein ligaments or proximal attachments of the volar plate can be released as described by Watson, Light, and Johnson, (1979). Both these procedures are extra-articular but nevertheless can result in limitation of flexion as well as extension in older patients. If one or other of these procedures fails to gain extension, it is best to accept the contracture and hope that postopertive splinting will lessen it. Some type of soft tissue release at the proximal interphalangeal joint was performed in only 11 per cent of operations upon the fingers (Table 121–3). It is a procedure that must be performed carefully and only in carefully selected patients.

Types of Incisions and Methods of Wound Closure

One should first of all decide what type of operation is to be performed, i.e., a fasciotomy, a regional fasciectomy, or an extensive fasciectomy. Second, the incision is planned, and third, it is decided how the wound is to be closed.

Incisions are generally transverse or longitudinal. Surgeons make specific modifications according to their individual methods of exposure and dissection and their experience with the healing wound. It is pointless to discuss and compare the great variety of incisions; it is best to use incisions that have been learned in training or developed by experience. The incisions preferred by the author are illustrated in Figure 121–14.

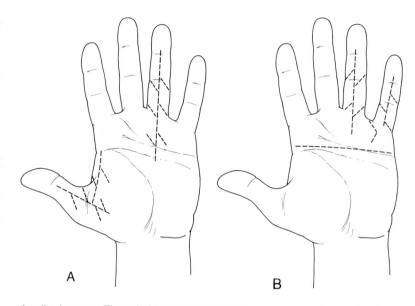

A

B

Figure 121–14. The author's preference for incisions. *A,* When a single finger is involved, a midline longitudinal incision is made from the proximal palm to just beyond the distal crease of the finger. At the completion of the dissection, three Z-plasties are designed, one near the middle crease of the finger, a second near the proximal crease of the finger, and a third near the distal crease of the palm. Disease of the thumb and thumb web can be removed through a longitudinal incision along the axis of the thumb, a longitudinal incision in the thumb web, or a combination of these two incisions. After removal of the diseased fascia, the incisions are closed, utilizing Z-plasties as required. *B,* If more than one finger is involved, a transverse incision is usually made in the palm near the distal crease. Through this transverse incision two, three, or four pretendinous cords can be excised. The fascia in the involved fingers is removed through a longitudinal incision. If it is difficult to expose the diseased fascia at the base of the finger, the longitudinal and transverse incisions are joined.

Most wounds are closed by suture. The wound may be modified by Z-plasty or V-Y advancement before closure in order to gain length. If a skin graft is required to close the wound, a full-thickness skin graft, removed from the inner arm or elbow crease, is preferred to a split-thickness skin graft because there is less contraction. Transverse wounds in the palm and the finger may be left open, after the method of McCash (1964).

Postoperative Management

There is a trend toward more outpatient surgical procedures. Most operations for Dupuytren's disease are of the magnitude of an outpatient procedure. However, the author prefers to have the patient in the hospital at least one and preferably two nights after surgery so that the hand and arm are sure to be elevated. Swelling, stiffness, and sympathetic dystrophy are unlikely to occur if the hand is elevated for the first 48 hours. During this time the patient is fitted with a thermoplastic splint (McFarlane and Albion, 1984), which is more comfortable than a bulky dressing and permits use of the uninvolved digits. It can be removed to allow active and passive movements of the involved digits. A static splint maintains the extension gained at surgery during the healing phase; it can

also be used to gain more extension at the proximal interphalangeal joint than was obtained at surgery. Patients are unlikley to gain maximal extension and regain full flexion until four to six weeks after the operation. They should be advised to wear a splint at night for about three months postoperatively even if full proximal interphalangeal extension has been obtained sooner. One cause of persistent flexion contracture at the proximal interphalangeal joint is postoperative scar contracture caused by the trauma of the operation. This can be controlled to some extent by prolonged splinting. However, these patients are of an age group in which they make their own decisions and often are not concerned about 20 or 30 degrees of flexion contracture at the proximal interphalangeal joint. They frequently discard the splint early in the postoperative period.

COMPLICATIONS

Complications are common after surgery, occurring in about 20 per cent of patients (Table 121–4). Hematoma, skin loss, and infection are a triad of associated problems often following in sequence. Hematoma is preventable by the liberal use of a bipolar coagulator, by wearing loupes during dissection so that even small vessels are seen and

Table 121–4. Frequency of Complications After Surgery for Dupuytren's Disease

Hematoma, skin loss, infection:	3%
Nerve and arterial division:	3%
Loss of flexion:	6%
Reflex sympathetic dystrophy:	5%
Overall:	19%

coagulated, and by release of the tourniquet before wound closure so that hemostasis is ensured. Skin loss occurs from an underlying hematoma, from excessive undermining of the skin, or from raising skin flaps that are very thin. The blood supply to the palmar skin is abundant so that it can be undermined extensively, especially if some of the vessels that perforate the palmar aponeurosis are preserved. The skin near the distal palmar crease may be attached to nodules and drawn into pits and folds; it may be very thin when dissected from the underlying disease and of doubtful viability. It may be prudent to excise the skin and apply a skin graft to the wound. In the finger it is often necessary to dissect the skin through the dermis in order to separate it from the diseased fascia. Again, it is better to excise the skin and apply a skin graft than to leave the skin to become necrotic. However, the skin can be treated as a free skin graft and held with a bolus dressing, as illustrated in Figures 121–16*H* and 121–20*E*. Usually, infection occurs secondary to hematoma and skin loss. One should be sure of the cleanliness of the skin in patients with severe and long-standing contracture or in patients with intertrigo of the web spaces from contracture of the natatory ligament. If the skin cannot be cleansed or the intertrigo controlled, a preliminary fasciotomy is advisable to gain access to the infected areas.

To prevent division of a digital nerve or artery, each neurovascular bundle should be exposed the entire length of the wound. This is best done with loupe magnification and usually is not difficult because there is a plane of dissection between the neurovascular bundle and the fascia. Division of nerve and artery occurs most frequently in the region of the web space in the presence of severe metacarpophalangeal and proximal interphalangeal contracture. The dissection can be made somewhat easier if the pretendinous cord is incised to correct the metacarpophalangeal contracture and the adjacent fingers are abducted to place the neurovascular bundles on tension. If either the nerve or the artery is divided, it should be repaired: the nerve to prevent neuroma formation, and the artery to restore needed circulation to the digit of an older person.

Loss of flexion is the most common complication, more common than the 6 per cent incidence in patients noted in Table 121–4 who had permanent loss of flexion. Usually the patient has full digital flexion before surgery (this should be recorded). All patients must be followed closely in the early postoperative period. The surgeon and therapist should be as concerned about patients regaining flexion as about their maintaining extension. Swelling is to be avoided and movements of the involved digits should be guarded until the wounds are healed. The incidence of this complication is related to the severity of the operation, so the surgeon should modify the surgery according to the anticipated response of the patient.

Every patient operated upon for Dupuytren's disease is a candidate for reflex sympathetic dystrophy. This complication is five times more common in women after surgery for Dupuytren's disease. Minor degrees of dystrophy are common but can usually be aborted by close observation of the patient, correction of swelling by elevation and hand therapy, and appropriate sedation. The problem may not become apparent for two or three weeks after surgery. Limitation of shoulder or elbow movement is an early sign and should be evaluated at each visit. An established dystrophy, with burning pain in the palm and fingers, swelling, and limitation of movement needs aggressive treatment that is best provided by readmission to the hospital.

RESULTS

To appraise results properly one should obtain subjective impressions from the patient, evaluate pre- and postoperative function, and also record objective improvement in the range of movement of the digits. Only the latter data are readily available. Table 121–2 shows the results obtained by digit and by joint in a large series of patients operated on in many different ways by several surgeons. The impressive figures are that invariably the contracture at the metacarpophalangeal joint is corrected whereas it is not at

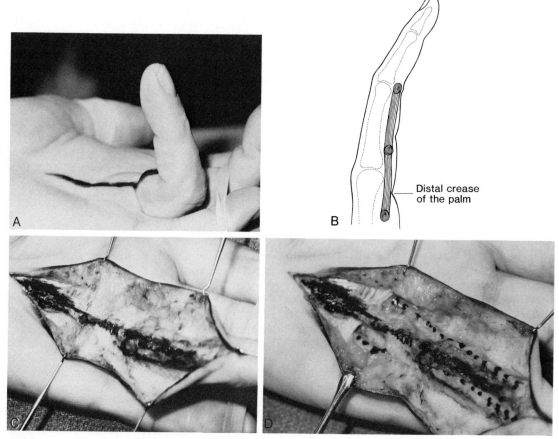

Figure 121–15. The author's method of treatment when one finger is involved. See text.

the proximal interphalangeal joint, particularly in the little finger. There are many reasons why the little finger does not do as well as the other fingers, such as the fact that it often contains much more disease than other digits and the tissue is not completely removed. Also, there is an inherent tendency for the little finger to flex when injured, and the trauma of the operation to correct Dupuytren's disease is indeed a form of trauma.

CASES TO ILLUSTRATE THE AUTHOR'S METHODS OF TREATMENT

WHEN A SINGLE FINGER IS INVOLVED

E.I.: a 64 year old male radiology clerk who first noted Dupuytren's disease in the left hand about ten years before. He was right-handed, had a negative family history, and had no associated diseases or ectopic deposits

of Dupuytren's tissue. In the left hand the disease was limited to the ring finger ray as a pretendinous cord continuing into a central cord. The metacarpophalangeal joint was contracted to 35 degrees and the proximal interphalangeal joint to 25 degrees. In the right hand there was a small nodule in the palm in the line of the ring finger ray.

The significant steps of the operation are illustrated in Figure 121–15. A midline longitudinal incision was made from the proximal palm to beyond the distal crease of the ring finger. Beginning proximally, the incision was deepened to expose the diseased fascia. In the proximal palm there is a good amount of subcutaneous fascia that can be left attached to the skin and therefore ensure its viability. As the dissection proceeds distally, however, the skin flaps become thinner because the fascia inserts into the skin just beyond the distal crease of the palm. In the finger, the diseased fascia is usually intimately adherent to the skin, and therefore

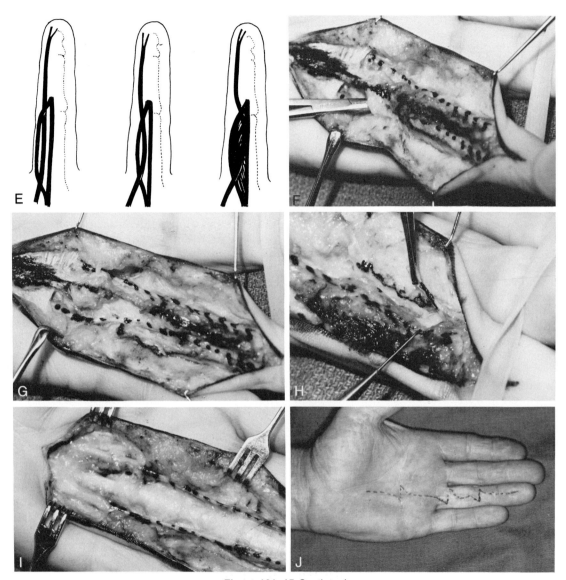

Figure 121–15 *Continued*

the skin must be dissected in the plane of the deep dermis. This important step in exposure is illustrated in Figure 121–15*B* and by the completed exposure of the disease in Figure 121–15*C*. The diseased fascia is marked by black ink. Proximally the pretendinous cord is wide because of the presence of a large nodule. The cord narrows at the distal crease of the palm where some of the fibers attach to the skin while other fibers (not shown) pass deeply as spiral bands on either side of the metacarpophalangeal joint. The cord then continues into the finger as a central cord that lies more on the ulnar side of the finger. Note that the skin that has been dissected

from this tissue is extremely thin compared with the skin on the radial side, which still has some subcutaneous tissue attached to it. In the palm, the skin flaps have been dissected just enough to expose the apparently normal pretendinous bands on each side of the ring finger ray. In the finger the skin flaps have been dissected to about the midlateral line. It is necessary to extend the incision beyond the distal crease of the finger in order to expose the diseased fascia that attaches to the tendon sheath just distal to the proximal interphalangeal joint.

The next step in the operation is to expose both neurovascular bundles and thereby protect them from injury during excision of the fascia. It is easiest to find the neurovascular bundle distally, where it is covered by a scant amount of fascia, and then expose it from distal to proximal. In Figure 121–15D the radial neurovascular bundle is completely exposed, as indicated by the dotted line. The ulnar neurovascular bundle has been exposed from the distal part of the finger to the base of the finger, but it then disappears into a mass of diseased fascia. It is again exposed in the palm. At this point one should be concerned that the ulnar neurovascular bundle has been displaced toward the midline by a spiral cord. It is not possible to palpate or predict the presence of a spiral cord preoperatively. A spiral cord is present and the mechanism of the displacement is explained in Figure 121–15E. In this illustration both a central cord and a spiral cord are involved. Originally these cords developed separately, but as the disease progresses the cords blend into a single mass of diseased tissue with the neurovascular bundle encased. There is, however, a plane of cleavage between the neurovascular bundle and the disease, as illustrated in Figure 121–15F. By blunt dissection it is possible to follow the neurovascular bundle through this tissue both proximally and distally, and then simply divide the disease to expose the neurovascular bundle, as illustrated in Figure 121–15G. The diseased tissue can now be excised methodically by removing all the disease between the neurovascular bundles and then all the disease lateral to the neurovascular bundles. Finally, retrovascular disease should be sought; in this patient there was a thick retrovascular cord deep to the radial neurovascular bundle (Fig. 121–15H). The radial neurovascular bundle is held toward the midline with a nerve hook. The cord was removed distal to the distal interphalangeal joint even though there was no flexion contracture at the joint.

The completed dissection is shown in Figure 121–15I. Both neurovascular bundles are shown, and all the diseased fascia has been excised. This included not only the disease of the ring finger ray but also the apparently normal pretendinous bands to the adjacent middle and little fingers. The transverse fibers of the palmar aponeurosis were excised. It is not necessary to excise these fibers but it is technically easier to do so when excising a pretendinous cord. The tourniquet was re-

leased and bleeding controlled before the wound was closed. Three Z-plasties were inserted into the longitudinal incision at the time of wound closure. The Z-plasties were not designed until the time of wound closure. This is an important technical point: if a Z-plasty is created at the initial incision the surgeon may find that the flaps of the Z are in an area where the skin is extremely thin, and the flaps may not survive. Although it is desirable to place the Z-plasties in or near a flexion crease, it is more prudent to place them where the skin is likely to be viable. Three Z-plasties are usually designed. One is placed near the middle crease of the finger, another at the proximal crease, and a third near the distal crease of the palm. It is not necessary to place a Z-plasty at the distal crease of the finger because a midline longitudinal scar across the distal crease never contracts. As noted in Figure 121–15J, the three Z-plasties are close to the creases but not in them because they were placed where the skin was most viable. This patient was last seen three years after surgery at which time he had full flexion and extension of the digits of his left hand and no evidence of recurrence or extension of disease.

WHEN MORE THAN ONE FINGER IS INVOLVED

J.V.: A 53 year old male retail salesman who noted Dupuytren's disease in both hands about two years before. He had no family history of Dupuytren's disease and no associated diseases or ectopic deposits of Dupuytren's tissue. Examination of the right hand revealed pretendinous cords in the little, ring, and middle finger rays with a nodule at the base of the little finger and a large nodule in the proximal segment of the little finger. There was 40 degrees of flexion contracture at the metacarpophalangeal joint and 15 degrees at the proximal interphalangeal joint of the little finger. Examination of the left hand revealed a small nodule in the palm and a developing pretendinous cord in the little finger ray.

The treatment of the disease in the right hand is illustrated in Figure 121–16. A transverse incision was made in the distal crease of the palm from the ulnar border of the hand to beyond the middle finger ray. Through this incision the pretendinous cords to the little, ring, and middle fingers were exposed. The

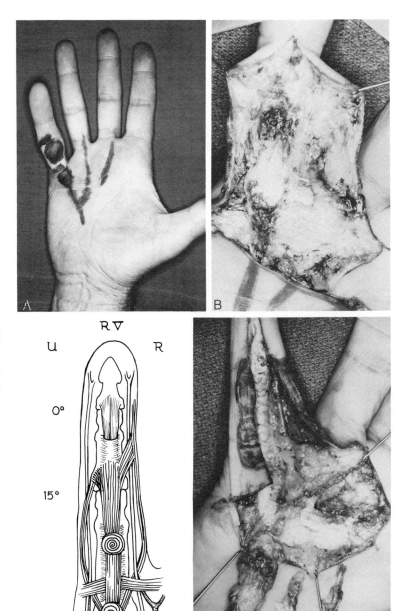

Figure 121–16. The author's method of treatment when more than one finger is involved. See text.

Illustration continued on following page

disease in the little finger (illustrated in Figure 121–16C) proved to be a pretendinous cord, a central cord, and spiral cords on each side that were diseased but had not yet shortened sufficiently to displace the neurovascular bundles. Note that the spiral cord on the ulnar side has taken the usual course deep to the neurovascular bundle to reach the side of the finger, and then passed superficial to the neurovascular bundle to attach to the tendon sheath and bone just distal to the proximal interphalangeal joint. The spiral cord on the radial side joined the fibers of the lateral cord and continued distally. Diseased fibers of Grayson's ligament are illustrated passing from the flexor tendon sheath to the lateral cord. One can imagine that with progressive disease, this complex would foreshorten and produce a typical spiral cord that would displace the neurovascular bundle toward the

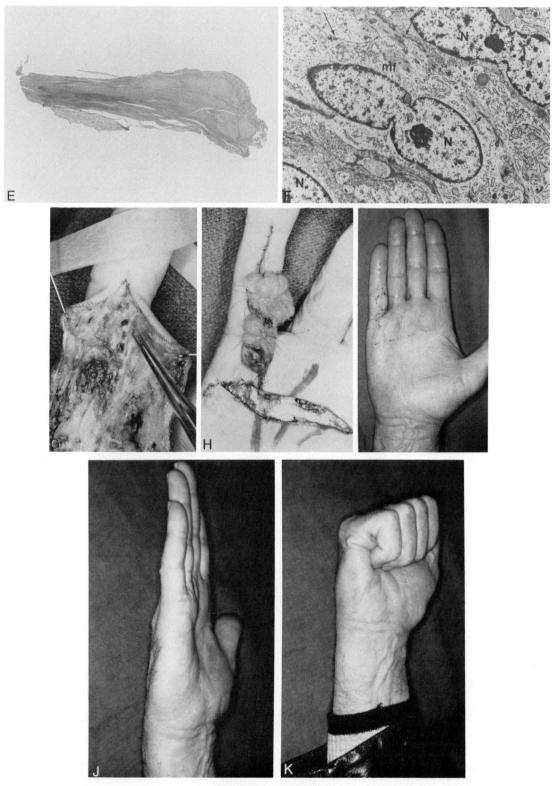

Figure 121–16 *Continued*

midline. Note the location of the nodules in the pretendinous and central cords and the attachment of the central cord to the flexor tendon sheath just beyond the proximal interphalangeal joint. The natatory ligament was diseased. This mass of tissue was removed, as shown in Figure 121–16D. The transverse fibers of the palmar aponeurosis were retained. In Figure 121–16E a longitudinal section of the disease in the little finger is illustrated under low power magnification (× 13). There are many nodules throughout the diseased tissue and not simply the two nodules that were noted clinically. Figure 121–16F is a transmission electron microscope photograph that demonstrates the features of the myofibroblast shown in Figure 121–2. Three nuclei are shown, two of them with the typical indentations of the myofibroblast nucleus. The arrows identify sites of intercellular junctions that permit a synchronous contraction of the myofibroblasts.

Again, both neurovascular bundles were completely exposed before the tissue was excised. In Figure 121–16G a retrovascular cord is shown at the end of the forceps dorsal to the radial neurovascular bundle. The longitudinal incision in the little finger was closed with a Z-plasty near the middle crease and another near the proximal crease of the finger. These skin flaps were very thin and were therefore treated as free full-thickness skin grafts by applying a bolus dressing over them. The transverse incision in the palm was left open to heal by second intention after the method of McCash. The wound was healed within four weeks of surgery at which time the patient had full extension and almost full flexion of his fingers. Figure 121–16I, J, and K shows views taken six years after surgery. He has full extension and flexion of the digits and there is no evidence of recurrence or extension of disease.

THUMB AND THUMB WEB

G.B.: A 55 year old white male laboratory technician who noted Dupuytren's disease in both hands about five years previously. He had an operation on both hands two years before and another on the right hand one year before. His general health was satisfactory but he complained of painful erections due to Peyronie's disease. When first seen he was placed on vitamin E, 1600 units per day for six months. The Peyronie's disease im-

proved so that he no longer complained of painful erections, but the Dupuytren's disease progressed. One year after he was first seen the right hand was operated on for recurrent disease. Two years later the left hand was operated on because of increasing contraction of the little finger and adduction contraction of the thumb (Fig. 121–17A). There was a longitudinal scar on the radial border of the thumb, so presumably fascia had been excised previously from the thumb. There was a nodule at the proximal crease of the thumb, a pretendinous cord, and a cord from the termination of the fibers of the superficial transverse ligament of the palm. The disease was exposed through a T-shaped incision, as illustrated in Figure 121–17B. The amount of tissue removed is shown in Figure 121–17C; also, the two digital nerves to the thumb and the radial digital nerve to the index finger are marked by dotted lines to show their relationship to the diseased fascia. Postoperatively there were no complications. When last seen three years after surgery he had normal movement of the thumb and no evidence of recurrence. The Peyronie's disease was present but was not painful.

SUBCUTANEOUS FASCIOTOMY

E.G.: A 56 year old white male who one year previously had a coronary artery bypass operation. He complained of difficulty using his left hand because of increasing contraction of the ring finger. Examination revealed disease localized to the ring finger with 40 degrees of contracture at the metacarpophalangeal joint and 35 degrees at the proximal interphalangeal joint. He was operated on under local anesthesia. A longitudinal incision was made over the pretendinous cord at the level of the distal crease of the palm, and the cord was incised. The patient was able to extend the metacarpophalangeal joint. The separation of the divided ends of the pretendinous cord is shown in Figure 121–18A. A Z-plasty was designed over the proximal segment of the finger, as shown in Figure 121–18B. The neurovascular bundles were identified and the diseased fascia incised with the bundles in view. Again, he was able to fully extend the proximal interphalangeal joint. Both wounds were closed by transposing the flaps of the Z-plasties, as shown in Figure 121–18C. Note that the transverse incision of the Z-plasty in the finger did not approxi-

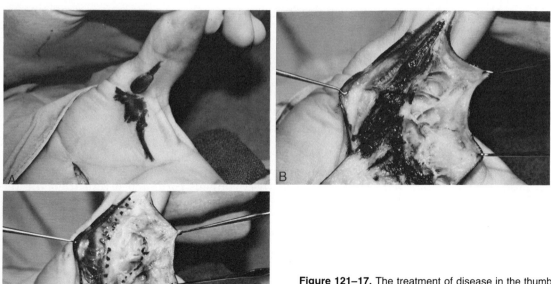

Figure 121–17. The treatment of disease in the thumb and thumb web. See text.

mate, so it was left open to heal secondarily. Postoperatively the patient regained full extension and did not lose flexion. Figure 121–18D, E, and F shows views taken one year after surgery during a hospitalization for further cardiac investigation. In this patient a better result was obtained at the proximal interphalangeal joint than is customary with this operation.

HYPEREXTENSION AT THE DISTAL INTERPHALANGEAL JOINT

Hyperextension at the distal joint occurs only with severe and long-standing contracture at the proximal interphalangeal joint. It occurs in all fingers, but most commonly in the little finger. It is not due to disease on the dorsum of the finger, but rather is secondary to flexion at the proximal interphalangeal joint. Landsmeer's ligament is not involved in the disease process, but becomes foreshortened because of proximal interphalangeal joint contracture. If the patient has passive flexion at the distal interphalangeal joint, the hyperextension deformity can be overcome by correcting the proximal interphalangeal joint flexion. If the hyperextension is not passively corrected, as illustrated

in Figure 121–19B, division of Landsmeer's ligaments or division of the extensor mechanism at the distal interphalangeal joint will improve the hyperextension. The patient shown in Figure 121–19 is a 60 year old male quality control inspector who had had Dupuytren's disease for at least 20 years. He had had one previous operation on the right hand and two previous operations on the left hand. He had no ectopic deposits of Dupuytren's tissue and no diabetes or epilepsy, but had been treated for bilateral cataracts. He admitted to drinking two to four bottles of beer each day. Examination of his left hand revealed multiple scars from previous operations and recurrent disease in the thumb web and the middle, ring, and little fingers. As noted in Figure 121–19A, he did not have recurrent metacarpophalangeal joint contracture, but rather recurrent proximal interphalangeal joint contracture of the little and ring fingers. At surgery, a dermofasciectomy of the skin and fascia of the proximal segment of the little finger was performed. This corrected the proximal interphalangeal joint contracture but did not correct the distal interphalangeal joint hyperextension. A tenotomy of the extensor tendon was carried out, as illustrated in Figure 121–19C and D.

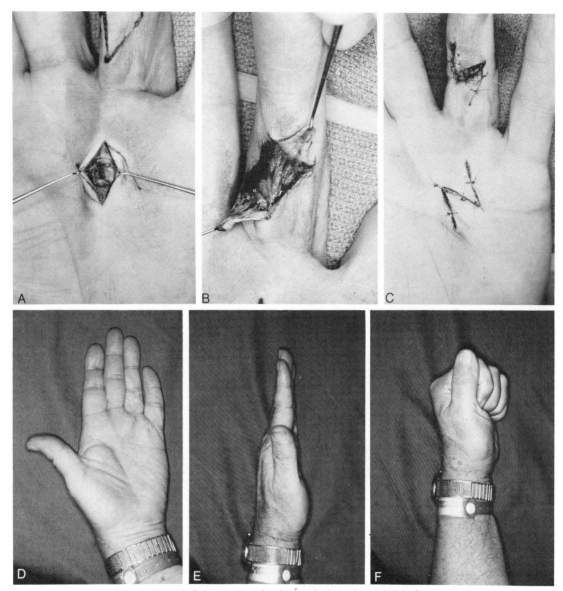

Figure 121–18. Subcutaneous fasciotomy in the palm and digit. See text.

Postoperatively the skin graft and the other wounds healed satisfactorily, and within one month the patient requested that the other hand be operated on. When last seen three years after surgery he had a flexion contracture of 45 degrees at the proximal interphalangeal joint of the little finger but was able to flex the distal joint about 10 degrees (Fig. 121–19*E* and *F*).

RECURRENT DISEASE

Most of the time, recurrent contracture is due to inadequate removal of diseased tissue at the first operation. At the second operation it is much more difficult to remove the diseased tissue because it is interspersed with scar tissue, and it is much more difficult to dissect and preserve the neurovascular bundles. In this regard it is wise to test for sensation in the digit before surgery. If a digital nerve was divided at the previous operation, one should assume that the artery was also divided. It would then be essential to preserve the remaining artery, otherwise the finger might be lost. If the skin is firmly fixed to the underlying scar and recurrent disease, it should be removed with the fascia

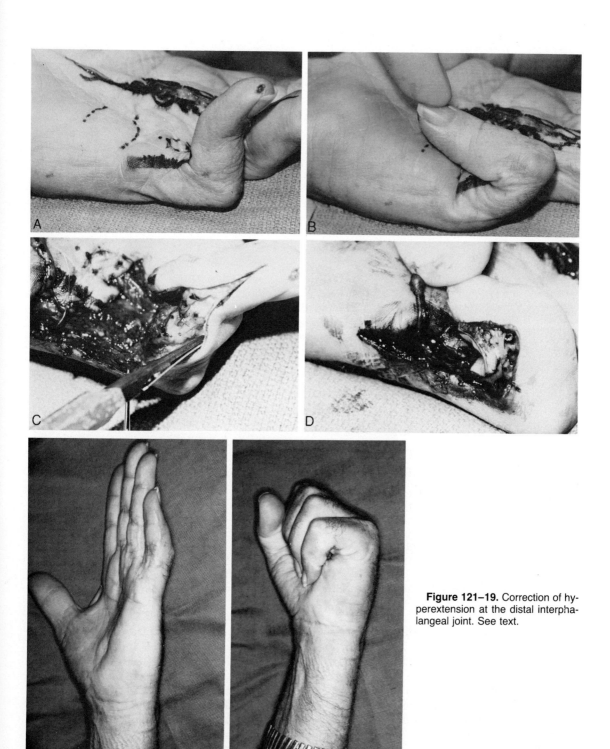

Figure 121–19. Correction of hyperextension at the distal interphalangeal joint. See text.

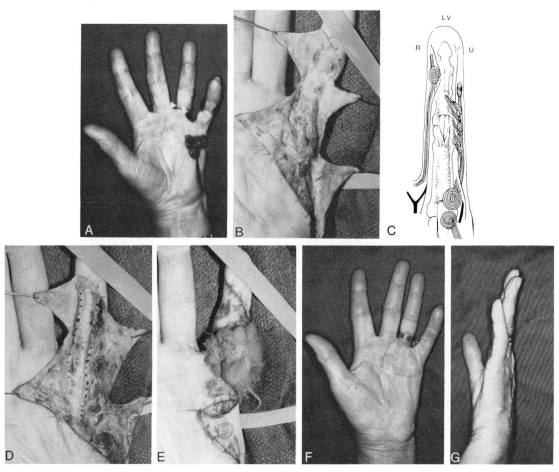

Figure 121–20. Correction of recurrent disease. See text.

as a dermofasciectomy. If the disease recurs in spite of an adequate initial operation, a dermofasciectomy is clearly the treatment of choice. The following cases illustrate these points.

J.P.: A 58 year old female nurse who suffered a left Colles' fracture two years previously. She had a below elbow cast applied for six weeks and during that time complained of numbness in her thumb. She noticed a thickening of the palmar fascia when the cast was removed. One sister had Dupuytren's disease and diabetes, but the patient was in good health and did not have knuckle pads or plantar fibromatosis. The right hand was not involved. She was operated on one year later because of progressive contraction of the little finger and disease in the thumb web. Three years after surgery she had recurrent contracture at the proximal interphalangeal joint of the little finger, and a large deposit of Dupuytren's tissue at the base of the little

finger, as illustrated in Figure 121–20*A*. At a second operation the previous incisions were opened and extended distally to beyond the distal crease of the finger and proximally onto the hypothenar area, as shown in Figure 121–20*B*. The skin flaps were extremely thin because they were dissected from the underlying disease tissue as well as scar tissue. The involvement within the little finger (illustrated in Fig. 121–20*C*) consists of a hypothenar cord that terminated in a large nodule at the level of the metacarpophalangeal joint, a large nodule at the insertion of the abductor digiti minimi tendon that extended distally as a spiral cord. Also, there was lateral cord tissue on both sides of the finger, a large nodule at the level of the distal interphalangeal joint on the radial side, and a smaller nodule proximal to this on the ulnar side. All this tissue was excised, preserving both neurovascular bundles (Fig. 121–20*D*). It was felt that the skin flaps would survive, and the most precarious one was supported by a bolus dressing, as illustrated in Figure 121–20E. Note that the transverse portion of the incision in the palm has been left open to heal secondarily. The patient was last seen six years after surgery, at which time she had full flexion of the fingers but lacked 30 degrees of extension at the proximal interphalangeal joint of the little finger. There was no evidence of recurrence or extension of the disease, although in the interval she developed palpable disease in the palm of the other hand.

S.J.: A 55 year old male civil engineer who had noticed Dupuytren's disease in the right hand about two years previously. He had a negative family history and was in good health. When first seen he lacked hyperextension at the metacarpophalangeal joint of the right ring finger. There was some fascial thickening in the palm. One year later there was progress of the disease in the right hand but no metacarpophalangeal joint contracture. There was evidence of disease in the left ring finger ray. Three years later the patient had 30 degrees of contracture at the metacarpophalangeal joint of the right ring finger and was operated on. Five years after he was first seen the left hand was operated on. He did not gain extension at the proximal interphalangeal joint after surgery and further developed increasing flexion contracture. The appearance of his hand three years after the initial operation is shown in Figure 121–21A. There is a large recurrent mass of tissue occupying much of the proximal segment of the finger. A dermofasciectomy was performed, as shown in Figure 121–21B, and a full-thickness skin graft was applied to the defect (Fig. 121–21C). When last seen three years after surgery, there was no evidence of recurrence or extension of the disease in either hand. There was still a 20 degree flexion contracture at the proximal interphalangeal joint of the ring finger. Presumably the recurrent disease in this patient was due to Dupuytren's tissue being left on the skin at the time of the initial exposure. This is less likely to occur if the dissection is carried out with the aid of loupe magnification.

E.C.: A 45 year old white housewife who noted lumps in both palms about three years previously. Since then she developed progressive finger contracture but her main complaint was burning pain and tenderness in her hand and fingers. Because of the discomfort and burning sensations in her hands, she was investigated for possible scleroderma or erythralgia. She had no family history of Dupuytren's disease nor ectopic deposits of Dupuytren's tissue and was otherwise in good health. The left hand was operated on to remove disease in the little and index finger rays and from the thumb web. Three years later she presented with recurrent disease in the areas of operation as well as new disease in the middle finger, as shown in Figure 121–22A. A dermofasciectomy of the recurrent disease of the little and index fingers was performed, as well as an extensive fasciectomy in the middle finger (Fig. 121–22B). Full-thickness skin grafts, removed from the groin, were applied to the defects of the little and index fingers and the thumb, and the middle finger was closed with Z-plasties. When seen two years after surgery the patient had 45 degrees of flexion contracture at the proximal interphalangeal joint of the little finger, but was able to make a firm fist (Fig. 121–22C and D). She still complained of tenderness and burning pain in the affected areas indicative of a vasculitis. This patient had a phenotype of Dupuytren's disease in which the fibromatosis was associated more with vascular symptoms than joint contracture. Correction of the joint contracture and removal of the diseased tissue did not control the symptoms. Perhaps this patient would have been improved by adventitial stripping of the digital vessels as recommended by Duschoff (1976).

A.P.: A 64 year old foreman who noticed bilateral finger contractures about ten years previously. He was an insulin dependent diabetic and had had one cataract operation. His only brother and one uncle also had Dupuytren's disease. On examination, he had extensive disease of both hands with severe flexion contractures of all metacarpophalangeal joints and of the proximal interphalangeal joints of the little, ring, and middle fingers of the right hand. The left hand had less involvement but contracture at all metacarpophalangeal joints and the proximal interphalangeal joint of the little finger. The left hand was operated on first. A transverse incision in the palm removed the pretendinous cords to the four fingers. The disease of the little finger was removed through a longitudinal incision. In Figure 121–23A, the extension gained in the little finger with the postoperative splint is illustrated. Within two

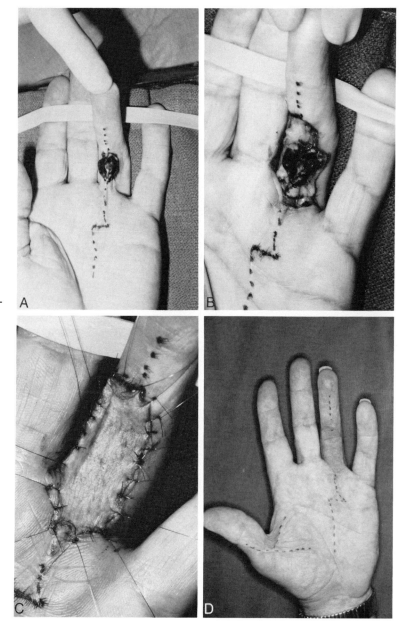

Figure 121–21. Correction of recurrent disease. See text.

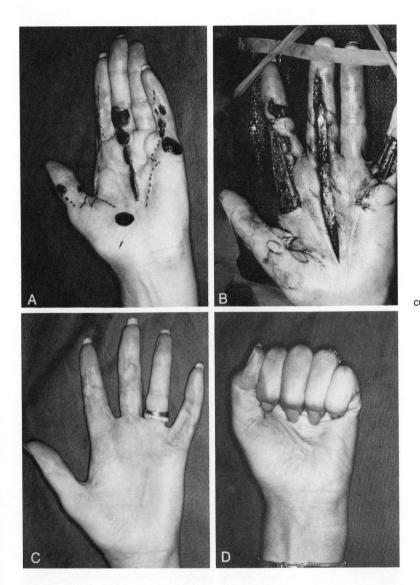

Figure 121–22. Correction of recurrent disease. See text.

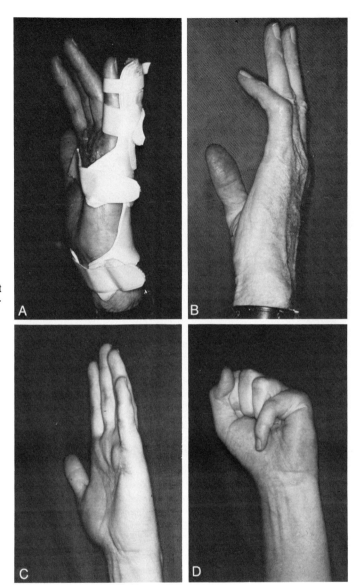

Figure 121–23. Correction of persistent flexion contracture by replacement arthroplasty. See text.

years, the proximal interphalangeal joint was flexed to 70 degrees even though there was no palpable Dupuytren's disease in the finger. Presumably the proximal interphalangeal flexion was due to scar contracture. The patient requested correction of this troublesome contracture, and a replacement arthroplasty was performed. Through a lateral incision on the ulnar side of the finger, the condyle of the proximal phalanx was removed and a Swanson implant inserted. By shortening the finger in this manner, it was possible to extend it. The patient regained full active extension but did not regain full flexion, as shown in Figure 121–23C and D. A replace-

ment arthroplasty is a reasonable alternative to amputation in a finger that is severely contracted because of scar contracture rather than by Dupuytren's contracture.

CONCLUSIONS

Within a very few years the etiology and pathogenesis of Dupuytren's disease should be clear. Therapy will be modified accordingly, although there will always be a need for surgical treatment of some sort. Until then established principles of treatment should be respected. Metacarpophalangeal

joint contracture is readily corrected by regional fasciectomy. The correction of proximal interphalangeal joint contracture is less
predictable but is best managed by extensive
fasciectomy within the finger.

REFERENCES

Ariyan, S., Enriquez, R., and Krizek T.: Wound contraction and fibroconnective disorders. Arch. Surg.,
113:1034, 1978.
Azzarone, B., Failly-Crepin, C., Daya-Grosjean, L., Chaponnier, C., and Gabbiani, G.: Abnormal behavior of
cultured fibroblasts from nodule and nonaffected aponeurosis of Dupuytren's disease. J. Cell Physiol.,
117:353, 1983.
Badalamente, M. A., Stern, L., and Hurst, L. C.: The
pathogenesis of Dupuytren's contracture: contractile
mechanisms of the myofibroblasts. J. Hand Surg.,
8:235, 1983.
Bailey, A. J., and Duance, B. C.: Collagen in acquired
connective tissue diseases: an active or passive role?
Eur. J. Clin. Invest., *10*:1, 1980.
Bailey, A. J., Sims, T. J., Gabbiani, G., Bazin, S., and
LeLous, M.: Collagen of Dupuytren's disease. Clin. Sci.
Mol. Med., *53*:499, 1977.
Barsky, H. K.: Guillaume Dupuytren—A Surgeon in His
Place and Time. New York, Vantage Press, 1984.
Barton, N. J.: Dupuytren's disease arising from the
abductor digiti minimi. J. Hand Surg., *9B*:265, 1984.
Bazin, S., LeLous, M., Duance, V. C., Sims, T. J., Bailey,
A. J., et al.: Biochemistry and histology of the connec-
tive tissue of Dupuytren's disease lesions. Eur. J. Clin.
Invest., *10*:9, 1980.
Bennett B.: Dupuytren's contracture in manual workers.
Br. J. Indust. Med., *39*:98, 1982.
Bowser-Riley, S., Bain, A. D., Noble, J., and Lamb, D.
W.: Chromosome abnormalities in Dupuytren's dis-
ease. Lancet, *2*:1282, 1975.
Brickley-Parsons, D., Glimcher, M. J., Smith, R. J.,
Albin, R., and Adams, J. P.: Biochemical changes in
the collagen of the palmar fascia in patients with
Dupuytren's disease. J. Bone Joint Surg., *63A*:787,
1981.
Brody, G. S., Peng, S. T. J., and Lawdel, R. F.: The
etiology of hypertrophic scar contracture: another
view. Plast. Reconstr. Surg., *67*:673, 1981.
Chiu, H. F., and McFarlane, R. M.: Pathogenesis of
Dupuytren's contracture: a correlative clinical-patho-
logical study. J. Hand Surg., *3*:1, 1978.
Chow, S. P., Luk, K. D. K., and Kung, T. M.: Dupuytren's
contracture in Chinese. A Report of three cases. J. R.
Coll. Surg. Edinb., *29*:49, 1984.
Crisp, A. J., and Heathcote, J. G.: Connective tissue
abnormalities in diabetes mellitus. J. R. Coll. Physi-
cians Lond., *18*:132, 1984.
Critchley, E. M. R., Vakil, S. D., Hayward, H. W., and
Owen, V. M. H.: Dupuytren's disease in epilepsy: result
of prolonged administration of anticonvulsants. J.
Neurol. Neurosurg. Psychiatry, *39*:498, 1976.
Curtis, R. M.: Capsulectomy of the interphalangeal joints
of the fingers. J. Bone Joint Surg., *36A*:1219, 1954.
Delbrück, A., Reimers, E., and Schönborn, I.: A comparative study of the activity of lysosomal and main

metabolic pathway enzymes in tissue biopsies and
cultured fibroblasts from Dupuytren's disease and palmar fascia. On the pathobiochemistry of connective
tissue proliferation, I. J. Clin. Chem. Clin. Biochem.,
19:931, 1981.
Delbrück, A., and Schröder, H.: Metabolism and proliferation of cultured fibroblasts from specimens of human palmar fascia and Dupuytren's contracture. The
pathobiochemistry of connective tissue proliferation,
II. J. Clin. Chem. Clin. Biochem., *21*:11, 1983.
Dupuytren, G.: De la Retraction des doigts par suite
d'une affection de l'apponeurose palmaire. J. Univ.
Med. Chir. Paris., *5*:352, 1831.
Duschoff, I. M.: Personal communication, 1976.
Early, P. F.: Population studies in Dupuytren's contrac-
ture. J. Bone Joint Surg., *44B*:602, 1962.
Egawa, T.: Personal communication, 1983.
Ehrlich, P. H., Brown, H., and White, B. S.: Evidence for
type V and I trimer collagens in Dupuytren's contrac-
ture palmar fascia. Biochem. Med., *28*:273, 1982.
Enzinger, F. M., and Weiss, S. W.: Fibromatosis. *In* Soft
Tissue Tumors. St. Louis, C.V. Mosby Company, 1983,
p. 45.
Flint, M. H.: Personal communication, 1985.
Flint, M. H., Gillard, G. C., and Reilly, C.: The glycos-
aminoglycans of Dupuytren's disease. Connect. Tissue
Res., *9*:173, 1982.
Gabbiani, G., Chaponnier, C., and Huttner, I.: Cyto-
plasmic filaments and gap junctions in epithelial cells
and myofibroblasts during wound healing. J. Cell Biol.,
76:561, 1978.
Gabbiani, G., and Majno, G.: Dupuytren's contracture:
fibroblast contraction? Am. J. Pathol., *66*:131, 1972.
Gelberman, R. H., Amiel, D., Rudolph, M. R., and Vance,
R. M.: Dupuytren's contracture. An electron microscopic, biochemical, and clinical correlative study. J.
Bone Joint Surg., *62A*:425, 1980.
Gonzalez, R. I.: Dupuytren's contracture of the fingers: a
simplified approach to the surgical treatment. Calif.
Med., *115*:25, 1971.
Ham, A. W., and Cormack, D. H.: The Origins, morphol-
ogies and functions (including immunological functions) of the cells of loose connective tissue. *In* Histol-
ogy. 8th Ed. Philadelphia, J.B. Lippincott Company,
1979, p. 225.
Hamamoto, H., Ueba, Y., Sudo, Y., Sanada, H. Yama-
muro, T., and Takeda, T.: Dupuytren's contracture:
morphological and biochemical changes in palmar fas-
cia. Hand, *14*:237, 1982.
Hanyu, T., Tajima, T., Takagi, T., Sasaki, S., Fujimoto,
D., et al.: Biochemical studies on the collagen of the
palmar aponeurosis affected with Dupuytren's disease.
Tohoku J. Exp. Med., *142*:437, 1984.
Houghton, S., Holdstock, G., Cockerell, R., and Wright,
R.: Dupuytren's contracture, chronic liver disease and
IgA immune complexes. Liver, *3*:220, 1983.
Hueston, J. T.: Dupuytren's contracture and specific
injury. Med. J. Aust., *1*:1084, 1968.
Hueston, J. T.: Dupuytren's contracture. *In* Flynn, J. E.
(Ed.): Hand Surgery. 3rd Ed. Baltimore, Williams &
Wilkins Company, 1982a, p. 797.
Hueston, J. T.: Dorsal Dupuytren's disease. J. Hand
Surg., *7*:384, 1982b.
Hueston, J. T.: Some observations on knuckle pads. J.
Hand Surg., *9B*:75, 1984.
Hunter, J. A. A., and Ogdon, C.: Dupuytren's contracture
II—scanning electron microscope observations. Br. J.
Plast. Surg., *28*:19, 1975.

Jung, Y., Hohmann, T. C., Gerneth, J. A., Novak, J., Wasserman, R. C., et al.: Diabetic hand syndrome. Metabolism, 20:1008, 1971.

Kischer, C. W., and Speer, D. P.: Microvascular changes in Dupuytren's contracture. J. Hand Surg., 9A:58, 1984.

Lagier, R., and Meinecke, R.: Pathology of "knuckle pads." A study of four cases. Virchows Arch. [Pathol. Anat.], 365:185, 1975.

Larsen, R. D., Takagishi, N., and Posch, J. L.: The pathogenesis of Dupuytren's contracture. J. Bone Joint Surg., 42A:993, 1960.

Law, P., and McGrouther, D. A.: The dorsal wrinkle ligaments of the proximal interphalangeal joint. J. Hand Surg., 9B:271, 1984.

Lawson, P. M., Maneschi, F., and Kohner E. M.: The relationship of hand abnormalities to diabetes and diabetic retinopathy. Diabetes Care, 6:140, 1983.

Ledderhose, G.: Zur Pathologie der Aponeurose des Fusses und der Hand. Arch. Klin. Chir., 55:694, 1897.

Legge, J. W. H., Finley, J. B., and McFarlane, R. M.: A study of Dupuytren's tissue with the scanning electron microscope. J. Hand Surg., 5:482, 1981.

Ling, R. S. M.: The genetic factors in Dupuytren's disease. J. Bone Joint Surg., 45B:709, 1963.

Lubahn, J. D., Lister, G. D., and Wolfe, T.: Fasciectomy and Dupuytren's disease. A comparison between the open palm technique and wound closure. J. Hand Surg., 9A:53, 1984.

Luck, V. J.: Dupuytren's contracture. J. Bone Joint Surg., 41A:635, 1959.

MacCallum, P., and Hueston, J. T.: The pathology of Dupuytren's contracture. Aust. N.Z. J. Surg., 31:2, 1962.

Majno, G., Gabbiani, G., Hirschel, B. J., Ryan, G. B., and Stratkov, R. R.: Contraction of granulation tissue in vitro. Science 173:548, 1971.

Matthews, P.: Familial Dupuytren's contracture with predominantly female expression. Br. J. Plast. Surg., 32:120, 1979.

McCash, C. R.: The open palm technique in Dupuytren's contracture. Br. J. Plast. Surg., 17:271, 1964.

McFarlane, R. M.: Patterns of the diseased fascia in the fingers in Dupuytren's contracture. Displacement of the neurovascular bundle. Plast. Reconstr. Surg., 54:31, 1974.

McFarlane, R. M.: The anatomy of Dupuytren's disease. Bull. Hosp. J. Dis. Orthop. Inst., 44:318, 1984.

McFarlane, R. M.: Unpublished Data from the Dupuytren's Disease Committee of the International Federation of Societies for Surgery of the Hand, 1985.

McFarlane, R. M., and Albion, U.: Dupuytren's disease. In Hunter, J. M., Schneider, L., Mackin, E., and Callahan, B. (Eds.): Rehabilitation of the Hand. 2nd Ed. St. Louis, C.V. Mosby Company, 1984, p. 617.

McGrouther, D. A.: The microanatomy of Dupuytren's contracture. Hand, 14:215, 1982.

McIndoe, A., and Beare, R. L. B.: Dupuytren's contracture. Am. J. Surg., 95:2, 1958.

Meister, P., Gokel, J. M., and Remberger, K.: Palmar fibromatosis—"Dupuytren's contracture." A comparison of light electron and immunofluorescence microscopic findings. Pathol. Res. Pract., 164:402, 1979.

Mennen, U., and Gräbe, R. P.: Dupuyten's contracture in a negro: a case report. J. Hand Surg., 4:451, 1979.

Menzel, E. J., Piza, H., Zielinski, C., Endler, A. T., Steffen, C., and Millesi, H.: Collagen types and anti-collagen—antibodies in Dupuyten's disease. Hand, 11:243, 1979.

Mikkelsen, O. A.: The prevalence of Dupuytren's disease in Norway. Acta. Chir. Scand., 138:695, 1972.

Mikkelsen, O. A.: Dupuytren's disease—the influence of occupation and previous hand injuries. Hand, 10:1, 1978.

Noble, J., and Harrison, D. H.: Open palm technique for Dupuytren's contracture. Hand, 8:272, 1976.

Noble, J., Heathcote, J. G., and Cohen, H.: Diabetes mellitus in the aetiology of Dupuytren's disease. J. Bone Joint Surg., 66B:322, 1984.

Nyberg, L. M., Jr., Bias, W. B., Hochberg, M. C., and Walsh, P. C.: Identification of an inherited form of Peyronie's disease with autosomal dominant inheritance and association and Dupuytren's contracture and histocompatibility B7 cross reacting antigens. J. Urol., 128:48, 1982.

Parsons, D., Adams, S., Smith, R., and Glimcher, M. J.: Collagen polymorphism in Dupuytren's disease. Abstr., Arth. Res. Society, Jan., 1985.

Pojer, J. Radivojevic, M., and Williams, T. F.: Dupuytren's disease. Its association with abnormal liver function in alcoholism and epilepsy. Arch. Intern. Med., 129:561, 1972.

Ravid, M., Dinai, Y., and Sohar, E.: Dupuytren's disease in diabetes mellitus. Acta Diabetol. Lat., 14:170, 1977.

Rosenbloom, A. L.: Skeletal and joint manifestations of childhood diabetes. Pediatr. Clin. North Am., 31:569, 1984.

Rowley, D. I., Couch, M., Chesney, R. B., and Norris, S. H.: Assessment of percutaneous faciotomy in the management of Dupuytren's contracture. J. Hand Surg., 9B:163, 1984.

Rudolph, R., Guber, S., Suzuki, M., and Woodward, M.: The life cycle of the myofibroblast. Surg. Gynecol. Obstet., 145:389, 1977.

Ryan, G. B., Cliff, W. J., Gabbiani, G., Irle, C., Montandon, D., et al.: Myofibroblasts in human granulation tissue. Hum. Pathol., 5:55, 1974.

Sabiston, D. W.: Cataracts, Dupuytren's contracture, and alcohol addiction. Am. J. Ophthalmol., 76:1005, 1973.

Salamon, A., and Hamori, J.: Possible role of myofibroblasts in the pathogenesis of Dupuytren's contracture. Acta Morphol. Acad. Sci. Hung., 28:71, 1980.

Seemayer, T. A., Lagace, R., Schurch, W., and Thelmo, W. L.: The myofibroblast: biologic, pathologic, and theoretical considerations. Pathol. Annu. 15:443, 1980.

Sergovich, F. R., Botz, J. S., and McFarlane, R. M.: Nonrandom cytogenetic abnormalities in Dupuytren's disease. N. Engl. J. Med., 308:162, 1983.

Skoog, T.: Dupuytren's contracture: pathogenesis and surgical treatment. In Hueston, J. T., and Tubiana, R. (Eds.): Dupuytren's Contracture. Edinburgh & London, Churchill Livingstone, 1974, p. 433.

Slack, C., Flint, M. H., and Thompson, B. M.: Glycosaminoglycan synthesis by Dupuytren's cells in culture. Connect. Tissue Res., 9:263, 1982.

Stack, G. H.: The Palmar Fascia. Edinburgh & London, Churchill Livingstone, 1973.

Su, C. K., and Patek, A. J., Jr.: Dupuytren's contracture. Its association with alcoholism and cirrhosis. Arch. Intern. Med., 126:278, 1970.

Thomine, J. M.: The development and anatomy of the digital fascia. In Hueston, J. T., and Tubiana, R. (Eds.): Dupuytren's Disease. Edinburgh & London, Churchill Livingstone, 1974, p. 1.

Tonkin, M. A., Burke, F. D., and Varian, J. P. W.: Dupuytren's contracture: a comparative study of fasciectomy and dermofasciectomy in one hundred patients. J. Hand Surg., *9B*:156, 1984.

Tubiana, R., and Defrenne, H.: Les localisations de la maladie de Dupuytren a la partie radiale de la main. Chirurgie, *102*:989, 1976.

Watson, J. D.: Fasciotomy and Z-plasty in the management of Dupuytren's contracture. Br. J. Plast. Surg., *37*:27, 1984.

Watson, H. K., Light, T. R., and Johnson, T. R.: Checkrein resection for flexion contracture of the middle joint. J. Hand Surg., *4*:67, 1979.

Windsor, J.: Permanent contraction of the fingers. Lancet, *2*:501, 1834.

Thumb Soft Tissue Injury Management

COMMON MINOR INJURIES

VOLAR SKIN TRANSFERS
    V-Y Advancement Flap
    Volar Advancement Flap
    Neurovascular Island Flap

DORSAL SKIN TRANSFERS
    Heterodigital
        Noninnervated
        Innervated (dependent on juncture between flap
            nerve and thumb nerve)
        Innervated (dependent on radial nerve translocation)
    Homodigital
        Noninnervated
        Innervated

Minor thumb injuries require no special treatment in comparison to the other digits. However, unique methods may be called for in managing more serious volar soft tissue and distal amputation injuries because of the thumb's important role in hand function. The general management of fingertip injuries is dealt with extensively elsewhere in this book and only briefly here. The indications, technical points, and results of the methods most indicated for serious thumb injuries are the primary focus of this chapter.

COMMON MINOR INJURIES

Although few injuries seem minor to those who sustain them, this term may be used to indicate simple and complex lacerations without tissue loss as well as skin loss without significant damage to pulp, bone, or nail bed. Careful repair of even very extensive lacerations often yields gratifying results (Fig. 122–1).

When volar skin loss has occurred, one must be sure that adequate pulp remains to pad the bone. If pulp loss is not excessive, the treatment choice lies between healing by secondary intention and skin grafting. As a general rule, wounds comprising up to 20 per cent of the volar surface distal to the interphalangeal joint crease may be allowed to heal by contraction and epithelization. Surprisingly large wounds heal relatively fast in this manner and the patient gains by the simplicity of the method, the rapid return to work, and a good final result (Fig. 122–2).

Skin grafting is used for larger wounds. A hairless full-thickness skin graft from the groin area is often preferred. The donor wound can be closed primarily and is in an inconspicuous location. In addition to defatting the graft, a variable amount of the dermis can be taken as well. Thus, the graft can be left as full thickness or converted to thick or thin split thickness as desired. It is immobilized with a tie-over bolster dressing. In blacks, Hispanics, and patients with dark complexions in general, there may be a severe color mismatch between the groin graft and the surrounding pink volar skin, yielding a poor esthetic result (Fig. 122–3). Defects in these patients may be covered with a split-thickness graft from the hypothenar eminence: this provides durable skin coverage with an excellent color match, and results in minimal scarring and no significant morbidity at the donor site (Fig. 122–4). Plantar skin may also be used in patients with an adequate arch (Fig. 122–5). There is much less reliable graft survival when amputated

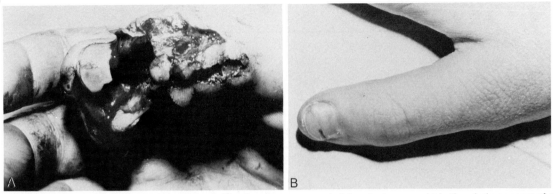

Figure 122–1. Complex thumb laceration. *A,* The thumb was severely injured when caught in the chain support of a swing from which the child fell. Although badly lacerated, no tissue was lost. *B,* Result several months after the distal phalangeal fracture was reduced and the soft tissue wounds were carefully repaired.

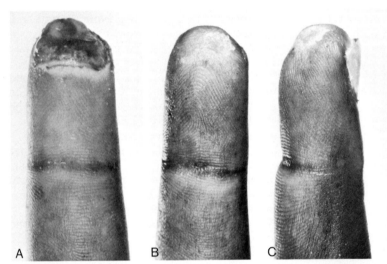

Figure 122–2. Healing by secondary intention. *A,* Open fingertip injury in a 60 year old patient. *B, C,* Six weeks later without surgical intervention.

Figure 122–3. Poor skin graft color match and inadequate padding mar this fingertip reconstruction done at an industrial medicine clinic. The graft was replaced with a thenar flap.

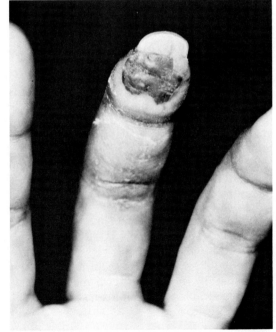

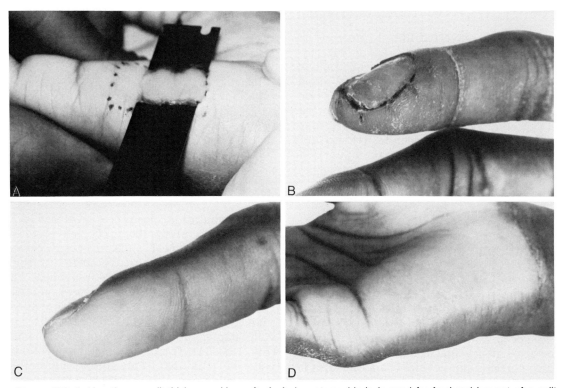

Figure 122–4. Hypothenar split-thickness skin graft. *A,* A dermatome blade is used for freehand harvest of a split-thickness graft of palmar skin from the hypothenar eminence. *B,* Grafted fingertip at six weeks. *C,* The same fingertip at four months. *D,* Donor site at four months.

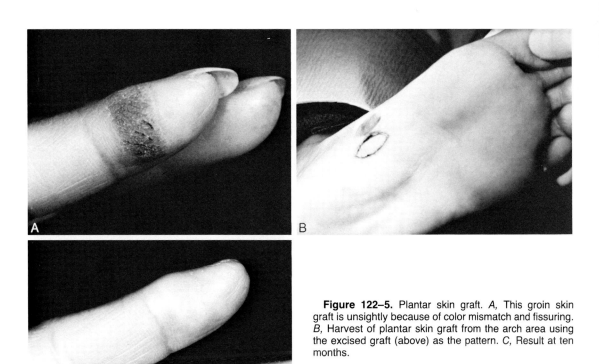

Figure 122–5. Plantar skin graft. *A,* This groin skin graft is unsightly because of color mismatch and fissuring. *B,* Harvest of plantar skin graft from the arch area using the excised graft (above) as the pattern. *C,* Result at ten months.

volar skin is converted into a graft and returned to the injury site.

As mentioned above, more severe injuries with loss of pulp substance and distal amputations often call for more complex flap reconstructive procedures. There should be clear and specific reasons for choosing one of these methods, as they add complexity and may compound the morbidity from the injury. The relevant methods are discussed below.

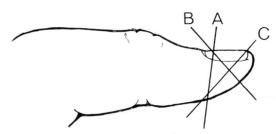

Figure 122–6. The angle of amputation is important in choosing a method of repair. *A, B,* and *C* represent different amputation injuries.

VOLAR SKIN TRANSFERS

V-Y Advancement Flap

This method allows certain tip amputations to be closed without further shortening the injured digit. This distal shift of volar tissues may be done as a flap from either side (Kutler, 1947) or as a large single flap from the volar surface (Atasoy and colleagues, 1970). The Kutler technique is often appropriate for transverse amputations (Fig. 122–6, *Line A*). The skin and soft tissue that might otherwise be excised as a "dog-ear" in a simple trans-

verse amputation closure is advanced over the tip. This allows bone shortening to be minimized. The most important design caveat is to not make the flaps too small. Atasoy's volar flap is used much more frequently. For the volar V-Y advancement flap to be effective the volar skin edge should be more distal than the dorsal one (Fig. 122–6, *Line B*). The volar flap should be of generous dimensions (Fig. 122–7A). The body of the flap should be wide, but the distal end at the amputation site should narrow to about nail width so that the reconstructed tip tapers normally and is not too boxy. In the typical distal tip ampu-

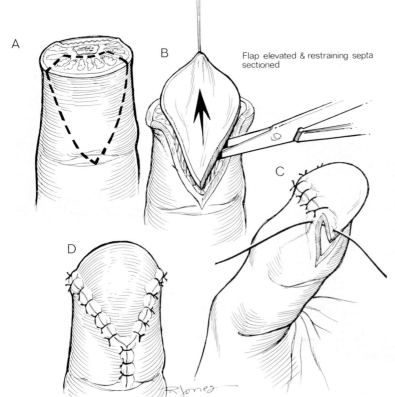

Flap elevated & restraining septa sectioned

Figure 122–7. V-Y advancement flap. *A,* The flap dimensions should be generous though not unduly wide distally. *B,* Ginger flap mobilization using fine scissor tips to section the restraining fibrous bands. *C,* Offset suturing of the flap to the wound edge helps draw the flap distally. *D,* Immediate result.

tation the proximal end of the flap (the bottom of the V) usually comes to the interphalangeal joint crease.

Tourniquet control and loupe magnification are used during the dissection of this flap. The deep plane between the subcutaneous tissue and the distal phalanx or tendon sheath is cleared. The skin is incised and the subcutaneous tissues are exposed. Gentle distal traction is exerted on the flap so as to pull taut the restraining fibrous septa. Fine scissors are used to feel and then section these bands one by one (Fig. 122–7B). The flap is thus progressively mobilized until it advances easily. Extensive freeing of the flap is preferable to forcibly dragging an unwilling, incompletely dissected flap into place. As the flap is sewn into its new position the sutures along the side are angled so as to pull the

flap out distally with each stitch (Fig. 122–7C). Good circulation throughout the flap should be present when the tourniquet is released. A stitch or two may have to be removed if severe blanching is present. A bulky soft dressing is adequate to protect the reconstructed fingertip (Fig. 122–7D). A clinical example is shown in Figure 122–8.

The results obtained with this method are generally excellent. The reconstructed fingertip has close to normal sensibility, a good contour, fine scars, and perfect color match. Careful testing reveals these flaps to be slightly hypoesthetic and, on application of firm pressure, often mildly dysesthetic. This technique, however, has stood the test of widespread use over a number of years and has become quite popular.

Some variations on the indications and flap

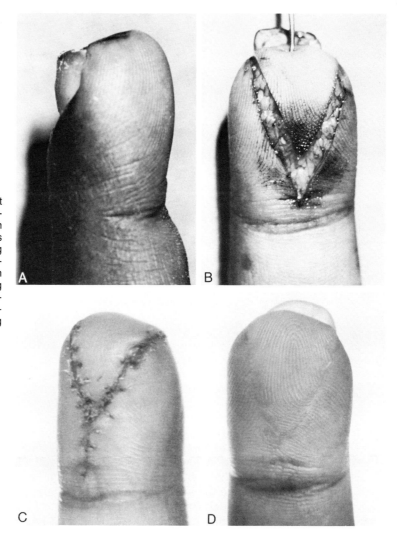

Figure 122–8. V-Y advancement flap—clinical case. A, Old tender fingertip amputation covered with an unsightly graft. The volar edge is longer than the dorsal edge, making this a favorable case for a V-Y advancement flap. B, The flap has been mobilized and advanced. C, Healing wounds show the degree of flap advancement. The relatively narrow distal end keeps the tip from looking squared off. D, Result at one year.

A   B

C   D

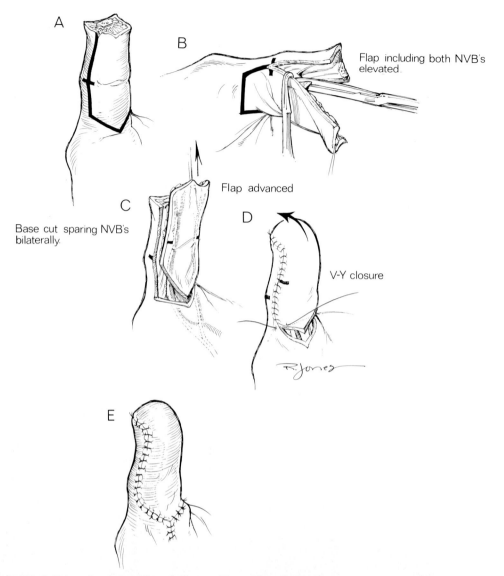

Figure 122–9. Volar advancement flap. *A,* Flap markings. Bilateral midaxial line incisions will be joined as a "V" at the base. The crosshatch serves to demonstrate the degree of advancement. *B,* Elevation of the flap to include all tissues volar to the phalanges and flexor tendon sheath. *C,* The base cut allows further flap advancement. The neurovascular bundles (NVB's) are spared. *D,* Wound closure. *E,* Immediate result.

design are occasionally appropriate. For instance, off-center defects can be treated with flaps that are offset. Also, a large, single, laterally placed V-Y advancement flap can be used for resurfacing oblique amputation injuries (Venkatasvoami and Subramanian, 1980; Shepard, 1983). The triangle used here has three unequal sides, unlike the isosceles triangle employed by the Atasoy method. Occasionally, a pair of these large lateral flaps can be used to manage the volar oblique injury with pulp loss in which the usual V-Y technique does not have a place.

Volar Advancement Flap

This method involves elevation and distal shifting of all the thumb's volar soft tissues superficial to the flexor tendon sheath (Moberg, 1964; Snow, 1967; Keim and Grantham, 1969; Posner and Smith, 1971; Millender, Albin, and Nalebuff, 1973). It is extremely useful for covering amputation injuries of the distal thumb (see Fig. 122–6, *Line A*) without having to further shorten the skeleton.

A midaxial incision is made on either side

of the thumb from the amputation site to the proximal portion of the proximal phalanx (Fig. 122–9). Cleland's ligaments are incised, and the dissection is carried across the thumb dorsal to the neurovascular bundles and superficial to the flexor tendon sheath. All of the skin and subcutaneous tissues and both neurovascular bundles are included in the flap. Several options are available for handling the flap base (Fig. 122–10). It can be left intact if the flap can be adequately advanced. Added advancement can be gained by cutting the base of the flap transversely, sparing the neurovascular bundles. A full-thickness skin graft is used to fill the proximal defect (O'Brien, 1968). Bilateral Z-plasties at the proximal portions of the midlateral incisions have also been recommended (House, 1982; Chase, 1984). This would seem to lengthen the flap laterally but still leave the central portion tethered. A V-Y method at the flap base is quite effective. The base of the flap is cut near the metacarpophalangeal joint in a V-shape, the flap is advanced, and the secondary defect is closed in a Y-fashion. This technique gives good distal advancement yet obviates the need for a graft on the anterior thumb surface. After the volar flap is advanced and sewn into its new location, the interphalangeal joint is splinted in flexion, occasionally with the help of a transarticular Kirschner wire. After ten days the splint and wire are removed and the patient then gently works the joint back to full range of motion. The ability to hyperextend the interphalangeal joint may be lost. A clinical example is shown in Figure 122–11.

Excellent results can be obtained with this technique. Sensation is essentially normal and there are no scars on the volar pad of the thumbtip. Some late observations of these flaps are relevant: (1) release of all volar soft tissue attachments results in poor fixation of these tissues to the underlying skeleton, so that there is abnormal sliding of the soft tissues on firm pinch; (2) the closure may seem somewhat tight initially, but after a year or so the tissues may loosen and require secondary tailoring; (3) the distal flap should be shaped to avoid a "squared-off" tip; and (4) bits of germinal nail bed can be buried and subsequently form subcutaneous cysts. These cysts and nail remnants may be difficult to eradicate.

Two modifications of the basic method are worth noting. An "extended palmar advancement flap" has been described (Dellon, 1983) that is carried across the metacarpophalangeal joint crease and down the thenar eminence to a point near the midpalm. Subsidiary flaps are used to fill gaps that develop on either side when the main flap is advanced. Although this advancement can be prodigious (up to 3 cm), significantly more dissection is necessary to achieve it. Second, when this flap was adapted for use in the fingers, a certain incidence of dorsal skin necrosis was noted (Nicoletis and Morel-Fatio, 1969; Shaw, 1971). This was due to the sectioning of vessels running from the volar surface to the dorsal skin during flap mobilization. This problem can be obviated by carefully preserving these vessels during the dissection (Macht and Watson, 1980). Although skin necrosis has not been a problem in the thumb, where most of the dorsal blood supply is longitudinally oriented, bridging vessels should be preserved when possible.

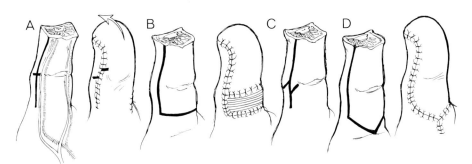

Figure 122–10. Methods of treating the base of the volar advancement flap. *A,* The base may simply be left intact. *B,* A transverse cut sparing the neurovascular bundles with full-thickness graft to the resulting defect. *C,* Bilateral lengthening Z-plasties placed in the midaxial incisions. *D,* V-Y advancement method.

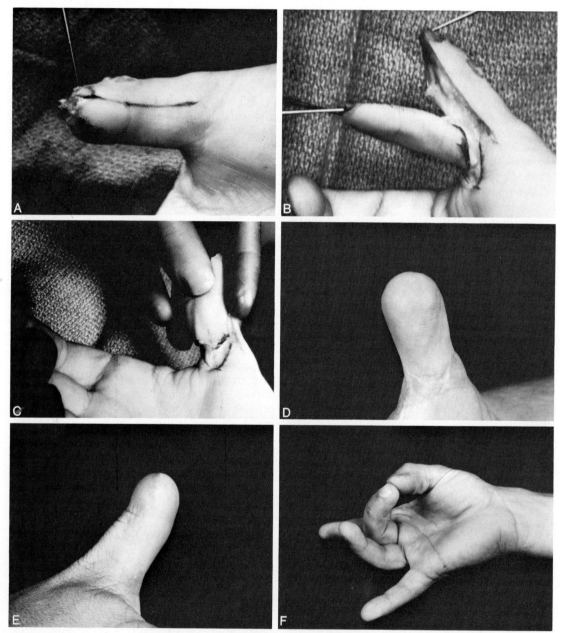

Figure 122–11. Volar advancement flap—clinical case. *A,* A distal transverse thumbtip amputation with exposed bone. *B,* The flap elevated with "V" cut to the base. *C,* The flap can easily be advanced distally. *D, E, F,* Result at three years with an intervening minor revision.

Neurovascular Island Flap

In this procedure (Moberg, 1955; Littler, 1960; Tubiana and DuParc, 1961), volar tissues from another digit are raised as an island flap on a neurovascular pedicle and passed subcutaneously across the palm to resurface all or a portion of the volar thumb. The volar skin coverage thus provided is well vascularized, innervated, and padded. In most cases the donor defect is closed with a full-thickness skin graft. Occasionally, when a small flap is used, the defect may be closed primarily. Success with this procedure demands rigorous attention to detail in design, execution, and aftercare and is not for the occasional hand surgeon.

There are three main indications for use of this flap: (1) for severe pulp defects in which skeletal length is to be maintained and sensibility is critical—it can be used acutely, but more commonly is chosen as a secondary procedure; (2) to provide a sensate working surface to complete an osteoplastic thumb reconstruction, i.e., for thumbs reconstructed by a bone graft covered with an abdominal or groin flap; and (3) to provide thumb sensation in hands suffering from irreparable median nerve lesions.

The ulnar, i.e., noncontact, aspect of the middle finger is usually chosen as the flap donor site (Fig. 122–12). Use of the long finger increases the flap's pedicle length and therefore its arc of rotation. This allows an easier reach to the thumb with less tension on the pedicle. Keeping within the median nerve territory also may make sensory reeducation and cortical reorientation easier for the patient. In cases of irreparable median nerve damage, the ulnar side of the ring finger (ulnar nerve distribution) should be chosen as the donor site. An Allen test should be performed on the donor and ring digits to confirm patency of all digital arteries.

A pattern of the defect is made to aid in planning the flap. In an acute injury, some allowance should be made for the natural gaping of the wound by designing the flap somewhat smaller than the defect. The distal end of the flap should be about 1.5 cm past the distal interphalangeal joint crease, thereby sparing the very tip of the donor digit. The width of the flap should fall between the confines of the volar midline and the lateral midline of the digit. The proximal edge of the flap typically falls somewhere over the middle phalanx. Generous darts should be used at joint creases to break up the straight lines of the flap donor defect and thereby lessen the possibility of a flexion contracture. A midlateral incision is used proximally to the web and then continued in a zigzag fashion to the midpalm.

In secondary reconstructive procedures the volar thumb skin or scar to be replaced is outlined but not removed until the flap has been elevated and its circulation judged to be adequate. The flap is elevated to include all the tissues volar to the flexor tendon sheath, including the neurovascular bundle, which is ligated at the distal margin of the flap. At the proximal edge of the flap the neurovascular pedicle is identified and traced into the midpalm. The radial proper digital artery to the ring finger is ligated and the epineurium of the common digital nerve is incised, thus allowing that nerve to be split proximally. The vascular pedicle and the nerve are freed to the level of the superficial palmar arch. Once it is ascertained that the pedicle is of sufficient length to reach the thumb defect without tension, a subcutaneous tunnel is made from the midpalm to the thumb defect. The tourniquet is released and hemostasis is obtained. If flap circulation appears satisfactory, the thumb defect is made and the flap is passed to it through the subcutaneous tunnel. The flap should be handled gently. If difficulty is experienced in passing the flap, the tunnel must be widened, or a counterincision made along its course, or the entire path may be opened. The flap is sewn loosely into the defect. Its circulation at this point often appears somewhat congested. The other wounds are closed and a full-thickness skin graft is sutured to the donor defect and held in place with a tie-over bolster. As mentioned, in some small flaps, primary closure of the donor site may be an option. Figure 122–13 shows a clinical case.

This flap is well padded and has good vascularity. However, opinions are mixed on the quality of the sensory results. The major issues are the maintenance of sensory acuity (typically measured by two-point discrimination), the development of hyperesthesia, and the ability to achieve cortical reorientation so that stimulation of the flap is perceived as arising from the thumb rather than the donor finger.

Sensory Acuity and Hyperesthesia. Tubiana and DuParc (1961), in their original

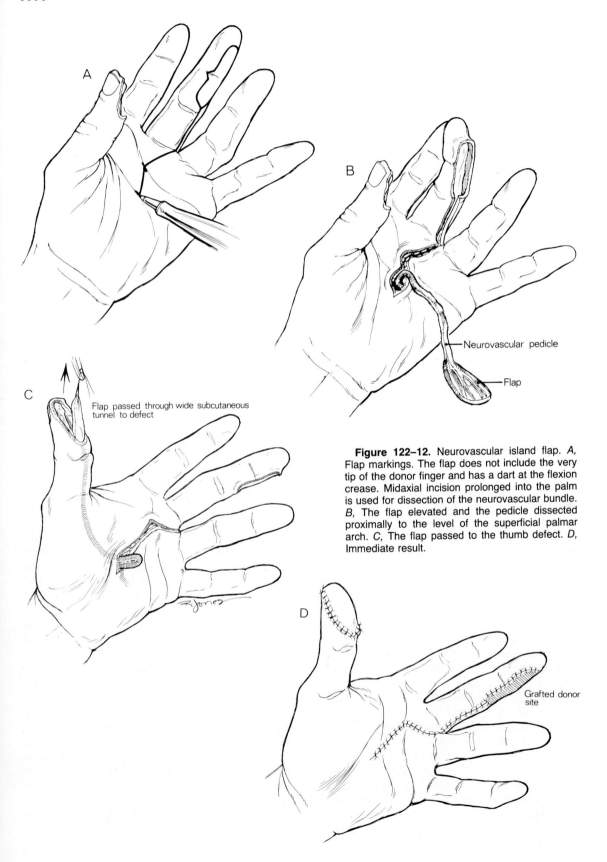

Figure 122–12. Neurovascular island flap. *A,* Flap markings. The flap does not include the very tip of the donor finger and has a dart at the flexion crease. Midaxial incision prolonged into the palm is used for dissection of the neurovascular bundle. *B,* The flap elevated and the pedicle dissected proximally to the level of the superficial palmar arch. *C,* The flap passed to the thumb defect. *D,* Immediate result.

A

B

Neurovascular pedicle

Flap

C

Flap passed through wide subcutaneous tunnel to defect

D

Grafted donor site

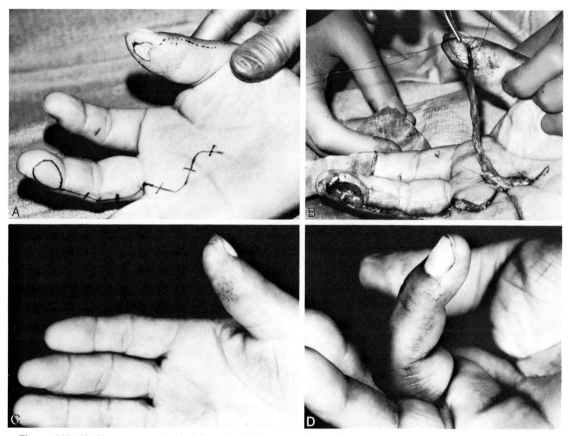

Figure 122–13. Neurovascular island flap—clinical case. *A,* A relatively small flap designed on the middle finger to replace skin and pulp destroyed over the volar thumbtip by a high pressure injection injury. Proximal tissue was not damaged sufficiently to warrant replacement but was unsuitable for advancement. B, The flap elevated and the pedicle dissected to the superficial palmar arch. *C,* Result at six months. Cortical reorientation had not occurred. *D,* The donor area closed without a graft (which is unusual).

paper on the method, and Chase (1971), in a symposium discussion, reported excellent results. Reid (1966), Murray, Ord, and Gavelin (1967), McGregor (1969), Omer and associates (1970), and Krag and Rasmussen (1975) have all presented patient series in which sensory problems such as hyperesthesia or progressive hypoesthesia with loss of meaningful two-point discrimination have predominated. Markley (1977) proposed two solutions to help counteract these problems. First, take the flap from the donor finger as distally as possible. This allows one to start with the most sensate skin, and also gives a longer pedicle and therefore less tension on the nerve after flap transfer. Second, make a continuous incision from the midpalm to the thumb and lay the neurovascular bundle in it rather than passing it through a tunnel. This method is designed to avoid unrecognized kinking and tension on the pedicle. Most surgeons seem to prefer the tunnel.

Cortical Reorientation. Very few patients appear to reorient the source of stimulation from the donor finger to the thumb. Peacock (1971) was not convinced that any make the reorientation, and Chase (1971) thought that those who did would convert back under stress. In a group of 15 patients (Murray, Ord, and Gavelin, 1967), only four—the youngest and most intelligent—reoriented after periods ranging from one and one-half to eight years after the surgery. A possible solution to this problem (in patients other

than those being treated for irreparable median nerve injury) would be to section the flap's nerve and join it to the severed end of a thumb digital nerve. Doing this at the time of flap transfer could be hazardous to the flap's circulation. However, even as a secondary procedure one exchanges the problem of cortical reorientation for the unpredictable sensory return following nerve repair.

The bolster is removed from the donor finger skin graft a week after surgery, and gentle motion and physical therapy are begun. The harvest of a large flap inflicts an injury on that digit which can result in permanent stiffness and disabilty. The patient, surgeon, and therapist must be persistent in their efforts to regain full motion in that finger.

DORSAL SKIN TRANSFERS

There are a host of flap transfers in which dorsal skin of either the same or another digit is moved to the volar surface of the thumb. Some are innervated and some are not. A classification of these flaps follows.

Heterodigital

NONINNERVATED

Cross Finger Flap (Fig. 122–14). This flap has proved a reliable option for digital resur-

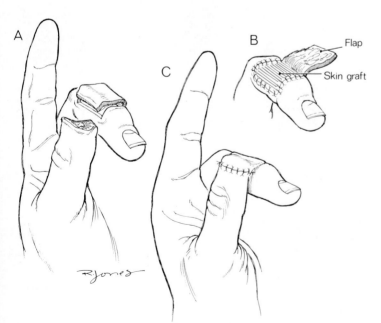

Figure 122–14. Cross finger flap. *A,* The flap elevated from the middle finger for coverage of a thumbtip amputation defect. *B,* A full-thickness graft used for the flap donor site. *C,* The flap sewn in place. Tape will be used to maintain apposition of the digits without tension on the flap.

facing (Gurdin and Pangman, 1950; Cronin, 1951; Curtis, 1957; Hoskins, 1960). Its greatest use is for injuries in which pulp loss predominates (Fig. 122–6, *Line C*).

The dorsal aspect of the middle phalanx of the long or ring fingers is the usual donor site for coverage of thumbtip defects. For larger pulp losses, the dorsal aspect of the index finger proximal phalanx can provide abundant tissue. The flap should be planned with a pattern that comfortably covers the defect. Typically, most or all of the entire dorsum of the chosen phalanx is used. In the case of the long or ring fingers, the flap generally is hinged on the ulnar midlateral border. In the case of the large index finger flap from over the proximal phalanx, it is hinged on the radial midlateral border of the digit.

The free borders of the flap are incised and the flap is elevated across the dorsum in the plane of the paratenon. A full-thickness skin graft from the groin, secured by a flat bolster, is used to cover the donor defect. After the flap is sewn into place, benzoin is painted on the digits, and multiple strips of narrow adhesive tape are used to stabilize the fingers in apposition. Kirschner wire fixation of the donor and recipient digits is not necessary. Gauze is tucked between the fingers to minimize skin maceration, and a bulky dressing, supplemented with a plaster splint, is applied to the entire hand. Frequent office visits for dressing changes and wound inspection are important in the two to three week period before division of the flap base. At that operation, very little dissection of the flap is done and the inset consists of only a few loosely placed sutures. After flap division, emphasis is placed on regaining full motion in the donor and recipient digits as rapidly as possible.

The cross finger flap is reliable and has a reasonably wide latitude in the details of its design and execution. All dorsal to volar flap transfers suffer functionally and esthetically to some degree because of the innate differences in the skin at the two sites. The esthetic shortcomings are most pronounced in dark-skinned patients because of the marked color contrast with the surrounding volar skin. Sensory return is variable and depends on nerve ingrowth from the bed and margins of the wound. The development of the innervated cross finger flap (described below) has resulted in better sensation and, therefore,

improved function. Color mismatch, slight hollowing, and hypertrophic scarring can occur at the grafted donor site. The donor finger is also prone to residual stiffness because of the immobilization and donor site skin graft. Aggressive physical therapy can minimize this in most cases.

Dorsal Hand to Thumb Flap: Noninnervated. Extensive thumb defects can be resurfaced with a random pattern flap consisting of dorsal hand skin from the space between the first and second metacarpals and based distally at the web space (McFarlane, 1962). The donor site is skin grafted. This noninnervated flap can cover the entire volar thumb. Alternative procedures for these larger defects are distant two-stage pedicle flaps (groin, abdominal, deltopectoral, or arm) or innervated single-stage free flaps (May and associates, 1977; Morrison and associates, 1978).

INNERVATED (DEPENDENT ON JUNCTURE BETWEEN FLAP NERVE AND THUMB NERVE)

Innervated Cross Finger Flap (Fig. 122–15). This technique (Berger and Meissl, 1975; Cohen and Cronin, 1983) is an extension of the basic cross finger flap method and can be used on any of the digits. A dorsal sensory nerve branch from the proper digital nerve innervates the skin over the middle phalanx used for the cross finger flap. Sensory return to the flap is enhanced by bringing this nerve with the flap and joining it to a thumb digital nerve.

When used for thumb defects, the free border of the flap is typically the radial side of the middle segment of the middle finger. The dorsal sensory nerve to the flap is isolated, sectioned proximally, and dissected in continuity with the flap. The end of the transected thumb digital nerve is isolated through a proximal incision at the defect, and joined to the flap nerve with the aid of the operating microscope at the time of flap transfer. Subsequent management and flap division do not differ from that of the standard cross finger flap. Figure 122–16 shows a clinical case.

Sensory return is significantly better in patients treated with this technique than in those treated with standard cross finger flaps. Cortical reorientation is not a problem as the flap nerve is joined to the appropriate recipient nerve.

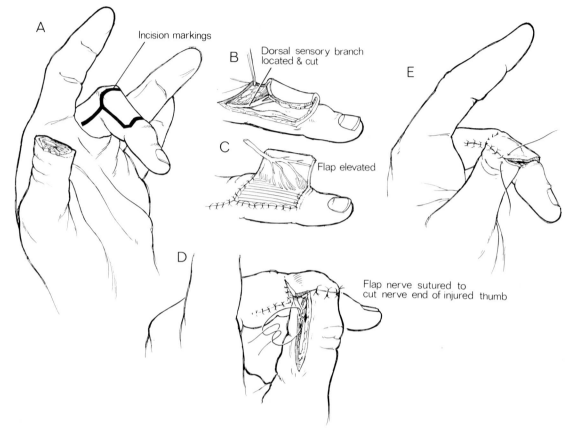

Figure 122–15. Innervated cross finger flap. *A,* Markings are similar to the standard cross finger flap but include a proximal incision for identification of the dorsal sensory nerve branch to the flap. Not visible is a planned short incision on the thumb to identify the distal ulnar digital nerve. *B,* The dorsal sensory nerve is found and a 2 to 3 cm segment is freed to the point that it enters the flap. The digital nerve in the donor finger is not disturbed. *C,* The nerve is sectioned proximally and is elevated with the flap. A skin graft is applied to the flap donor site. *D,* Flap to thumb sutures stabilize the digits as the neurorrhaphy is performed between the flap nerve and the amputated end of the thumb digital nerve. This is done with the aid of an operating microscope. *E,* The flap inset completed.

INNERVATED (DEPENDENT ON RADIAL NERVE TRANSLOCATION)

There are a variety of designs within this group, but all share two common features: they are taken from the dorsum of the proximal phalanx of the index finger, and the innervating radial nerve fibers are left intact and rerouted so as to accompany the flap transfer to the thumb. There are three major variations on this concept.

Flaps with a Permanent Skin Pedicle (Fig. 122–17). Holevich (1963) transposed a racquet-shaped flap in one stage to resurface the tip and a strip along the length of the thumb. The flap carries the underlying radial nerve fibers and vascular supply and thus brings sensate skin along the entire length of the thumb. Its primary use is for osteoplastic thumb reconstruction and irreparable

median nerve lesions. The "flag" flap of Iselin (1973) and Vilain and Dupuis (1973) is much the same flap.

Island Flap (Fig. 122–18). Foucher and Braun (1979) described a "kite" or island flap from the dorsal index finger for coverage of either dorsal or volar thumb defects. The neurovascular pedicle is composed of the first dorsal metacarpal artery, dorsal veins, and radial nerve fibers. The flap was successfully transferred in 12 consecutive cases. The authors were not enthusiastic about the use of this flap for restoration of thumb sensibility. Lesavoy (1980) reported a good result in one case in which this same technique was used. He noted that it would be difficult to reach the tip of a thumb of normal length with this method.

Cross Finger Flap (Fig. 122–19). This flap is hinged on the radial midlateral border of

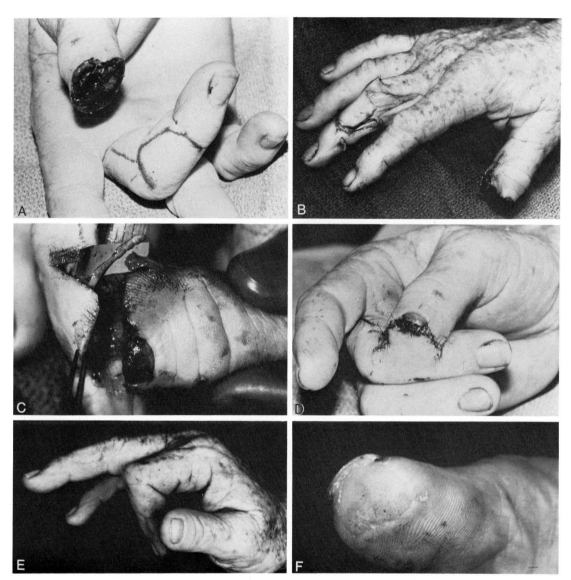

Figure 122–16. Innervated cross finger flap—clinical case. *A,* Incisions are marked for obtaining coverage of a distal volar oblique thumbtip amputation. Note the proximal extension for finding the flap nerve. *B,* The flap and its nerve are dissected. The thumb's ulnar digital nerve is exposed and prepared for junction. *C,* The thumb and flap are brought into apposition. Nerves to be joined lie adjacent to one another. *D,* The nerve junction and flap inset completed. *E, F,* Result at two years. The tip has a good contour and the flap, which has good sensation and is not tender, is calloused from use. (Reproduced by permission from Cohen, B. E., and Cronin, E. D.: An innervated cross finger flap for fingertip reconstruction. Plast. Reconst. Surg., *72*:688, 1983.)

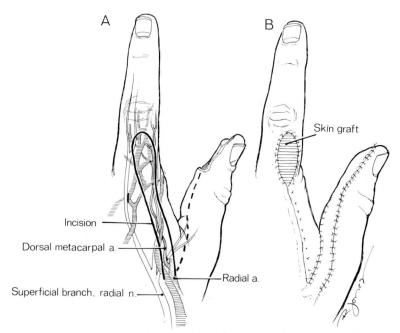

Figure 122–17. Radial innervated dorsal skin flap. *A,* This axial pattern flap carries the underlying vasculature and radial nerve fibers with it to the thumb defect. An incision along the length of the thumb will receive the flap when it is transposed. *B,* The transferred flap creates a sensate strip along the length of the thumb.

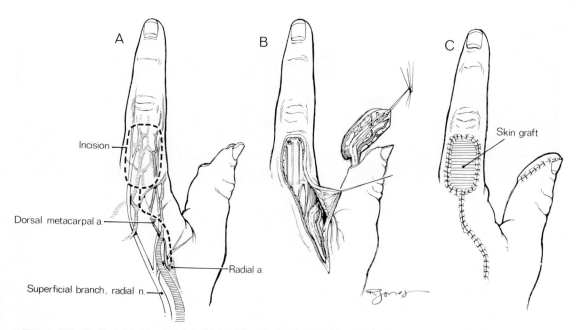

Figure 122–18. Radial innervated dorsal island flap. *A,* A skin island from the dorsal index proximal phalanx is planned. It is supplied by a proximal neurovascular pedicle. *B,* The flap and pedicle are passed subcutaneously to the thumb defect. *C,* The flap sewn in place. A skin graft covers the flap donor defect.

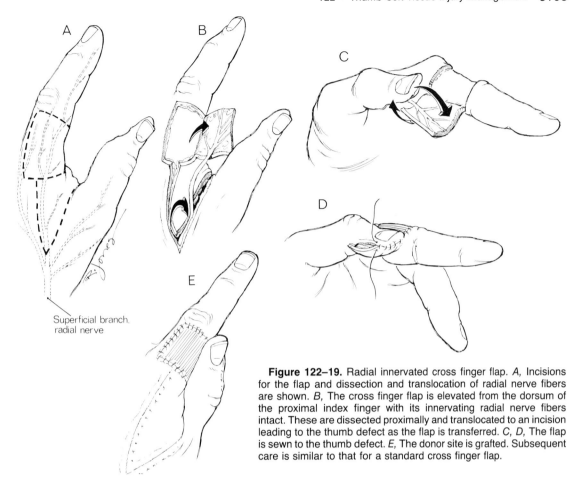

Figure 122–19. Radial innervated cross finger flap. *A,* Incisions for the flap and dissection and translocation of radial nerve fibers are shown. *B,* The cross finger flap is elevated from the dorsum of the proximal index finger with its innervating radial nerve fibers intact. These are dissected proximally and translocated to an incision leading to the thumb defect as the flap is transferred. *C, D,* The flap is sewn to the thumb defect. *E,* The donor site is grafted. Subsequent care is similar to that for a standard cross finger flap.

the index proximal phalanx (Adamson, Horton, and Crawford, 1967; Gaul, 1969; Walker, Hurley, and May, 1986). One stays as proximal as possible to maximize the radial nerve fiber density in the flap. The radial nerve branches entering the flap are identified proximally and transposed via a connecting incision to the thumb. At the second operation the flap base is divided and inset in the usual manner. Bralliar and Horner (1969), employing the same concept, used a proximal base flap and transposed the nerve at the second operation when the flap was divided.

This technique works best for the shortened thumb. It creates problems of cortical reorientation, as does the volar neurovascular island flap, and it has not given a high level of sensory acuity in most cases.

Homodigital

NONINNERVATED

Ogunro (1983) described a dorsal transposition flap for resurfacing oblique thumb amputations (Fig. 122–20). The flap, based on

Figure 122–20. Dorsal thumb flap—noninnervated. *A,* A transversely oriented dorsal thumb flap based near the proximal edge of an oblique thumb amputation is marked. *B,* After flap transfer, an incision is marked for dorsal skin advancement. *C,* The dorsal skin advances to close the flap donor defect. *D,* All wounds closed.

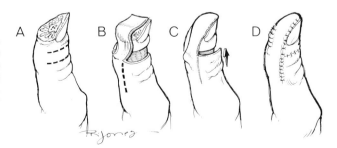

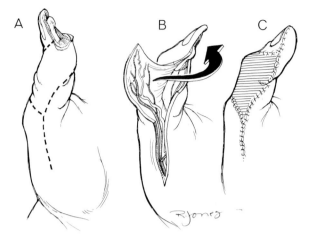

Figure 122–21. Dorsal thumb island flap–innervated. *A,* This flap based on dorsal neurovascular branches from the main bundle is outlined. *B,* The flap is elevated anteriorly, and if circulation is adequate, the incision around the island is completed. *C,* The flap is transferred to the defect. The donor site is grafted.

the side of the amputation and oriented transversely across the dorsal thumb, is rotated through 90 degrees to the wound. The donor defect is closed by dorsal skin advancement or a skin graft.

INNERVATED

Neurovascular branches from the volar to the dorsal aspect of the thumb allow innervated dorsal tissue to be isolated and transferred to the volar aspect of the same digit. Flint and Harrison (1965) used these branches as the basis of a long oblique flap with the skin base intact, which was rotated to the anterior aspect of the same digit. Iselin (1973) proposed a local "flag" flap that could be isolated from the dorsal thumb and used to close an amputation defect of the same digit.

Joshi (1974) and Pho (1979) described dorsal vascularized and innervated skin islands that were moved by a combination of transposition and advancement to cover defects over the radial-volar aspect of the thumb (Fig. 122–21).

All these procedures bring sensate skin to the thumb. Staying within the same digit is both an advantage and a disadvantage. Problems of cortical reorientation should be fewer and other parts of the hand are not immobilized, but use of the same digit as a flap source does inflict additional trauma on an already injured part.

CONCLUSION

Clearly, the thumb is the most important digit of the hand. Because injuries to it impact markedly on the function of the entire extremity, sophisticated reconstructive efforts are distinctly worthwhile. In all cases, the decision to use a particular method should be made with thoughtfulness, and the procedure should be carefully planned and executed.

REFERENCES

Adamson, J. E., Horton, C. E., and Crawford, H. H.: Sensory rehabilitation of the injured thumb. Plast. Reconstr. Surg. *40:*53, 1967.

Atasoy, E., Ioakimidis, E., Kutz, J. E., and Kleinert, H. E.: Reconstruction of the amputated fingertip with a triangular volar flap. J. Bone Surg., *52A:*921, 1970.

Berger, A., and Meissl, G.: Innervated skin grafts and flaps for restoration of sensation to anesthetic areas. Chir. Plast., *3:*33, 1975.

Bralliar, F., and Horner, R. L.: Sensory cross-finger pedicle graft. J. Bone Joint Surg., *51A:*1264, 1969.

Chase, R. A.: Island pedicle gymnastics (discussion). *In* Cramer, L. M., and Chase, R. A. (eds.): Symposium on the Hand. Vol. 2. St. Louis, C. V. Mosby Company, 1971, p. 221.

Chase, R. A.: Skin and soft tissue. *In* Atlas of Hand Surgery. Vol. 2. Philadelphia, W. B. Saunders Company, 1984, p. 15.

Cohen, B. E., and Cronin, E. D.: An innervated cross finger flap for fingertip reconstruction. Plast. Reconstr. Surg., *72:*688, 1983.

Cronin, T. D.: The cross finger flap: a new method of repair. Am. Surg., *17:*419, 1951.

Curtis, R. M.: Cross finger pedicle flaps in hand surgery. Ann. Surg. *145:*650, 1967.

Dellon, A. L.: The extended palmar advancement flap. J. Hand Surg., *8:*190, 1983.

Flint, M. H., and Harrison, S. H.: A local neurovascular flap to repair loss of digital pulp. Br. J. Plast. Surg., *18:*156, 1965.

Foucher, G., and Braun, J. B.: A new island flap transfer from the dorsum of the index to the thumb. Plast. Reconstr. Surg., *63:*344, 1979.

Gaul, J. S.: Radial innervated cross finger flap from index to provide sensory pulp to injured thumb. J. Bone Joint Surg., *51A:*1257, 1969.

Gurdin, M., and Pangman, W. J.: Repair of surface defects of fingers by transdigital flaps. Plast. Reconstr. Surg., 5:368, 1950.

Holevich, J.: A new method of restoring sensibility to the thumb. J. Bone Joint Surg., 45:496, 1963.

Hoskins, H. D.: The versatile cross finger pedicle flap: a report of twenty-six cases. J. Bone Joint Surg., 42A:261, 1960.

House, J. H.: Modification of volar advancement flap. ASSH Newsletter. No. 1982:14, February, 1982.

Iselin, F.: The flag flap. Plast. Reconstr. Surg., 52:374, 1973.

Joshi, B.: A local dorsolateral island flap for restoration of sensation after avulsion injury of fingertip pulp. Plast. Reconstr. Surg., 54:175, 1974.

Keim, H. A., and Grantham, S. A.: Volar flap advancement for thumb and fingertip injuries. Clin. Orthop., 66:109, 1969.

Krag, C., and Rasmussen, K. B.: The neurovascular island flap for defective sensibility. J. Bone Joint Surg., 57:495, 1975.

Kutler, W. : A new method for fingertip amputation. J.A.M.A., 133:29, 1947.

Lesavoy, M. A.: The dorsal index finger neurovascular island flap. Orthop. Rev., 9:91, 1980.

Littler, J. W.: Neurovascular skin island transfer in reconstructive hand surgery. In Transactions of the International Society of Plastic Surgery, Second Congress, London, 1959. London, E. S. Livingstone, 1960, p. 175.

Macht, S. D., and Watson, H. K.: The Moberg volar advancement flap for digital reconstruction. J. Hand Surg., 5:372, 1980.

Markley, J. M.: The preservation of close two-point discrimination in the interdigital transfer of neurovascular island flaps. Plast. Reconstr. Surg., 59:812, 1977.

May, J. W., Chait, L. A., Cohen, B. E., and O'Brien, M. C.: Free neurovascular island flap from the first web of the foot in hand reconstruction. J. Hand Surg., 2:378, 1977.

McFarlane, R. M., and Stromberg, W. B. Jr.: Resurfacing of the thumb following major skin loss. J. Bone Joint Surg., 44A:1364, 1962.

McGregor, I. A.: Less than satisfactory experiences with neurovascular island flaps. Hand, 1:21, 1969.

Millender, L. H., Albin, R. E., and Nalebuff, E. A.: Delayed volar advancement flap for thumb tip injuries. Plast. Reconstr. Surg., 52:635, 1973.

Moberg, E.: Discussion of the place of nerve grafting in orthopaedic surgery, by Donal Brooks. J. Bone Joint Surg., 37A:305, 1955.

Moberg, E.: Aspects of sensation in reconstructive surgery of the upper extremity. J. Bone Joint Surg., 46A:439, 1964.

Morrison, W. A., O'Brien, B. M., McLeod, A. M., and Gilbert, A.: Neurovascular free flaps from the foot for innervation of the hand. J. Hand Surg., 3:235, 1978.

Murray, J. F., Ord, J. V. R., and Gavelin, G. E.: The neurovascular island pedicle flap. J. Bone Joint Surg., 49A:1285, 1967.

Nicoletis, C., and Morel-Fatio, D.: Etranges necroses. Ann. Chir. Plast., 14:56, 1969.

O'Brien, B.: Neurovascular island pedicle flaps for terminal amputations and digital scars. Br. J. Plast. Surg., 21:258, 1968.

Ogunro, O.: Dorsal transposition flap for reconstruction of lateral or medial oblique amputations of the thumb with exposure of bone. J. Hand Surg., 8:894, 1983.

Omer, G. E., Day, D. J., Ratliff, H., and Lambert, P.: Neurovascular cutaneous nerve sensibility. J. Bone Joint Surg., 52:1181, 1970.

Peacock, E. E.: Island pedicle gymnastics (discussion). In Cramer, L. M., and Chase, R. A. (Eds.): Symposium on the Hand. Vol. 2. St. Louis, C. V. Mosby Company, 1971, p. 218.

Pho, R. W. H.: Local composite neurovascular island flap for skin cover in pulp loss of the thumb. J. Hand Surg., 4:11, 1979.

Posner, M. A., and Smith, R. J.: The advancement pedicle for thumb injuries. J. Bone Joint Surg., 53A:1618, 1971.

Reid, D. A. C.: The neurovascular island flap in thumb reconstruction. Br. J. Plast. Surg., 19:234, 1966.

Shaw, M. H.: Neurovascular island pedicled flaps for terminal digital scars—a hazard. Br. J. Plast. Surg., 24:161, 1971.

Shepard, G. H.: The use of lateral V-Y advancement flaps for fingertip reconstruction. J. Hand Surg., 8:254, 1983.

Snow, J. W.: Use of a volar flap for repair of fingertip amputations. Plast. Reconstr. Surg., 40:163, 1967.

Tubiana, R., and DuParc, J.: Restoration of sensibility in the hand by neurovascular skin island transfer. J. Bone Joint Surg., 43B:474, 1961.

Venkatasvoami, R., and Subramanian, N.: Oblique triangular flap: a new method of repair for oblique amputations of the fingertip and thumb. Plast. Reconstr. Surg., 66:296, 1980.

Vilain, R., and Dupuis, J. F.: Use of the flag flap for coverage of a small area on a finger or the palm. Plast. Reconstr. Surg., 51:397, 1973.

Walker, M. A., Hurley, C. B., and May, J. W.: Radial nerve cross-finger flap differential nerve contribution in thumb reconstruction. J. Hand Surg., 11A:881, 1986.

Vincent R. Hentz

Congenital Anomalies of the Thumb

FAILURE OF FORMATION (THUMB APLASIA OR
 HYPOPLASIA)
 Principles of Operative Management

FAILURE OF DIFFERENTIATION (ABNORMALITY OF
 THUMB POSTURE)
 Congenital Trigger Thumb
 Thumb-in-Palm or Clasped Thumb Deformities
 Adducted Thumb
 Abducted Thumb
 Hypoplastic or Absent Thumb

DUPLICATION OF PARTS (PREAXIAL POLYDACTYLY)
 Classification of Thumb Polydactyly
 Principles of Operative Management
 Type 7 (Preaxial Polydactyly—Triphalangeal Thumb)
 High Degrees of Polydactyly ("Mirror Hand")

Those congenital anomalies that most frequently involve the thumb include disorders classified under the first three categories of the system (Swanson, 1976) adopted by the International Federation of Hand Surgery Societies (Table 123–1):

I. Failure of formation of parts.

II. Failure of differentiation of parts.

III. Duplication of parts.

This chapter discusses the presentation and management of the most common thumb disorders within these categories. See Chapter 128 for further congenital thumb disorders.

For most congenital anomalies that involve the thumb, the functional and cosmetic stigma is great. "On the length, strength, and free lateral motion and perfect mobility of the thumb, depends the power of the human hand. The thumb is called pollex because of its strength and that strength is necessary to

the power of the hand being equal to that of all the fingers" (Bell, 1832).

Thumb deformity imposes a proportionally greater functional liability than does deformity of any other digit. As the radial pillar of manual dexterity, the need to provide an opposable thumb assumes supreme importance. The normal thumb is a biomechanical marvel composed of a series of interrelated bony segments connected by special joints and retinacular (restraining) systems. These modify and abet the action of intrinsic and extrinsic muscular systems to provide the infinite variations of the thumb's prime functions of prehension, position, stability, strength, and sensibility. Pollical agenesis as in thumb aplasia, or severe hypoplasia or ineffectiveness as in severe first web space syndactyly, pentadactyly, or "mirror hand," renders the hand considerably more primitive.

FAILURE OF FORMATION (THUMB APLASIA OR HYPOPLASIA)

Congenital absence usually consists of anomalies of all first ray elements, including

**Table 123–1. Congenital Anomalies
of the Thumb**

I.	Failure of formation of parts (arrest of development)
II.	Failure of differentiation (separation) of parts
III.	Duplication of parts
IV.	Overgrowth (gigantism)
V.	Undergrowth (hypoplasia)
VI.	Congenital constriction band syndrome
VII.	Generalized skeletal abnormalites

Modified from Swanson, A. B.: A classification for congenital limb malformations. J. Hand Surg., *1*:8, 1976.

scaphoid, trapezium, and phalangeal elements. The hypoplastic thumb is generally attached to the radial side of the hand farther distally; its attachment may be a tenuously small skin bridge ("pouce floutant," Fig. 123–1), so frail as to endanger its own blood supply by twisting on its pedicle (Fig. 123–2). Fortunately, most radial deficiency states are terminal and four normal fingers are present. If additional radial or preaxial deficiency exists, as in so-called radial "clubhand," the remaining digits, particularly the radialmost, are distorted by the muscle-tendon imbalance incident to the radiovolar deviation of the hand.

In spite of thumb aplasia or marked hypoplasia, children may use their hands skillfully, even when lacking pulp to pulp prehension. In an effort to simulate form and a more refined grasping (pinching) mechanism, the child naturally sooner or later turns to the next most independent and usually radial situated digit. This programmed adaptation of pinch and grasp between existing digits is inevitable and has nothing to do with satisfying a nonexistent area of thumb representation in the cerebral cortex. Reconstructive surgery should do nothing more or less than recognize this natural attempt and help in its attainment. Normally it is to the index finger that the child turns (Fig. 123–3). With use it will attain considerable abduction and pronation with associated widening of the first cleft. Pollicization of the index finger to provide a functionally and esthetically acceptable thumb seems the only logical choice when the first ray is absent and four normal fingers exist.

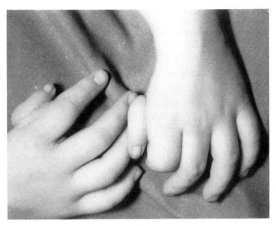

Figure 123–2. If the pedicle is threadlike and the part very diminutive, it should be ablated early in infancy in case parent and child attach undue emotional importance to the part. Occasionally the part can be better secured to the adjacent digit, to be preserved as a source of bulk in the restoration of a more esthetic thenar eminence at the time of pollicization.

Other considerations become important when a hypoplastic thumb is present. A rudimentary thumb precariously attached ("pouce floutant") should be deleted in early

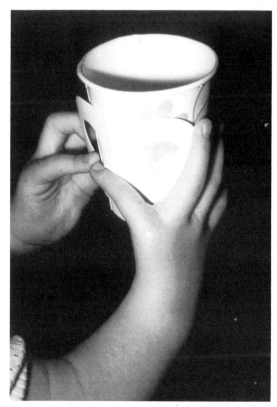

Figure 123–3. With time and use, the index digit will become abducted and rotated as the child attempts to use this next most radial digit as a thumb.

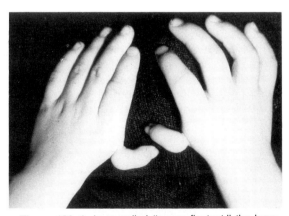

Figure 123–1. In so-called "pouce floutant," the hypoplastic thumb may be attached by only a tenuous skin bridge.

infancy before emotional attachment occurs. Although conservation of tissue and skilled deployment of parts are basic concerns to the reconstructive surgeon, it is rare that even a firmly attached hypoplastic thumb, especially a distally attached one, can contribute toward thumb reconstruction. Rather than a long and time-consuming series of operations being attempted to position and power such a digit, even with good sensibility, it is suggested that its subdermal soft tissue elements might be buried in the thumb position to provide thenar bulk at the time of or prior to the formal index pollicization. The hand with five normally located fingers is the obvious candidate for thumb reconstruction (Fig. 123–4). Thumb reconstruction in the four-fingered hand is rarely resisted by parents, especially if the absence is bilateral and if surgery is regarded as a more strategic digital deployment.

There is still considerable controversy over the timing of thumb reconstruction. Buck-Gramcko (1971) and others suggest reconstructive surgery even during early infancy, usually at less than 1 year of age; Buck-

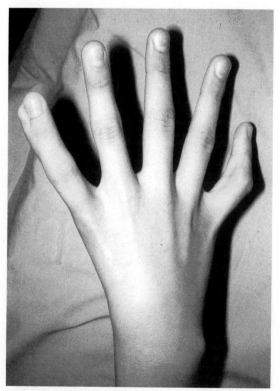

Figure 123–4. In pentadactyly, the additional digit is located more distally than a normal thumb. This condition represents a clear indication for pollicization.

Gramcko reports an operation on an 11 week old infant. He states that there is no significant difference in the rate of improvement at different ages. However, the index finger is influenced by functioning in the thumb position so that its structure becomes more thumblike in morphologic development; i.e., it develops a much larger metacarpal. It is problematic whether this hypothetic gain offsets the difficulties inherent in repositioning such small structures. A later optimal age of 1½ to 3 years (certainly before the beginning of school) takes into account a knowledge of neuromuscular maturation (McGraw, 1943), greater ease of precision surgery, and some cooperation of the child that could not be expected of an infant.

Principles of Operative Management

The transposition of the index finger by neurovascular pedicle technique, as a definitive method of thumb reconstruction, was originally developed to replace the amputated digit. The imaginative contributions of Gosset (1949) and Hilgenfeldt (1950) culminated in the precision techniques of Littler (1952, 1966, 1974) (Fig. 123–5). Spurred by the thalidomide tragedy, Buck-Gramcko (1971) and others developed further technical modifications for digital transfer in congenital absence. Ignorance of refined technique led to some poor results that fostered criticism of the procedure (Brooks, 1964). However, the large series published by Buck-Gramcko (1971) demonstrated that when the techniques are properly performed, results can be excellent both functionally and esthetically.

It is a recognized fact that good function is almost synonymous with appeal. Our reconstructive plan should encompass both aspects, for one generally embraces the other. Applied to thumb reconstruction with neurovascular index pollicization, this implies creation of a radially positioned opposable digit of proper length and stability. The normal size of the index ray requires that articular reduction play a significant role. Proper length is attained by resection of most of the index metacarpal, the head of the metacarpal acting as a trapezium. To prevent subsequent overgrowth, the metacarpal epiphysis is destroyed. With first metacarpal aplasia the radial component of the normal semicircular

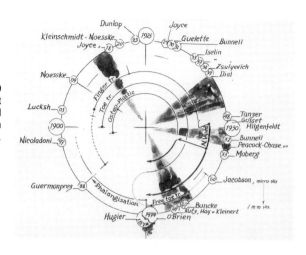

Figure 123–5. Littler, in his classic article detailing 100 years of effort at reconstruction of the thumb, gives credit to the many innovative surgeons who have developed and refined the techniques of thumb reconstruction. (From Littler, J. W.: On 100 years of thumb reconstruction. J. Hand Surg., 1:35, 1976.)

carpal arch is lacking (Fig. 123–6) and a diametric placement of the transposed digit for true opposition with the ulnar digits is impossible. This is significant because the stable opposition achieved by the normal thumb, although contributed to by intrinsic muscles, is more a part of the configuration of the carpometacarpal joint and its ligaments. The thumb is guided unerringly to the correct rotation (Napier, 1966). In the absence of the trapezium, the radial pillar of the arch (Littler, 1966), the repositioned finger is fixed to its own metacarpal base. Each index finger joint then becomes a correspondingly more proximal one, corresponding to those of the thumb. Four congruous movements of the transposed index finger must be accurately controlled for optimal results. Recession is accomplished by accurately predicting and utilizing the length of index finger necessary for appropriate thumb length. Rotation of the index finger on its long axis is necessary to provide proper axial alignment for optimal pulp to pulp pinch. Approx-

imately 100 to 120 degrees of rotation are necessary. Rotation of only 90 degrees results in key-type pinch against the adjacent finger. Radial abduction and palmar abduction must be controlled by proper fixation of the index metacarpal neck or head to its metacarpal base in the basic mean thumb projection of 20 degrees' radial abduction and 35 degrees' palmar abduction. This skeletal readjustment must occur in conjunction with the other equally important operative components: skin incisions, control of the neurovascular pedicle, and muscular rebalancing.

The skin incision must allow adequate exposure for freeing of the metacarpal from its ligamentous restraint, yet preserve dorsal veins and be situated to avoid a compromising scar within the first web space. The neurovascular pedicle is developed by ligating the proper digital artery to the radial side of the long finger and separating the common digital nerves sufficiently proximal to avoid tension when the index finger is recessed. Vascular anomalies, e.g., constrictions, are

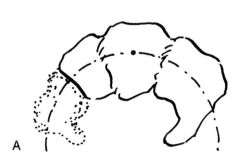

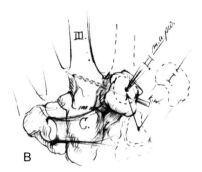

Figure 123–6. In radial aplasia, the trapezium, normally the radial pillar of the semicircular arch, is lacking (A). Either the base of the second metacarpal or the trapezoid serves to determine the mean thumb projection illustrated in B as the mean axial projection (m. a. pro).

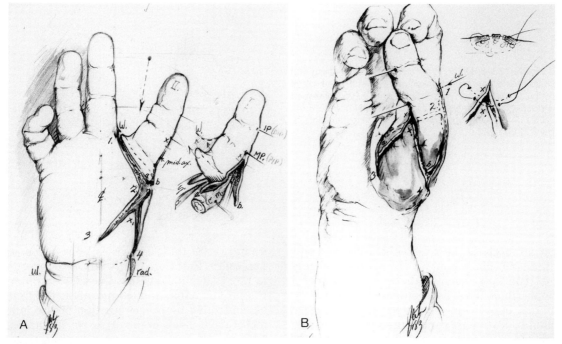

Figure 123–7. *A, B,* Skin incisions must allow sufficient exposure for dissection and permit the reconstruction of an adequate first web space. Scars should fall along the borders of the normal tetrahedral space so as not to cause later compromise. The smaller palmar flap (X_1) helps cover the additional bulk of the relocated abductor indicis, now abductor pollicis brevis muscle *(B)*.

frequent, and the absence of the radial digital vessel must be kept in mind. Muscular stabilization utilizes the abductor indicis (there is no first dorsal interosseous in thumb aplasia) advanced to insert on the proximal phalanx as the abductor pollicis brevis. The volar interosseous serves as the adductor pollicis. The tendon extensor indicis proprius is adjusted surgically, while the flexor tone will equalize postoperatively. Stability is more important than mobility.

OPERATIVE STEPS

Incisions (Fig. 123–7). Properly designed incisions are mandatory for functional and esthetic success. In contrast to traumatic amputations of the thumb, adequate radial skin cover is typically present in thumb agenesis. Occasionally, the cutaneous envelope of a rudimentary thumb can provide supplemental skin through carefully designed incisions (Fig. 123–8). The need for additional skin

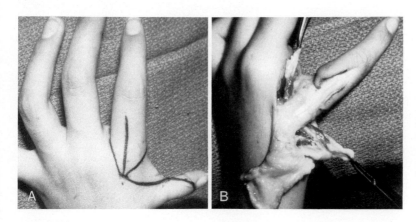

Figure 123–8. *A, B,* If the part to be deleted is of sufficient size, a portion can be maintained, deepithelized, and buried to augment the soft tissue deficiency in the thenar eminence. In this case, additional skin and subcutaneous tissue were preserved from the hypoplastic element and used to add bulk to the point of attachment of the pollicized index digit.

cover in the form of a full-thickness skin graft usually signifies incorrect placement of incisions.

Soft Tissue Dissections. Through generous skin flaps, precise dissection allows identification and preservation of the radial and ulnar neurovascular bundles to the index finger. The important neural and arterial bifurcation to the radial aspect of the middle finger is identified. Attention is then turned to the intrinsic muscle cone about the index finger. The proximal phalangeal attachment of the abductor indicis and volar interosseous muscles is isolated, the muscles elevated from the index metacarpal for subsequent repositioning (Fig. 123–8B). On the volar surface of the hand, the intervolar plate ligament between the index and adjacent metacarpal is divided. This maneuver allows significant freedom in approaching the volarly located neurovascular bundles. The proximal volar plate pulley is opened to allow flexor tendons to approach the proximal interphalangeal joint at a better angle and permit adequate recession of the phalanx (Fig. 123–9). On the dorsal aspect of the hand, the dorsal veins and dorsal radial sensory nerves to the index finger are isolated and preserved. Finally, both extensors to the index finger, the extensor indicis and the common extensor, are isolated. The extensor communis is sectioned proximally and dissected distally (Fig. 123–10.)

Skeletal Reduction and Bony Fixation. Once the soft tissue dissection is completed, the skeleton can be safely shortened (Fig. 123–11) and the neopollex properly positioned. In congenital deficiency, the metacar-

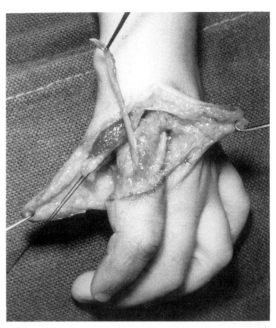

Figure 123–10. The common extensor tendon (EDC) is sectioned proximally and dissected distally. It will eventually serve as a point of attachment of the abductor indicis muscle.

pophalangeal joint of the recessed finger serves as the basal (trapezium-metacarpal) joint. The ovoid or ginglymoid joint of the finger substitutes only imperfectly for the universal saddle or toroidal joint of the thumb. This ovoid metacarpophalangeal, now basal, joint permits the proximal phalanx, now serving as the metacarpal, mobility in several planes but not the refined conjunct rotation of the normal thumb carpometacarpal joint (Fig. 123–12).

If the trapezium is absent, the base of the index metacarpal must serve as the trapezium. The index metacarpal is sectioned just distal to its basal flare. Distally, in order not to transfer the epiphysis of the index metacarpal, the metacarpal head is sectioned through the growth plate, destroying this. Abnormally long growth of the pollicized digit is thus avoided. The digit can now be recessed and properly positioned on the base of the second metacarpal now serving as the trapezium (see Fig. 123–11).

Three specific motions are involved in achieving normal thumb projection: at least 100 degrees of pronation of the head of the metacarpal; approximately 35 degrees of palmar flexion of the index finger proximal phalanx relative to the third metacarpal; and

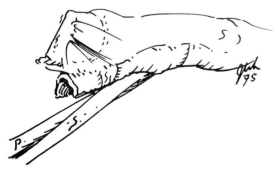

Figure 123–9. Littler suggested releasing the proximal portion of the flexor sheath pulleys to allow the flexor tendon to bowstring volar to the axis of rotation of the joint, and thus have a better mechanical advantage at the previous metacarpophalangeal, now carpometacarpal joint, and allow adequate recession of the phalanx.

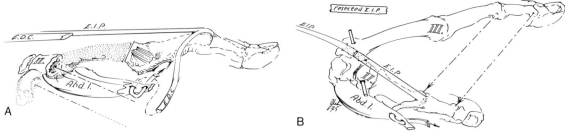

Figure 123–11. It is very important to shorten the second metacarpal adequately *(A)* and to ablate the epiphysis within the metacarpal head to avoid too many growth centers, and ultimately too long a thumb. *B,* The relationships of the shortened skeleton are rebalanced and transferred tendons are depicted. Note the manner in which the tendon of the EDC is used to anchor the repositioned abductor indicis muscle in its new location. EIP = extensor indicis proprius; EDC = extensor digitorum communis; Abd. I = abductor indicis.

approximately 20 degrees of radial abduction of the ray.

The normal ovoid metacarpophalangeal joint of the index finger demonstrates hypermobility in extension occasionally exceeding 90 degrees. Buck-Gramcko has been credited with the simple but elegant maneuver of positioning the metacarpal head (now the

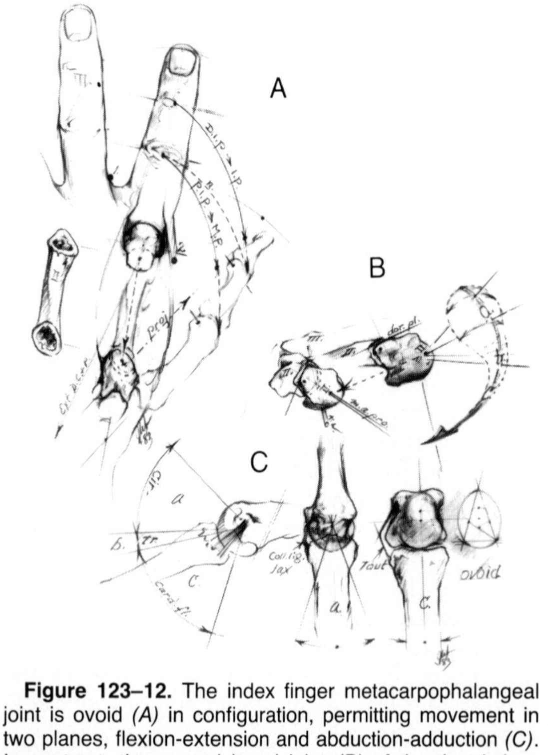

Figure 123–12. The index finger metacarpophalangeal joint is ovoid *(A)* in configuration, permitting movement in two planes, flexion-extension and abduction-adduction *(C).* In contrast, the normal basal joint *(B)* of the thumb is a sellar or toroidal (saddle) joint. With flexion of the thumb metacarpal, there occurs simultaneous axial or conjunct rotation of the metacarpal that inclines the thumb pulp toward the pulps of the index and middle digits. The ovoid metacarpophalangeal joint substitutes only imperfectly for the normal basal joint.

trapezium analogue) in a flexed position relative to the long axis of the digit (Fig. 123–13), to avoid instability, especially into hyperextension. This maneuver diminishes excessive extension. Small Kirschner wires can be used to fix this flexed metacarpal head onto its own metacarpal base. The best functional results have occurred when a true stable bony union has been achieved, as opposed to a somewhat mobile fibrous pseudarthrosis.

Rebalancing of Intrinsic and Extrinsic Muscle Forces. A redistribution of muscle forces is essential for stability and movement of the thumb substitute (Fig. 123–14). The child must be able to stabilize, through intrinsic muscles, the basal joint (formerly the metacarpophalangeal joint) and the metacarpophalangeal joint (formerly the proximal interphalangeal joint) in order to utilize ex-

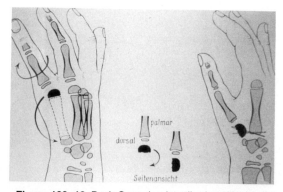

Figure 123–13. Buck-Gramcko described positioning the metacarpal head in a flexed position in relation to the longitudinal axis of the digit. When fixed in this position the former metacarpophalangeal, now basal, joint can be flexed but will not extend any farther than a distance equal to the long axis. Reproduced from Buck-Gramcko, D.: Pollicization of the index finger. J. Bone Joint Surg., *53A*:1065, 1971.

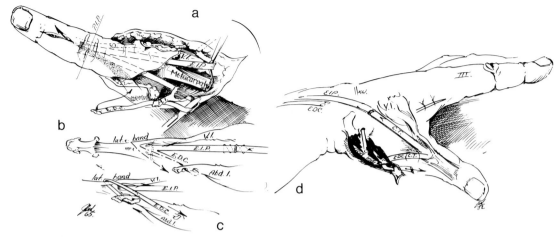

Figure 123–14. Rebalancing extrinsic-intrinsic motor forces is critical to functional success for several reasons. The skeleton has been considerably shortened and several intrinsic muscles will serve slightly different functions. The extensor indicis proprius *(EIP)* will serve as the prime extrinsic extensor of the thumb ray *(a)*. It is shortened in accordance with the magnitude of skeletal reduction. The distal tendon of the extensor digitorum communis *(EDC)* is used to attach the previously mobilized abductor indices *(Abd. I)* to a more distal site of insertion near the radial border *(b)* of the now rotated and shortened index ray, where it will serve as the abductor pollicis brevis, stabilizing the neopollex in palmar abduction. The volar interosseous will serve as the adductor pollicis. It is mobilized only as necessary to allow recession and rotation of the digit *(c)*. In *d* the attachment and new position of the abductor pollicis brevis are illustrated.

trinsic flexion-extension control of the terminal phalanx. The basic requirement for proper positioning of the index finger into the thumb projection is stability at the basal joint, formerly the index finger metacarpophalangeal joint. The interosseous muscles, both radial and ulnar, are used for this purpose. The abductor indicis is advanced to simulate the abductor pollicis brevis, providing palmar abduction and flexion-pronation for the transposed digit. The volar interosseous serves as the adductor pollicis, providing additional stability against hyperextension at the metacarpophalangeal (formerly proximal interphalangeal) joint. The abductor indicis is secured over the proximal phalanx of the thumb (formerly the middle phalanx of the index finger), utilizing the distal attachment of the common extensor tendon previously divided. The volar interosseous muscle is adjusted separately and is attached into the lateral band of the index finger extensor mechanism. Segmental resection of a proper length of the extensor indicis and end to end suture complete the dorsal rebalancing. The flexor tendons are allowed to shift volarly by sectioning of the A1 and A2 portions of the retinacular system, and will adjust in length as time passes and growth occurs. Such is not the case with the extensor mechanism and these tendons must be properly shortened.

In spite of what would appear to be adequate rebalancing, there still exists no prime flexor of the thumb metacarpal, formerly the index finger proximal phalanx. Some basal joint hyperextension may be inevitable and, if excessive, may require secondary tendon transfers such as transfer of the ring finger superficialis tendon or transfer of the abductor digiti minimi to stimulate the function of the short flexor and opponens pollicis for flexion and pronation (Pellegrini, Hentz, and Littler, 1986).

Skin Closure and Dressings. Some adjustment of the skin closure may be necessary to position scars properly so that any contraction that occurs does not lead to dysfunctional contracture. In those cases in which a thumb remnant has been present, some approximation of thenar muscle bulk can be achieved by burying the subcutaneous elements of this remnant in the proper position (see Fig. 123–8).

A dressing is carefully molded about the part and reinforced with a full-length plaster shell worn for five to six weeks. Kirschner wires placed to stabilize the metacarpal head to its new "trapezium" may be left in place if they are causing no trouble. The child is allowed to begin exercises after six weeks and generally no specific retraining is necessary.

One acknowledges the simple fact that a

finger can never be a true thumb (Hentz, 1985). It can never meet the full anatomic and functional characteristics of the normal thumb because of circumferential differences, curvature, axial joint length relationships, and terminal pulp volume. With well-established procedures and exacting surgery, such a transfer can substitute very well as the prime digit in opposing the other fingers for pinch and grasp, approaching both esthetically and functionally the normal thumb (Fig. 123–15).

A somewhat more limited procedure is occasionally useful in dealing with certain congenital thumb absences, e.g., when only one hand is affected and the other is completely normal, especially in the female child (Hentz, 1977). This limited procedure involves mini-

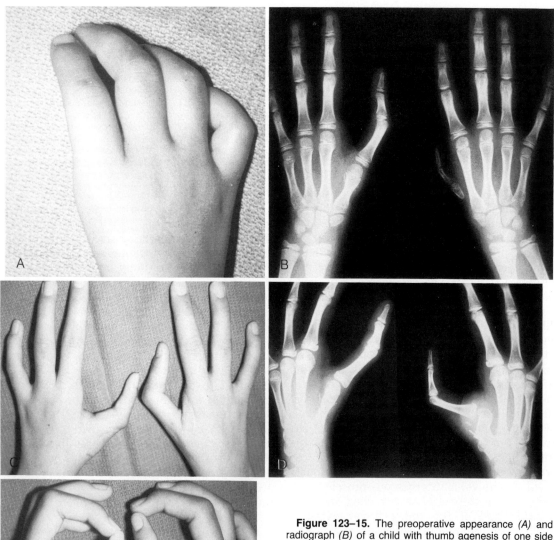

Figure 123–15. The preoperative appearance *(A)* and radiograph *(B)* of a child with thumb agenesis of one side and hypoplasia of the other. The postoperative radiograph *(C)* and appearance of both hands *(D, E)* are demonstrated. On the left hand, it was possible to utilize the soft tissue elements of the hypoplastic digit to augment the bulk of the reconstructed thenar eminence (see Fig. 123–8). The left side was shortened slightly more than the right, lending it less the appearance of a finger and more that of a thumb.

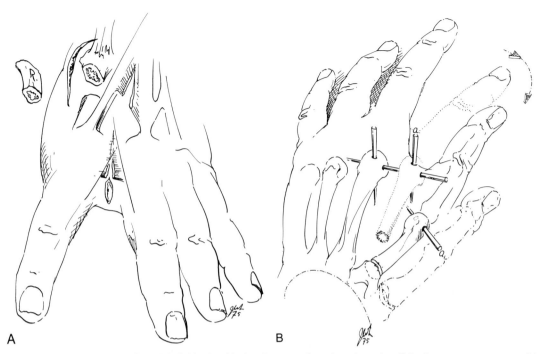

A   B

Figure 123–16. In some selected individuals with thumb agenesis, a less formal pollicization may serve to provide a more functional key pinch between the pulp of the index and the next most radial digit rather than a side to side pinch, but still maintaining the appearance of four digits. This limited recession-rotation of the metacarpal is accomplished through two small incisions *(A)*. Key steps include sectioning of the intervolar plate ligament and excision of approximately 1.5 cm of metacarpal. The metacarpal is recessed, rotated approximately 75 to 90 degrees, and slightly palmarly angulated *(B)*.

mal scarring and less exacting surgery. The operation is designed to take advantage of the usually well-developed first cleft between index and long finger, which frequently has widened considerably as a consequence of the patient's efforts at opposition with the next most radial digit. The procedure incorporates much of the mechanisms of the more formal operation without the need for rebalance of intrinsic and extrinsic motors or shifts of local tissue (Fig. 123–16). A limited metacarpal recession in association with rotation and palmar angulation of the metacarpal is combined with division of the intervolar plate ligament, dorsal and interosseous fascia, and palmar fascia. Because minimal incisions are employed, scarring is limited. The procedure may be performed when the patient is 3 to 4 years of age and then again several years later after further adaptation of the part. The very limited incisions are designed so that formal pollicization can be performed subsequently if indicated. The index finger becomes a more functional unit for opposition, yet in repose the hand still resembles one with four fingers, rather than the three fingers of the formal index pollicization (Fig. 123–17).

FAILURE OF DIFFERENTIATION (ABNORMALITY OF THUMB POSTURE)

There are several varieties of congenital deformities of thumb posture. Causes range from absent or vestigial extensor tendons or flexor tendon nodules to neuromuscular hypoplasia or arthrogryposis.

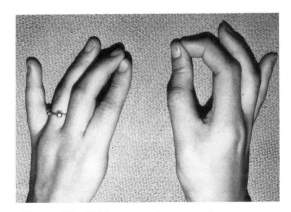

Figure 123–17. The pre- and postoperative appearance following limited pollicization is demonstrated.

Congenital Trigger Thumb

This least complex deformity was described by Notta (1850), and the nodule on the flexor pollicis longus tendon bears the title "Notta's node." At birth, the hand of the infant is maintained in a state of primitive grasp. This includes a thumb positioned in palmar adduction and flexion but overlapped by the flexed remaining digits. The deformity may not be recognized until the infant is 3 to 4 months of age when normally a more proficient grasp involving extension of the thumb as well as the fingers is attempted (Fig. 123–18).

Flatt's text on congenital anomalies (1977) pictures a child and a mother with similar congenital trigger thumb, demonstrating the occasional inherited tendency of this deformity. Because the normal posture of the infant's thumb is one of flexion, the diagnosis is frequently missed until the parent notices that the child cannot actively extend the thumb, or (more commonly) resistance is felt on forceful passive extension, although the tendon rarely produces a snapping effect.

On examination, the nodule on the flexor tendon may slide through the contracted fibrocartilaginous portion of the pulley on passive extension, or the deformity may be fixed and the interphalangeal joint cannot be passively extended.

MANAGEMENT

If the interphalangeal joint can be passively extended, it is worthwhile to splint the thumb in full extension for several weeks. Frequently, on renewed motion, the thumb again becomes fixed in flexion at the interphalangeal joint. A period of further splinting may be attempted, but success is variable. Durham and Meggitt (1974) suggested that trigger thumbs present at birth can be essentially ignored, since 30 per cent resolve spontaneously. If diagnosis is made later in life, an additional period of observation is still helpful, because the problem may resolve spontaneously in a few patients even at this late date. Durham and Meggitt recommended, however, that a child presenting after the age of 3 years should undergo a surgical release of the involved flexor sheath. Even children operated on after age 4 years did not appear to develop permanent flexion contractures.

Surgery is usually performed on an outpatient basis under general anesthesia. Through a transverse incision at the metacarpophalangeal joint crease, with care taken to avoid the nearby digital nerves, the flexor sheath over the metacarpophalangeal joint is exposed and opened longitudinally. There is disagreement over whether or not to reduce in size the nodule on the flexor tendon. The skin can be closed with absorbable sutures and the interphalangeal joint splinted in full extension for several weeks while wound healing occurs. It is often helpful to involve the parents in postoperative exercises to maintain free movement of the flexor pollicis longus tendon and assist in overcoming any volar soft tissue contractures.

Thumb-in-Palm or Clasped Thumb Deformities

Tamplin (1846) described a case of flexion adduction deformity. Absence of one or all extrinsic abductor or extensor tendons to the thumb has been described (Zadek, 1934; Miller, 1943; Crawford and Adamson, 1966).

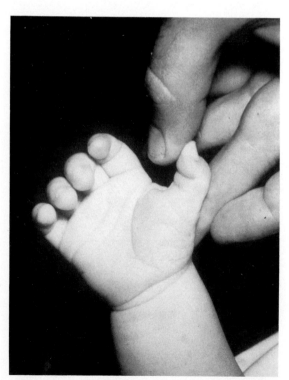

Figure 123–18. Congenital trigger thumb. The terminal joint of the thumb cannot be fully extended and a palpable nodule is present at the base of the proximal phalanx.

With congenital clasped thumb, the short thumb extensor is most often abbreviated or absent and the thumb is flexed at the metacarpophalangeal joint (Fig. 123–19). With the long abductor affected also, all three bony segments may be adducted and flexed across the palm. This frequently hereditary trait is usually bilateral and symmetric. It must be differentiated from trigger thumb, arthrogryposis, and some upper motor neuron spastic conditions associated with so-called "clasped thumb." Weckesser (Weckesser, 1955; Weckesser, Reed, and Heiple, 1968) identified various causes of the deformities and grouped them accordingly. Group I demonstrated deficient extension only felt secondary to a defect in the extensor muscles or tendons. An X-linked recessive pattern of inheritance has been suggested. Group II is characterized by flexion contractures of the thumb and other digits with associated deficient extension. A muscular rather than a neural mechanism is suggested. Group III is characterized by hypoplasia of all the structures of the thumb and appears to be a variant of hypoplasia or undergrowth. Group IV is distinguished by preaxial polydactyly with deficient extension.

MANAGEMENT

When the condition is suspected in infancy, prevention of soft tissue contraction should be accomplished by splinting and by parental manipulation or stretching of the first web

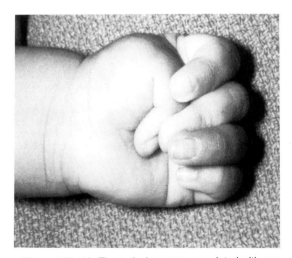

Figure 123–19. The typical posture associated with congenital clasped thumb, or thumb-in-palm deformity, is demonstrated. One or all of the extensor-abductor muscle tendon units to the thumb may be deficient.

space. Surgery should be postponed until the child has attained an age associated with a more complex grasping movement including thumb extension and pronation, usually achieved by 3 years of age. Even in older children, splinting may overcome some soft tissue capsular tightness. In their report, Weckesser, Reed, and Heiple (1968) suggest prolonged plaster of Paris splinting, the splint being changed as necessary to allow for growth of the hand. They advocate a long period of immobilization, up to six months, and report long-term maintenance of the correction in patients with a good response to splinting. When the deformity is not amenable to simple splinting, surgical correction may involve release of volar soft tissue contractions using skin grafts or Z-plasties, as well as release of a first web space soft tissue adduction contracture. Here, procedures such as palmar release of the adductor or short thumb flexors has been advocated (Verdan, as reported by Crawford and Adamson, 1966). The long thumb flexor can also be a restraining force requiring release.

If the deformity recurs after splinting or responds favorably to splinting, surgical correction is indicated. In most cases, lack of success with conservative measures implies complete absence of the extensor pollicis brevis and/or extensor pollicis longus tendons. Surgical correction usually involves a tendon transfer to provide power to the extensor or abductor tendons of the thumb. Kelikian (1974) reports using the extensor carpi ulnaris extended by a free graft. Other useful motors mentioned include the extensor indicis proprius or brachioradialis. Very frequently, a tendon graft is necessary because, on exploration, the extensor mechanism may be represented only by a thin amorphous collagenous sheet or a tiny, threadlike tendon. Prolonged postoperative splinting is frequently necessary, otherwise the powerful flexor muscles stretch out or disrupt the transfer.

The congenitally clasped hand may also exhibit the flexion deformities of some or all remaining fingers. Frequently, absence of extensors is implicated. In others, they may be present but of limited amplitude. The author (Hentz and Littler, 1977a,b) has treated several cases of congenital absence of digital extensors by tendon transfer using a superficialis tendon. The superficialis tendons to the middle, ring, and little fingers are utilized. These are passed subcutaneously either radially or ulnarly across the wrist, inserting into the extensor hood over the proximal phalanx of the finger or thumb, maintaining the normal finger cascade. This provides a tenodesis effect with wrist flexion. There has been no problem with recurvature deformity at the proximal interphalangeal joint secondary to sacrifice of the superficialis. This procedure provides improved balance between strong flexor and weak extensor forces.

Adducted Thumb

Anomalies of thumb posture include deformities characterized by an adducted thumb, caused either by problems of the first web space or by absence of the thenar intrinsic muscles. The condition also may represent one variation of the hypoplastic thumb. Many of these children also demonstrate absence of the flexor pollicis longus or weakness of this muscle-tendon unit. The thumb is usually somewhat short but positioned correctly relative to the remaining digits. For patients presenting with problems of the first web space, many creative procedures have been

described, including various dorsally based flaps rotated into the web space to deepen the space, and variations of Z-plasty techniques including the four-flap Z-plasty. These techniques are similar to those described for release of first web space contractures secondary to burns or paralytic deformities.

Those thumbs adducted secondary to hypoplasia or aplasia of the radially placed intrinsic muscles are best managed by traditional so-called opponens tendon transfers, described elsewhere.

Occasionally, the thumb is held in adduction by virtue of syndactyly between the thumb and index finger. This is a common occurrence in certain types of cleft or split hand deformities. In conditions with first web space adduction contracture, the goal is an adequate first cleft with a properly aligned first ray to oppose with a more centralized (ulnarly placed) index digit assuming a position intermediate between the normal index and middle fingers. Whether one or two stages are required depends on the degree of syndactyly existing between the thumb and index finger and the severity of the adduction contracture (Fig. 123–20) (Hentz, 1977). The management of this condition is discussed in detail in the section on cleft hands.

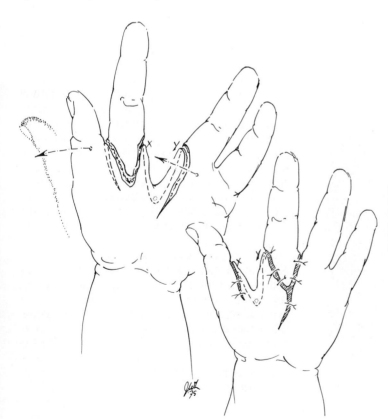

Figure 123–20. An adduction contracture between thumb and index occasionally exists as part of cleft hand deformity. In this case the additional skin of the abnormal cleft can be used to reconstruct the defect that follows release of the first web space.

Abducted Thumb

A rare but interesting deformity is characterized by extreme abduction of the thumb. The patients described by Tupper (1969) all appeared to have an aberrant flexor pollicis longus tendon, which crossed the metacarpophalangeal joint on the radial side, acting as a radial deforming force. Suggested management includes release of the deforming forces and strengthening of the weakened ulnar collateral ligament at the metacarpophalangeal joint of the thumb.

Hypoplastic or Absent Thumb

Categorized as having "failure of differentiation," the thumb in this condition may be severely or only slightly hypoplastic. Blauth (1967) classified hypoplasia of the thumb into five categories (Table 123–2). The thumb is frequently involved in such associated conditions as congenital amputations or so-called congenital constriction band syndromes. Typically, the thumb is the least involved digit in both these conditions. Various residual lengths of the thumb may be present. This general condition is discussed elsewhere (see Chap. 128); therefore, only those aspects related to management of the deformed thumb in this condition are discussed here.

Because the degree of hypoplasia can vary from minimal shortening to one of near-complete absence, this category somewhat bridges two of the categories of congenital

Table 123–2. Hypoplasia and Aplasia of the Thumb

Grade I	Minor hypoplasia, in which all elements are present, the thumb being overall somewhat smaller than normal
Grade II	Adduction contracture of first web space; laxity of ulnar collateral ligament of metacarpophalangeal joint; hypoplasia of thenar muscles; normal skeleton with respect to articulations
Grade III	Significant hypoplasia, with aplasia of intrinsics, rudimentary extrinsic tendons (if any); skeletal hypoplasia, especially of carpometacarpal joint, which is vestigial
Grade IV	Floating thumb (pouce floutant), a vestigial, totally uncontrolled digit attached just proximal to metacarpophalangeal joint of index finger
Grade V	Total absence

Modified from Lister, G.: The Hand: Diagnosis and Indications. Edinburgh, Churchill Livingstone, 1984, p. 340.

Table 123–3. Subclassification of the Short Thumb

Metacarpal (short and slender)
  Isolated variant
  Associated with anomalies of spine and cardiac and
    gastrointestinal systems
  Hematopoietic system (Fanconi's syndrome)
  Holt-Oram syndrome
  Juberg-Hayward syndrome
Metacarpal (short and broad)
  Cornelia de Lange's syndrome
  Hand-foot-uterus syndrome
  Dystrophic dwarfism
  Myositis ossificans progressiva
Proximal phalanx (short and broad)
  Brachydactyly
Distal phalanx (short and broad)
  Brachydactyly
  Rubinstein-Taybi syndrome
  Apert's syndrome
  Carpenter's syndrome

From Dobyns, J. H., Wood, V. E., and Bayne, L. G.: Congenital hand deformities. *In* Green, D. P. (Ed.): Operative Hand Surgery. 2nd Ed. New York, Churchill Livingstone, 1988, p. 386.

anomalies, failure of formation and failure of differentiation. This section will concentrate on hypoplasia other than complete absence or floating thumbs best treated by pollicization and discussed earlier in this chapter. Defects discussed below include the underdeveloped or short thumb that does not extend to the level of the proximal interphalangeal joint of the index finger. Table 123–3 (Dobyns and associates, 1982) catalogues many of the syndrome states associated with short thumbs (Edgerton, 1965).

Many types of congenitally short thumb require no specific treatment, since very little functional deficit is present. Shortened thumbs that are malpositioned with respect to the other digits do require treatment. Such anomalies as the adducted or abducted thumb are examples and have been discussed earlier. The adducted and hypoplastic thumb may appear to have a more radial placement on the hand (Fig. 123–21). Frequently some element of syndactyly exists between the thumb and index finger, causing the first web space to extend more distally. Strauch and Spinner (1976) stressed the frequency of absent thenar muscles. Principles of treatment include correction of a deficient first web space, as discussed in the section on congenitally clasped thumb, followed by opposition transfers such as that of the abductor digiti minimi. Often the flexor pollicis longus is also deficient.

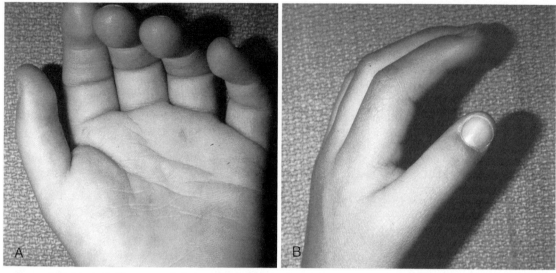

Figure 123–21. *A, B,* The congenitally hypoplastic thumb often appears to be placed more radially and distally on the hand.

MANAGEMENT

The management of the hypoplastic thumb is influenced primarily by its bone and soft tissue relationships. Occasionally, there is significant soft tissue redundancy. A relatively well-formed metacarpal may be present on top of which is a substantial soft tissue element but one lacking in sufficient skeletal support (Fig. 123–22). Simple procedures such as bone grafts from rib, hip, or toe phalanx transferred to this soft tissue pocket and secured to the thumb metacarpal stabilize the redundant soft tissue elements of the thumb and provide some additional functional length. The fate of bone grafts placed in this terminal position is somewhat varia-

ble and further growth unpredictable. The procedure frequently has to be repeated as the child grows.

In contrast, many infants with transverse terminal deficiencies or congenital amputations affecting the thumb present with no disproportion between soft tissue envelope and underlying skeleton. When there is a normal complement of adjacent digits, pollicization of one of these adjacent digits must be strongly considered. In instances in which adjacent digits are themselves hypoplastic, several procedures have been proposed, including microvascular free toe transplants (Gilbert, 1982) or skeletal distraction lengthening techniques (Kessler, Baruch, and Hecht, 1977; Matev, 1979). The transfer by

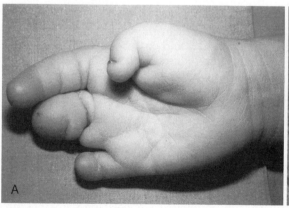
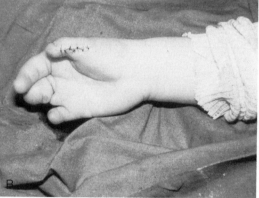

Figure 123–22. Many hypoplastic thumbs lack the necessary skeletal support for the terminal soft tissues *(A)*. A bone graft has been placed with the soft tissue envelope to relatively lengthen this thumb and provide a more stable thumbtip *(B)*.

microvascular methods of composite tissues such as toes to replace congenitally absent fingers is still in its infancy. An insufficient number of children have been observed over a long enough period to establish the rightful place of this technique in the surgical armamentarium. The technical aspects are discussed elsewhere (see Chap. 128).

There is, however, renewed interest in applying the skeletal distraction lengthening techniques developed for the management of lower limb length discrepancies to congenitally shortened thumbs and fingers (see Chap. 128). The ideal candidate would appear to be a child with a first metacarpal plus or minus some portion of the proximal phalanx and associated metacarpophalangeal joint (Fig. 123–23A,B). A sufficient length of bone must be present to allow four transversely oriented pins to be placed serially along the metacarpal. The operative procedure involves a dorsal radial incision exposing the metacarpal, the placement through separate stab wounds of four transversely directed fixation pins, the attachment of a stabilizing distraction frame, and sectioning of the metacarpal between the two sets of pins. Sectioning of the periosteal sleeve allows easier and more rapid distraction. There are several commercially available devices suitable for distraction lengthening of small digits. Most involve some screw or worm-drive mechanism allowing controlled steady distraction of the part while the proper axial alignment is maintained. Typically, the mechanism is adjusted to lengthen the part 0.5 to 1 mm per day until the predetermined length is gained (Fig. 123–23C,D). At a second operative procedure, the apparatus is removed and a bone graft of sufficient size, harvested from the hip or rib, is inserted into the gap. This bone graft can be wired into place using the preexisting drill holes in the metacarpal, drilling additional holes in the bone graft. Alternatively, the thumb may be maintained in the rigid stabilizing device until new bone spontaneously bridges the gap, or the device may be removed and the pins incorporated in a plaster cast to await similar spontaneous bony union. If more than 2 cm of length has been attained through distraction, it is preferable to bone graft the defect at a second operation.

When distraction lengthening has been applied to the metacarpal, the first web space typically migrates distally. The first web space can be deepened by any one of several methods at the time of insertion of the bone graft. The four-flap Z-plasty methods seem preferable. Because the lengthened thumb will not grow proportional to the other digits, the procedure may need to be repeated, typically during the immediate preteenage years. The place of this procedure in the surgical armamentarium awaits further study.

DUPLICATION OF PARTS (PREAXIAL POLYDACTYLY)
(See also Chap. 128)

When the normally pentadactylous hand presents with excess digits, the condition is termed polydactyly or supernumerary digits. Early authors viewed polydactylism as an expression of atavism or reversion of a part to a more primitive evolutionary state, e.g., the multiray extremity of an earlier animal. Indeed, Darwin (1896) considered this idea of a malformation representing a persistent phylogenetic form to be logical. Present teratologic research indicates that polydactylism is the result of an excess of longitudinal segmentation, probably representing an increased folding of the apical ectodermal ridge, inducing supernumerary digit formation. With syndactyly it represents the most common hand anomaly, and it is the most common hand malformation in the black population. More frequently inherited than syndactyly, its mode of transmission is via an irregular dominant gene with variable expression.

The exact incidence is difficult to determine because small pedunculated masses of skin along border digits that represent the least expression of the anomaly are often removed at the time of birth by the obstetrician or pediatrician. However, Shapiro and associates (1958) found an incidence of one in 400 in a study of 30,000 consecutive births. Border digits are by far the most commonly affected, and preaxial duplication requires more reconstructive procedures than do ulnar border anomalies.

Studies demonstrated that postaxial polydactyly was more frequent than preaxial polydactyly. Postaxial polydactyly was 11 times more common in the black population, whereas preaxial polydactyly was equally common in both races (0.08 in 1000). The large number of anatomic varieties of preaxial polydactyly

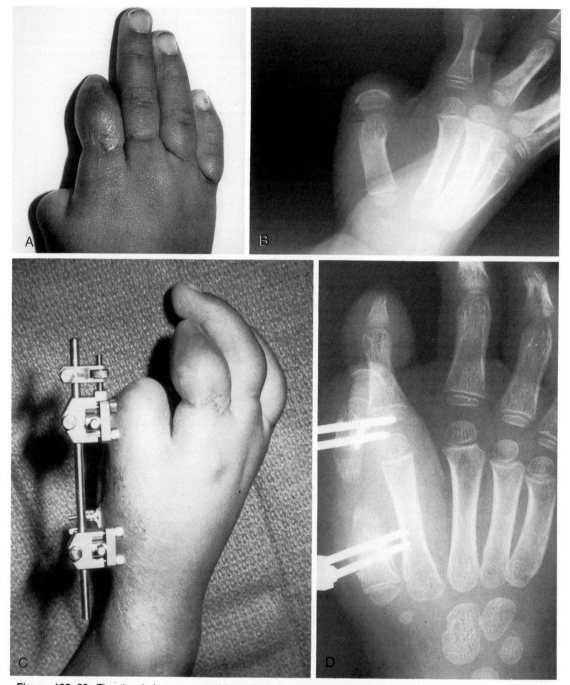

Figure 123–23. The thumb is represented by only a hypoplastic metacarpal *(A, B)*. Following application of the distraction device *(C)* the thumb metacarpal is slowly lengthened, typically about 0.5 to 1 mm a day. Even though the periosteum has been sectioned, new bone will bridge the defect, or the defect can be bone grafted if the defect is sizable *(D)*.

indicate its genetic heterogeneity. Temtamy and McKusick (1978) suggest two classifications of preaxial polydactyly that involve the thumb: thumb polydactyly and polydactyly of a triphalangeal thumb. Like syndactyly, preaxial polydactyly may be syndromic.

When preaxial polydactyly is an isolated malformation, its inheritance appears to be via autosomal dominant traits. When associated with syndrome states, preaxial polydactyly demonstrates various patterns of inheritance. The most common syndrome states are termed acrocephalopolysyndactyly. One of these, Noack's syndrome (Noack, 1959), is transmitted as a dominant trait; another, Carpenter's syndrome (Carpenter, 1901), is transmitted as a recessive trait. Preaxial polydactyly is infrequently associated with facial clefts, brachydactyly, and deafness. Polydactyly is usually represented by a soft tissue appendage attached to a pre- or postaxial border digit and arising close to the metacarpophalangeal joint. This may be complicated by the presence of osseous or cartilaginous elements with a more complex attachment to the metacarpal or phalanx; in this case, an extra articular facet often is present. Finally, there may be a separate, perfectly formed supernumerary digit with its own metacarpal neurovascular bundle flexor and extensor tendons.

Classification of Thumb Polydactyly

Wassel's classification (Wassel, 1969), after an analysis of patients seen at the University of Iowa, described seven different types based on the skeletal morphology, particularly the skeletal level of duplication (Fig. 123–24).

Principles of Operative Management

Aside from the reduction in the number of elements, the principal goal is the accurate establishment of the longitudinal skeletal axis.

When one part is clearly dominant in size and function, surgical decisions are easy. When both elements are more equal in size, the decision can be difficult. In these cases, careful and often prolonged observation of the child during play may be necessary.

Conservation of usable structures should be kept foremost in mind. Extensor or flexor tendons from the ablated segment may be used to reinforce remaining tendons or redirected to balance forces across the segment to be saved.

The surgeon must consider the prime function of the thumb, i.e., to be in opposition against the other digits, and the prerequisites for stable pinch, especially a stable metacarpophalangeal ulnar collateral ligament. Fortunately, the radial-most digit is usually the more hypoplastic, allowing conservation of the ulnar-most part and its important ulnar collateral ligament. The parents must understand that the remaining part is usually smaller than the normal side and that secondary imbalance is frequent. Secondary operative procedures also are often necessary.

The aim of surgery is usually one of cosmetic improvement. When polydactyly is represented only by a poorly attached extra digit, very early amputation is indicated. The morphologic hallmark of man's upper limb is a pentadactylous hand with one preaxial opposable member. Even though a supernumerary digit may enhance function somewhat (Fig. 123–25), the reconstructive aim is to-

Types: Wassel

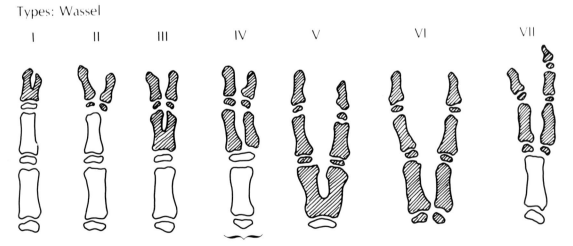

Most common

Figure 123–24. Wassel described seven different types of first ray duplications. (Adapted from J. Bone Joint Surg., 75:118, 1980.)

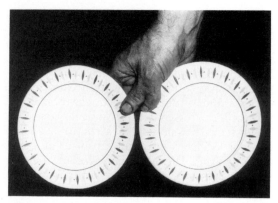

Figure 123–25. Occasionally, preaxial duplications are functionally useful to the patient. This man declined excision of his duplicated thumb.

ward normal morphology, and surgical re-creation of the normal state is indicated.

Surgical restoration of a more functional and esthetic unit has involved either amputation of the supernumerary digit or reducing and combining the two digits into one. In growing children, care should be taken to avoid injury to the epiphyses. It may be necessary to delay final correction until most growth is complete: even though epiphyses are uninjured, the resulting postsurgical scar may restrict normal development at the operative site. This is reflected in the deviation

of the remaining unit toward the radial side (since the more radial member is usually sacrificed) with subsequent growth. When deviation has resulted in an abnormal joint configuration, treatment is limited to straightening the deviation by interphalangeal fusion. If possible, this should be delayed until most growth has occurred.

OPERATIVE MANAGEMENT OF SPECIFIC TYPES OF PREAXIAL POLYDACTYLY

Types 1 and 2. In Types 1 and 2 preaxial polydactyly, there is a more or less complete duplication of the distal phalanx. A duplicated skeleton may be contained within a single skin envelope with only a slight indentation of the terminal skin and a ridge along the nail (Fig. 123–26A). Frequently the duplicated elements are of near-similar size. The preferred treatment is the so-called Bilhaut-Cloquet procedure (Bilhaut, 1890), resecting a central wedge of skin, nail, and bone, tapering each half, and bringing them together (see Fig. 123–31). If one element is much smaller, it can be deleted, perhaps preserving some nail margin from the part to be removed for attachment to the lateral aspect of the remaining nail plate (Fig. 123–26B). In Type 2 deformities (Fig. 123–27), reconstruction of the interphalangeal joint ligament is neces-

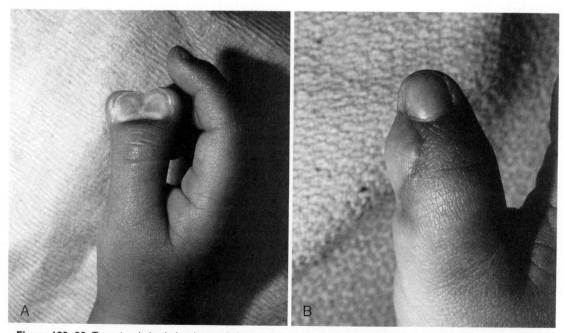

Figure 123–26. Type 1 polydactly involves only incomplete separation of the terminal phalanx *(A)*. In this example, the radial half was ablated, preserving some skin to restore more normal contour to the nail and distal phalanx *(B)*.

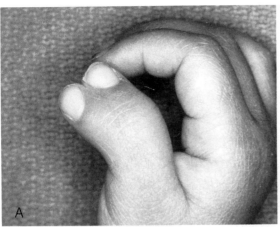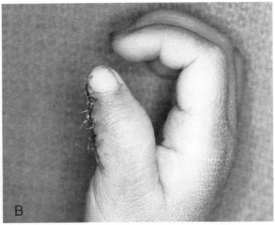

Figure 123–27. Type 2 polydactyly. There is complete duplication of the terminal phalangeal elements *(A). B,* Postoperative appearance following excision of the radial-most element. A small dorsally based flap of skin taken from the ablated part was used to reconstruct the nail margin.

sary. It is usually possible to conserve the ligament on the side to be excised, and reattach this ligament, preferably through drill holes placed in the phalanx. A small pin placed across the interphalangeal joint assists in maintaining the reduction and protects the ligament repair during the early postoperative period. Incomplete motion at the interphalangeal joint is a less significant problem than lateral instability. For this reason, prolonged postoperative splinting with a padded malleable external splint is very helpful. In spite of these precautions, there is a high incidence of late deviation toward the side of the amputated segment (Fig. 123–28). Persistent deviation results in articular remodeling, soft tissue contracture, and extensor and flexor tendon imbalance. These secondary deformities are difficult to correct (Miura, 1977) by soft tissue repositioning alone, and typically fusion of the interphalangeal joint with restoration of proper axial alignment is necessary once epiphyses are closed.

Type 3. Type 3 deformities are typically managed by ablating one element, usually the radial-most (Fig. 123–29A,B). Others have extended the Bilhaut-Cloquet operation to this more proximal level of duplication (Karchinov, 1962). Excision of the less normal component, as determined by careful examination and observation of the function of the digit, is the procedure of choice (Kleinert, Grundberg, and Kutz, 1973). Careful consideration is given to the placement of incisions. As opposed to syndactyly, where a skin defect is always present, polydactyly, particularly

the preaxial condition, involves an excess of skin. The bony or cartilaginous components are removed by filleting the extra digit (Fig. 123–29C). A carefully outlined Z-plasty can then be created with loose closure of the flaps (Fig. 123–29D). A straight midaxial line of closure is assiduously avoided to reduce the restraint that scar causes to subsequent growth. Lateral deviation may be lessened or avoided, provided epiphyseal damage has not occurred. Extensor and flexor tendons to the ablated part must be dissected from these parts. If present, they may be transected flush with the remaining tendons or used to rebalance forces about the remaining joints.

Type 4. Type 4 deformities may present with complete duplication of the distal and proximal phalanges, the elements well separated in separate skin envelopes (Fig. 123–30A), or more or less contained within a single skin envelope (Fig. 123–30B,C), with or without ungual union. The articular surface of the head of the metacarpal is always abnormally wide; however, the inclination of the duplicated elements from the longitudinal axis of the metacarpal is determined by the relative position of the two articular facets of the enlarged metacarpal head. The proper choice of operative procedure hinges somewhat on the axial alignment of the duplication. When the head of the metacarpal possesses partially separated articular facets, there is great divergence of the two proximal phalanges and frequently reciprocal convergence of the distal phalanges, particularly when the skin envelope is not itself well

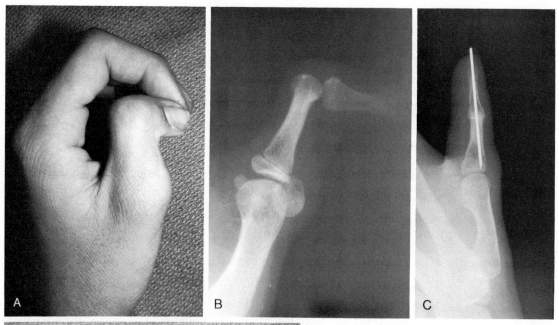

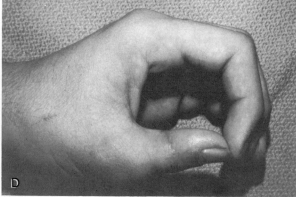

Figure 123–28. Fifteen years previously this teenage boy had had excision of a Type 2 polydactyly. Loss of ulnar collateral stability and abnormal growth caused progressive radial deviating of the terminal phalanx *(A, B)*. The interphalangeal joint was fused and the skin redistributed to allow proper alignment of the digit *(C, D)*.

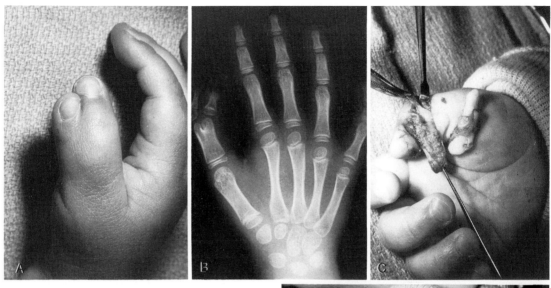

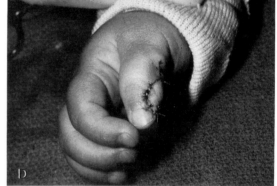

Figure 123–29. Type 3 polydactyly. The radial-most elements *(A, B)* were to be deleted. The skeletal and cartilaginous tissues are excised *(C)*. A careful search is made for flexor and extensor tendon elements to the parts to be deleted. The skin and subcutaneous tissues are used to augment the contour of the remaining parts *(D)*.

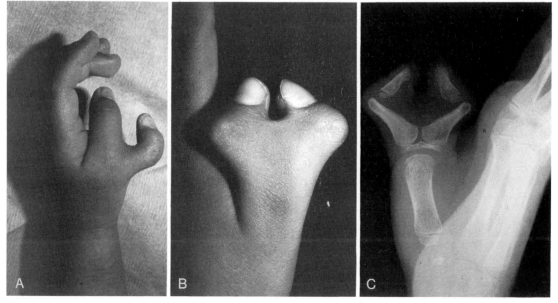

Figure 123–30. Type 4 polydactyly. The duplicated parts may be quite separated *(A)* or contained within a more or less single skin envelope *(B, C)*.

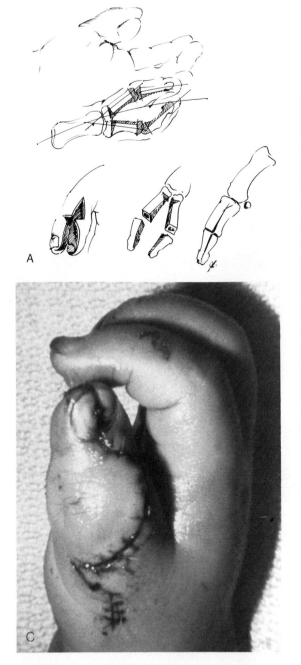

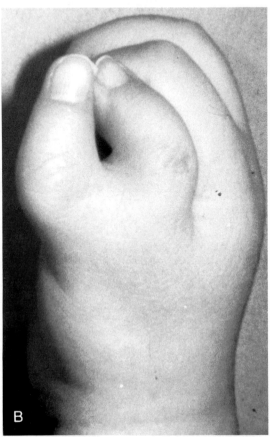

Figure 123–31. Bilhaut and Cloquet described a procedure that is occasionally useful in Type 4 abnormalities such as that pictured in Figures 123–30*B, C* and 123-31*B, C*. However, the bone carpentry necessary to achieve proper skeletal reduction and axial alignment is very difficult to perform on diminutive parts. Likewise, it is difficult to fashion symmetric articular surfaces at the interphalangeal joint if the parts differ in size.

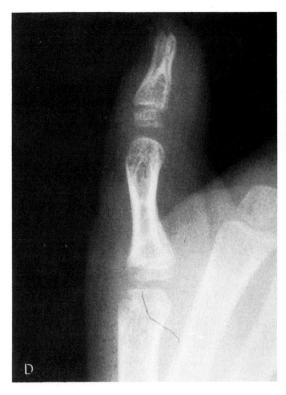

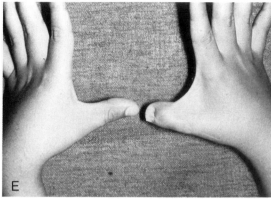

Figure 123–31 *Continued* With time and growth, some remodeling of this surface occurs *(D, E)*. (Case of Relton McCarroll, M.D.)

duplicated. If the metacarpal articular facets are located more side by side, the two distal elements are more often parallel and have better axial alignment. In the latter case, ablation seems most indicated. In the former, ablation of one element leaves a zigzag alignment of the remaining parts. Axial alignment of the misdirected phalanges is difficult to achieve by soft tissue reconstruction alone, and some type of closing or opening wedge osteotomy of metacarpal or proximal phalanx, or both, is required. In such instances, some modification of the Bilhaut-Cloquet procedure may be helpful in creating reasonable axial alignment (Fig. 123–31). The principal esthetic drawback, that of a longitudinal split in the nail, can be obviated by using the nail from one of the elements to reconstruct the entire remaining nail plate. In those cases amenable to ablation of the lesser element (Fig. 123–32), the metacarpophalangeal musculoligamentous complex on the side of the ablation must be reconstructed. The metacarpophalangeal joint collateral ligament can be dissected at the subperiosteal level from the proximal phalanx to be discarded, and then securely attached to the base of the proximal phalanx to be retained. A bony insertion is far more secure than an insertion of this important ligamentous complex into soft tissues. The intrinsic muscles, either abductor pollicis brevis or adductor pollicis attachment, must also be preserved from reattachment. In all cases, the extensor and/or flexor mechanisms have unusual sites of attachments and these systems must be explored completely. Following skeletal reduction, a search for residual deforming structures must be made. These include abnormal flexor or extensor tendons, as mentioned above, or intrinsic tendon insertions, fascial bands about the neurovascular bundles, or abnormal position of collateral ligaments. Failure to recognize these potentially deforming forces will result in progressive deviation and joint imbalance as growth continues.

Types 5 and 6. When more complete duplication exists, one element is almost always predominant. The more diminutive element is ablated, taking into account the precautions regarding deforming forces just discussed.

Type 7. Triphalangeal thumb is discussed as a separate entity below.

SECONDARY SURGERY

The most common sequela of the surgical reconstruction of preaxial polydactyly is either lack of motion at the interphalangeal

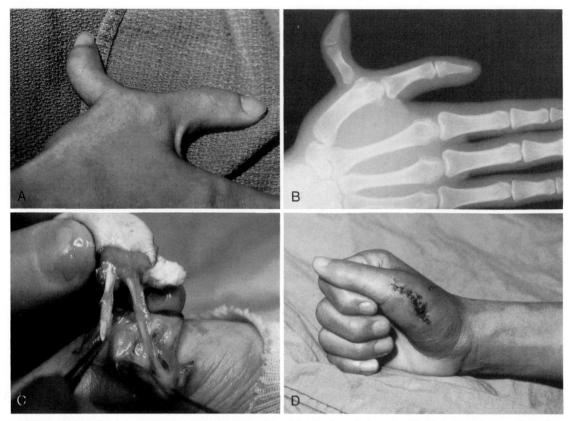

Figure 123–32. Type 4 polydactyly with great separation of the duplicated elements *(A)*. Through a dorsoradial incision *(B)*, the duplicated flexor and extensor tendons to the part to be ablated are dissected *(C)* and excised or used to help balance the remaining forces about the remaining part. The immediate postoperative appearance is depicted in *D*.

joint, deviation of growth away from the normal longitudinal axis, or instability at either the interphalangeal or metacarpophalangeal joint or both. The result of secondary surgery for these deformities is often disappointing. Attempts to correct deviation or instability by secondary soft tissue procedures frequently fail, and fusion is often required. Lack of motion at the interphalangeal joint is most often secondary to adherence of portions of flexor or extensor tendons previously attached to the now amputated part (Fig. 123–33). If these divided ends are attached proximal to the interphalangeal joint, they will check rein the function of the interphalangeal flexor-extensor system. Likewise, if the flexor or extensor systems have not been centralized at the time of initial reconstruction, subsequent growth of the part may result in greater and greater deviation of these tendons off the longitudinal axis and loss of mechanical advantage. If axial alignment is relatively good but motion of the interphalangeal joint is limited, exploration and tenolysis or tendon repositioning can succeed in pro-

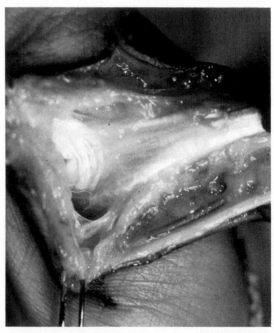

Figure 123–33. A duplication of the extensor aponeurosis. If this is left long it can attach to bone or soft tissues and restrict the excursion of the remaining extensor tendons.

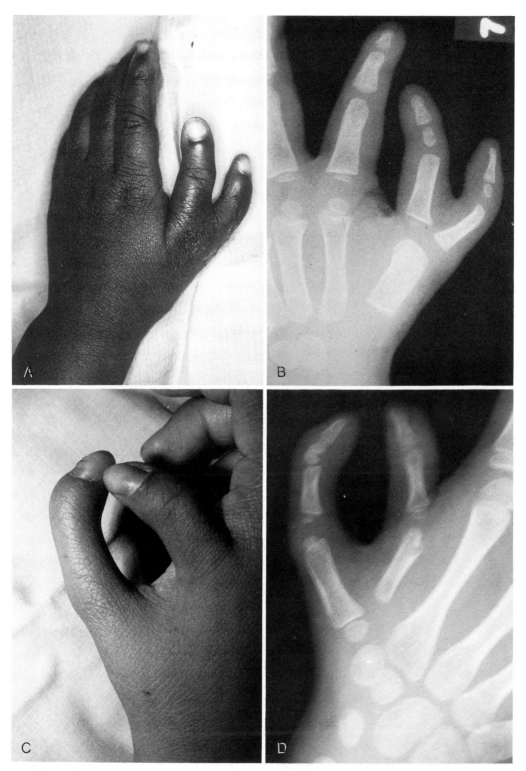

Figure 123–34. Type 7 polydactyly, or triphalangeal thumbs. When duplicated, both parts can be triphalangeal *(A, B)* or only one of the two elements may have three phalanges *(C, D).*

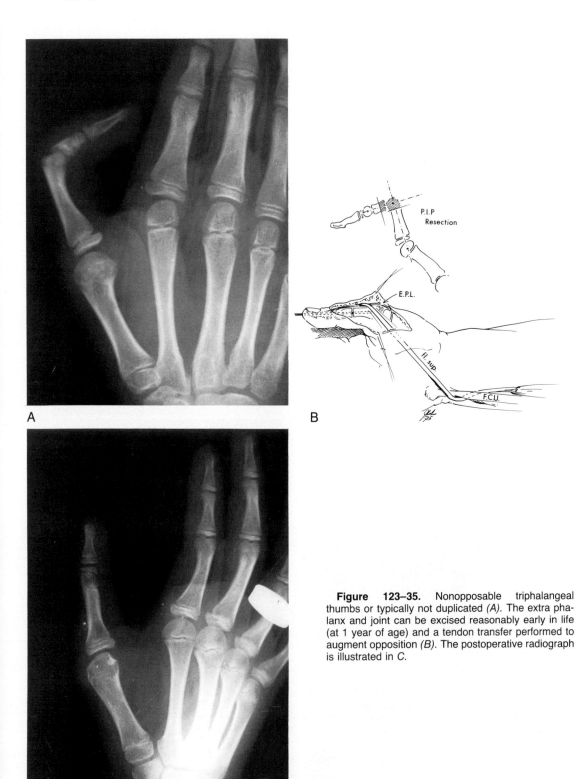

Figure 123–35. Nonopposable triphalangeal thumbs or typically not duplicated (A). The extra phalanx and joint can be excised reasonably early in life (at 1 year of age) and a tendon transfer performed to augment opposition (B). The postoperative radiograph is illustrated in C.

viding additional interphalangeal joint motion. When deviation of the phalanx and poor motion function coexist, the results of soft tissue procedures are disappointing.

Type 7 (Preaxial Polydactyly—Triphalangeal Thumb)

In Wassel's series (1969), triphalangeal thumbs were the second most commonly seen form of duplication. While pollical triphalangism is occasionally seen as an isolated entity (Lapidus, 1943), it more frequently occurs in association with preaxial polydactyly. Commonly, both duplicated parts are triphalangeal (Fig. 123–34A,B). Occasionally, one thumb is triphalangeal while the other has the normal skeletal complement (Fig. 123–34C,D). Triphalangeal thumbs are typically opposable or nonopposable. Those incapable of opposition are often singular and have more the appearance of an extra finger, termed pentadactyly. This condition is discussed in the section on pollicization. Triphalangeal thumb may present with different manifestations. Theories regarding the origin of this malformation include (1) an arrest in development (Haas, 1939) with persistence of the middle phalanx that normally fuses with the distal phalanx; (2) persistence of a remnant of one of the phalanges (Lapidus, 1943) of an incompletely duplicated distal phalanx of the thumb; or (3) in some cases, duplication of the index finger and absence of the thumb. It may be associated with an abnormal first metacarpal; Temtamy and McKusick (1978) also mention several syndromes associated with triphalangeal thumb.

Opposable triphalangeal thumbs are most often associated with preaxial polydactyly (Fig. 123–34). Typically, one element is dominant and preserved, while the other is ablated. Flatt (1977) urges caution in deciding which element to discard, especially in cases in which one element is triphalangeal and the other biphalangeal. He suggests considering saving the member with the normal number of skeletal elements even if it is slightly more hypoplastic. In so doing, one may avoid the problems of joint instability and progressive deviation common to most triphalangeal thumbs.

The extra phalanx, typically felt to be the middle phalanx, may be well formed, large, or small; when triangular in shape, it is termed delta phalanx. If the child is seen early in life, generally under 1 year of age, the accessory middle phalanx should be excised in association with ligament reconstruction and tendon rebalancing (Fig. 123–35). With time and continued growth, the axial directed forces assist in remolding the new joint faces. In older, untreated children, excision still may be performed, but secondary fusion of the two remaining phalanges will probably be necessary. It seems preferable to maintain the distal interphalangeal joint if well fashioned and fuse the base of the middle phalanx to the properly determined length of the base of the proximal phalanx. As in pollicization, the flexor tendon accommodates over time to this change in length. The extensor tendon should, however, be appropriately shortened surgically.

High Degrees of Polydactyly ("Mirror Hand")

These are rare types of polydactyly typically associated with duplication of more proximal elements. An associated condition involves a "mirror hand," sometimes called ulna duplication or ulnar dimelia. Here the normal preaxial structures are replaced by a mirror image of the postaxial digits, including duplication of the ulna. Some rounding of the distal ulnar articulation may cause it to resemble a radius, but an x-ray film of the elbow will demonstrate two olecranon processes. This condition is rare. Treatment involves amputation of extra radial digits, except one, which is pollicized. Entin (1959) and Davis and Farmer (1958) syndactylyzed two weak digits to fashion a strong thumb.

In conclusion, there is rarely an indication to simply amputate an extra thumb. In every instance, care must be taken to avoid the unhappy sequelae of a poorly planned and executed procedure.

REFERENCES

Bell, C.: The Hand. Its Mechanics and Vital Endowments as Evincing Design. 3rd Ed. London, W. Pickering, 1832.

Bilhaut, M.: Guérison d'un pouce bifide par un nouveau procédé opération. Cong. Fr. Chir., 4:576, 1890.

Blauth, W.: Der hypoplastische Daumen. Arch. Orthop. Unfall-chir., 62:225, 1967.

Brooks, D.: _In_ Wynn Perry, C. B. (Ed.): Rehabilitation of the Hand. 2nd Ed. London, Butterworth, 1964, pp. 336–348.

Buck-Gramcko, D.: Pollicization of the index finger. J. Bone Joint Surg., _53A_:1065, 1971.

Carpenter, G.: Two sisters showing malformations of the skull and other congenital anomalies. Rep. Soc. Study Dis. Child. London, _1_:110, 1901.

Crawford, H., and Adamson, J.: Congenital aplasia and hypoplasia of the thumb and extensor tendons. J. Bone Joint Surg., _48A_:82, 1966.

Darwin, C.: The Variation of Animals and Plants Under Domestication. Vol. 1. New York, D. Appleton & Company, 1896.

Davis, R. G., and Farmer, A. W.: Mirror hand anomalies. Plast. Reconstr. Surg., _21_:80, 1958.

Dobyns, J., Wood, M., Bayne, L., and Frykman, G.: Congenital hand deformities. _In_ Green, D. P. (Ed.): Operative Hand Surgery. New York, Churchill Livingstone, 1982.

Durham, J., and Meggitt, B.: Trigger thumbs in children. J. Bone Joint Surg., _56_:153, 1974.

Edgerton, M. T.: Surgical treatment of congenital thumb deformities. J. Bone Joint Surg., _47A_:1453, 1965.

Entin, M. A.: Reconstruction of congenital abnormalities of the upper extremity. J. Bone Joint Surg., _41A_:681, 1959.

Flatt, A. B.: The Care of Congenital Hand Anomalies. St. Louis, C. V. Mosby Company, 1977.

Gilbert, A.: Toe transfers for congenital hand defects. J. Hand Surg., _7_:118, 1982.

Gosset, J.: La pollicisation de l'index. J. Chir., _65_:403, 1949.

Haas, S. L.: Three-phalangeal thumbs. Am. J. Roentgenol., _42_:677, 1939.

Hentz, V. R.: Conventional techniques for thumb reconstruction. Clin. Orthop., _195_:129, 1985.

Hentz, V. R., and Littler, J. W.: The surgical management of congenital hand anomalies. _In_ Converse, J. M. (Ed.): Reconstructive Plastic Surgery. 2nd Ed. Philadelphia, W. B. Saunders Company, 1977a, pp. 3306–3349.

Hentz, V. R., and Littler, J. W.: Abduction-pronation and recession of the second (index) metacarpal in thumb agenesis. J. Hand Surg., _2_:113, 1977b.

Hilgendeldt, O.: Operativer Daumenersatz. Stuttgart, Ferdinand Enke Verlag, 1950.

Karchinov, K.: The treatment of polydactyly of the hand. Br. J. Plast. Surg., _15_:362, 1962.

Kelikian, H.: Congenital Deformities of the Hand and Forearm. Philadelphia, W. B. Saunders Company, 1974.

Kessler, I., Baruch, A., and Hecht, O.: Experience with distraction lengthening of digital rays in congenital anomalies. J. Hand Surg., _2_:394, 1977.

Kleinert, H. E., Grundberg, A. B., and Kutz, J. E.: Treatment of the reduplicated thumb (Abstr.). J. Bone Joint Surg., _55A_:874, 1973.

Lapidus, P. W.: Triphalangeal thumb. Report of 6 cases. Surg. Gynecol. Obstet., _77_:178, 1943.

Littler, J. W.: Subtotal reconstruction of the thumb. Plast. Reconstr. Surg., _10_:215, 1952.

Littler, J. W.: Current Practice in Orthopaedic Surgery. Vol. 3. St. Louis, C. V. Mosby Company, 1966, pp. 157–172.

Littler, J. W.: Restoration of the amputated thumb. Symposium on Reconstructive Hand Surgery. Vol. 9. St. Louis, C. V. Mosby Company, 1974, p. 202.

Matev, J.: Thumb reconstruction in children through metacarpal lengthening. Plast. Reconstr. Surg., _64_:665, 1979.

McGraw, M.: The Neuromuscular Maturation of the Human Infant. New York, Hafner Publishing Company, 1943, pp. 93–101.

Miller, J. W.: Pollex varus. Univ. Hosp. Bull. Ann Arbor, _10_:10, 1943.

Miura, T.: An appropriate treatment for postoperative Z-formed deformity of the duplicated thumb. J. Hand Surg., _2_:380, 1977.

Napier, J. R.: Functional aspects of the anatomy of the hand. _In_ Rob, C., and Smith, R. (Eds.): Clinical Surgery. London, Butterworth, 1966, p. 19.

Noack, M.: Ein Beitrag zum Krankheitsbild der Akrocephalosyndaktylie. Arch. Kinderheilkd., _160_:168, 1959.

Notta, A.: Recherche sur une affection particulière des gaines tendineuse de la main. Arch. Gen. Med., _24_:142, 1850.

Pellegrini, V. D., Hentz, V. R., and Littler, J. W.: Thumb reconstruction. _In_ McFarland, R. W. (Ed.): Unsatisfactory Results in Hand Surgery. Edinburgh, J. B. Lippincott Company, 1987.

Shapiro, R. N., Eddy, W., Fitzgibbon, J., and O'Brien, G.: The incidence of congenital anomalies discovered in the neonatal period. Am. J. Surg., _96_:396, 1958.

Strauch, B., and Spinner, M.: Congenital anomalies of the thumb. Absent intrinsics and flexor pollicis longus. J. Bone Joint Surg., _58A_:115, 1976.

Swanson, A. B.: A classification for congenital limb malformations. J. Hand Surg., _1_:8, 1976.

Tamplin, R. W.: Lecture on the nature and treatment of deficiencies. London, Longman, Brown, Green. Longman and Roberts, 1846, pp. 256–267.

Temtamy, S., and McKusick, V.: The Genetics of Hand Malformations. Volume XIV. New York, Alan R. Liss, 1978, p. 364.

Tupper, J. W.: Pollex abductus due to congenital malposition of the flexor pollicis longus. J. Bone Joint Surg., _51A_:1285, 1969.

Wassel, H. D.: The results of surgery for polydactyly of the thumb. Clin. Orthop., _64_:175, 1969.

Weckesser, E. C.: Congenital flexion-adduction deformity of the thumb. J. Bone Joint Surg., _37_:977, 1955.

Weckesser, E. C., Reed, J. R., and Heiple, G.: Congenital clasped thumb. J. Bone Joint Surg., _50_:1417, 1968.

Zadek, I.: Congenital absence of the extensor pollicis longus of both thumbs. J. Bone Joint Surg., _16_:432, 1934.

J. William Littler

Finger Pollicization for Traumatic Loss

HISTORICAL NOTE

NEUROVASCULAR PEDICLE METHOD OF DIGITAL
    TRANSFER

LEVELS OF THUMB AMPUTATION

RECONSTRUCTION OF THUMB BY FINGER
    TRANSFER
    Technique for Index Finger Transposition

Salvage of the severed thumb through primary microvascular reanastomosis has dramatically reduced the need for any secondary finger or toe transposition or osteoplastic reconstruction. But the congenitally thumbless child depends on finger pollicization alone for a more useful hand.

Traumatic thumb loss through the metacarpal with preservation of an intact carpometacarpal (CMC) joint with some intrinsic muscle control was for many years, during and following World War II, successfully managed by a one-stage finger (preferably the index) transposition. Even with total traumatic thumb loss at the carpal level, simulating somewhat that of agenesis, an intact index finger substitutes effectively for the thumb when its proximal phalanx is fused directly to the carpus in strategic projection. In most recession finger transpositions, only the extensor tendons require primary length adjustment.

A toe or finger, substituting for lost phalangeal length, can in selected cases restore strong pinch and supplement grasp. The transfer of free partial toe is preferred to that of a finger, unless damaged, for subtotal thumb reconstruction.

Sacrifice of a normal finger for only phalangeal thumb loss is extravagantly injudicious; the one-stage composite toe osteoplastic reconstruction method introduced by Foucher and associates (1980) and Morrison, O'Brien, and MacLeod (1980) is now the method of choice (see Chaps. 125 and 126).

Most thumb amputations are at the metacarpophalangeal (MCP) level or beyond. Normally destruction of this joint, which has extremely variable ranges of movement, allows fusion of the severed phalangeal portion or of a subsequent transposed part to the metacarpal with some shortening but little significant loss of essential function. Cantilever stability of the metacarpal–proximal phalangeal unit enhances active interphalangeal joint movement.

It is not the full length of the thumb, nor its great strength and movement, but rather its strategic position relative to the fingers and the integrity of the specialized terminal pulp tissue that determine its prehensile status.

HISTORICAL NOTE

During the late nineteenth century, the critical disability imposed by a thumb amputated at the metacarpophalangeal level caught the surgical attention of Huguier (1874), who reported improving hand function through the creation of an interosseous cleft, a procedure later referred to as first metacarpal "phalangization" by Klapp (1912). In 1887 the imaginative surgeon Guermonprez suggested transferring an adjacent finger for thumb loss.

It was not until 1897, however, that Nicoladoni presented his case, of six years before, wherein he had completely resurfaced the divested right thumb of a young factory worker with a left pectoral skin flap. Although the resurfacing was redundant and retained the nipple, and despite poor sensibility, the patient was able to continue his work (Fig. 124–1A). Nicoladoni (1897) introduced the osteoplastic method for thumb reconstruction and also suggested that a toe or a finger from the opposite hand be substituted for thumb loss. In 1900 he reported three successful toe to thumb position transfers and in 1903 analyzed the results. This complicated distant digital transfer met, understandably, with little contemporary surgical enthusiasm, and the more reasonable but less spectacular and less precarious transposition of an adjacent digit, as first suggested by Guermonprez, then gained some favor. Nicoladoni had no occasion to transfer a finger. This rarely indicated procedure was left for Joyce (1918) of England, who utilized a contralateral ring finger in three cases. Bartlett, Moses, and May (1986), using neurovascular anastomosis, transferred a damaged finger to reconstruct loss of a right thumb.

Just before and during World War I, the foundation was laid for more successful methods of thumb reconstruction; noteworthy is the paper of Noesske (1920), who established basic techniques for thumb reconstruction (see Littler, 1974). Iselin (1937) devoted special attention to the problem of traumatic thumb loss and presented fundamental ideas on the desirable features of reconstruction, espousing the transfer of the independent index finger. Zsulyevich (1938) achieved an especially fine thumb restoration, following Iselin's suggestions, by uniting the proximal phalanx of a transposed index finger to the thumb metacarpal remnant through an intramedullary bone graft (Fig. 124–2). In 1930 a somewhat discouraging note was sounded by the French surgeon Gueulette, who decried the transfer of an intact index finger for thumb loss; "Has not the hand found its function diminished by the transplant of a healthy digit?"

Hilgenfeldt (1950), working independently in Germany during World War II, developed a relatively free method for transposing a finger on intact nerves and blood vessels beneath a slender but nonessential palmar skin bridge; in most cases the long finger was selected for thumb substitution (see Fig. 124–

6). His results were analyzed in an excellent monograph (1950), regrettably untranslated. Similar but less sophisticated thumb work was also done in the United States Army Hand Surgical Centers, where osteoplastic (Nicoladoni) reconstructions were at first popular. However, the generally unsatisfactory functional and esthetic results (i.e., rigidity, redundant unstable coverage, and poor sensibility and circulation) (see Fig. 124–1A,B), led finally to the less complicated but technically unperfected finger transfer (Greeley, 1946; Kelikian and Bintcliffe, 1946; Tanzer and Littler, 1948; Dehne, 1952). The cleft resulting from the radiopalmar shifting of the finger routinely required a pedicle skin flap for closure.

In 1949 the French surgeon Jean Gosset introduced a neurovascular pedicle technique for digital transfer, quite similar to that of Hilgenfeldt but using the independent index finger for thumb amputation substitution as suggested earlier by his countryman Iselin. This method, free of any skin bridge, allowed ease of transfer to thumb position for any finger with good circulation and sensibility. The introduction of the palmodigital neurovascular pedicle shifting of composite tissue enabled a high degree of freedom and surgical precision in local reconstruction for treatment of not only traumatic thumb amputation but also agenesis (Littler, 1952, 1953, 1966) (see Chap. 123).

Peacock (1966) and Chase (1969) reported a number of excellent results of thumb reconstructions from their experience with traumatic loss during the Korean War; many papers and several monographs dealing with the problems of traumatic and congenital thumb loss have since swelled the surgical literature (Hage, 1966; Simonetta, 1975). A renewed interest in toe transfer and primary reunion for thumb and finger amputation followed the precise microsurgical neurovascular work of Bunke (1973) and O'Brien and associates (1975).

NEUROVASCULAR PEDICLE METHOD OF DIGITAL TRANSFER

Thumb loss imposes a critical hand disability by deprivation of a refined and powerful pinch and grasp mechanism. However, through a carefully planned and skillfully

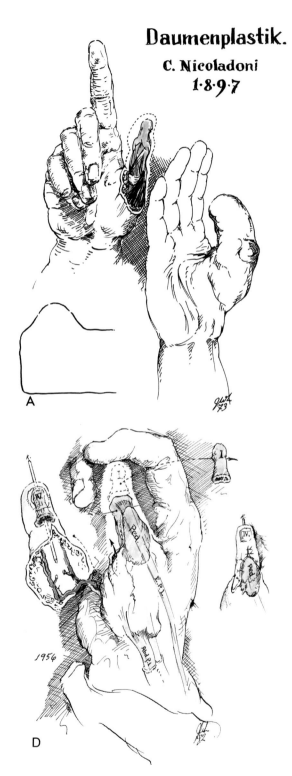

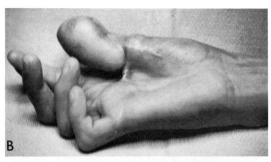

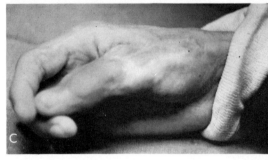

Figure 124–1. *A,* Nicoladoni's (1897) first "Daumen-plastik" for an extensive skin avulsion of a young man's right thumb, leaving musculotendinous and skeletal structures intact. When seen on the day following injury, the full active movement of the denuded joints created "an odd impression." Salvage was made through a pedicle skin flap from the left pectoral region. The resultant thumb was thick, covered like a "mitten," and flexed at the interphalangeal joint by volar bridging suture line scar. The left nipple was present on the radial aspect of the thumb. The patient continued to work; the thumb had considerable strength, and, although tactile sensibility was minimal, it was protective. Temperature was lower than that of the other digits. A reduction in volume, excision of the nipple, and a neurovascular skin island transfer from the ulnar aspect of the long finger would have provided an excellent result. *B,* The condition of a worker's right hand after a crush burn avulsion injury of the right thumb and palm. A primary abdominal pedicle flap was utilized to preserve the thumb. Despite skeletal preservation, the nature of the coverage rendered the thumb useless as an opponent for the intact index and long fingers. *C,* An exceptionally useful thumb was restored by substituting the terminal phalanx of the ring finger distal to its extensor and flexor insertions on its intact neurovascular pedicle. The investing skin of the ring finger was transferred with the distal segment, thus eliminating the redundant coverage. *D,* Ring finger components transferred for reconstruction of divested thumb. Example of an early neurovascular transfer operation presaging the free toe wrap-around osteoplastic operation of Foucher and associates (1980) and Morrison, O'Brien, and MacLeod (1980). E.P.L. = Extensor pollicis longus; K. = Kirschner wire.

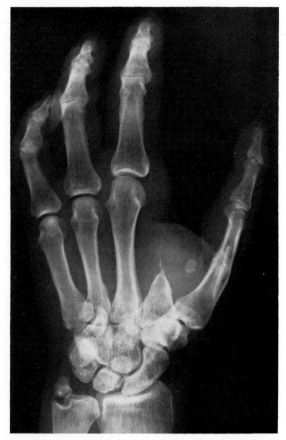

Figure 124–2. X-ray film demonstrating intramedullary bone graft for skeletal fixation of the transposed index digit, maintaining the longitudinal arch of the "thumb."

executed finger transfer or toe osteoplastic-neurovascular skin island reconstruction, a near-normal phalangeal thumb substitute is possible. Selection of cases appropriate for surgery depends on the functional loss, some understanding by the patient of what can be accomplished, and a desire for the operation. Despite the discouraging opinion of some that loss of even a dominant thumb, with the other hand remaining normal, constitutes no indication for reconstruction, particularly by digital transfer, experience and a relatively high degree of result predictability can alter this attitude and provide better hands for some patients (Fig. 124–3).

Correct length, strategic position, and stability are the mechanical requisites, and movement and sensibility are the physiologic ones, for a successful thumb reconstruction. Excessive length, as noted in many early restorative attempts, detracts both functionally and esthetically, but with the method

presented below length is not a problem. Strong flexion-adduction and full extension-abduction along a cardinal oblique radiopalmar plane are the prime movements for the new thumb. Basal stability is essential either through the integrity of an intact carpometacarpal joint under control of some intrinsic musculature or through fusion of the transferred digit to the carpus or metacarpus (in an optimum [fist] projection) (Fig. 124–4).

All degrees of loss are encountered, and obviously the best functional result is achieved when at least a basal part of the first metacarpal and its intrinsic muscles remain, preserving stability and the unique rotatory movement of the carpometacarpal joint. The precise incisional design and calculation of skin and skeletal finger length necessary to complement the loss can be accurately established with the neurovascular pedicle transfer method. Because of the variegated nature of injury, incisional modification (because of cicatrix) is often necessary, further complicating the procedure.

LEVELS OF THUMB AMPUTATION

There are two major categories of thumb loss.

1. *Total amputation*—at the carpal level. It is traumatic or congenital. There is loss of skin commissure, intrinsic musculature, and basal joint.

2. *Subtotal amputation*—at the metacarpophalangeal level, proximal or just distal to the joint. The commissure, intrinsic musculature, and basal joint are usually preserved.

RECONSTRUCTION OF THUMB BY FINGER TRANSFER

In both categories of thumb amputation, the adjacent index finger is often damaged—proximally, as a rule with total loss, or distally, with subtotal radial-oblique loss. If length reduction is required when transposing a finger, it is preferable to resect a basal segment rather than the more important distal phalanx as advocated by Gosset (1949). For a total traumatic thumb amputation, the proximal phalanx of the transferred finger is joined to the carpus (trapezium) or, in con-

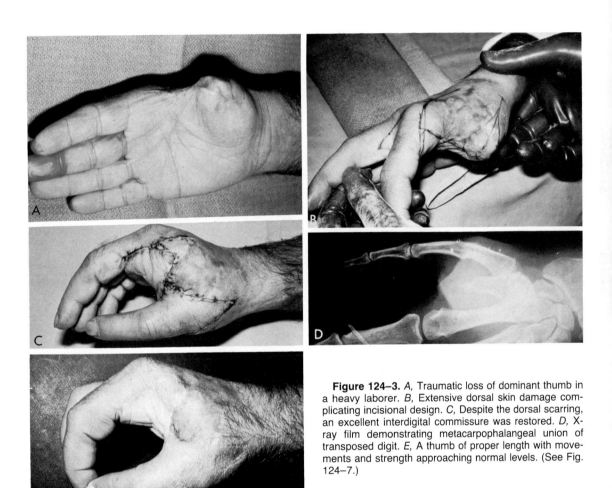

Figure 124–3. *A,* Traumatic loss of dominant thumb in a heavy laborer. *B,* Extensive dorsal skin damage complicating incisional design. *C,* Despite the dorsal scarring, an excellent interdigital commissure was restored. *D,* X-ray film demonstrating metacarpophalangeal union of transposed digit. *E,* A thumb of proper length with movements and strength approaching normal levels. (See Fig. 124–7.)

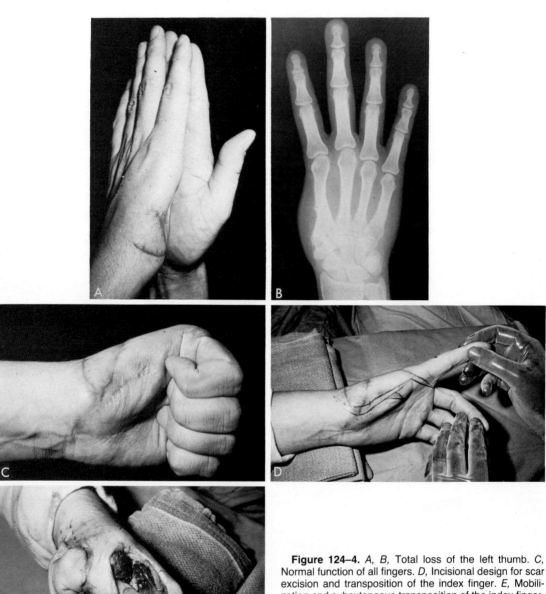

Figure 124–4. *A, B,* Total loss of the left thumb. *C,* Normal function of all fingers. *D,* Incisional design for scar excision and transposition of the index finger. *E,* Mobilization and subcutaneous transposition of the index finger.

Figure 124–4 *Continued F, G,* Fixation of proximal phalanx to trapezium in mean thumb projection. *H,* Flexion-extension along a cardinal plane provided excellent pinch and grasp.

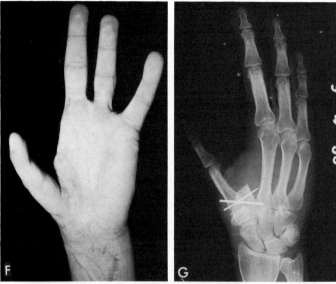

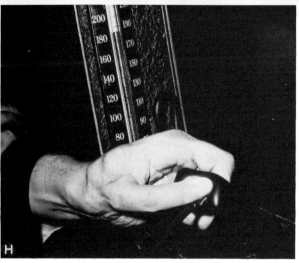

genital thumb absence, if basal stability of the recessed index metacarpophalangeal joint cannot be maintained, to its index metacarpal base in a fixed mean functional projection.

For a subtotal thumb amputation at or proximal to the metacarpophalangeal joint, an appropriate phalangeal segment of either the index or the ring finger, or possibly another damaged finger, may be transferred. However, when the thumb metacarpophalangeal joint is present, especially in the young patient, a ring finger unit (middle and distal phalanges) is preferred (Figs. 124–5 and 124–6) (Hilgenfeldt, 1950; Le Tac, 1952; Gosset and Sels, 1964) unless a damaged finger can be used. An osteoplastic reconstruction may be more applicable in this situation, especially in the younger adult, and the Foucher-Morrison toe procedure, though difficult to perform, is probably the best.

Any finger can be transferred to thumb position on its palmar neurovascular pedicle. When the index finger is selected, a dorsal vein can be preserved, assuring a more adequate venous return; if congestion complicates the transfer, an anastomosis between a previously isolated dorsal phalangeal vein and a wrist radial vein should be considered. The proximal phalangeal base of the finger segment is fixed either to the carpus or to the thumb metacarpal remnant by an intramedullary bone graft, Kirschner wires, or both. Adjustment of tendon length is confined principally to the extensors, since in the case of the index the relatively independent excursion of the flexors is generally sufficiently accommodating to preserve function despite recession. In some instances, the flexors may require secondary shortening; even better, the proximal long thumb flexor remnant* is transferred to the liberated profundus tendon at the wrist or distal forearm level (Fig. 124–7), thereby bringing flexion of the terminal phalanx under normal cortical control. Here, also, the independent superficial flexor tendon may require segmental shortening for more effective action. When the proximal phalanx of a recessed finger is united to the first metacarpal remnant, its proximal interphalangeal (PIP) joint remains under control of the superficial flexor, now simulating flexor pollicis brevis action.

---

*Sufficient excursion for the flexor pollicis longus is preserved if, after injury, it adheres just beyond the radiocarpal joint.

Full terminal phalangeal flexor independence resides only in the index finger and is successively lost ulnarward, even though the median innervated superficial flexors are all independent. When a digit other than the index is transferred, its deep flexor tendon must be isolated and empowered by an independent motor, preferably the flexor pollicis longus (see above) or a superficial flexor. In traumatic thumb loss, the long flexor (or extensor) tendon may be avulsed, requiring at least a shortening and radial shift of the independent extensor indicis proprius—now substituting for the extensor pollicis longus.

The position and relative independence of the index finger favor it as a substitute for most traumatic thumb amputations and certainly when agenesis is the problem. In traumatic loss, when the proximal phalanx of the transferred finger is united to the thumb metacarpal remnant, the proximal sellar, ginglymoid interphalangeal joint substitutes for the thumb metacarpophalangeal joint but lacks its axial, lateral, and conjunct rotatory characteristics. Therefore, when uniting the thumb metacarpal remnant to the finger proximal phalanx, it is essential that the phalangeal segment be pronated somewhat to compensate for the normal metacarpophalangeal axial rotation. Finger transposition may restore the correct length but not the normal thumb interaxial joint-length relationship (see Figs. 124–7 and 124–10).

Technique for Index Finger Transposition

Moving the independent index finger into thumb position is simpler and less precarious than moving either the long or the ring finger, despite the not infrequent damage to the index lateral neurovascular bundle, specifically the radialis indicis artery, which generally originates from the princeps pollicis. Tandler (1897) and Coleman and Anson (1961) made extensive studies of arterial variations; these were important contributions in vascular anatomy for the hand surgeon. Pulsation of the proper palmar digital vessels and intact sensibility on either side of the finger indicate integrity of the neurovascular bundle. Normal color and temperature are reassuring, and Allen's test determines patency of the vascular system. In doubtful

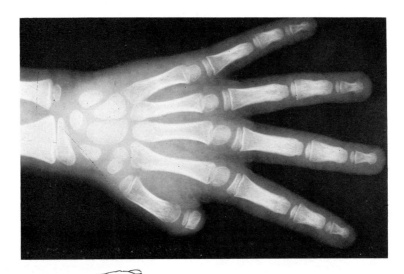

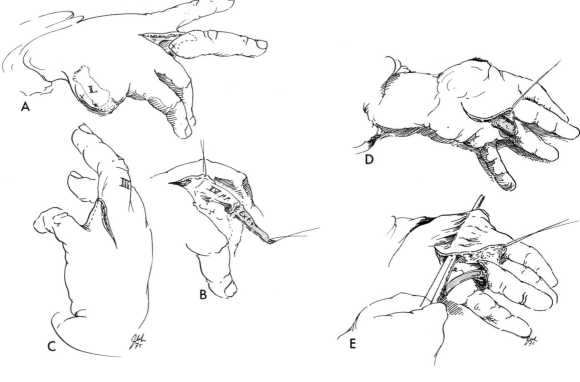

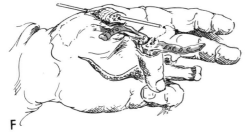

Figure 124–5. X-ray film of rope avulsion of left thumb of 7 year old boy. *A,* Incisional design for ring finger (middle and terminal phalangeal) transfer. *B,* Isolation of common extensor tendon (Ext. t.) and resection of proximal phalanx (p.p.). *C,* Web closure, dorsal aspect. *D,* Isolation of neurovascular bundles (see Fig. 124–6). *E,* Sectioned profundus tendon; development of subfascial tunnel to thumb amputation site. *F,* Transarticular Kirschner wire for intramedullary fixation of transferred digit.

Illustration continued on the following page

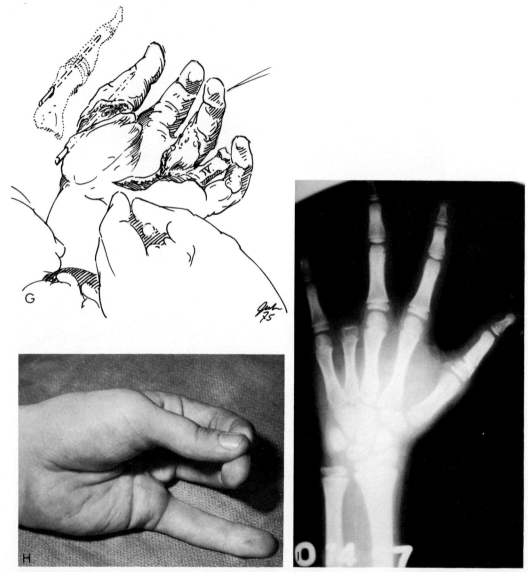

Figure 124–5 *Continued G,* Fixation of ring phalangeal segments to remnant of proximal phalanx of thumb. *H,* Three months later, because of avulsion of the flexor pollicis longus, the ring flexor digitorum profundus was motored by the fourth flexor digitorum superficialis. *I,* With time the third interosseous space was narrowed owing to growth arrest of the fourth metacarpal. Hand function was excellent; the patient became a Marine. Little fingers have also been used for thumb reconstruction (see Herndon, Littler, and Watson, 1975.)

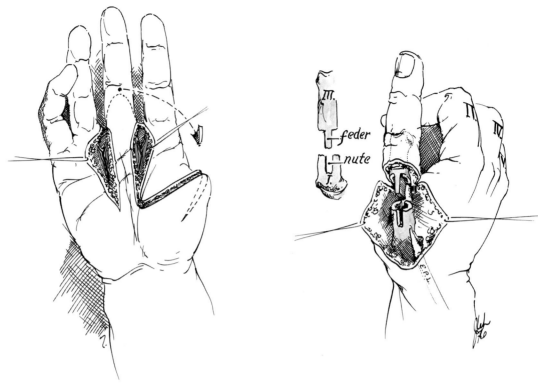

Figure 124–6. "Operativer Daumenersatz." Hilgenfeldt's transposition of the long finger on neurovascular pedicles for thumb loss. The palmar skin bridge is unnecessary because circulatory jeopardy may possibly complicate the transposition. Although the long finger has more appropriate phalangeal size and length for thumb substitution, its use results in an undesirable central cleft. The index or ring finger, depending on the degree of thumb loss, is a more desirable transfer. Intramedullary bone graft fixation, rather than mortise and tenon juncture, possibly allows for a more adjustable metacarpophalangeal positioning of the transposed finger segment.

cases an arteriogram may be obtained but is rarely necessary. The author has, under unanticipated duress, transferred one index finger on a single (the second) intermetacarpal artery, and another via the collateral circulation of the adjacent long finger. These problems are readily managed by microvascular anastomosis or grafting.

The operation of finger transposition, performed in a bloodless field with refined surgical technique, embodies five basic steps for mobilization and secondary fixation of the finger into the thumb position.

1. *Skin incisions.* Two incisions, one placed elliptically at the cicatrized amputation site and the other at the base of the index finger, are joined diagonally to form proximally based dorsal and palmar triangular flaps, which allow full exposure yet retain the commissure if minimal damage is present. Local scarring not infrequently necessitates a variation of this basic incisional scheme (see Figs. 124–3 and 124–4), and occasionally preliminary resurfacing is necessary—possibly with a pedicle skin flap.

An exact representation of the thumb loss is plotted on the index finger; that part sufficient to restore thumb length is determined by skeletal and dorsal and palmar skin measurements (Fig. 124–8A). Extreme care in dissection is necessary at the palmar base of the finger when isolating the neurovascular bundles that lie just beneath the skin and superficial fascia; these are easily damaged, and the operation's success is obviously based on their integrity. With completion of the incisions, a major dorsal (indicis) vein is isolated and preserved; the two triangular flaps are elevated, exposing the extensor tendons (extensor digitorum communis and extensor indicis proprius), the second metacarpal, and the first dorsal interosseous muscle. The junctura tendinum and fascia lying between the extensor communis of the index and long fingers are divided.

2. *Preparation of neurovascular pedicles.*

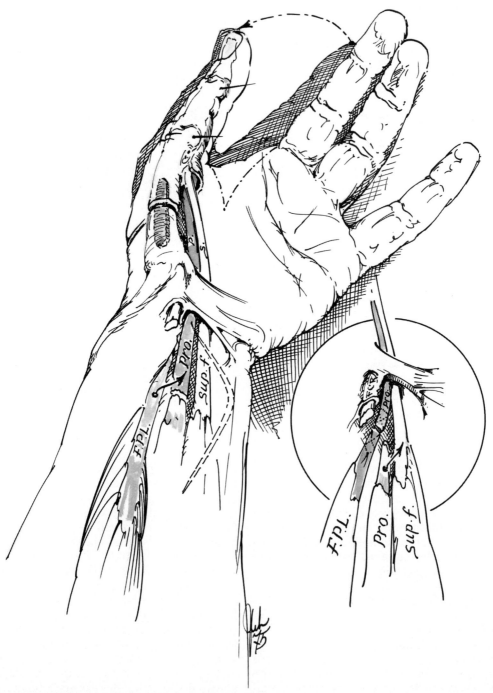

Figure 124–7. Transfer of flexor pollicis longus (F.P.L.) to flexor profundus (Pro.) of transposed index. If traction on the profundus at the wrist level flexes the "thumb" independently of the adjacent long finger terminal phalanx, the flexor pollicis longus juncture may be made into it under appropriate tension. If not, the second profundus must be isolated from the third. This is generally accomplished by sectioning and withdrawing the second profundus through a proximal palmar incision, with extreme caution being paid to the median nerve, and then returning the profundus tendon to the wrist, where it is sutured end to end to the flexor pollicis longus. Sup. f. = superficial flexor.

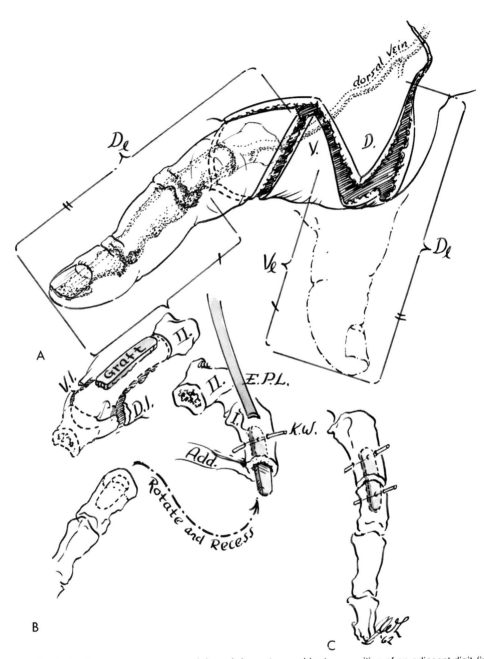

Figure 124–8. Restoration of thumb amputated through its metacarpal by transposition of an adjacent digit (index). *A,* Skin and skeletal measurements correspond precisely to the extent of thumb loss. V and D indicate palmar and dorsal skin flaps, respectively (modified by any existing scars). D_e = Dorsal skin length; V_e = palmar skin length. *B* and *C,* Metacarpophalangeal resection allowing an index phalangeal unit of a skeletal length necessary to restore the thumb loss. This is joined to the first metacarpal remnant in 10 degrees of pronation by intramedullary bone graft and Kirschner wire (K.W.) fixation. E.P.L. = Extensor pollicis longus.

The neurovascular pedicles are further isolated by careful dissection at the base of the finger, with special care being taken to preserve the vulnerable (especially when distended) accompanying veins. It is necessary to section the compartmental vertical septa of the palmar fascia to provide freedom for the radial shift of the nerves, the vessels, and the flexor tendons. The bifurcation of the common palmar artery is joined by the dorsal interosseous artery at the distal border of the interpalmar plate (intermetacarpal) ligament. The oblique fascial septum separating the second dorsal and palmar interosseous muscles is longitudinally divided, further exposing the interosseous artery and the interpalmar plate ligament with its deep palmar fascial extension proximally, which is sectioned. Here the artery to the radial side of the long finger is divided and ligated (Fig. 124–9). The common palmar nerve to the index and long fingers normally bifurcates more proximally than the artery, but it can be separated further if necessary to provide

more freedom. Congestion of the finger is avoided if a dorsal vein with its subcutaneous tissue, lymphatics, and dorsal nerve branches can be preserved. Although the common palmar and proper digital arteries have accompanying veins proximally, they are small and may be overburdened.

3. *Mobilization of the finger.* The first dorsal interosseous muscle is detached from its broad insertion at the radiovolar base of the proximal phalanx. This exposes the sagittal restraining bands of the central extensor tendon encircling the metacarpal head, beneath which lies the sturdy radial collateral ligament.

A careful subcutaneous separation of the central tendon from the lumbrical and palmar interosseous lateral bands exposes the base of the proximal phalanx. The second metacarpal is then subperiosteally obliquely resected at its base and detached distally from the proximal phalanx by sectioning the collateral ligaments and joint capsule. Whether the donor index finger is normal or has suf-

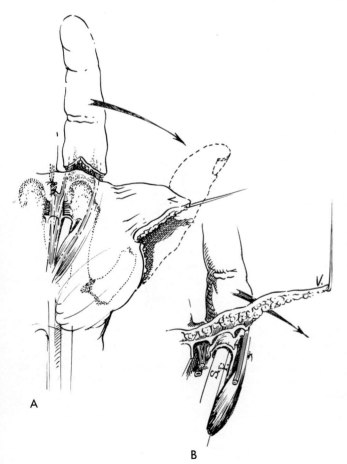

Figure 124–9. *A,* Ligation of proper palmar digital artery to adjacent long finger; division of metacarpophalangeal interpalmar plate ligament and deep proximal palmar fascia. *B,* Section of palmar fascial septa to permit radial shift of digit. V. = Palmar flap.

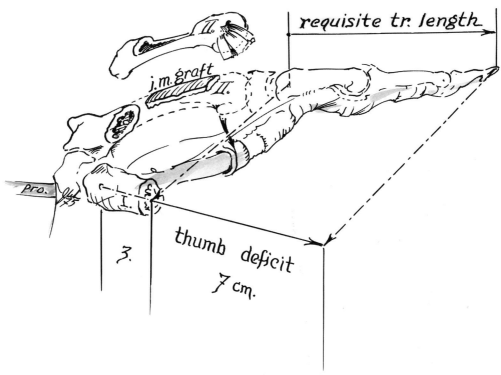

Figure 124–10. Flexor tendon assembly released from base of proximal phalanx. This allows a more normal approach for the flexor system to the index proximal interphalangeal joint, which is now at the metacarpophalangeal level of the new "thumb." Recession and fixation of the index phalangeal segment are also facilitated by this maneuver (see Fig. 124–7).

fered a loss of length will determine in part the level of section, either proximal or distal to the metacarpophalangeal joint (see Fig. 124–8*A*), so that the length of segment transferred is a near skeletal duplication of the thumb loss. The normal thumb extends nearly to the level of the proximal interphalangeal joint of the index finger and, when fully developed, has an average metacarpophalangeal length of approximately 9 to 11 cm. Requisite length measurement can be determined from the opposite hand or one of like size.*

4. *Fixation of the transposed finger.* When a part of the first metacarpal is present and either the index metacarpal of a distally damaged, shortened finger or the proximal phalanx is to be united to it, fixation is securely gained through an intramedullary bone graft taken from the resected portion of the second metacarpal. The graft is doweled into the first metacarpal remnant and transfixed with a

Kirschner wire; the index unit is then impaled on the graft and transfixed at the desired degree of pronation (Fig. 124–8*B,C*). This simple, stable intramedullary bone graft and Kirschner wire fixation has been used with ease in the author's cases, rather than the more difficult mortise and tenon juncture advocated by Gosset (1949) and Hilgenfeldt (1950).

5. *Adjustment of tendons.* If the finger has been appreciably recessed (approximately 5 cm when a fully developed finger of normal length is used), the slackened long extensor tendons must be corrected primarily; any flexor tendon adjustment is done secondarily. The flexor mechanism is released from the proximal phalanx by sheath section to allow recession and ease of fixation to the metacarpal remnant (Fig. 124–10). In most cases, the lateral (radial) angulation and shortening of the extensors (extensor digitorum communis and extensor indicis proprius) negate their function; adjustment is made by dividing the extensor digitorum communis proximally and making an end to end juncture between it and the extensor pollicis longus (Fig. 124–11). If the extensor pollicis longus has been

---

*A first metacarpal residual base length of 3 cm requires 7 to 8 cm of index skeletal length to complement the average length loss of the fully developed adult thumb.

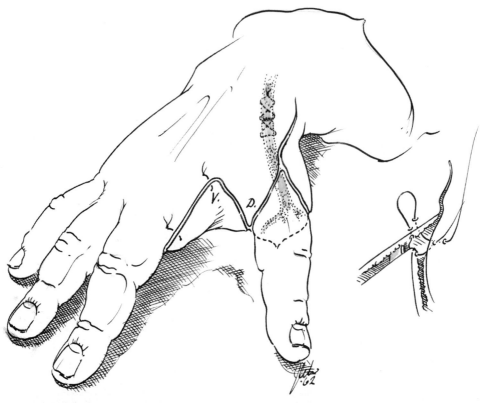

Figure 124–11. Index transfer to thumb position, with closure of palmar (V) and dorsal flaps restoring interdigital commissure. Figure-of-eight suture uniting thumb and index extensors. *Inset,* Apical suture.

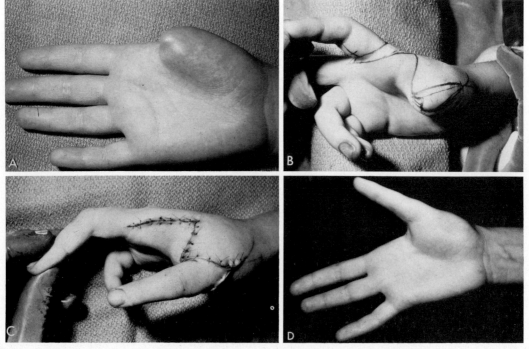

Figure 124–12. *A,* Amputation of right thumb through metacarpophalangeal joint in a 19 year old female. *B,* Incisional design (see Fig. 124–8*A*). *C,* Closure (see Fig. 124–11). *D,* Functional and esthetic result.

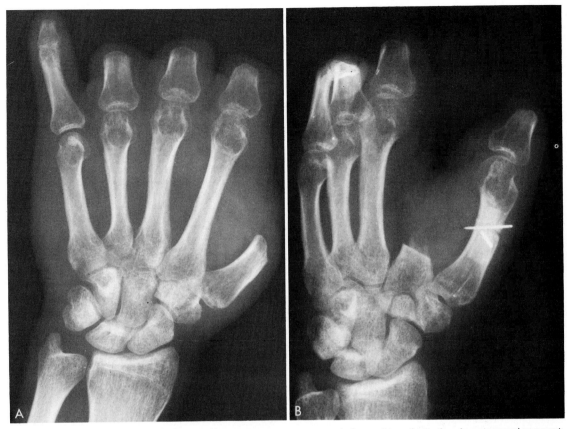

Figure 124–13. *A,* Subtotal amputation of hand. *B,* Index metacarpophalangeal transfer to thumb metacarpal remnant. Resection and transfer created an adequate cleft and a thumb of substantial length, movement, and strength.

avulsed, it is necessary to sever the extensor indicis proprius at its metacarpophalangeal juncture with the common extensor, withdraw it proximal to the dorsal carpal ligament, and transfer it, more radialward, subcutaneously in the normal path of the extensor pollicis longus, where it is reunited to the extensor digitorum communis at a balanced tension.* With thumb agenesis, this radial rerouting of the extensor mechanism is unnecessary.

A meticulous closure with everting interrupted skin sutures at the base of the transposed finger is essential, and great care must be taken not to damage subjacent neurovascular bundles. Correct placement of the midpalmar incision at the base of the finger will be indicated by the apex of the skin triangle at the palmar base of the thumb remnant; this last refinement gives some added flare and volume to the finger as it joins the basal remnant of the thumb (Fig. 124–12).

Immobilization with the wrist moderately extended and the thumb projected in line with the radius is maintained for six to eight weeks after postoperative suture removal at two to three weeks. With time and use the transposed digit will assume thumb characteristics; more normal function can be further enhanced (Littler, 1952) if the long thumb flexor is sutured to the flexor profundus of the transposed finger (see Fig. 124–7). A number of variations on the above procedure will be necessary when transferring any other finger or its components to thumb position in extensive and complex injuries of the entire hand (Fig. 124–13). Proficiency in the careful assessment of what can be saved and then redistributed for the reconstruction of a prehensile unit constitutes one of the outstanding qualities of the experienced hand surgeon.

REFERENCES

Bartlett, S. P., Moses, M. H., and May, J. W., Jr.: Thumb reconstruction by free microvascular transfer of an injured index finger: a case report. Plast. Reconstr. Surg., 77:660, 1986.

---

*The extensor indicis proprius can also be used to reinforce intrinsic (palmar interosseous) interphalangeal extension (Littler, 1953).

Bunke, J.: Thumb replacement: great toe transplantation by microvascular anastomosis. J. Plast. Surg., *26*:194, 1973.

Chase, R. A.: An alternate to pollicization in subtotal thumb reconstruction. Plast. Reconstr. Surg., *44*:421, 1969.

Coleman, S. S., and Anson, B.: Arterial patterns in the hand based upon a study of 650 specimens. Surg. Gynecol. Obstet., *113*:409, 1961.

Dehne, E.: Operativer Ersatz des Daumens. Chirurgie, *23*:566, 1952.

Foucher, G., Merle, M., Maneaud, M., and Michon, J.: Microsurgical free partial toe transfer in hand reconstruction. A report of 12 cases. Plast. Reconstr. Surg., *65*:616, 1980.

Gosset, J.: La pollicisation de l'index. J. Chir., *65*:403, 1949.

Gosset, J., and Sels, M.: Technique, indications et résultats de la pollicisation du 4ᵉ doigt. Ann. Chir., *18*:1005, 1964.

Greeley, P. W.: Reconstruction of the thumb. Ann. Surg., *124*:60, 1946.

Guermonprez, F.: Notes sur quelques résections et restaurations du pouce. Paris, P. Asselin, 1897.

Gueulette, R.: Pollicisation de l'index: étude critique des procédés de restauration du pouce. J. Chir., *36*:1, 1930.

Hage, J.: Het tot duim van de wijbvinger volgens Littler. Doctoral thesis, Rijksuniversiteit te Groningen, 1966.

Herndon, J. H., Littler, J. W., and Watson, F. M.: Traumatic amputation of the thumb and three fingers: treatment by digital pollicization. J. Bone Joint Surg., *57A*:708, 1975.

Hilgenfeldt, O.: Operativer Daumenersatz. Stuttgart, Ferdinand Enke Verlag, 1950.

Huguier, P. L.: Remplacement du pouce par son métacarpien, par l'agrandissement du premier espace interosseux. Arch. Gén. Méd., *1*:78, 1874.

Iselin, M.: Reconstruction of the thumb. Surgery, *2*:619, 1937.

Joyce, J. L.: A new operation of the substitution of a thumb. Br. J. Surg., *5*:499, 1918.

Kelikian, H., and Bintcliffe, E. W.: Functional restoration of the thumb. Surg. Gynecol. Obstet., *83*:807, 1946.

Klapp, R.: Uber einige kleinere plastische Operationen an Fingern und Hand. Dtsch. Z. Chir., *188*:479, 1912.

Le Tac, R.: Reconstitution du pouce détruit par pollicisation de l'annulaire ou de 5ᵉ doigt. Mem. Acad. Chir., *78*:262, 1952.

Littler, J. W.: Subtotal reconstruction of the thumb. Plast. Reconstr. Surg., *10*:215, 1952.

Littler, J. W.: Neurovascular pedicle method of digital transposition for reconstruction of the thumb. Plast. Reconstr. Surg., *12*:303, 1953.

Littler, J. W.: Digital transposition. *In* Adams, J. P. (ed.): Current Practice in Orthopaedic Surgery. St. Louis, MO, C. V. Mosby Company, 1966.

Littler, J. W. (ed.): Symposium on Reconstructive Hand Surgery. Vol. 9. St. Louis, MO, C. V. Mosby Company, 1974.

Morrison, W. A., O'Brien, B. McC., and MacLeod, A. M.: Thumb reconstruction with a free neurovascular wraparound flap from the big toe. J. Hand Surg., *5*:575, 1980.

Nicoladoni, C.: Daumenplastik. Wien. Klin. Wochenschr., *10*:663, 1897.

Nicoladoni, C.: Daumenplastik und organischer Ersatz der Fingerspitze (Anticheiroplastik und Daktyloplastik). Arch. Chir., *6*:606, 1900.

Nicoladoni, C.: Weitere Erfahrungen über Daumenplastik. Arch. Klin. Chir., *69*:697, 1903.

Noesske, H.: Uber Ersatz des bamt Metacarpus verlorenen Daumens durch operative Umstellung des Zeigefingers (mit Lichtbildern). Münch. Med. Wochenschr., *16*:465, 1920.

O'Brien, B. McC., MacLeod, A. M., Sykes, P. J., and Donahoe, S.: Hallux-to-hand transfer. Hand, *7*:128, 1975.

Peacock, E. E., Jr.: Reconstruction of the thumb. *In* Flynn, J. E. (ed.): Hand Surgery. Baltimore, Williams & Wilkins Company, 1966.

Rank, B. K., Wakefield, A. R., and Hueston, J.: Surgery of Repair As Applied to Hand Injuries. 4th Ed. New York, Longman, 1973.

Simonetta, C.: Chirurgie réparatrice des pertes de substance et des amputations du pouce. Doctoral thesis, Lausanne, 1975.

Tandler, J.: Zur Anatomie der Arterien der Hand. Anatomische Hefte, *7*:263, 1897.

Tanzer, R. C., and Littler, J. W.: Reconstruction of the thumb by transposition of an adjacent digit. Plast. Reconstr. Surg., *3*:533, 1948.

Zsulyevich, I.: Ein Fall von plastischem Daumenersatz. Chirurgie, *10*:433, 1938.

James W. May, Jr.

Microvascular Great Toe to Hand Transfer for Reconstruction of the Amputated Thumb

On the length, strength, free lateral motion, and perfect mobility of the thumb depends the power of the human hand. The thumb is called pollex because of its strength and that strength is necessary to the power of the hand being equal to that of all the fingers.

SIR CHARLES BELL

The thumb is fundamentally important in hand function and makes up 40 to 50 per cent of the functional capacity of the hand. It is for this reason that through the eons of time surgeons have toiled and struggled with thumb reconstruction.

Over the past 15 years since the introduction of elective microvascular reconstructive surgery, many improvements have been made in the armamentarium of the reconstructive hand surgeon. No operation in all of microvascular reconstructive surgery has added a greater degree of improvement to the level of its predecessor operations than microvascular reconstructive toe to hand transfer in replacing the traumatically amputated thumb.

Of all mammals, only primates have an opposable thumb (Boyes, 1970). As man evolved, so the thumb has shifted from being a digit of cylinder grasp to a digit of opposition (Bell, 1833). This provides for improved object manipulation and single hand prehension. The presence of an opposable thumb has set the stage in human development for the ability to manipulate objects, and the ability of a superior central nervous system to contemplate use of those objects.

As stated by Sir Charles Bell (1833), "Some animals have horns, some have hoofs, some teeth, some talons, some claws, some spurs, and beaks—man hath none of these, but is weak and feable and sent unarmed into the world—why, a hand, with reason to use it, supplies the use of all these."

The thumb represents the strongest of our digits, and one that allows three different aspects of prehension, making possible strong manipulation, and fine manipulation of objects. In thumb opposition, the thumb is brought into pulp pinch with the index and middle fingers to allow fine and delicate manipulation of small objects, whereas a more powerful chuck three-point pinch is used between the thumb, index, and middle finger pulp to grasp and hold objects more firmly. In adduction pinch, the thumb is pulled into juxtaposition to the radial border of the index finger, which provides a much more firm and powerful grasping unit. This is commonly termed "key pinch". Finally, the thumb plays an important locking or stabilizing factor in hand-digital cylinder grasp. These various degrees of function are dependent on sensibility, mobility, length, and strength (Bunnell, 1931; Tanzer and Littler, 1948), all features that Bunnell has described as being fundamental to and characteristic of a normal thumb.

Nicoladoni (1897, 1900) popularized the toe to hand transfer method of thumb reconstruction, having in 1898 transferred the second toe in a 5 year old boy, to reconstruct the thumb. This pedicle type of transfer was awkward but successful, and was repeated on a number of occasions (Clarkson and Furlong, 1949) subsequent to this first procedure. Gueullette (1930) reviewed 17 cases of nonmicrovascular toe transfers, and Davis (1964) described his experience with 40 such operations.

Jacobson and Suarez (1960) awakened the world of reconstructive surgery by publishing their findings on anastomoses of small blood vessels. Before this time Kleinert, Kasdan, and Romero (1963), using larger needles and sutures, were able to rejoin traumatically divided digital vessels in fingers, and led the way in the hand surgery world toward an appreciation and realization of the merits of small blood vessel repair. In 1965 Buncke (Buncke, Buncke, and Schulz, 1966) successfully transferred the great toe of a monkey to the thumb position with a living free tissue transfer after repairing both arteries and veins to make possible the viability of this digit. The first clinical case was reported by Corbett (1969), who in 1968 performed great toe to hand transfer in a 32 year old man who had traumatically lost his thumb. Despite the need for reexploration in this operation, the toe ultimately survived completely, and this became the first successful toe to hand transfer in man. After this case report, Buncke and O'Brien (O'Brien and associates, 1975) began a substantial series of toe to hand transfers and started to make significant refinements in the technique of this operation, which we use today. As microtechnique has become an integral part of the armamentarium of all contemporary hand surgeons, so toe to hand transfer with variations has taken its eminent and deserved role as an important method of thumb restoration in traumatic cases in which thumb replantation cannot be performed.

INDICATIONS

Although immediate toe to hand transfer reconstruction has been reported after an amputation injury (Rose and Hendel, 1981), it is currently the author's preference to use elective methods of thumb reconstruction only for patients who have a well-healed thumb stump, and to whom a detailed explanation of the procedure and all alternatives has been given. This provides patients and their families with an appropriate time for all questions to be answered. One should not underestimate the risk of tissue loss and the recovery time required after reconstructive surgery.

If the thumb has been amputated at a distal level, sensibility and strength are very often preserved, in which case no reconstruction may be necessary (Strickland, 1988). This is particularly true in thumbs in which a portion of the distal phalanx is intact and full carpometacarpal and metacarpophalangeal joint motion exist.

If the thumb is amputated near the interphalangeal joint, and further length is felt to be desirable, thumb metacarpal distraction lengthening is the treatment of choice. This is also chosen for patients with more proximal amputation levels if microvascular toe to hand transfer or index finger pollicization cannot be performed for other reasons (see Chap. 127). This procedure is often followed by a first web deepening procedure.

In thumbs that have been amputated distal to the metacarpophalangeal joint, pollicization (see Chaps. 123, 124), thumb lengthening (see Chap 127), and bone augmentation with partial toe pulp microvascular techniques may be indicated (Gilbert, 1976; May and associates, 1977; Morrison, 1978; Strauch and Tsur, 1978; Morrison, O'Brien, and MacLeod, 1980; Doi and associates, 1981; Doi, 1982; Minanni, 1984; Doi, Kuvata, and Kawai, 1985; Nunley, Goldner, and Urbaniak, 1985; Urbaniak, 1985; Yu and He, 1985).

Pollicization (see Chap. 124) remains the treatment of choice in patients who have thumb reconstructive needs, and who have an amputated index finger at or near the level of the proximal interphalangeal joint. This is particularly true if the patient finds the index finger awkward, and it is believed by the patient and the surgical team that an improvement in hand function would be gained by removal of the index ray, in addition to thumb reconstruction. Index finger pollicization is also our treatment of choice for congenital absence of the thumb (May, Smith, and Peimer, 1981) (see Chapter 123), when the patient has four normal digits. Great toe to hand transfer is functionally more powerful than pollicization when normal thenar muscles remain in the hand, although the functional power comparison between index finger thumb reconstruction and great toe to hand transfer thumb reconstruction is related primarily to the strength of the intrinsic muscles that remain in the hand, rather than anything intrinsic to the method of reconstruction itself. In congenital absence of the thumb, toe to hand transfer has been performed (O'Brien and associates, 1978), but is perhaps best suited to those circumstances in which pollicization is not suitable (May, Smith, and Peimer, 1981).

If the thumb has been lost at or near the metacarpophalangeal joint, a number of fundamental decisions must be made. If the articular surface of the metacarpal head can be maintained, a great toe metatarsophalangeal joint disarticulation can take place, and thus allow a functional metacarpophalangeal joint to exist in the thumb after appropriate capsuloplasty and repair. Here the sesamoids remain in the foot. If the thumb amputation has occurred proximal to the metacarpophalangeal joint, the metatarsophalangeal joint of the foot is transferred to the hand to convert it to a functional joint in the hand, leaving the sesamoids on the foot. If the amputation has taken place distal to the metacarpophalangeal joint, and if interpha-

langeal joint motion is considered a desirable feature in the hand, the toe is amputated just distal to the metatarsophalangeal joint of the foot with an osteosynthesis in the hand done at the proximal level of the thumb proximal phalanx, allowing the normal metacarpophalangeal joint in the hand to function as an anatomically normal joint. If interphalangeal joint motion is not a goal, a partial toe (Gilbert, 1976; May and associates, 1977; Morrison, 1978; Strauch and Tsur, 1978; Minanni, 1984) or wrap-around (Morrison, O'Brien, and MacLeod, 1980; Doi, 1982; Doi, Kuvata, and Kawai, 1985; Nunley, Goldner, and Urbaniak, 1985; Urbaniak, 1985; Yu and He, 1985) type of procedure plus bone graft (see Chap. 126) may be the best procedure selection.

Great toe to hand transfer is also the author's favored procedure if the thumb has been amputated at the level of the carpometacarpal joint or further proximally. In this case it is preferable to transfer the great toe with the metatarsophalangeal joint left intact to function as a neocarpal metacarpal joint. In many patients in this category, the index finger ray will also have been damaged or lost if the thumb amputation level is quite far proximally, and thus a somewhat foreshortened thumb can be very well tolerated as long as a generous web space and fully mobile remaining fingers exist (see Fig. 125–43B). The more digital loss that is seen in the radial side of the hand, the greater is the web space after thumb reconstruction and web resurfacing. In the mutilated hand, great toe to hand transfer can greatly upgrade hand function, and in some patients the great toe, after successful transfer and innervation, will be the best digit in the hand (see Fig. 125–43C).

Second toe to hand transfer is preferred by some authors (Leung, 1985); the major advantage of this operation is the avoidance of a cosmetically significant donor site in the foot (see Chap. 95). However, the author prefers in almost all cases to offer the patient great toe to hand transfer as the primary microvascular procedure, because the esthetic (May and Daniel, 1978; May and Rohrich, 1987) and functional attributes of the great toe are much more similar to those of the normal thumb. In our northeastern society in the United States, shoes or foot apparel are worn to cover the cosmetic abnormality in the donor site a great deal of the time by most patients.

Each of these methods can be extraordinarily successful in carefully selected and counseled patients. It is the author's current preference to explain the relative advantages and disadvantages of each method to each individual patient, and thus to allow a significant degree of patient input. If a patient has lost the thumb near or at the metacarpophalangeal joint, and if metacarpophalangeal joint motion is a goal of ultimate reconstruction, great toe to hand transfer is usually the method of choice. If under unusual circumstances the patient has an adjacent injured useless digit or one such on the opposite hand (Bartlett, Moses, and May, 1986), it may be possible to transfer such a digit, improving the donor site as well as the recipient site. It is important for hand reconstruction surgeons to be familiar with the orthopedic and plastic surgical aspects of all methods of thumb reconstruction (Reid, 1960; Littler, 1976), so that an appropriate procedure can be carefully tailored and selected for the individual patient. It is best to select the procedure for the patient rather than vice versa (May, 1987a). All the methods mentioned above can provide a satisfactory result to patients who are well informed and have played an active role in the selection of the procedure.

Great toe to hand transfer is technically demanding even for the most experienced surgeon (May, 1981, 1987a). Because the vascular loss of a great toe during a toe to hand transfer procedure is a tragedy, every effort must be made through patient selection (May and Rohrich, 1987) and procedure organization and execution (Greenberg and May, 1988) to avoid such an event. The organization of the microsurgical team, patient selection, patient information, and technical completion of the operation with appropriate postoperative management all lead ultimately to a successful outcome. The orchestration of this endeavor, however, can test the skill of the most competent hand surgeon and hand surgical team. Thus, a thorough understanding of the anatomy of the donor and recipient sites is fundamentally important for successful completion of these procedures. The facility afforded the operating team in fresh cadaver dissection cannot be overemphasized, since this adds a significant level of confidence through anatomic familiarity for surgeons carrying out this operation.

COMPARATIVE ANATOMY OF FOOT AND HAND

Skin

Nowhere in the body is pulp tissue similar to the thumb pulp found except in the hand and foot. The natural relationship between the fibrous septal anatomy of the thumb pulp and the anatomy of the toe pulp is similar, and thus the adherent skin overlying the transferred bone anatomy of the great toe mimics the thumb in every way. At the base of the normal thumb, the flexible first web space skin must be reproduced after thumb reconstruction by toe transfer, if full mobility of the carpometacarpal joint, allowing positioning of the new thumb, is to be achieved (Figs. 125–1 to 125–6). This cannot be stressed too highly and should be accomplished before or at the time of toe transfer for best results. This allows proper tendon, vascular, and nerve tension to be established with a generous web space (Fig. 125–6) rather than trying to create it later. If a significant amount of hand radial flap tissue is needed, the author prefers to reconstruct the radial side of the hand with an initial staged flap (May and Bartlett, 1981). If the amount of skin needed is small (4 to 6 sq cm), this can often be added with a full-thickness skin graft placed at the time of toe transfer over well-perfused pedicle tissues (Figs. 125–7 to 125–9) (May, 1987a). A full-thickness skin graft is preferred to a split-thickness graft, because the wound contraction characteristics after healing appear to favor increased flexibility and motion of the full-thickness graft (see

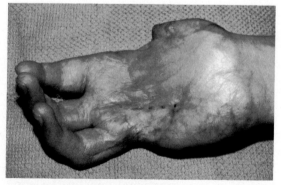

Figure 125–1. The right hand of an 18 year old male who sustained thumb and small finger amputations in a devastating hot plastic molding machine accident.

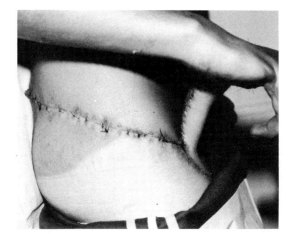

Figure 125–2. The right hand in a groin flap prior to toe to hand transfer. Note that the tube has resurfaced the radial side of the hand and allowed for thumb metacarpal-adductor contracture release prior to toe to hand transfer.

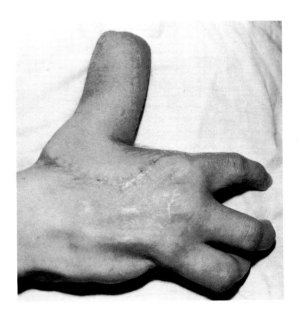

Figure 125–3. The right hand with the groin flap banked prior to toe to hand transfer.

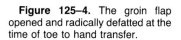

Figure 125–4. The groin flap opened and radically defatted at the time of toe to hand transfer.

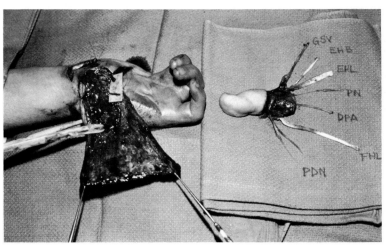

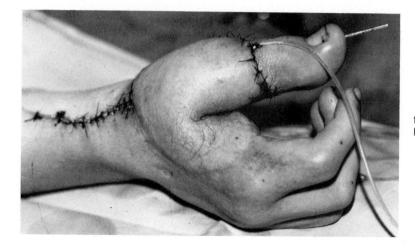

Figure 125–5. New thumb and flap after tailoring. Note that very little flap has been discarded.

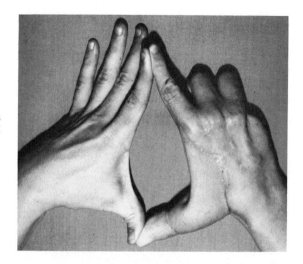

Figure 125–6. Flap application prior to toe transfer has produced a web space comparable with that of the normal hand.

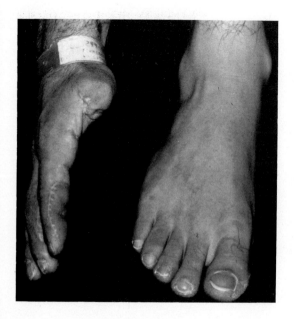

Figure 125–7. A 20 year old male prior to toe to hand transfer with well-healed skin overlying the thumb metacarpal. Here only a full-thickness skin graft will be needed.

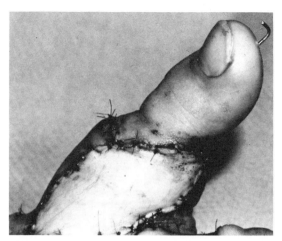

Figure 125–8. Full-thickness skin graft applied over a perfused soft tissue pedicle covering the web side of the dorsal thumb after transfer.

Figs. 125–2, 125–3). In the pulp tissues the skin innervation organelles (including free nerve endings, Meissner's corpuscles, Merkel's discs, and pacinian corpuscles), although somewhat different in density, are similar in make-up in the thumb and great toe. Although the great toenail inherently grows more slowly than the thumbnail, the general anatomic relationship between the toenail and the toe distal phalanx is similar to that in the thumb, and provides a stable pulp and an esthetic nail and nail bed compared with the normal thumb. Interestingly, the great toe in many patients is variable in size in comparison with the thumb, and often has a lateral bulge to the pulp tissues, which is an esthetic disadvantage compared with the normal thumb. In addition, on the lateral view (Fig. 125–10) the vertical height of the great toe in some patients is significantly greater than the height of the pulp in the normal thumb. Both these features may be taken into consideration in ultimate secondary procedures, if necessary.

Bone

The bone anatomy of the great toe, compared with that of the normal thumb is interesting (Fig. 125–10), since one can see the normal great toe, as a result of the wearing of shoes over time, laterally deviates at the metatarsophalangeal and the interphalangeal joint. It is for this reason that the ipsilateral great toe is usually chosen for

transfer, because it will thus deviate toward the index and middle fingers rather than away from these digits. In addition, from the metatarsophalangeal joint to the distal bony phalanx, the great toe in most adults is approximately 5 mm longer than its thumb counterpart (Fig. 125–11). This is surprising to most surgeons; however, if the metatarsophalangeal joint of the foot is to be disarticulated during the process of toe transfer, the reconstructed thumb will be slightly longer than the normal thumb. In addition, the width of the toe phalanx, both proximal and distal, is greater than that of the thumb in most patients (Fig. 125–11).

The great toe interphalangeal joint often has slightly less range of motion with a lesser degree of hyperextension than the normal thumb. The metatarsophalangeal joint of the great toe, as compared with the metacarpo-

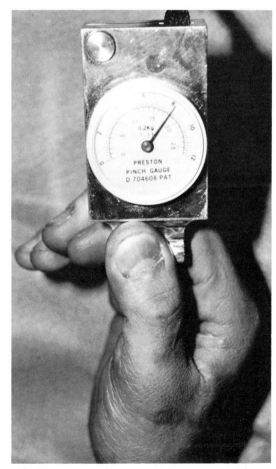

Figure 125–9. One year postoperatively with adequate web space and 20 lb adduction pinch (patient shown in Fig. 125–8).

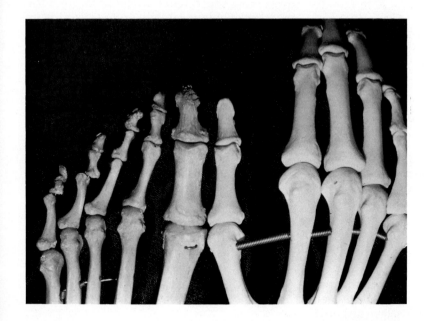

Figure 125–10. Comparative bony anatomy between the left great toe and right thumb.

Figure 125–11. Comparative lengths of the thumb *(left)* and great toe *(right).*

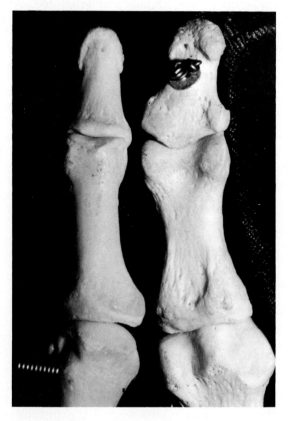

phalangeal joint, is primarily an extension rather than a flexion joint (Fig. 125–12). For the metacarpophalangeal joint of the foot to be transferred to the hand and converted functionally into a hyperflexion joint, several considerations must be made. If a new combination metacarpophalangeal joint is to be made, the volar plate must be shortened at the time of transfer to prevent hyperextension of the metacarpophalangeal joint in the hand position, but at the same time to allow full flexion (Fig. 125–13). On the other hand, if the metacarpophalangeal joint of the foot is transferred to the hand, an oblique osteotomy must be carried out (Fig. 125–14) from a dorsal to plantar direction, to allow the metacarpophalangeal joint when it is fixed in the hand to be actually placed in a hyperextended position. With an oblique osteotomy, this hyperextended toe joint position translates into the neutral position of the new thumb metacarpophalangeal joint, and thus allows the new thumb metacarpophalangeal joint to flex in the hand position (Fig. 125–15). At the same time, a volar plate shortening and stabilization must be carried out to prevent hyperextension (Fig. 125–16). Under ideal circumstances the sesamoids are left in the foot, and thus the division of the volar plate just distal to the sesamoids in the foot provides a shortening of the volar plate when the joint is transferred. Some volar plate or volar fibrous tissues should be dissected and maintained on the volar surface of the thumb metacarpal in the hand to provide for secure suture placement. This is an important step

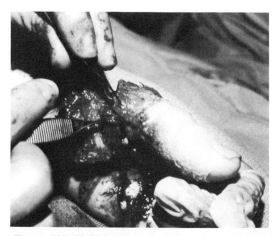

Figure 125–13. Volar plate plasty is performed by separating the sesamoids from the volar plate in the foot and, after transfer, attaching the shortened volar plate of the toe to the dissected scar plate of the volar metacarpal in the hand. Tension should be adjusted to avoid new metacarpophalangeal joint hyperextension.

and must be considered as bone exposure is being dissected in the hand.

Tendon

The ipsilateral great toe and the thumb are relatively similar in tendon anatomy, with some notable exceptions. The normal thumb has two extrinsic extensor tendons, the extensor pollicis longus (EPL) and the extensor pollicis brevis (EPB), while the great toe has the extensor hallucis longus (EHL) and extensor hallucis brevis (EHB). However, in the ipsilateral great toe, the EHB lies lateral to the EHL while in the ipsilateral thumb the EPL lies ulnar to the EPB. This means that when the great toe is transferred to the hand, if an ipsilateral toe transfer is carried out, the EPB must be routed beneath the EHL to be repaired to its EPB counterpart (Fig. 125–

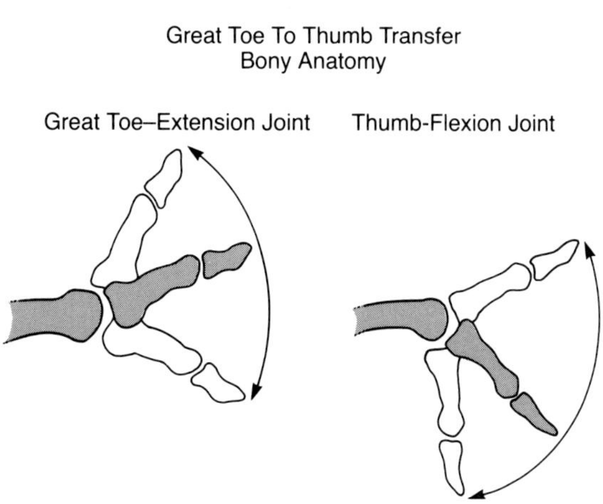

Great Toe To Thumb Transfer
Bony Anatomy

Great Toe–Extension Joint   Thumb-Flexion Joint

Figure 125–12. The thumb metacarpophalangeal joint is primarily a flexion joint, whereas the great toe metatarsophalangeal joint is primarily an extension joint.

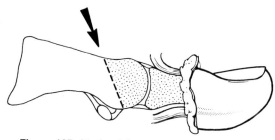

Figure 125–14. An oblique osteotomy (45 degrees) *(arrow)* is carried out to allow the new metacarpophalangeal joint to be a flexion joint rather than an extension joint.

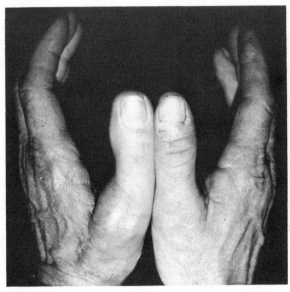
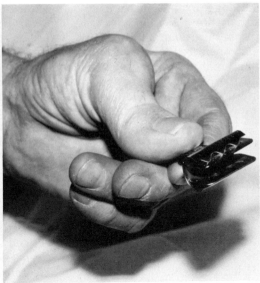

Figure 125–15. Note the metacarpophalangeal extension *(A)* and flexion *(B),* three years after a left toe to hand transfer.

17). Conversely, some other extra motor extensor tendon, such as the extensor indicis proprius (EIP), can be repaired to the EHB in the hand if such a tendon is available. In addition, to prevent drooping of the interphalangeal joint of the thumb, the normal thenar intrinsic muscles should be connected to the interphalangeal joint extensor mechanism after toe transfer (Fig. 125–18). Thus, the normal interphalangeal joint extension mechanism provided by the abductor pollicis brevis (APB) and the adductor can be reestablished after toe transfer as long as the

thumb thenar intrinsic muscles are relatively normal. This repair in full interphalangeal joint extension allows these intrinsic muscles to provide for thumb interphalangeal joint extension. It is probably more important to have thumb interphalangeal joint extension than flexion, since pulp to pulp digital prehension is far superior to thumbnail to pulp contact. If the thumb interphalangeal joint is allowed to drop into flexion, the metacarpo-

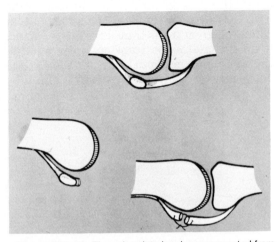

Figure 125–16. The volar plate has been separated from the sesamoids, which remain on the foot. Tension is being adjusted to tighten the volar plate and to prevent hyperextension of the new metacarpophalangeal joint.

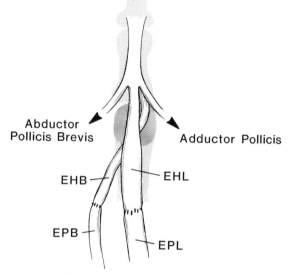

Figure 125–17. Tendon anatomy of the right great toe after transfer to the right hand.

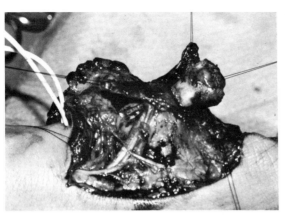

Figure 125–18. The intrinsic abductor pollicis brevis in preparation for repair to a split slip of the extensor hallucis longus tendon after toe to hand transfer in the right hand. This step helps to prevent flexion deformity of the interphalangeal joint of the thumb by provision of an intrinsic mechanism for active thumb interphalangeal joint extension.

phalangeal joint over time usually hyperextends, creating a zigzag deformity of the thumb. The reverse sequence can occur if the metacarpophalangeal joint volar plate repair is inadequate and allows the new metacarpophalangeal joint to hyperextend, thus permitting the interphalangeal joint to drop into flexion. By preventing metacarpophalangeal joint hyperextension and thumb interphalangeal joint flexion, the hand surgeon can thus avoid this deformity and upgrade overall thumb function. The flexor hallucis longus (FHL) tendon is slightly larger in diameter than the flexor pollicis longus (FPL), and in the foot this tendon is frequently adherent to the common toe flexors. Although it is occasionally possible to retrieve the FHL tendon from behind the medial malleolus, the author has found that in most cases midfoot incision is necessary to identify the tendon and free it, thus provding division and delivery of the tendon into the distal operative field. Making a midfoot incision for this maneuver provides enough FHL tendon length to allow tenorrhaphy in the transferred position proximal to the wrist, and thus avoids adhesions of the tenorrhaphy within the hand. Tenorrhaphy must be done far enough proximally in the wrist to allow full thumb abduction and extension without impingement of the repair at the carpal tunnel. The abductor hallucis tendon stump can be left on the thumb during toe to hand transfer, as this tendon stump can allow ultimate opposition transfer attachment or similar thumb positioning transfers where needed.

Nerve

Two-point discrimination studies between the lateral pulp of the great toe and the normal thumb have been carried out in 50 hospitalized patients (May and associates, 1977). In this study the two-point discrimination of the lateral great toe averaged a mean 11.3 mm, that of the normal thumb being approximately 3 to 4 mm. Thus, the great toe two-point discrimination in this study exceeded the dorsal foot and second toe two-point discrimination, and was the best innervated foot skin studied for use in hand reconstruction. The great toe innervation potential provides a very thumblike structure for ultimate thumb replacement. Ultimate sensibility after nerve repair may require three to five years for full recovery (Ome, 1962). Sensibility in the 9 to 12 mm two-point discrimination range (May, Smith, and Peimer, 1981) can often be expected. The deep peroneal nerve accompanies the dorsalis pedis artery beneath the dorsal foot retinaculum, and courses from proximal to distal to innervate the proximal dorsal first web tissues between the great and second toes (see Fig. 125–8).

The superficial peroneal nerve frequently has fibers that crosscommunicate with the deep peroneal nerve, and innervate the dorsal foot skin tissues up near the level of the interphalangeal joint of the great toe (Kosniski, 1926; Mileen, 1959; May and associates, 1977). As many of these nerve fibers as possible are taken with the toe transfer to allow repair of the radial nerve to these nerve fibers. In the hand the dorsal radial nerve normally innervates dorsal thumb tissues up to the level of the interphalangeal joint of the thumb, and sometimes distal to this point. Thus, repairing fibers of the deep peroneal and occasional superficial peroneal fibers of the toe to the unsatisfied distal ends of the sensory radial nerve fibers can create a satisfactory reinnervation pattern after great toe transfer. The cross section of the radial nerve fibers in the hand usually exceeds significantly that of the superficial and deep peroneal nerves of the great toe. In the palmar digital nerve area, the two digital nerves of the thumb coursing from the radial aspect of the median nerve are very similar to the plantar digital nerves of the great toe. The cross sectional area of the hand digital nerves is greater than that of the toe digital nerves in many patients. In toe dissection, considerable nerve length must be taken on the toe digital nerves to avoid the need for a nerve graft at the time of toe transfer. It is thus important to measure the distance over which the plantar digital nerves to the great toe must be dissected, in order to provide a tension-free neurorrhaphy in the hand when the great toe is transferred. In uncommon circumstances the median nerve may be unsuitable for recipient nerve repair. Here the dorsal radial nerve unsatisfied fibers can provide very useful total thumb innervation, and at the same time decrease the risk of a problematic end radial nerve neuroma in the hand.

Arterial

In the hand, the radial artery travels from a palmar to a dorsal location, as the artery courses deep to the abductor pollicis longus (APL) tendon and comes up beneath the EPL and EPB tendons, deeply within the first web space of the hand. It is in this location that the radial artery is ideally suited for receiving an end to end or end to side arterial anastomosis from the dorsalis pedis artery (Fig. 125–19). In most patients the dorsalis pedis artery is slightly larger than the radial artery at this position. Although the former may be slightly thicker than the latter, the vascular anastomosis usually involves the repair of vessels that are at least 2 mm in

diameter (Greenberg and May, 1988), and thus the repair is very likely to remain patent after careful microvascular anastomosis.

The blood vessel anatomy of the great toe and its similarities to the thumb has been the subject of great interest in previous dissection work (Adochi, 1928; Huber, 1941; Edwards, 1960; Koster, 1968; Gilbert, 1976; May and associates, 1977; Leung, 1985). The great toe is generously supplied by both the dorsal and plantar supplies of the distal foot (Greenberg and May, 1988). Dorsally the dorsalis pedis artery courses from proximal to distal, providing the first dorsal metatarsal artery, which courses from its origin from the dorsalis pedis artery distally, in the first web of the foot, to course dorsal to the transverse metatarsal ligament, and then through a distal communicating branch to join with the plantar arterial system (Fig. 125–20). In 78 per cent of 50 cadaver feet dissected (May and associates, 1977), this first dorsal metatarsal artery came from the dorsalis pedis artery dorsal to the midaxis for the metatarsals, and coursed within the first web space in a relatively superficial Type I pattern (Fig. 125–20). In 22 per cent of feet dissected this vessel emerged from a more deep location and coursed through the web space deeply, originating deep to the midaxis of the metatarsal (Fig. 125–21). However, in all feet dissected some contribution was noted by the first dorsal metatarsal artery passing dorsal to the

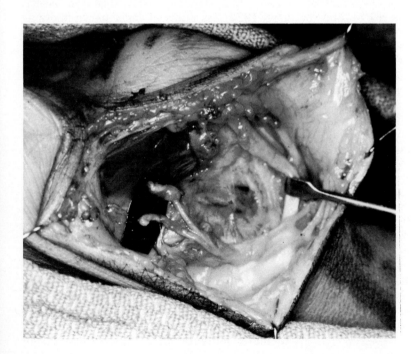

Figure 125–19. Radial artery and accompanying veins coming beneath the long thumb extensor in the left hand of a 9 year old patient. Note the radial nerve neuromas in preparation for repair to the deep peroneal nerve lying on top of the intact and functional adductor pollicis muscle.

Anatomy of First Dorsal Metatarsal Artery

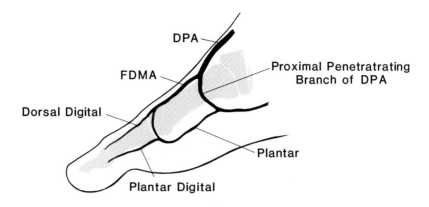

Type I 78%

Figure 125–20. Lateral view of the arterial anatomy of the foot first web in the most common Type I pattern.

transverse metatarsal ligament, and ultimately connecting through the distal communicating artery into the plantar system. Other investigators (Urbaniak, 1985) found this vascular anatomy less consistent in clinical patients, although at the Massachusetts General Hospital the dorsal inflow system has been used, whether Type I or Type II, in over 90 per cent of patients undergoing great toe to hand transfer (Greenberg and May, 1988). In the anatomic dissections (May and associates, 1977), the first dorsal metatarsal artery in general was slightly smaller than

the first plantar metatarsal artery, but tracing its connection into the dorsalis pedis system allowed the dorsalis pedis artery to actually be the repaired arterial inflow vessel. This simplifies both the dissection, and the microanastomosis repairing a large foot vessel into a large hand vessel (usually the radial artery). As the distal communicating artery connects into the plantar system, a single large plantar digital artery is given off to the lateral great toe, which should be preserved as the major outflow vessel perfusing the great toe. Thus, the dorsal inflow system perfuses the plantar dominant outflow system within the toe in most patients (Greenberg and May, 1988).

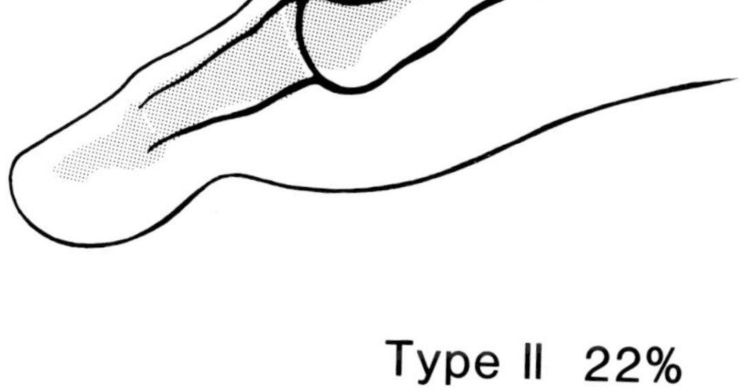

At the Massachusetts General Hospital, biplane preoperative angiography has been found very helpful in determining the size and location of the foot and hand arterial anatomy (May, Athanasoulis, and Donelan, 1977) and thus in planning for the arterial dissection (Fig. 125–22) (Greenberg and May, 1988). No matter how carefully one plans, however, it is necessary to be flexible and prepared to use whichever arterial inflow system is needed to provide safe, high flow vessel repairs, even if vein grafts are needed.

Venous

A knowledge of the venous anatomy of the dorsum of the foot and the drainage of the great toe is very important to an understand-

Type II 22%

Figure 125–21. Lateral view of the arterial anatomy in the less common Type II vascular pattern.

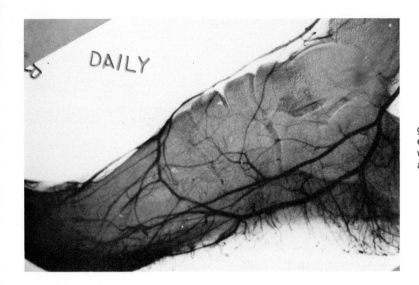

Figure 125–22. Lateral foot angiogram demonstrating the presence of the dorsalis pedis artery with takeoff of the first dorsal metatarsal artery in a Type I pattern.

ing of the transfer. There are multiple discernible venous layers of the dorsum of the foot (Koster, 1968; Jacobson, 1970; Askar, Kassem, and Shannel, 1975); the largest and deepest of these layers is the one upon which the venous outflow of the great toe transfer is based. This involves tracing the greater saphenous vein from proximally in the foot distalward until it curves across the distal forefoot, creating the deep dorsal transverse venous arch (Fig. 125–23). On occasion, branches of this deep transverse venous arch and the venae comitantes of the first dorsal metatarsal artery intercommunicate. Once this venous anatomy is identified, a large vein extending down into the first web space of the foot can usually be seen (Fig. 125–23) joined by a contribution from the more medial side of the great toe, joining this vein several centimeters proximal to the metatarsopha-

langeal joint of the foot. If these two large veins can be left intact with the intervening soft tissues between them, this perfused tissue at the time of toe transfer allows a full-thickness skin graft (see Fig. 125–8) to be placed upon it, and thus can allow a very useful degree of soft tissue skin augmentation at the time of transfer. When this deep venous anatomy has been identified and preserved, all more superficial veins can be left in the flaps surrounding the great toe, which will remain in the foot.

The goal of venous anatomic identification is to create a large venous conduit (the greater saphenous vein), and to preserve several major channels draining into this vein from the portion of the great toe that will be ultimately transferred. A second important goal is to leave all other veins in the dorsal foot flaps intact to prevent foot skin slough.

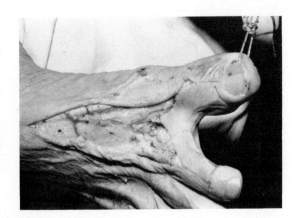

Figure 125–23. Dorsal cadaver foot dissection. Note the proximal transverse venous arch with the larger intermetatarsal branch draining the great toe.

In the hand, several large branches of the cephalic vein are seen over the radial side. These branches usually are slightly smaller and less thick than the greater saphenous vein, but a direct end to end vascular anastomosis can usually be accomplished with vessels that are in the 3 to 4 mm diameter range. If significant discrepancy in size is noted, end to side vein repair is a good alternative. It provides an excellent caliber vascular outflow for the toe to hand transfer, and has never presented a problem in any patient at the Massachusetts General Hospital. Rarely, veins on the ulnar side of the hand may need to be used if radial side hand trauma has been extensive.

OPERATIVE STEPS

Since great toe to hand transfer is a complex procedure, it is best to have two teams of surgeons involved in the organization of the operation who are conversant in the detailed anatomy described above. On the author's teaching service, when possible, a cadaver dissection is carried out preoperatively to familiarize all team members with the full aspects of hand and foot anatomy.

Before operation, any and all soft tissue flap procedures will have been done to the radial side of the hand. This sets the stage for a well-positioned thumb metacarpal, which will have been covered with soft pliable tissues (see Figs. 125–1 to 125–6). In patients who have had significant damage to the radial side of the hand, this usually requires flap coverage before toe to hand transfer.

Although some investigators do not perform routine preoperative angiography before toe to hand transfer (Morrison, O'Brien, and MacLeod, 1980; Lister, Kalisman, and Tsai, 1983; Gordon and associates, 1985), the author has found a preoperative transfemoral angiogram very useful in demonstrating both the arterial anatomy of the donor foot (anterior, posterior, and lateral views) and that of the recipient hand (Fig. 125–24) (Greenberg and May, 1988). The angiography will have been performed 48 hours before toe transfer to avoid any bleeding complications at the site of angiography, if patient heparinization is necessary at the time of surgery. It has been documented experimentally (Yaremchuk and associates, 1981) that angiographic contrast media do not adversely affect the

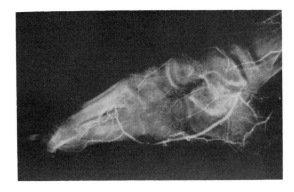

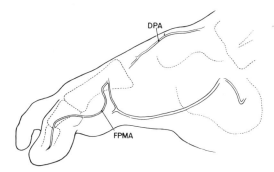

Figure 125–24. Lateral foot angiogram demonstrating lack of an adequate dorsal inflow system in this previously damaged foot donor site.

patency of microvascular anastomoses, unless the concentration of contrast media far exceeds those currently in clinical use. The night before surgery, the patient is given an enema to evacuate the distal colon, and has respiratory therapy education where appropriate. Since the operation may last eight or more hours in some patients, the anesthesia service will have been previously notified, and will be aware of the importance of patient positioning and body temperature maintenance. In addition, the anesthesia team will be familiar with the use of tourniquets in both the arm and leg, and with the systemic vascular impact of multiple tourniquet application and release.

Very importantly, the operating room nursing team will have been informed of the instruments needed for the procedure, and the combined length of the foot dissection and hand dissection, in addition to the transfer itself. In most patients the operating microscope is used primarily at the time of transfer for blood vessel and nerve repairs, and the foot and hand dissections are done with loupe magnification.

The night before surgery the patient is

given oral aspirin, which is continued post-operatively for approximately six weeks.

The morning of surgery, after general anesthesia is obtained, the patient is positioned on an inflatable air mattress, so that pressure points can be alternated to avoid any pressure necrosis. Tourniquet placement is chosen and applied by the surgeons. Finally, a Foley catheter is inserted to allow the anesthesia team better patient monitoring and to simplify the early postoperative recovery.

Foot Dissection

The foot dissection is initiated under tourniquet control, but without venous blood evacuation by Esmarch. This dissection is usually initiated an hour or so before hand dissection is begun, since the foot dissection usually takes rather longer than the hand dissection.

At the time of foot dissection, in the operating room, anteroposterior and lateral angiographic views of the foot are available to help guide the surgical team in proper inflow arterial vessel dissection. Before the foot skin incision, the major branch of the greater saphenous vein is identified, and the dorsalis pedis area of vessel palpation is also identified. A line is then drawn between these two vessels from proximal to distal, joining the great toe over the EHL tendon (Fig. 125–25). The incision is intentionally deviated from lateral to medial at the most distal end, as it is in this location that medial foot flap slough occurs most often. Although it seems unnatural to place the incision directly over the EHL tendon in this location, it must be remembered that this tendon will no longer

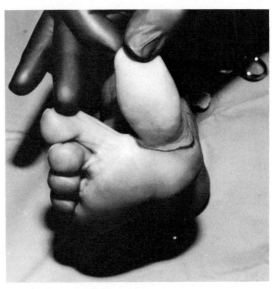

Figure 125–26. Circular completion of the toe incision, care being taken to leave ample pushoff flap tissues on the plantar pushoff area.

exist at the time of foot donor site closure. Thus, the laterally based flap created by this maneuver in the foot will be better perfused in most patients than the medially based flap, which will get its blood supply ultimately from nonincised proximal and plantar tissues. A circular incision (Fig. 125–26) around the base of the great toe is placed on the plantar surface of the great toe at the proximal toe flexion crease. This leaves the important plantar pushoff thick skin and foot fat pad tissues on the foot. This should provide for a well-healed pushoff surface for the great toe metatarsal, which remains in the foot.

The foot incision is thus made from proximal to distal and around the base of the great toe. Dissection should begin at the level of the greater saphenous vein from proximal to distal, and every effort should be made to preserve as much of the vascular anatomy of the flaps remaining on the foot as possible, keeping the dissection at the level of the greater saphenous vein and the major branches that will ultimately supply the great toe. A great mistake can be made at this point in tracing anatomically each of the superficial veins of the foot toward the great toe, and thus separating these branches from the foot flap. It will ultimately be discovered that these veins are not necessary, and thus their role in draining the remaining flaps on the foot will have been lost. After the junction

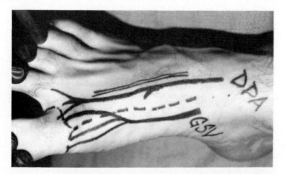

Figure 125–25. Dorsal foot prior to incision. The dotted line (planned incision) is located between the greater saphenous vein and the palpable dorsalis pedis artery.

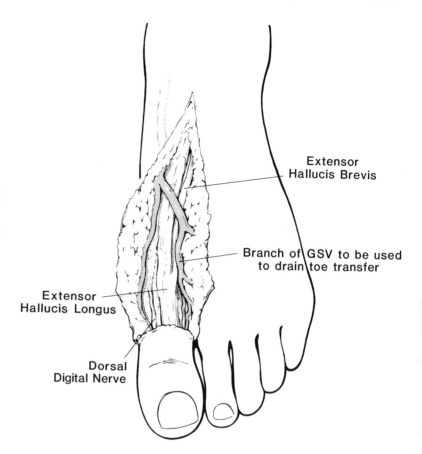

Figure 125–27. Dissection view of the foot with flaps elevated just superficial to the large deep veins. The dorsalis pedis pedicle and the first dorsal metatarsal artery are just deep to the extensor hallucis brevis tendon. GSV = greater saphenous vein.

Extensor Hallucis Brevis

Branch of GSV to be used to drain toe transfer

Extensor Hallucis Longus

Dorsal Digital Nerve

of the greater saphenous vein to the major venous branches draining the toe has been identified, the EHL tendon should be seen and traced from distal to proximal to the level of the EHB muscle tendon junction. At this point, the EHB can be divided to allow reflection of the proximal stump proximally and the distal stump distally. Here, with tendon distraction and retraction, the deep peroneal nerve and the first dorsal metatarsal artery can usually be seen coming from the dorsalis pedis artery (Fig. 125–28). It is convenient in toe dissection to take each of the divided structures and fold them distally to be wrapped in a saline moist Kling gauze, placed circumferentially around the toe (Fig. 125–29). This gauze is periodically irrigated with iced saline to keep the toe and all dissected structures as cool and wet as possible. The superficial peroneal nerve branches are usually seen superficial to the dorsal retinaculum, intermingling with the greater saphenous vein branches as they course from proximal to distal. As soon as a large branch of the superficial peroneal nerve can be identified, it is divided and the nerve is dissected

and turned distally over the great toe. This level of nerve division must be made with consideration for the level of the superficial radial nerve fibers existent in the hand. Any error should be made on the side of too much nerve length, because a tension-free neurorrhaphy both dorsally and on the palmar surface must be provided.

The dorsalis pedis artery and its two venae comitantes usually are easily identifiable. The dorsalis pedis artery is dissected and controlled with vascular loupes. With the tourniquet still remaining elevated, this dorsalis pedis artery is then dissected from proximal to distal, and the first dorsal metatarsal artery is identified. The deep continuation of the dorsalis pedis artery is then divided. At this point it is useful to correlate the surgical and angiographic findings. The division of the dorsalis pedis artery takes place deep within the first web space of the foot, and of course distal to the place where the first dorsal metatarsal artery branches from the dorsalis pedis artery. The first dorsal metatarsal artery, as it continues from the dorsalis pedis artery, is then dissected from proximal

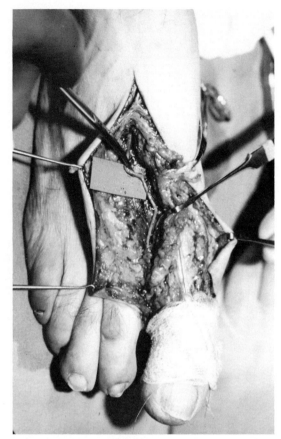

Figure 125–28. In this clinical case the right great toe is dissected. The first dorsal metatarsal artery is of the Type I pattern. The background is behind the artery. The deep peroneal nerve has been divided and is turned distally over the Kling gauze.

to distal, and the venae comitantes are discarded and ligated. As much as possible, bipolar coagulation is used. If vessel branches are 1 mm or larger in diameter, small 5-0 silk ligatures are used to avoid axial arterial damage. The first dorsal metatarsal artery frequently lies within some fibers of the interosseous muscles, but usually dorsal to the midaxis of the metatarsals themselves (May and associates, 1977). The vessel is then traced distally over the transverse intermetatarsal ligament, and further distally into the region of its bifurcation into the plantar digital vessels of the first web. The plantar digital vessel going to the second toe is ligated with 5-0 silk tie, and the junction between the distal communicating artery distally and the major plantar digital artery to the great toe is identified. At this junction the major plantar common digital artery is seen coming from a proximal direction, and contributing

to the plantar circulation of the great toe itself. This vessel should be ligated with a small cuff of length preserved with the toe to provide a vascular "bail out" in case a vein graft augmentation to the arterial blood supply of the great toe becomes necessary. (This maneuver was needed in only one patient in the author's series.) The EHL tendon is traced, divided, and turned distally, and attention is then turned to the plantar dissection. If it has been determined that the dorsal system will not be useful, the arterial anatomy must be dissected from the plantar surface.

A vertical plantar incision (Fig. 125–30) is made between the great toe and second toe, to allow exposure of the plantar digital nerves

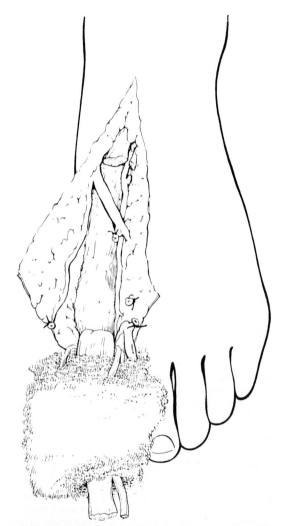

Figure 125–29. Dorsal left foot view. Here all the structures supplying the left great toe have been divided and turned distally under the Kling gauze except the arterial inflow.

the division of the digital nerves in the foot. These digital nerves from the foot are then divided to provide adequate digital nerve length, and also to avoid painful neuroma formation within the foot over a pressure surface more distally. The digital nerves are folded over the Kling gauze in the foot, and the FHL tendon is dissected and divided through a separate incision made in the midfoot, slightly proximal in the instep area (Fig. 125–31). This dissection must be done carefully, as digital nerves can be inadvertently encountered, in addition to the long flexor tendons to the remaining toes. Once the FHL has been divided (Fig. 125–32) the tourniquet is released in the leg. This usually requires an approximately two hour tourniquet run, which is the maximal length of tourniquet run currently used in the leg. If dissection problems have been encountered and the tourniquet must be relieved before this time, this is now done, and at least a 20 minute interval of leg perfusion is provided before reelevation of the foot tourniquet.

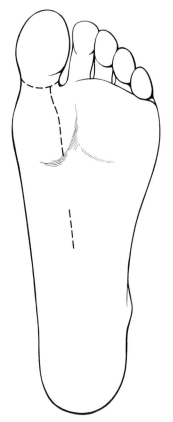

Figure 125–30. Plantar left foot incision length varies, depending on the difficulty of the dissection and the length of the structures needed.

and some exposure of the FHL tendon. It is deceptive how deeply the digital nerves are located. As far as possible, all the pushoff fat pad should be left on the plantar surface of the foot during this dissection (Fig. 125–31). The dissection should be initiated at the level of the tendon sheath overlying the great toe proximal phalanx and metatarsophalangeal joint. As much as possible the pulley of the FHL should be left intact to provide a pulley mechanism in the hand after the toe transfer. The plantar skin flap, which will be proximally and medially based, is then elevated at this deep level, and the great toe digital nerves come into view lying near the midaxis of the toe itself (Fig. 125–31). Once the medial and the lateral digital nerves are identified, they are dissected as far proximally as possible. At this point the hand team should be consulted as to recipient site requirements. It is important to use the operating microscope in making the digital nerve division determination in the hand, so that good fascicular anatomy has been seen and confirmed before

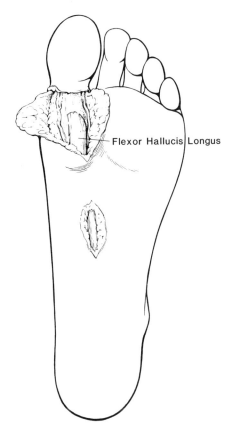

Flexor Hallucis Longus

Figure 125–31. Plantar view; note the sheath of the flexor hallucis longus and the digital nerves. Note the fat left on the exposure flaps to remain in the push area of the forefoot.

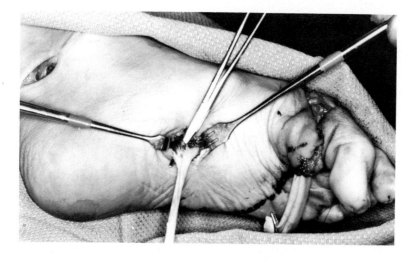

Figure 125–32. In this patient extra flexor hallucis longus tendon was needed and an incision was made behind the medial malleolus to obtain additional tendon length. Routinely, only the midfoot incision is needed.

After a 20 minute perfusion time in the foot, great care is taken to observe how well the great toe pulp has been perfused. If there is a problem at this stage with great toe perfusion, the arterial and venous anatomy should be bathed in 2 per cent lidocaine (Xylocaine). The patient's body temperature and overall systolic blood pressure should also be checked to make toe perfusion optimal. Vessel spasm and lack of great toe perfusion at this stage are a signal that something is wrong, and a painstaking microdissection along the arterial vascular path may be needed to identify the point of vessel spasm or obstruction.

After tourniquet reelevation, the dorsalis pedis artery and the greater saphenous vein are divided and irrigated with heparin saline. These vessels are then very carefully dis-

sected from proximal to distal, and folded under the wet Kling gauze over the great toe. If the great toe is to be taken without the articular surface of the metatarsal, a capsulotomy is carried out with division of the volar plate immediately distal to the location of the sesamoids beneath the great toe metatarsal head. The toe is then transferred to the hand (Fig. 125–34). If the metatarsophalangeal joint is to be transferred from the foot to the hand, a 45 to 60 degreee oblique osteotomy is carried out from proximal to distal, allowing a significant portion of the articular surface of the metatarsal head to go with the transferred toe (Fig. 125–34), but at the same time allowing the sesamoid bones to stay with the remaining volar portion of the metatarsal head within the foot. When this osteotomy has been carried out with a sagittal saw, it

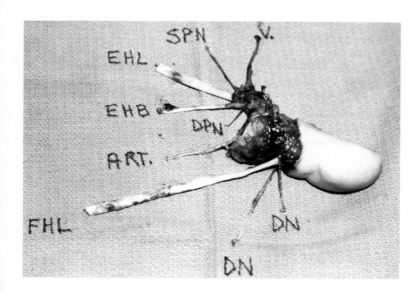

Figure 125–33. Labeled toe structures ready for repair in the hand.

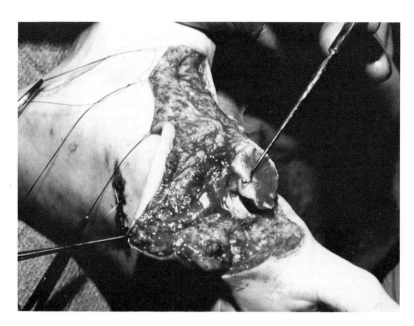

Figure 125–34. In this case a 45 degree osteotomy has been completed and the toe is transferred to the hand.

provides enough subchondral bone and bone stock to permit fixation of the great toe metatarsal head on the prepared metatarsal within the hand, and yet an adequate amount of volar plate exists with the transferred toe to allow a volar plate shortening and plasty within the hand. A wet gauze is placed over the donor site, and the tourniquet is released from the leg to allow adequate foot perfusion before foot donor site closure is undertaken. All foot flaps should be released from their retracted position to avoid flap ischemia during the toe transfer. An experienced member of the team should begin foot wound closure as soon as possible to avoid excessive swelling.

Hand Dissection

The dorsal and palmar incisions in the hand will have been positioned to allow for structure repair in the hand. In the hand, the first web space incision should be positioned to allow a radial and volar perfused flap to become directly juxtaposed to the plantar surface of the great toe. Other issues related to skin and soft tissue have been discussed under Skin (see p. 5156). It should be kept in mind that incision placement is dictated by perfusion viability requirements and postoperative scar contracture considerations. Exposure incisions should be placed volarly only where they cross flexion creases obliquely. In the hand, full exposure must be obtained to

both the digital nerve stumps of the thumb, which are located preoperatively by the site of the percussible Tinel's sign, and the stump of the divided FPL tendon.

Additionally in the hand, the stumps of the EPL and EPB are prepared and dissected outside of local scar, and their excursions are confirmed along with the excursion of the FPL. If FPL excursion is less than 1.5 to 2 cm or if it has been avulsed, the flexor digitorum superficialis of the index finger at the level of the wrist can be used to motor the new thumb flexor.

If the thumb metacarpophalangeal joint is to be made by a combination of thumb and toe joints, volar capsular tissues are preserved to attach to the volar plate after sesamoid resection and toe transfer. If the metacarpophalangeal joint is to be reconstructed in the hand by total transfer of the joint from the foot, similar tissues are preserved again to attach to the volar plate after the metatarsal head has been fixed in the hand. Occasionally, bone fragments from the distal metacarpal head can be saved for a bone graft. The metacarpal in the hand is prepared by sagittal saw osteotomy so that a flush, edge to edge osteosynthesis can be achieved.

Before transfer, and after the toe is removed from the foot, a longitudinal medium Kirschner wire (K-wire) is placed from the osteotomized segment of the metatarsal distally through the metatarsophalangeal joint and interphalangeal joint exiting from the tip of the great toe. This is then used to secure the toe longitudinally into the shaft of the metacarpal, once the transfer has been carried out.

Transfer and Repair

When the toe is transferred to the hand, the longitudinal K-wire is driven into the shaft of the metacarpal just short of the carpometacarpal joint. It may be useful to place the volar plate securing sutures (Fig. 125–35) prior to K-wire fixation of the toe into place, because exposure may be difficult after the toe is in place. Usually No. 26 interosseous wiring is used to fix the great toe metatarsal head onto the metacarpal within the hand, and these twistdown wires are placed volarly to allow the bulk of the wire to be hidden in a more volar position rather than a dorsal position with the overriding extensor mechanism. Once the great toe has been transferred, the extensor pollicis to extensor hallucis longus repair is done using a side to side overlapping repair technique with 4-0 nylon. This is done distal to the wrist retinaculum, and proximal to the osteosynthesis site near the base of the thumb metacarpal. The EPB is repaired to the EHB by routing the EHB underneath the EPL (see Fig. 125–17). If the EPB has no excursion, the EHB can be repaired to the EIP or not repaired at all. The intrinsic APB and adductor tendons are then attached to the EHL tendon by turning down side slips of the latter

both radially and ulnarly to allow these muscle tendon units to hold the interphalangeal joint in full extension (see Fig. 125–17). This repair is also done with 4-0 nylon. After the extensor tendons have been repaired, the FHL is brought across the wrist by suturing it to a previously placed pediatric feeding tube, which is led through the bed of the FPL. The FHL is then repaired by Pulvertaft weave into the FPL or the flexor digitorium superficialis well proximal to the volar transverse carpal ligament. Finally, the greater saphenous vein is repaired end to end employing the operating microscope using 10-0 nylon suture into a cephalic vein branch, and the dorsalis pedis artery is brought into the dorsal web space area and repaired end to side into the radial artery (Fig. 125–36). Microvascular clamps are released and the color of the toe is observed. During the entire toe transfer process, great care must be given not to allow desiccation of the blood vessels. Once the vascular perfusion is restored, care must be taken not to damage the artery or vein until wound closure. At this point the superficial and deep peroneal nerve neurorrhaphies to the proximal end of the radial nerve are carried out using the operating microscope, and finally the digital nerves of the great toe are repaired in their reperfused state to appropriate branches of the median nerve. Wound closure after toe to hand transfer is of critical importance, since any delayed wound healing and ultimate sepsis can lead to delayed vessel thrombosis. It has not been

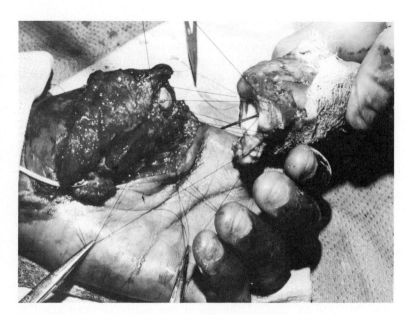

Figure 125–35. A combination new metacarpophalangeal joint is being constructed by combining the good metacarpal articular surface of the remaining thumb remnant with the toe proximal phalanx articular cartilage. Here the volar plate sutures have been placed and left long before fixing the toe in place via the pre-positioned K-wire.

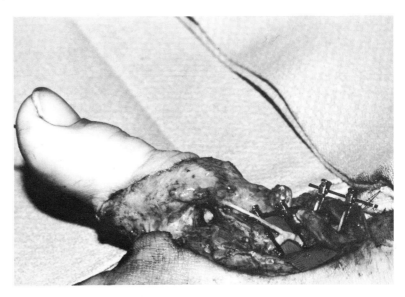

Figure 125–36. "T" dorsalis pedis artery repair into a defect of the radial artery in left toe to hand transfer.

the author's routine to carry out any tendon transfers at the time of primary toe transfer, although it is possible to leave a silicone rod behind, which can ultimately act as a pathway through which thumb opposition transfer can be later placed (Fig. 125–37).

If a groin flap has preceded the toe transfer, the flap can be tailored and split into whatever configuration is necessary for ultimate wound closure. It is surprising how much surgical manipulation these tissues will tolerate once they have regained blood supply from the hand recipient site. If any significant dead space is left at the time of great toe wound closure, small suction catheter drains are left behind, and removed at a formal dressing change five to seven days after toe transfer. Finally, superficial thermocouples are placed on the pulp of the thumb (see Fig. 125–5) and on the adjacent index or middle

finger as a control thermocouple. These probes are secured to the pulp with either sutures or Steritapes, and are led through the hand dressing to avoid being avulsed in the postoperative period. The final dressing on the hand is a form-fitting, supportive, forearm multilayered splint, which positions the thumb in full first web space expansion, but in a position in which the color of the thumb pulp can be easily seen.

Foot Closure

Foot wound closure is an important part of the procedure; it is often neglected, which can lead to difficulties. Hemostasis must be achieved in the cancellous bleeding area of the great toe osteotomized metatarsal. Usually medial metatarsal and dorsal metatarsal

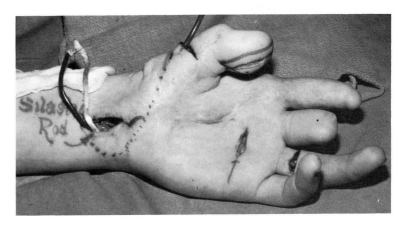

Figure 125–37. Flexor digitorum superficialis opposition transfer after toe to hand transfer. Note the silicone rod used as a spacer placed at the time of toe transfer; this avoids secondary dissection around vital nerve and vessel repairs. Pulp plasty is also being completed.

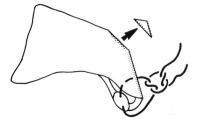

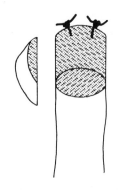

Figure 125–38. Note the narrowing of the metatarsal and sesamoid bone fixation. The arrow indicates the removal of the dorsal bony metatarsal prominence.

edges should be smoothed with a pineapple bur, to allow a tension-free closure (Fig. 125–38). Two small vertical drill holes are placed in the volar lip of the great toe metatarsal, and through these holes the sesamoid–volar plate unit is attached to the metatarsal lip and pushoff surface with 3-0 nylon. This gives the medial foot a rather smooth surface with which to apply force, and prevents descent of the metatarsal head (Fig. 125–38). Hemostasis is carefully checked and a large Jackson Pratt drain is brought in from the proximal end of the foot wound into the cleft between the great toe metatarsal and second metatarsal, to avoid any hematoma collection in this area. The foot flaps are then tailored and closed without tension (Fig. 125–39). The plantar wounds are also closed with interrupted sutures (Fig. 125–40), and the foot is very carefully supported with a full 6 inch plaster posterior splint, brought just distal to the knee. It is sometimes necessary to splint the second toe in a medial direction to take tension off the wound closure. This splinting force is removed at the time of formal dressing change.

POSTOPERATIVE MANAGEMENT

In the recovery room the color and perfusion characteristics of the great toe are monitored and recorded together with the patient's vital signs and urinary output. It is critical to use the thermocouple temperature monitor system as a back-up to clinical observation and not as a replacement for it. This cannot be emphasized too strongly. For the first 24 hours, the same surgical team should look at the thumb without alternating various observers in an around-the-clock

shift. This allows the same individual to see the toe and to recognize any subtle changes in color. It is for this reason that an intensive care unit setting is ideal for early postoperative observation of microvascular cases; excellent lighting is a critical part of this monitoring sequence. The hand should be modestly elevated and immobilized. The patient should be kept sedated, calm, warm, and well hydrated. Antibiotics are given in-

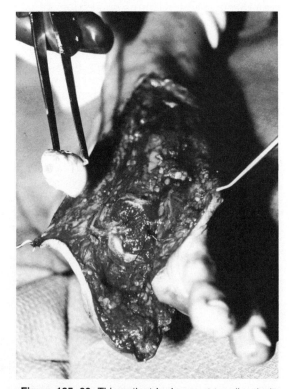

Figure 125–39. This patient had a great toe disarticulation with a combination joint reconstruction. At the time of foot closure, tension was noted. Thus, a dorsal oblique osteotomy was done to remove excessive dorsal metatarsal prominence, and tension was relieved. Healing was uneventful.

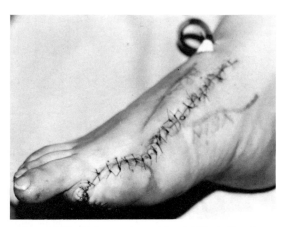

Figure 125–40. Appearance of the right foot after closure with a drain in place.

traoperatively, and again postoperatively for one week. Intravenous dextran, 30 ml per hour, plus aspirin are continued until the day after the drains are removed at the time of the first dressing change, one week postoperatively. Only aspirin, 300 mg orally each day, is continued after this time. Patients are kept off the donor foot for three weeks, but are allowed up in a wheelchair three to five days after toe transfer. Most patients are hospitalized for one week to ten days until any questionable areas of wound healing have become apparent; any alterations or modifications are made at the time of formal dressing change.

It is not uncommon at the time of the first dressing change to note some areas of scabbing and crusting, and also some areas of full-thickness skin graft that have not completely healed. These areas are treated very conservatively and are simply allowed to separate as much as possible on their own, as long as this does not inhibit hand rehabilitation. If an area of full-thickness skin loss on the foot is seen, it is best to excise and reclose the foot under local anesthesia to avoid a prolonged recovery period.

REHABILITATION

As in any complex hand surgical reconstruction, the caliber of the result can be no better than the quality of the rehabilitation (Leung, Wong, and Wan, 1981).

Two weeks after toe to hand transfer, the longitudinal K-wire is removed to allow early joint mobility and to permit early hand ther-

apy to begin. Two to three weeks postoperatively (Robbins and Reece, 1985), active flexion and extension are emphasized, the thumb being splinted at night in full extension with full first web space abduction (Fig. 125–41). Warm water soaks before each active exercise period, and Coban wraps between exercises to decrease swelling, are useful. At the end of the fifth week, gentle, passive range of motion exercises are added to the vigorous active range of motion exercise program, and by the sixth postoperative week rubber band traction is instituted to help strengthen the flexor and extensor muscles. Usually one month after toe to hand transfer, the Tinel's signs at the neurorrhaphy sites begin to move distally, and by six months after transfer sensibility is noted in the distal thumb. During this time sensory reeducation is useful (Dellon, Curtis, and Edgerton, 1974). Great care must be taken to avoid injury to the insensate thumb during the early rehabilitation period. At this time, two-point discrimination and stereognosis begin to improve, and usually within two to three years after toe to hand transfer the two-point discrimination is in the 9 to 12 millimeter range, with complete stereognosis and point stimulation orientation throughout the thumb. If the interphalangeal joint of the thumb begins to droop, a night splint, and a day extension

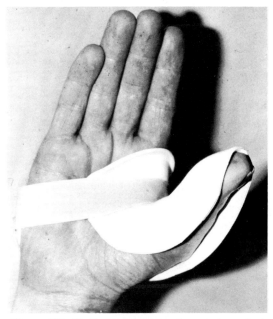

Figure 125–41. First web and thumb extension splint in place three weeks after right toe to hand transfer.

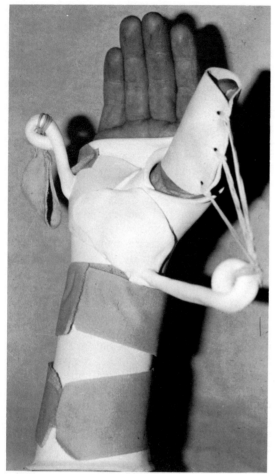

Figure 125–42. Rubber band dynamic exercises begin six weeks after right great toe to hand transfer.

splint between exercise periods, is instituted. All efforts must be made to maintain interphalangeal joint full extension, because a mallet flexion deformity at the interphalangeal joint and hyperextension at the metacarpophalangeal joint will decrease useful function.

TOE TO HAND TRANSFER FOR RECONSTRUCTION OF THE MUTILATED HAND

The restoration of a functional thumb with mobility and sensibility can upgrade the function of a mutilated hand in a remarkable way. The remaining digits can simply act as an innervated post, and as long as the mobile thumb retains restored sensibility, the hand can function with much greater sophistication than a prosthesis.

It is the author's preference to use the great toe to reconstruct the mutilated hand with a missing thumb, because the width of the great toe allows a more utilitarian pinch mechanism to develop (Fig. 125–43).

GAIT ANALYSIS

Foot functional deformity is an important issue to be considered when great toe to hand transfer is anticipated. At the Massachusetts General Hospital, 12 patients were studied in detail, both preoperatively and postoperatively, and detailed gait analysis was performed by Dr. Sheldon Simon at the Children's Hospital (Lipton, May, and Simon, 1987). The mean age of patients involved in this study was 29.3 years, with a mean clinical follow-up period of 30.3 months. Only one patient of the 12 exhibited a significant motion change postoperatively, which was a reduction in ankle plantar flexion at weight release of the operated foot during pushoff. The average cadence step length of the operated foot, the single and double limb stance times of each foot, and the step width did not significantly change. There was only a slight average reduction in stride length of 4.6 per cent, which resulted from a decrease in the step length of the unoperated foot. Nine patients had no clinical complaints whatsoever, and two had occasional mild discomfort near the second and third metatarsal heads. A single patient noticed occasional cold intolerance. It was concluded from this detailed pre- and postoperative gait analysis study that no major objective disturbance of foot function was seen after great toe to hand transfer, provided that the pushoff surface of the great toe metatarsal was left intact. Several of the patients in the author's toe to hand transfer series have continued jogging avidly and one patient has persisted as a semiprofessional baseball player. Another patient, six years after great toe to hand transfer, was successfully inducted into the Massachusetts state police force after a rigorous training period that involved significant hand dexterity and foot durability.

The author's findings are consistent with those of Poppen, Norris, and Buncke (1983), who studied ten patients with postoperative gait analysis alone after great toe to hand transfer, and others who noted no significant problem in ambulation after toe to hand transfer (O'Brien and associates, 1975; Lister, Kalisman, and Tsai, 1983).

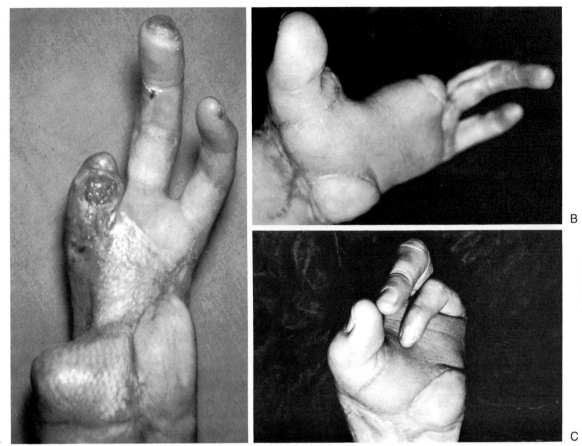

A

B

C

Figure 125–43. *A,* Note the condition of the left hand after a bomb blast injury in this young male. *B,* Three years after thumb reconstruction by great toe to hand transfer preceded by a groin flap. Note the size of the web space. *C,* The left hand in prehension-thumb opposition to the remaining ring finger.

SECONDARY PROCEDURES

In keeping with basic principles of reconstructive surgery, the surgeon and patient should continue to work closely together after a toe to hand transfer procedure to achieve a maximal functional and esthetic result. In most patients the new thumb circumference atrophies by 10 to 15 per cent within the first three years after transfer (Fig. 125–44). However, in almost all patients the thumb pulp is still larger than that of a normal thumb, and some patients may desire an esthetic improvement. A common procedure that many choose is a soft tissue pulp plasty of the reconstructed thumb designed to narrow the thumb and to decrease the profile of the thumb pulp height (Fig. 125–45). The pulp plasty usually is not performed earlier than one year postoperatively, and involves an elliptic excision of skin and subcutaneous tissues under local anesthesia, carried out on an outpatient basis (Fig. 125–45C). It is important that the pulp plasty should not disturb the digital nerves, and it therefore involves debulking only of the fibrofatty lobule of the center of the thumb pulp (Fig. 125–45D). After pulp plasty, a well-healed vertical scar is seen in the pulp of the thumb (Fig. 125–45E). This procedure has been carried out in over a dozen patients, and there appears to be no significant associated morbidity.

On occasion, extensor tendon or flexor tendon adhesions develop between the extensor or flexor mechanism and surrounding tissues. This can be relieved under intravenous regional anesthesia by a formal tenolysis procedure, as with any other adherent tendon (see Chap. 101).

Tendon transfer can be quite useful, particularly in patients who have had thumb reconstruction after mutilating avulsion denervation injury to the radial side of the hand.

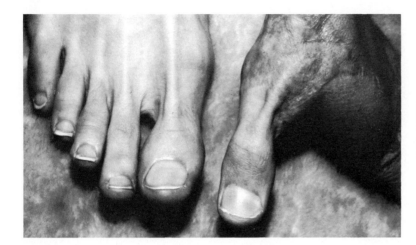

Figure 125–44. 24 year old male three years after toe to hand transfer. The new thumb has decreased 15 per cent in circumference compared with the normal great toe during follow-up.

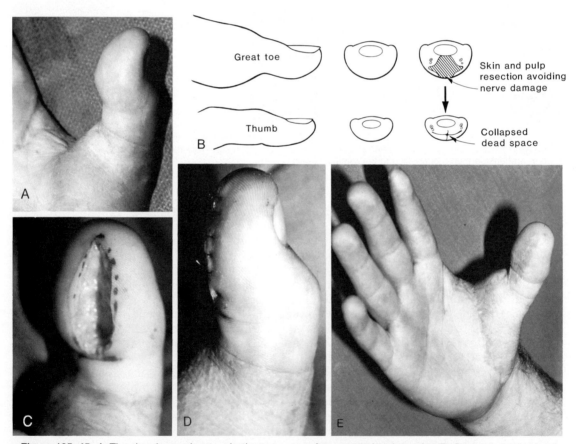

Figure 125–45. *A,* Thumb pulp prominent projection, one year after a toe to hand transfer. *B,* Comparison of great toe and thumb contour. Note the tissue removed in cross section during pulp plasty. *C,* Thumb reduction pulp plasty. *D,* Closure of pulp plasty. Note the normal thumb contour. *E,* Well-healed incision in the center of the thumb pulp.

The most common tendon transfers carried out are opposition transfers, using the ring finger superficialis tendon or the EIP tendon of the index finger brought around the ulnar side of the hand to aid in thumb opposition. If there has been ulnar nerve paralysis in the same hand and adductor function is also lacking, the extensor carpi radialis brevis prolonged by a plantaris tendon can be useful in augmenting and strengthening adduction pinch (see Chap. 114).

Finally, and uncommonly, the interphalangeal joint of the thumb droops into a flexed position because of the inadequacy of repair or the restoration of the intrinsic mechanism to maintain the interphalangeal joint in extension. Under these circumstances a decision must be made whether the extensor mechanism is reconstructable, or whether it is better to salvage function and appearance with fusion of the interphalangeal joint of the thumb. If fusion is carried out, the width of the joint can be narrowed to enhance the appearance.

FAILED TRANSFER AND FOOT COMPLICATIONS

Over the past 12 years at the Massachusetts General Hospital, 37 microvascular foot to hand transfers have been completed. In two patients the great toe failed to survive. In both the cause of failure was an inability to restore adequate arterial inflow to the great toe after transfer (Fig. 125–46*A, B*). Foot complications with delayed healing after toe to hand transfer have been seen in 10 per cent of the author's patients (Fig. 125–46*C*). However, in no patient has significant foot functional abnormality been encountered.

DISCUSSION

Great toe to hand transfer can provide a functional and esthetic replacement for the normal thumb in an otherwise uninjured hand (Fig. 125–47) and can greatly assist

Figure 125–46. *A, B,* This 12 year old boy underwent toe to hand transfer preceded by a groin flap after loss of the radial side of his hand in a bomb accident. The toe was lost because of an unrecognized arterial obstruction, but the groin flap was used to wrap around the avascular bony anatomy of the toe after soft tissue debridement. Note the motion of the thumb with some functional provision. *C,* Foot flap necrosis seen two weeks postoperatively. The flap slough was thought to be caused by improper thinning of the foot flaps. The wound went on to heal in six weeks with no gait disturbance.

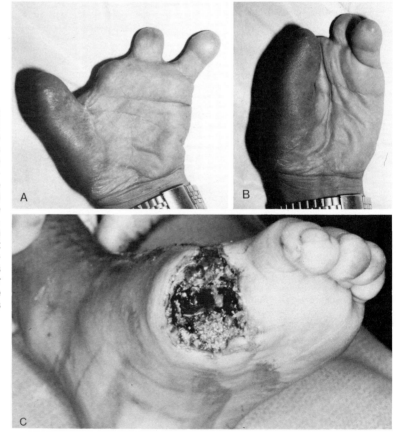

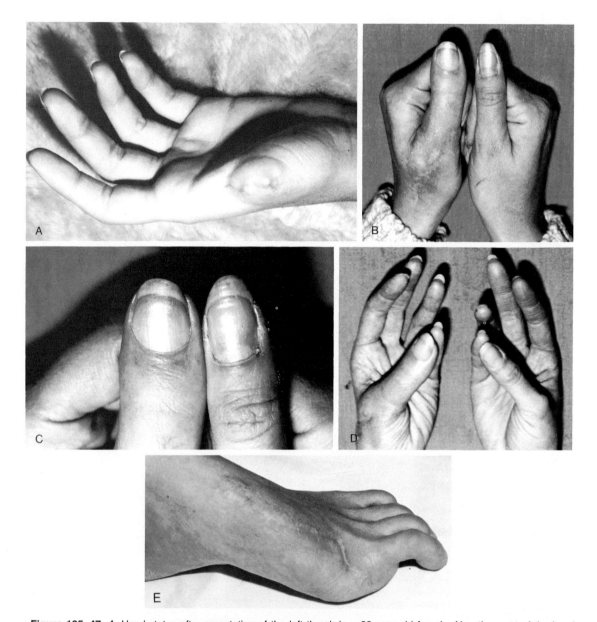

Figure 125–47. *A,* Hand status after amputation of the left thumb in a 28 year old female. No other part of the hand was injured. *B,* Three years postoperatively, acceptable symmetry in comparison with the opposite thumb is evident. *C,* After pulp plasty the new thumb is less than 1 cm larger than the normal thumb. This difference has not been of any significance. *D,* Thumb adduction and opposition pinch are similar to the opposite hand, as the left hand intrinsic muscles are normal. Thumb sensibility shows two-point discrimination of 12 mm. *E,* Appearance of the functional foot three years postoperatively.

the rehabilitation of a mutilated hand. This method of thumb reconstruction maximizes the concept of free tissue transfer, allowing a functionally complex composite of free tissue to be relocated to the important functional and esthetic thumb position. Several points must be reemphasized to optimize the esthetic and functional results of toe to hand transfer.

1. A detailed knowledge of the comparative anatomy of the hand and foot is essential in allowing the most functional and esthetic procedure to be carried out with as large a margin of safety as possible.

2. A team approach is preferable, because this allows an efficient use of time and manpower in what otherwise is a very arduous procedure. Despite the length of the operation, each step must be carried out carefully and safely, and patients should not be selected as optimal operative candidates unless they can tolerate eight to 12 hours of general anesthesia without undue risk.

3. The normal toe is slightly longer than the normal thumb. This length discrepancy must be taken into consideration when thumb reconstruction is completed.

4. The ipsilateral great toe is usually chosen, as it deviates slightly laterally, which is the optimal position for the reconstructive thumb in terms of contact with the index and middle fingers.

5. The skin incisions in the hand should be planned to allow volar and radial coverage over the flexor tendons and digital nerves, wound closure being optimally managed by a previously placed flap or by a full-thickness skin graft. The author does not consider it prudent to take extended tissues from the foot to reconstruct the web space in the hand, since these tissues are much more important to maintain a well-healed functional foot.

6. Joint imbalance after toe transfer is avoided by reconstructing the metacarpophalangeal joint in its conversion from a hyperextension joint to a hyperflexion joint, and by reattaching the intrinsic muscles of the thumb to extend the interphalangeal joint of the thumb.

7. If adequate motors for thumb opposition or adduction are not present, transfers can be provided at subsequent procedures.

8. Normal gait is seen after toe to hand transfer, if the pushoff surface of the great toe metatarsal and sesamoids can be left in an undisturbed position.

9. The institution of regimented specific hand therapy after toe to hand transfer maximizes the merits of thumb reconstruction.

10. The reconstructive surgeon and the patient should work together to add secondary and tertiary finishing touches to the toe to hand transfer to make it more esthetically and functionally acceptable. These procedures are done secondarily rather than at the time of transfer, because the author believes they can be performed more safely and definitively after initial tissue transfer and survival.

CONCLUSION

Great toe to hand transfer for thumb reconstruction is a procedure that has gone through the declaration and innovation phases, and is currently in the refinement phase of procedure development. The operation provides a major improvement in functional and esthetic quality to the hand, at the expense of an esthetic abnormality in the foot. There is no significant functional abnormality in the foot in walking after toe to hand transfer. A hand that looks better works better, and the reverse is also true. On the basis of these two major reconstructive goals (improvement in function and esthetic appearance), the author can confidently recommend this method of thumb reconstruction in carefully selected patients.

Acknowledgement: The author would like to acknowledge the assistance of the residents and fellows in Plastic and Reconstructive Surgery and the Hand Surgery Service for the care of all the patients treated by toe to hand transfer at the Massachusetts General Hospital. Specific appreciation is acknowledged for the help of Dr. Rodney Rohrich, Paula Zingarelli, and Marjorie Ciampa in preparation of this manuscript.

REFERENCES

Adochi, B. Das Arteriensystem der Japaner Kyoto: Imperial Japanese University, 1928, p. 285.

Askar, D., Kassem, K. A., and Shannel, A. A.: The venographic pattern of the foot. J. Cardiovasc. Surg., 16:64, 1975.

Bartlett, S. P., Moses M. H., and May, J. W., Jr.: Thumb reconstruction by free microvascular transfer of an injured index finger: a case report. Plast. Reconstr. Surg., 77:660, 1986.

Bell, Sir C.: The Hand. Its Mechanism and Vital Endowments as Evincing Design. London, William Pickering, 1833, pp. 107–109.

Boyes, J. H.: Phylogeny and comparative anatomy. Bunnell's Surgery of the Hand. 5th Ed. Philadelphia, J. B. Lippincott Company, 1970, p. 51.

Buncke, H. J., Buncke, C. M., and Schulz, W. P.: Immediate Nicoladoni procedure in the rhesus monkey, or hallux-to-hand transplantation, utilising microminiature vascular anastomoses. Br. J. Plast. Surg., *19*:332, 1966.

Bunnell, S.: Physiological reconstruction of a thumb after total loss. Surg. Gynecol. Obstet., *52*:245, 1931.

Clarkson, P., and Furlong, R.: Thumb reconstruction by transfer of the big toe. Br. Med. J., *2*:1332, 1949.

Cobett, J. R.: Free digital transfer: report of a case of transfer of a great toe to replace an amputated thumb. J. Bone Joint Surg., *51B*:677, 1969.

Davis, J. E.: Toe to hand transfers (pedochyrodactyloplasty). Plast. Reconstr. Surg., *33*:422, 1964.

Dellon, A. L., Curtis, R. M., and Edgerton, M. T.: Reeducation of sensation in the hand after nerve injury and repair. Plast. Reconstr. Surg., *53*:297, 1974.

Doi, K.: Microsurgical thumb reconstruction report of six cases with a wrap around free flap from the big toe and an iliac bone graft. Ann. Acad. Med. Singapore, *11*:225, 1982.

Doi, K., Hattori, S., Kawai, S., Nakamura, S., Kotani, H., et al.: New procedure on making a thumb—one-stage reconstruction with free neurovascular flap and iliac bone graft. J. Hand Surg., *6*:346, 1981.

Doi, K., Kuvata, N., and Kawai, S.: Reconstruction of the thumb with a free wrap-around flap from the big toe and an iliac bone graft. J. Bone Joint Surg., *67A*:439, 1985.

Edwards, E. A.: Anatomy of the small arteries of the foot and toes. Acta Anat., *41*:81, 1960.

Frykman, G. K., O'Brien, B. M., Morrison, W. A., and MacLeod, A. M.: Functional evaluation of the hand and foot after one-stage toe-to-hand transfer. J. Hand. Surg., *11A*:9, 1986.

Gilbert, A.: Composite tissue transfers from the foot; anatomic basis and surgical technique. *In* Donillier, A. J., and Strauch, B. (Eds.): Symposium on Microsurgery. St. Louis, C. V. Mosby Company, 1976.

Gordon, L., Leitner, D. W., Buncke, H. J., and Albert, B. S.: Hand reconstruction for multiple amputations by double microsurgical toe transplantation. J. Hand Surg., *10A*:218, 1985.

Greenberg, B. M., and May, J. W., Jr.: Great toe to hand transfer: role of the preoperative lateral arteriogram of the foot. J. Hand Surg., *13A*:411, 1988.

Gueullette, R.: Etude critique des procedes de restauration du ponce. J. Chir. (Paris), *36*:1, 1930.

Huber, J. F.: The arterial network supplying the dorsum of the foot. Anat. Rec., *80*:373, 1941.

Jacobson, B. H.: The venous drainage of the foot. Surg. Gynecol. Obstet., *131*:22, 1970.

Jacobson, B. H., and Suarez, F. L.: Microsurgery in anastomosis of small vessels. Surg. Forum, *11*:243, 1960.

Kleinert, H. E., Kasdan, M. L., and Romero, J. L.: Small blood vessel anastomosis for salvage of the severely injured upper extremity. J. Bone Joint Surg., *45A*:788, 1963.

Kosniski, C.: The course, mutual relations and distribution of the cutaneous nerves of the metatarsal region of the leg and foot. J. Anat., *60*:274, 1926.

Koster, G.: Anatomy of the veins of the foot. Surg. Gynecol. Obstet., *127*:317, 1968.

Leung, P. C.: Thumb reconstruction using the second-toe transfer. Hand Clin., *1*:285, 1985.

Leung, P. C., Wong, A., and Wan, C. Y.: A proposed programme of physical rehabilitation for patients undergoing toe to hand transfer operations. Br. J. Occup. Ther., *4*:187, 1981.

Lipton, H. A., May, J. W., Jr., and Simon, S.: Preoperative and postoperative gait analysis of patients undergoing great toe to thumb transfer. J. Hand. Surg., *12A*:66, 1987.

Lister, G. D., Kalisman, M., and Tsai, T. M.: Reconstruction of the hand with free microneurovascular toe-to-hand transfer: experience with 54 toe transfers. Plast. Reconstr. Surg., *71*:372, 1983.

Littler, J. W.: On making a thumb: one hundred years of surgical effort. J. Hand Surg., *1*:35, 1976.

May, J. W., Jr: Aesthetic and functional thumb reconstruction: great toe to hand transfer. Clin. Plast. Surg., *8*:356, 1981.

May, J. W., Jr.: Reconstruction of the amputated thumb by great toe-to-hand microvascular transfer. *In* Urbaniak, J. R. (Ed.): Microsurgery for Major Limb Reconstruction. St. Louis, C. V. Mosby Company, 1987a, pp 76–85.

May, J. W., Jr.: Thumb restoration by free great toe to hand transfer. *In* The Artistry of Reconstructive Surgery. St. Louis, C. V. Mosby Company, 1987b, pp 813–819.

May, J. W., Jr., Athanasoulis, C. A., and Donelan, M. D.: Preoperative magnification angiography of donor and recipient sites for clinical free transfer of flaps and digits. Plast. Reconstr. Surg., *64*:483, 1977.

May, J. W., Jr., and Bartlett, S. P.: Staged groin flap in reconstruction of the pediatric hand. J. Hand Surg., *3*:163, 1981.

May, J. W., Jr., Chait, L. A., Cohen, B. E., and O'Brien, B. M.: Free neurovascular flap from the first web of the foot in hand reconstruction. J. Hand Surg., *2*:387, 1977.

May, J. W., Jr., and Daniel, R. K.: Great toe to hand transfer. Clin. Orthop., *133*:140, 1978.

May, J. W., Jr., and Rohrich, R. J.: Free microvascular great toe-to-thumb reconstruction. *In* Green, D. P. (Ed.): Operative Hand Surgery. 2nd Ed. New York, Churchill Livingstone, 1987.

May, J. W., Jr., Smith, R. J., and Peimer, C. A.: Toe-to-hand free tissue transfer for thumb construction with multiple digital aplasia. Plast. Reconstr. Surg., *67*:205, 1981.

Mileen, M. R.: Patterns of cutaneous innervation of the human foot. Am. J. Anat., *105*:233, 1959.

Minanni, A.: Thumb reconstruction by free sensory flaps from the foot using microsurgical techniques. J. Hand Surg., *9B*:239, 1984.

Morrison, W. A.: Neurovascular free flaps from the foot for innervation of the hand. J. Hand Surg., *3*:235, 1978.

Morrison, W. A., O'Brien, B. M., and MacLeod, A. M.: Thumb reconstruction with free neurovascular wrap-around flap from the big toe. J. Hand Surg., *5*:575, 1980.

Nicoladoni, C.: Daumenplastik. Wein Klin. Wochenschr., *10*:663, 1897.

Nicoladoni, C.: Daumenplastik und organischer Ersatz der Fingerspitze (anticheiroplastik und daktyloplastik). Arch. Clin. Chri., *61*:606, 1900.

Nunley, J. A., Goldner, R. D., and Urbaniak, J. R.:

Thumb reconstruction by the wrap-around method. Clin. Orthop., *195*:97, 1985.

O'Brien, B. M., Black, M. J., Morrison, W. A., and MacLeod, A. M.: Microvascular great toe transfer for congenital absence of the thumb. Hand, *10*:113, 1978.

O'Brien, B. M., Brennen, M. D., and MacLeod, A. M.: Microvascular free toe transfer. Clin. Plast. Surg., *5*:223, 1978.

O'Brien, B. M., MacLeod, A. M., Sykes, P. J., and Donahoe, S.: Hallux-to-hand transfer. Hand, *7*:2, 128, 1975.

Ome, L.: Recovery of sensibility and sudomotor activity in the hand after nerve suture. Acta Chir. Scand. (Suppl.), 300, 1962.

Poppen, N. K., Norris, T. R., and Buncke, H. J., Jr.: Evaluation of sensibility and function with microsurgical free tissue transfer of the great toe to the hand for thumb reconstruction. J. Hand Surg., *8*:516, 1983.

Reid, D. A.: Reconstruction of the thumb. J. Bone Joint Surg., *42B*:444, 1960.

Robbins, F., and Reece, T.: Hand rehabilitation after great toe transfer for thumb reconstruction. Arch. Phys. Med. Rehabil., *66*:109, 1985.

Rose, E. H., and Hendel, P.: Primary toe to hand transfer in the acutely avulsed thumb. Plast. Reconstr. Surg., *67*:214, 1981.

Strauch, B., and Tsur, H.: Restoration of sensation to the hand by a free neurovascular flap from the first web space of the foot. Plast. Reconstr. Surg., *62*:361, 1978.

Strickland, J. W.: Thumb reconstruction. *In* Operative Hand Surgery. New York, Churchill Livingstone, 1988, p. 2175.

Tanzer, R. C., and Littler, J. W.: Reconstruction of the thumb by transposition of an adjacent digit. Plast. Reconstr. Surg., *3*:533, 1948.

Urbaniak, J. R.: Wrap-around procedure for thumb reconstruction. Hand Clin., *1*:259, 1985.

Yaremchuk, M. J., Bartlett, S. P., Sedacca T., and May, J. W., Jr.: The effect of preoperative angiography on experimental free flap survival. Plast. Reconstr. Surg., *68*:201, 1981.

Yu, Z. J., and He, H. G.: Thumb reconstruction with free big toe skin-nail flap and bones, joints, and tendons of second toe: report of cases. Chin. Med. J., *98*:863, 1985.

Wayne A. Morrison

Thumb Reconstruction by the Wrap-Around Technique

THUMB FUNCTION

Pollicodigital or pinch grip involves sensation, mobility, power, length, and stability. Mobility and power are essentially products of the proximal thumb, i.e., the metacarpal shaft, the carpometacarpal joint, and the thenar muscles. Subtotal thumb reconstruction distal to the metacarpal neck therefore needs to deal only with length, sensation, and stability.

A reconstructive method that provides these attributes with relatively little secondary defect is the wrap-around toe flap combined with iliac crest bone graft for the thumb skeleton (Morrison and associates, 1978, 1980, 1984). Functionally it offers unique glabrous skin, padded nonswivel pulp, and a nail. Sensation is restored by direct digital nerve repair to the proximal thumb nerves and is not dependent on island transfers from another digit. Esthetically it is potentially unsurpassed because of the ability to tailor the shape and size to the opposite normal

thumb. The procedure offers most of the functional and esthetic attributes of the hallux without the need to sacrifice it, so that the patient can retain all toes.

Because the thumb skeleton is constructed from an iliac crest bone graft, no joint is included in the reconstruction and the thumb has no growth potential. Ideally, therefore, the wrap-around method of thumb reconstruction is most suited to amputations distal to the metacarpophalangeal joint in young adults.

Long-term experiences with this flap have been reported (Morrison, O'Brien, and MacLeod, 1984). Other authors have developed similar techniques of thumb reconstruction using partial toe transfer (Foucher and associates, 1980) or have suggested modifications to the technique described here (Leung and Ma, 1982; Steichen, 1984; Doi, 1985).

PREOPERATIVE EVALUATION

The anatomic basis for all foot transfers, whether they be whole or partial toes, is the dorsalis pedis–first metatarsal arterial system. The venous drainage is via the long saphenous system (Fig. 126–1). In approximately 75 per cent of cases (Gilbert, 1976; May and associates, 1977) the dorsal metatarsal artery is superficial and large, and with the dorsalis pedis artery allows direct anastomosis to the radial artery at the wrist. Such favorable anatomy makes transfer simple, speedy, and above all safe. In the remaining cases the artery is deep, small, or absent and the transfer must be vascularized on the plantar system, which will be reciprocally

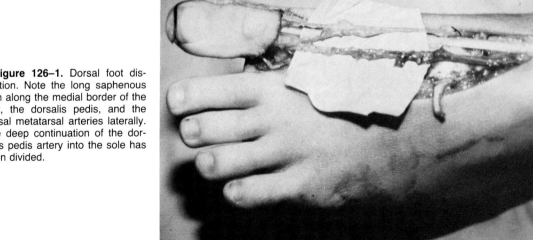

Figure 126–1. Dorsal foot dissection. Note the long saphenous vein along the medial border of the foot, the dorsalis pedis, and the dorsal metatarsal arteries laterally. The deep continuation of the dorsalis pedis artery into the sole has been divided.

large. However, the accessible plantar vessels are short and usually need a vein graft to allow anastomosis to the recipient radial artery at the wrist.

Clinical examination is almost always sufficient to evaluate the anatomy. An impalpable or weakly palpable dorsalis pedis artery does not have an appropriate dorsal metatarsal artery and it is necessary to use the plantar system. A palpable dorsalis pedis artery may not necessarily have a dorsal metatarsal artery of adequate size, and then again the plantar system must be used. However, neither of these situations precludes the use of the flap, so that preoperative arteriography is unnecessary and (unless done by peripheral selective techniques in the lateral view) is inadequate to show the dorsal metatarsal artery system in any case.

The ipsilateral toe is chosen so that the intact lateral aspect of the toe becomes the dominant ulnar side of the thumb. The suture line is along the radial border. The vascular pedicle also lies favorably along the first web space of the hand, leading to the radial vessels at the wrist.

The medial toe flap markings pass medial to the nail bed so that the whole of the toenail irrespective of its width is transferred, including its medial eponychial edge. One should aim to conserve plantar skin on the foot, ideally not extending more proximally than the web skin level, even if this means some compromise on the length of the reconstructed thumb.

Markings

A template of the opposite intact thumb is made, measuring its circumference and length. These measurements are transcribed onto the ipsilateral hallux, the difference in circumference of the two digits being the width of the intact skin flap that remains along the medial border of the tip of the toe (Figs. 126–2, 126–3). This skin flap usually measures about 1 to 1.5 cm in width at its proximal base, and tapers distally. It is innervated by a separate long and large dorsal branch of the medial plantar nerve, which arises just proximal to the metatarsophalangeal joint, and it courses dorsal to this joint.

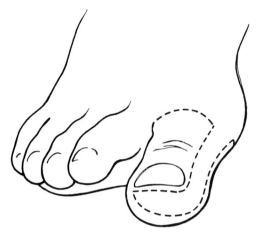

Figure 126–2. Markings for the wrap-around flap. Note the medial toe and tip skin bridge that is retained on the foot. The transferred flap involves the plantar, lateral, and dorsal skin including the nail.

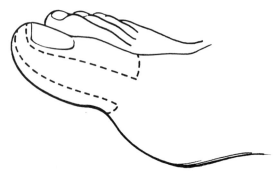

Figure 126–3. Toe markings demonstrating the retained medial skin flap. Note that the dorsal skin flap usually extends more proximally than the plantar one.

The dorsal venous drainage from the proximal margin of the toe flap should be marked out preoperatively by applying a venous tourniquet.

OPERATIVE TECHNIQUE

A straight incision is made on the dorsum of the foot just lateral to the course of the flexor hallucis longus tendon from the distal limit of the extensor retinaculum to the proximal limit of the toe flap markings, which are also incised. Superficial veins are dissected free emerging from the toe flap and traced proximally until a sufficient pedicle has developed, which drains to the long saphenous vein on the medial border of the foot. All large branches of the long saphenous vein are then ligated to the level of the proximal incision.

The dorsalis pedis artery and venae comitantes are next located at the lower level of the retinaculum just lateral to the flexor hallucis longus tendon between it and the flexor digitorum communis tendons. This pedicle is traced distally where it is crossed by the extensor hallucis brevis muscle and tendon, which should be divided for adequate exposure. The vessels are further dissected to the proximal limit of the first dorsal intermetatarsal space where they penetrate deeply through the foot into the sole. At this point the dorsal metatarsal artery should be identifiable branching from the main vessel and continuing distally in the metatarsal space (Fig. 126–4). In favorable cases it is large, approximately 1.0 to 2.0 mm in diameter, and it lies superficially or shallowly within the substance of the first dorsal interosseous muscle. In approximately 25 per cent of cases it is too small or absent and the dorsal arterial system must be abandoned for the shorter plantar one. Usually the dorsal metatarsal artery can be traced distally up to its bifurcation into digital vessels proper to the big and second toes. The dorsal metatarsal artery continues plantarward over and distal to the intermetatarsal ligament to join its plantar counterpart. It is from this arch that the digital vessels arise, both dorsal and plantar, but the plantar are dominant and usually the only branches identified. The division to the second toe is ligated. When the plantar system is dominant the plantar digital artery proper is easily identified via the dorsal exposure distal to the intermetatarsal ligament, where it lies dorsal to the large lateral digital nerve. By means of an extended plantar incision skirting the ball of the foot, the plantar artery and nerve are traced proximally as far as possible, but a vein graft is usually needed to lengthen the arterial pedicle.

The toe is now incised around its markings,

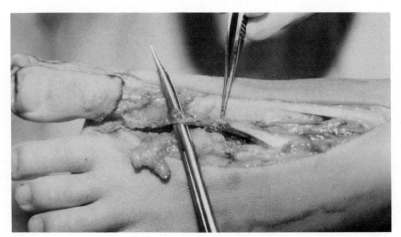

Figure 126–4. Dorsal vascular dissection of the wrap-around flap. Note the dorsalis pedis artery and venae comitantes proximally crossed by the tendon of the extensor hallucis brevis, and the dorsal metatarsal artery continuing distally to the first web space, demonstrated by the scissors.

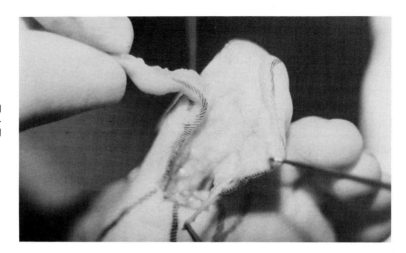

Figure 126–5. The tip and medial skin flap is elevated from the underlying distal phalanx to the level of the middle of the phalanx.

and the tip of the retained medial skin flap is elevated from the underlying phalanx around to the medial side as far proximally as the level of the proximal eponychial fold, i.e., approximately midway along the medial border of the distal phalanx (Fig. 126–5). The dorsal skin of the toe flap is now elevated in the plane deep to the veins, but care must be taken to preserve the joint capsule and paratenon over the extensor tendon insertion. The germinal matrix is elevated from the distal phalanx down to the level of the eponychial fold. At this level the phalanx is osteotomized and the distal segment remains attached to the dorsal segment of the transferred toe sleeve as a vascularized bone graft. Retention of the piece of bone in the flap not only supports and protects the nail bed but also helps vascularization of the free interposed bone graft that is used for the thumb skele-

ton, and reduces its potential for resorption. Elevation of the skin flap continues into the first web and around the lateral border of the phalanges to the plantar aspects.

It is now easier to recommence the dissection at the medial edge and elevate the plantar flap from medial to lateral. The medial digital nerve is located, dissected, and divided as far proximally as required by tunneling proximally underneath the intact plantar skin (Fig. 126–6). The flap is raised from the distal phalangeal segment and flexor tendon sheath, and the lateral plantar nerve and artery are defined, the nerve being plantar to the artery. Usually, sufficient length of nerve can be obtained without a plantar incision, but this latter may sometimes be required, especially if the plantar artery is the dominant vessel for transfer. Care must be taken in freeing the lateral plantar digital artery

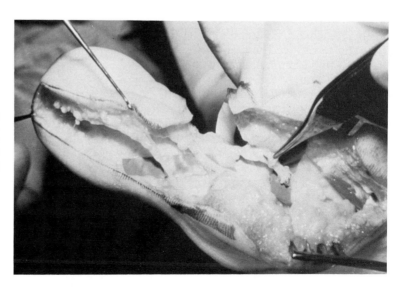

Figure 126–6. Plantar dissection of the wrap-around flap, demonstrating the medial and lateral plantar digital nerves and the plantar digital artery held in the dissecting forceps.

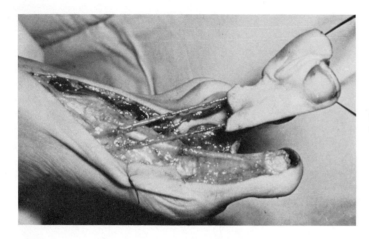

Figure 126–7. Wrap-around flap including the distal half of the distal phalanx mobilized on the dorsal vascular pedicle.

from the edge of the skeleton, as there is a constant large branch to the interphalangeal joint of the hallux, which arises proximal to the joint and passes deep to the flexor tendon. This must be clipped to allow final elevation of the flap.

Once the soft tissue has been completely separated except for the nail bed over the distal half of the distal phalanx, an osteotomy of the distal phalanx is performed at the level at or just proximal to the proximal eponychial fold. This is technically difficult and is best done with fine bone cutters.

The composite osteocutaneous sleeve now remains connected by the dorsalis pedis artery and long saphenous vein (Fig. 126–7). The tourniquet should now be released to allow a period of revascularization and to confirm that the vascular anatomy is intact.

Hand Dissection

Simultaneously a second surgeon prepares the hand to receive the transfer.

The thumb stump skeleton remnant is exposed by a transverse incision at the dorsal edge, which is reflected palmarward as a volar based flap. This augments skin closure on the palmar side where a conservative amount of plantar skin has been supplied in the toe flap to avoid problems with toe closure. The bony stump is squared off, taking care to preserve any remaining proximal phalanx so that metacarpophalangeal joint function will be retained.

At the ulnar aspect of the palmar flap the incision is continued proximally into the first web on the palmar side to expose the digital nerve stumps of the thumb.

A separate dorsal flap incision is made

overlying the snuffbox region to expose the cephalic vein and dorsal continuation of the radial artery. These vessels are stripped of branches, delivered into the wound, and prepared for microvascular repair. Good forward arterial flow is confirmed by release of the tourniquet.

A wide tunnel is created over the dorsum of the first metacarpal communicating the snuffbox incision with the exposed stump.

Bone Graft

Depending on the length of residual proximal phalanx, a free bone graft is usually required for insertion between the proximal phalanx and the vascularized bone segment in the flap. The bone graft should be as large as can be possibly accommodated within the toe sleeve and is appropriately taken from the iliac crest, including cortical and cancellous segments. A postoperative waisted appearance at the proximal phalangeal level is common after this method of reconstruction and is due to the fact that no tendons are included in the transfer or in the reconstructed thumb. The absence of this normal bulk plus the natural bulky terminal pulp of the hallux results in a relative narrowing or waisting of the proximal thumb. This must therefore be corrected by deliberately inserting as big a piece of bone as possible in this area without preventing skin closure.

Thumb Reconstruction

The toe flap is now detached from the foot, the artery being ligated first, and transferred to the hand. Where the nail of the toe is

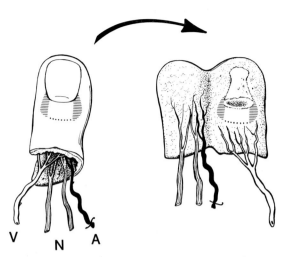

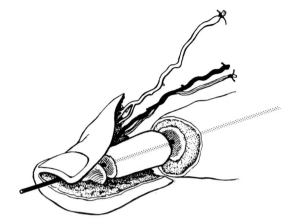

Figure 126–8. Resection of the corners of the germinal matrix from the undersurface of the toe flap. The area of resection is crosshatched.

Figure 126–9. Iliac crest bone graft inserted between the proximal and distal segments of vascularized bone.

obviously too wide to make a convincing thumb, it is a relatively simple matter to open up the two leaves of the sleeve flap and expose the undersurface of the germinal matrix. The corners at each side can be resected so that when the nail grows down it will be narrowed to the desired degree (Fig. 126–8). The bone graft is interposed between the flap bone fragment distally and the proximal phalangeal stump. It is transfixed in a shish kebab fashion with a longitudinal Kirschner wire inserted through the distal phalanx up into the metacarpal across the intact metacarpophalangeal joint. A further two small, crossed Kirschner wires are usually inserted to ensure the proximal osteosynthesis.

The vascular pedicle is tunneled proximally to the region of the radial vessels, care being taken to avoid kinking, twisting, and compression. The toe sleeve is now closed around the bone graft and sutured around the tip and along its radial border (Fig. 126–10).

The long saphenous vein is anastomosed to the cephalic vein or to a vena comitans of the radial artery, and the dorsalis pedis artery is anastomosed, usually to the dorsal continuation of the radial artery end to end.

Once vascularization has occurred the flap should be checked to ensure that too tight a closure has not been performed. Pallor is frequently observed at the distal radial corner of the nail bed, and some sutures may need release to avoid necrosis.

It should be reiterated that no tendon reconstruction is performed. A typical case fol-

Figure 126–10. The toe sleeve flap being wrapped around the bone graft and the vascular pedicle directed to the radial snuffbox.

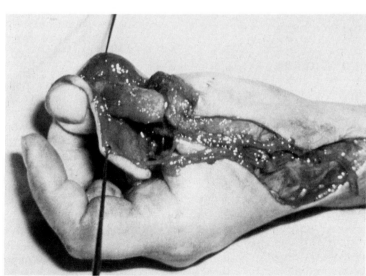

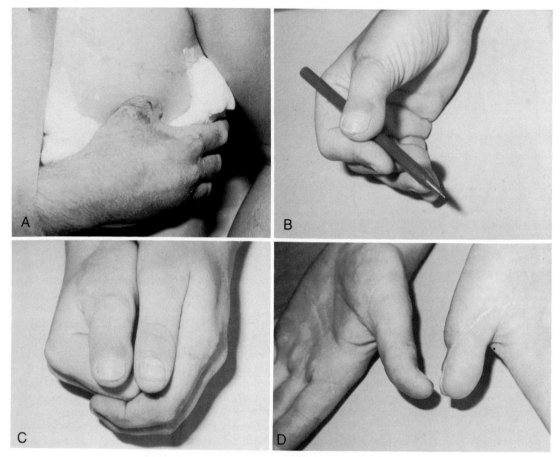

Figure 126–11. *A,* Preoperative view demonstrating a degloved thumb through the interphalangeal joint with skin degloved to the level of the metacarpophalangeal joint. Initial preservation of the exposed proximal phalanx is effected by insertion into a chest wall pocket. *B,* Postoperative result one year following wrap-around flap from the big toe. No iliac crest bone graft has been used in this case because sufficient length was obtained by approximation of the distal phalangeal toe segment to the residual proximal phalanx of the thumb. *C,* Postoperative result at one year comparing both thumbs; dorsal view. *D,* Palmar view.

lowing reconstruction is shown in Figure 126–11.

Foot Closure

Success of the procedure depends as much on the avoidance of foot morbidity as on the thumb reconstruction. In general the foot heals much more slowly than the hand, and the patient must remain with strict foot elevation for ten days to minimize the risk of complications. The stump of the distal phalanx is first trimmed smooth and the corners rounded off. The long tip flap is checked for viability and any suspicious skin is excised, even if this means further bone shortening for closure. The flap is then folded around the toe tip and along the lateral aspect of the toe

into the first web, where it is tacked into position.

A full length cross toe flap extending from the nail bed distally to the interdigital web proximally is raised from the dorsum of the second toe and based on its medial side. This is opened out to cover the whole of the plantar surface of the big toe defect.

The remaining dorsal defects on the big and second toes are covered with a thick split-thickness skin graft (Fig. 126–12). Any exposed cortical bone can be nibbled to cancellous bone and this readily accepts skin grafts. A tie-over dressing is applied.

The toes are separated any time after one month, and small split-thickness skin grafts to adjacent sides of the big and second toes after division will expedite healing. Figure 126–13 demonstrates the foot defect 12

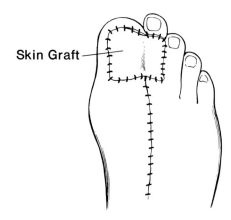

Figure 126–12. Method of closure of a toe defect. *Above*: thick split-thickness skin graft applied to the dorsum of the big and second toes. *Below*: large full width and full length cross toe flap from the dorsum of the second toe applied to the plantar surface of the hallux.

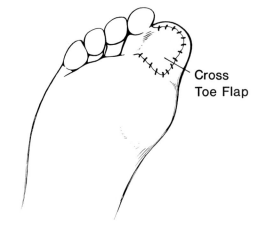

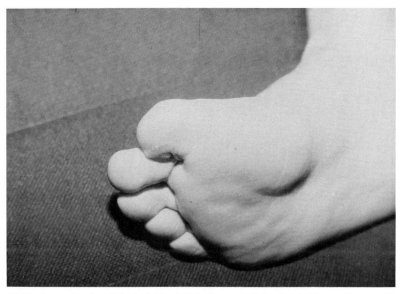

Figure 126–13. Secondary toe defect at 12 months (the case illustrated in Figure 126–11). Plantar view.

months postoperatively in the case illustrated in Fig. 126–11.

Modifications

Since the original publications (Morrison and associates, 1978, 1980), some modifications have been made. Because of concern over bone atrophy, the distal half of the distal phalanx of the hallux is incorporated in the transfer so that the nonvascularized iliac crest graft now lies between vascularized bone proximally and distally.

Sculpturing of the bone graft has been reduced to a minimum, aiming instead to fill up the toe sleeve cavity as much as possible.

The nail width is reduced not by a wedge-type excision, but by trimming the corners from the germinal matrix on the undersurface of the flap, as explained.

Finally, the cross toe flap now is a conventional dorsal one designed to cover the plantar defect of the hallux with flap skin, rather than a split skin graft, and this has greatly reduced the incidence of ulceration and hyperkeratotic reaction of the plantar aspect of the hallux.

REFERENCES

Doi, K., Kawata, N., and Kawai, S.: Reconstruction of the thumb with a wrap-around flap and an iliac crest bone graft. J. Bone Joint Surg. 67A:439, 1985.

Foucher, G., Merle, M., Meneaud, M., and Michon, J.: Microsurgical free partial toe transfer in hand reconstruction: a report of 12 cases. Plant. Reconstr. Surg., 65:616, 1980.

Gilbert, A.: Composite tissue transfers from the foot: Anatomic basis and surgical technique. In Daniller, A., and Strauch, B. (Eds.): Symposium on Microsurgery. Vol. 15. St. Louis, C.V. Mosby & Company, 1976, Chap. 25.

Leung, P.C., and Ma, F.: Digital reconstruction using the toe flap. Report of 10 cases. J. Hand Surg., 7:366, 1982.

May, J.W. Jr., Chait, L.A., Cohen, B., and O'Brien, B.M.: Free neurovascular flap from the first web space of the foot in hand reconstruction. J. Hand Surg., 2:387, 1977.

Morrison, W.A., O'Brien, B.M., and Hamilton, R.: Neurovascular free foot flaps in reconstruction of the mutilated hand. Clin. Plast. Surg., 5:265, 1978.

Morrison, W.A., O'Brien, B.M., and MacLeod, A.M.: Thumb reconstruction with a free neurovascular wrap-around flap from the big toe. J. Hand Surg., 5:575, 1980.

Morrison, W.A., O'Brien, B.M., and MacLeod, A.M.: Experience with thumb reconstruction. J. Hand Surg., 9B:223, 1984.

Steichen, J.: Modifications to the wrap around method of thumb reconstruction. Presented at Fifth A.O.A. International Symposium, "Limb reconstruction" Micro or Macrosurgery. Boca Raton, Florida, Nov., 1984.

Thumb Reconstruction by Bone Lengthening

During the last decade a new procedure of thumb reconstruction has been introduced into surgical practice. The procedure described uses the resources of the amputation stump for reconstruction. The first metacarpal bone is cut in the middle third, and by means of a special device it is gradually lengthened, together with the soft structures. The gap between the pulled apart fragments fuses through spontaneous osteogenesis or is bridged by a bone graft. The advantages of thumb reconstruction through distraction lengthening are the rationality of the procedure and the quality of skin coverage in the new thumb: the skin of the lengthened stump retains its normal pattern of sensibility.

Metacarpal bone lengthening proves to be a reliable and safe procedure for thumb re-construction in thumb hypoplasia and amputation of the thumb in children and adults. The drawback of this procedure is the rather prolonged term of treatment, the average being three months.

HISTORY

There are no data published on the use of the distraction lengthening method in thumb reconstruction before the May, 1967 Anglo-Scandinavian Symposium on Hand Surgery, held in Lausanne and Vienna, where Matev (1967) reported a 27 year old patient with amputation of the thumb through the meta-carpal head. Following osteotomy of the thumb metacarpal, the fragments were distracted gradually, and a bone graft was interposed between the fragments. A 2 cm lengthening of the metacarpal was achieved.

Thus, the principles of Putti (1921) and Codivilla (1904) for continuous traction and countertraction of the long bones, applied to the metacarpal of an amputated thumb, resulted in a new method of thumb reconstruction (Fig. 127–1).

During subsequent years a personal series of treated patients was reported (Matev, 1969, 1970, 1972, 1979, 1980, 1983). The distraction method is effective not only in thumb reconstruction, but also in finger lengthening and other hand disorders, such as palm shortening, clinodactyly, and dislocation. Successful results with the distraction lengthening method for thumb and finger reconstruction have also been reported by many authors, with the richest experience accumulated by Ulitzkii and Maligin (1971), Kessler (1976, 1977), and Cowen (1980). Other cases have been described by Ben-Hur (1980), Cugola,

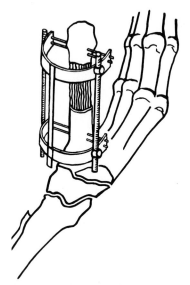

Figure 127–1. The method of thumb reconstruction by gradual distraction lengthening.

Colognese, and Marcer (1974), Manninger (1980), Neff (1981), and Vossman and Zellner (1980).

INDICATIONS

The distraction lengthening procedure is indicated for thumb amputation in the region of the metacarpophalangeal joint, i.e., the area of decompensated thumb amputation (Fig. 127–2).

The presence of the whole metacarpal bone or two thirds of its length is a prerequisite for realization of the procedure. The availability of at least 3 cm of the metacarpal shaft guarantees the successful outcome of thumb lengthening.

The second prerequisite is good condition of the stump's own skin. Scarring in the first web is a relative contraindication for the lengthening procedure, but it is always better to release the scars in advance by means of a skin plasty operation. Extensive scar involvement of the stump top has to be treated before the bone surgery is undertaken. One should not expect good skin coverage with adequate sensibility in the reconstructed thumb if the skin of the amputation stump is not good enough.

The thumb lengthening procedure is indicated for thumb amputation and thumb hypoplasia among teenagers, children, and adults. Application of distraction lengthening in children under 7 or 8 years of age is possible, but it should be done carefully in order to prevent damage to the epiphyseal plate, with ensuing disturbance of normal metacarpal growth. The best indication for the thumb lengthening procedure is the hypoplastic thumb with part of the metacarpal bone available, as well as thumb amputation in the metacarpophalangeal region with good skin in the stump and in the first web.

Limits of Distraction

Lengthening of the amputation stump by up to 50 per cent of the original length of the first metacarpal is easily achieved. Distraction of 70 to 80 per cent, which usually corresponds to 2.5 to 3 cm in length, equal to that of a thumb proximal phalanx, is accomplished without difficulties. A 100 per cent lengthening of the initial length of the metacarpal is not unusual, especially in children. This appears to be the limit for lengthening of an amputation stump in the hand through gradual distraction, for the soft tissues behave adequately and do not reveal obvious disorders in the blood supply or any other impairment (Fig. 127–3).

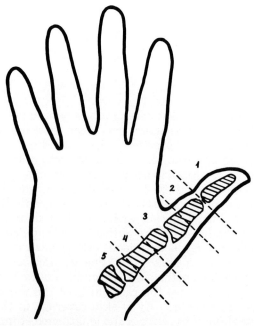

Figure 127–2. Schematic representation of the amputation levels: *1*, compensated amputation zone; *2*, partially compensated; *3*, decompensated; *4*, subtotal; *5*, total amputation zone.

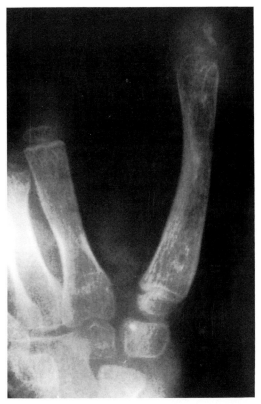

Figure 127–3. In this 10 year old boy a 100 per cent lengthening of the initial length of the first metacarpal is achieved without difficulty.

Distraction Device

An effective distraction device meets the following basic requirements:

1. It should be stable, thereby preventing deformation of the device by the distraction forces acting during the period of bone lengthening, and providing a strict immobilization of the pulled apart fragments during the fusion process.

2. It should be compact, preferably a one- or two-piece apparatus, for easy and quick application and handling by the surgeon.

3. The distraction device has to be simple and readily adjustable by the patient himself, or by the parents of the children undergoing treatment, during the period of gradual bone lengthening.

A good distraction device secures firm fixation of the pins crossing the fragments transversely. The weight of the device should not exceed 80 gm for children, and 150 gm for adults.

Drilling of the pins into the metacarpal bone is facilitated if a separate auxiliary guide is used (Fig. 127–4). The guide secures quick and accurate parallel driving of the pins in one or two planes of the bone. The pins the author uses are thick Kirschner wires.

THE OPERATION

Insertion of Pins. The operation begins with the transverse insertion (at a right angle) of four pins into the metacarpal. Under radiographic control one pair is driven through the proximal and the other through the distal third of the bone. Enough distance should be left between the inserted pairs of pins to facilitate the performance of the osteotomy. A 1 cm distance is the best one, but with several millimeters less the procedure can still be done without difficulties.

It is better to start with the most proximal pin, which should be inserted at a point about 1 cm distant from the first carpometacarpal joint. The proper position of this pin is essential, especially in children, in order to prevent damage to the epiphyseal plate, and thus secure normal metacarpal growth.

An accurate insertion of the pins into the metacarpal bone is achieved provided a guide is used.

In most of the author's patients the Kirschner wires were driven in a parallel fashion in one palmar plane (the longitudinal one). The pins may also be inserted parallelly in two closer palmar planes, or crossed in two transverse planes (Fig. 127–5).

Osteotomy. With the four pins driven into the bone, a 1.5 to 2 cm long skin incision is done on the dorsal surface, in the middle third of the first metacarpal. The periosteum is detached over a short distance through a small longitudinal incision. With a Bunnell hand drill the bone is pierced many times in a transverse plane at various angles, and the metacarpal is cut in the middle third using a small chisel (Fig. 127–6). It is preferable to carry out jagged osteotomy because the numerous tiny particles stimulate the osteogenesis in the gap between the fragments. The periosteum should not be cut transversely, otherwise an obvious retardation of the spontaneous bone production in the lengthened metacarpal takes place.

Application of Device. After wound clo-

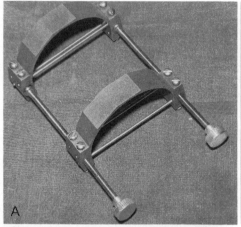
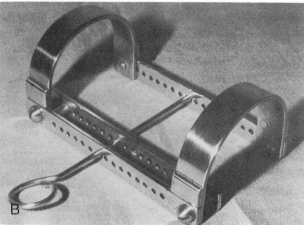
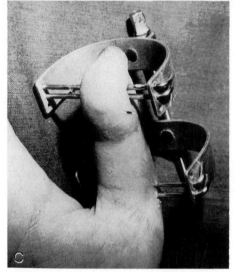

Figure 127–4. *A,* A one-piece distraction device for metacarpal bones. *B,* Detachable auxiliary guide for accurate insertion of the Kirschner wires. *C,* A smaller device for lengthening of the thumb proximal phalanx.

sure with one catgut suture for the periosteum and fascia, another one for the subcutis, and two stitches for the skin, the device is carefully mounted on the four pins. Each pin is firmly fixed to the device. The screws of the latter are turned several turns in order to achieve an initial lengthening of several millimeters. The distal two-thirds of the forearm, the wrist, the palm, and the first metacarpal are immobilized with the device for several days in a dorsal plaster of Paris splint.

Distraction Period

Gradual lengthening begins several days after the operation when the pain and postoperative edema subside. The screws of the distraction device are turned every day, providing 1 to 1.5 mm of elongation, which is very well tolerated by the patient. A greater lengthening causes discomfort and pain, and may delay or even compromise the treatment. In the device used by the author, one full turn of the screws corresponds to 1 mm lengthening of the bone.

Usually, to achieve 2.5 to 3.5 cm lengthening of the metacarpal, the distraction period lasts 25 to 35 days. A quicker distraction stimulates the spontaneous osteogenesis of the gap between the fragments. The metacarpal lengthening in children goes faster, and the average elongation attained is greater than that in adolescents and adults. In several 10 to 12 year old boys the author obtained an increase of up to 110 per cent to the original length of the metacarpal without any difficulty. Occasionally, during the sec-

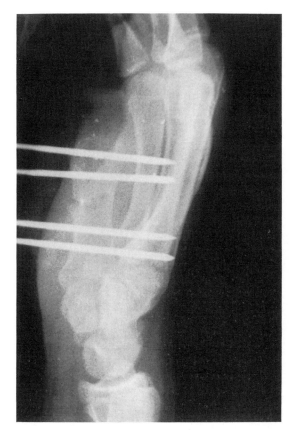

Figure 127–5. The Kirschner wires are inserted parallelly in one palmar plane and osteotomy is done; application of the device follows.

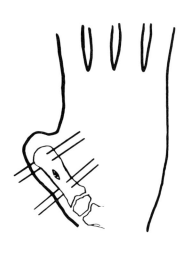

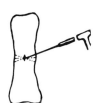

Figure 127–6. Schematic drawing of the skin incision and the mode of osteotomy.

ond half of the distraction period, a persistent pain occurs after the screws are turned. In such cases the lengthening should be discontinued for one to two days.

Firm pin fixation to the device is absolutely necessary during the whole treatment. There is no need to splint the hand in the distraction lengthening period. Rigid fixation of the fragments is not necessary. The author's experience shows that a certain degree of vibration of the fragments stimulates spontaneous ossification of the existing gap.

Tissue Response to Stretching

The considerable elongation does not cause visible disturbances in the soft tissues. The periosteum, muscles, neurovascular bundles, and skin run an uneventful course of slow and gradual distraction. During the second half of the distraction period, when the elongation goes beyond the 2.5 to 3 cm limit, a single distraction of 2 mm or more causes a sharp pain, accompanied by pallor and numbness on top of the stump. A 1 mm lengthening is tolerated well and causes no visible blood supply impairment. The rheograms taken at termination of the distraction period, immediately after turning the screws, show mild transient suppression in the blood supply to the stump top. It was not necessary to turn back the screws of the device in any of the author's cases. Electromyographic examination of the thenar muscles during the second phase of the distraction period disclosed slight quantitative changes in the activity of muscle fibers, which were not accompanied by qualitative alterations. The long-term EMG follow-up in patients with final lengthening of the first metacarpal in excess of 80 per cent to the original length showed no difference in the registered action potentials, in comparison with the ones elicited from the thenar muscles of the sound hand.

A slight transient depression in the sensibility of the tip skin is observed in the course of distraction. A prolonged numbness associated with hypoesthesia on the stump end may be observed after a more significant metacarpal elongation. These sensory disturbances usually disappear during the immobilization period. The quality of sensitivity on the surface of the reconstructed thumb depends mainly on the original state of the stump skin. If this is good the reconstructed thumb usually preserves a sensitivity that is qualitatively the same as that in the amputation stump before treatment.

Immobilization Period

Immobilization begins after the distraction has ended, and lasts two to three months until complete ossification of the interfragmental gap and solid bone fusion take place. The pulled apart fragments should be well immobilized; this is secured by the distraction device itself, but if necessary a plaster splint may also be used. Loosening of the pins should be avoided since it may result in an undesirable secretion from the bone canals. The patient's condition is checked at two week intervals, and serial radiographs show a gradual consolidation of the interfragmental gap. Spontaneous ossification is strictly kept within the frames of the periosteum. The consolidation period depends first on the degree of elongation, and second on the patient's age. In children aged 8 to 10 years, a 2.5 to 3.5 cm gap usually ossifies spontaneously within one and one-half to three months after cessation of the distraction. For teenagers the period required is longer, while in adults spontaneous fusion of the fragments occurs very rarely. The time of treatment is shortened considerably if the interfragmental gap is bridged with a bone graft, taken ideally from the iliac crest.

Filling the Gap

Spontaneous Osteogenesis. The consecutive x-ray films show a gradual filling of the interfragmental gap with bone substance (Fig. 127–7). An opacity between the fragments is usually visible at termination of the second distraction week. The increasing density in the gap assumes a longitudinal orientation. The ossification process lags significantly behind the distraction of the fragments, being less pronounced nearer the distal fragment. The central zone of the gap is the last one to be bridged (Fig. 127–8). Spontaneous ossification is limited within the frame of the periosteum and is never noted beyond the bony contour. The periosteum is the main, but by no means the sole, contributor to the ossifying process. The enormous

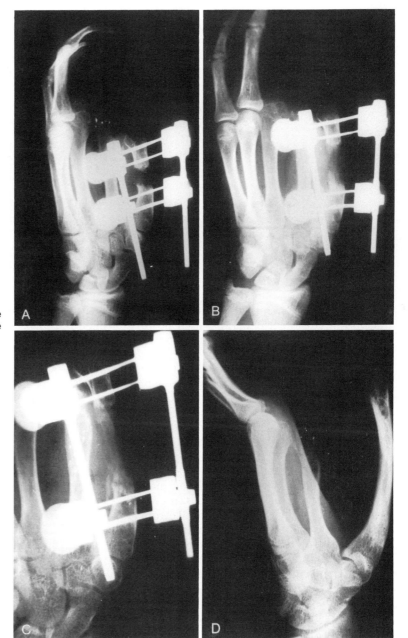

Figure 127–7. *A to D,* The course of spontaneous osteogenesis of the interfragmental space.

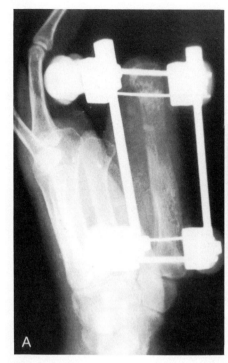

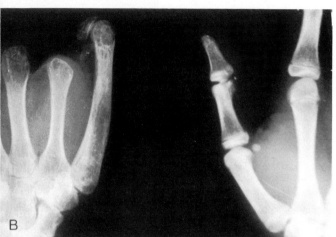

Figure 127–8. *A,* The central zone ossifies last. *B,* The same patient three months later.

stretching (over 2 cm) undoubtedly leads to disruption of the periosteum, which however does not interfere with the spontaneous ossification of a 3 to 3.5 cm gap in children and in many teenagers. In adults this is hardly possible owing to the reduced osteogenetic activity of the bone tissue (Fig. 127–9).

Stimulation of Spontaneous Osteogenesis. Acceleration of the spontaneous ossification of the gap may be achieved by bone growth electrostimulation. For this purpose a noninvasive electromagnetic or a semi-invasive needle bone growth stimulator may be used. During the last few years, in a greater number of the author's patients electromagnetic bone stimulation was applied in the first half of the distraction period, switching to the semi-invasive needle bone stimulator during the second half of the metacarpal lengthening (Fig. 127–10). In case a marked positive effect is recorded, bone growth stimulation should be continued during the immobilization period, since in younger patients subjected to bone growth stimulation, fusion of the fragments often occurs faster through the speeded-up spontaneous ossification, thereby sparing a bone grafting operation for the successful completion of treatment.

Bone Grafting of Gap. Spontaneous ossi-fication of the interfragmental gap may be expected in younger patients. A 3 cm or more gap in patients over 20 years of age should be filled by a bone graft without any delay, because spontaneous consolidation is very unlikely to occur.

The speed of spontaneous osteogenesis is clearly seen on serial radiographs taken during the distraction period. If during the last week of the lengthening, or during the first two weeks of the immobilization period, spontaneous ossification is not proceeding fast enough (i.e., is not seen to be progressing well radiographically), surgery should be undertaken without delay.

A periosteal-cortico-cancellous bone graft taken from the external half of the contralateral iliac crest is the best. Without removal of the distraction device, a longer skin incision is made on the dorsum of the lengthened metacarpal just overlying the previous surgical scar. The longitudinally arranged fibers filling the interfragmental space are excised and the bone graft is placed. It is fixed through firm wedging into longitudinal clefts of each of the fragments, usually without using Kirschner pins for additional stabilization of the graft. A plaster of Paris splint is applied for 45 days (Fig. 127–11).

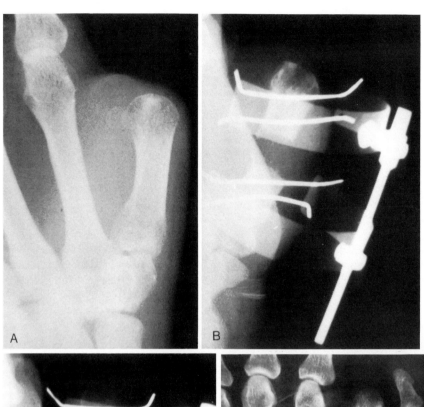

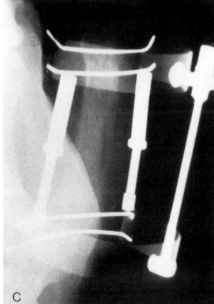

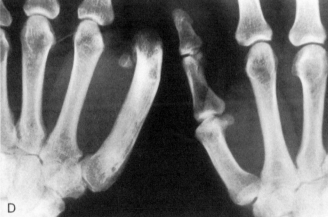

Figure 127–9. The oldest patient in the author's series, aged 39, with spontaneous fusion of the interfragmental gap. *A,* Before treatment. *B, C,* During treatment. *D,* Three years after completion of treatment. The metacarpal is lengthened by 3 cm, which equals the length of the proximal phalanx of the sound thumb.

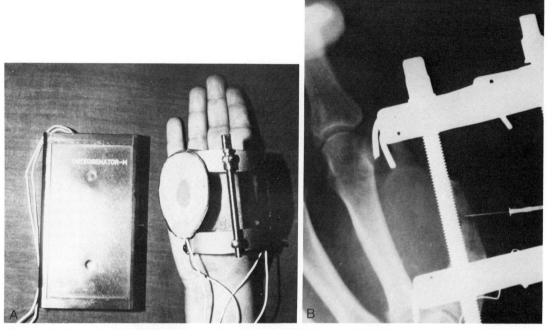

Figure 127–10. *A*, Noninvasive electromagnetic bone growth stimulation. *B*, Semi-invasive stimulation with an active needle electrode in the interfragmental space, and an external electrode on the skin. Stabilized pulsed current is produced by a pocket-size battery bone growth stimulator.

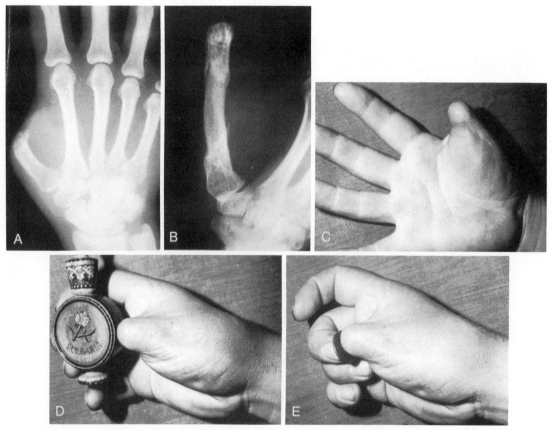

Figure 127–11. In this 28 year old patient the 3.5 cm interfragmental gap is bridged by an iliac crest graft. *A*, Radiograph before the osteotomy. *B to E*, Three years after the bone grafting procedure.

When to Remove Distraction Device

The device is removed when there is radiographic evidence of a complete union between the two fragments with ossification (spontaneous or by grafting) of the interfragmental gap along the full width of the metacarpal bone.

SECONDARY OPERATIONS

In some cases, after the distraction lengthening procedure, additional surgery has to be considered.

Deepening of First Cleft. During distraction lengthening of the metacarpal, the first web space is drawn in a distal direction together with the peripheral fragment. If the web skin is normal, it stretches enough for the interdigital web to prove adequately deepened. When scarring in the web is present, the skin remains tense with a crest displaced distally. Surgical correction is then necessary. Very often a Z-plasty is enough for deepening the interdigital web. In more severe cases the use of a rotational double innervated flap, taken from the dorsal side of the index, proves to be the optimal skin grafting procedure (Fig. 127–12). During the operation, all fibrous structures interfering with abduction of the first metacarpal should be cut.

Resurfacing of Palmar Surface of Reconstructed Thumb. In cases in which the skin of the lengthened metacarpal is thin and fibrotic, resurfacing of the palmar area of the thumb end is necessary. This procedure improves the sensibility and functional ability of the thumb and hand. In the author's experience the dorsal double innervated flap, taken from the index as a rotational or island flap, is an adequate solution of the problem (Fig. 127–13). The donor area is closed by a thick split-thickness free graft.

Raised as a rotational flap, the dorsal double innervated index flap covers both the grasping surface of the thumb and the bottom of the deepened first web, thus providing a better skin coverage of the two thumb areas that are functionally the most important.

COMPLICATIONS

Reconstruction of the thumb through gradual bone lengthening may give rise to complications.

Secretion from Openings of Pin Bone Channels. This happens seldom during the distraction period, but quite often during the immobilization period. When the pins are loose, conditions are created for movement of the bone fragments and of the distraction device frame itself along the length of the pins, and secretion starts. In the latter case the pins should be immediately fixed firmly to the distraction device, and the hand and forearm temporarily immobilized in a plaster of Paris splint. Secretion is never seen if stable fixation of the four pins to the distraction device is secured.

Angulation of Lengthened Metacarpal. This happens if the distraction device is taken off before the full ossification of the interfragmental gap in length and width. The lengthened metacarpal opposes the long-lasting compression forces of the distracted soft structures, and angulation of the elongated bone never results if the device and pins are removed after the interfragmental gap is fully ossified, and the graft (if used) is solidly integrated into the fragments. If, for such reasons as those clarified above, angulation of the lengthened metacarpal occurs, the distraction device should immediately be mounted once again, after manual correction of the angle between the fragments, and the treatment then should be continued (Fig. 127–14).

THUMB LENGTHENING IN CHILDREN

Distraction lengthening in children does not differ principally from that in adults. The distraction device is almost the same but is smaller and lighter (Fig. 127–15).

The operation is always undertaken under general anesthesia. Special care is taken during the insertion of the proximal pins, particularly the most proximal one, which should be sufficiently distant, at least 5 mm, from the epiphyseal plate. If the most proximal pin

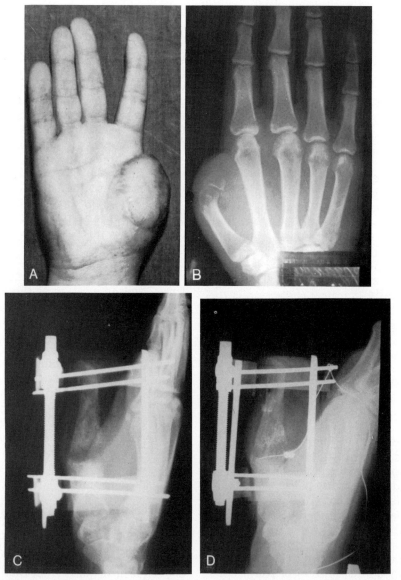

Figure 127–12. The patient sustained an amputation of the thumb with avulsion of the thenar and dorsal skin. The wound was covered by an abdominal flap. In the author's department the metacarpal was lengthened by 3 to 5 cm; the first cleft was deepened and covered with a dorsal, radially innervated rotational flap including both neurovascular bundles. A, B, Condition before the lengthening procedure. C, D, The interfragmental gap fused spontaneously with the help of semi-invasive bone growth stimulation.

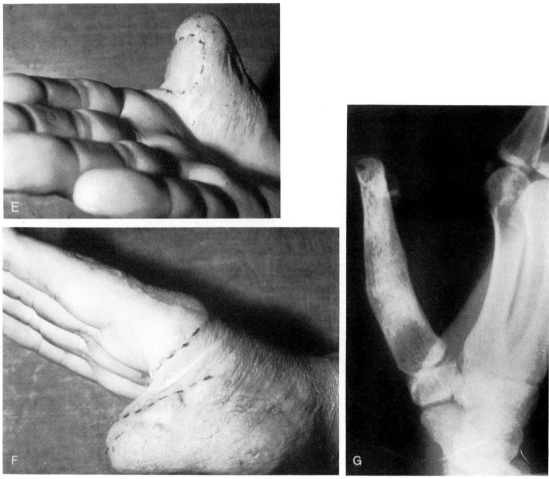

Figure 127–12 *Continued E, F,* After deepening of the first cleft; the radially innervated flap is dotted. *G,* Radiograph seven years after treatment.

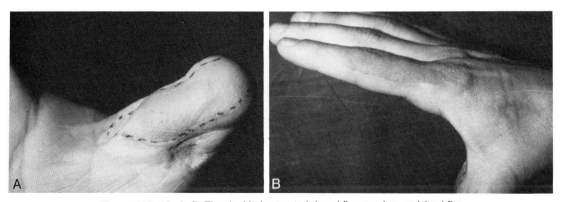

Figure 127–13. *A, B,* The double innervated dorsal flap used as an island flap.

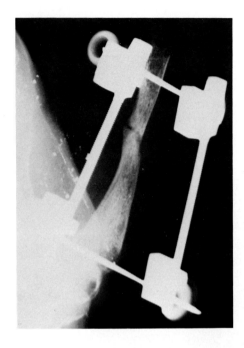

Figure 127–14. Metacarpal angulation followed early removal of the device. The latter is applied once again with only two Kirschner wires. The angle between the fragments is corrected. Fusion comes after 45 days.

Figure 127–15. In children a smaller device is used.

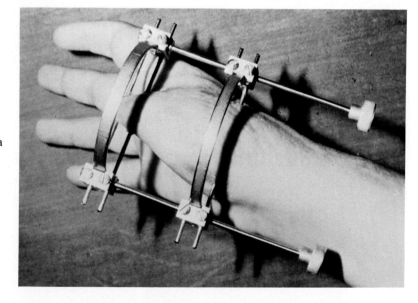

is driven closer to the epiphyseal plate, the pressing forces that the pin exerts on the bone during the distraction period may affect the epiphyseal plate. On the other hand, if loosening of the pins occurs and secretion starts during the long immobilization period, the inflammation of the bone channels may damage the adjoining epiphyseal plate. Insertion of a pin through the plate is a serious mistake that may prevent normal growth of the metacarpal bone.

Osteotomy is once again done transversely and subperiosteally in the middle of the metacarpal, through a small skin incision and minimal opening of the periosteum. After repeated piercing of the bone with a hand drill, the author usually very easily cuts the bone manually, i.e., performs an osteoclasis. This type of osteotomy keeps the hematoma within a closed periosteum cuff, and thus stimulates the ossification process.

Two to three days of rest after the operation are enough before the distraction is begun. A longer waiting period may result in fusion of the fragments and may render difficult the distraction lengthening of bone.

The bone lengthening rate in children goes 1 to 1.5 mm daily without problems. There are usually no complaints during the distraction period, which may last 25 to 40 days.

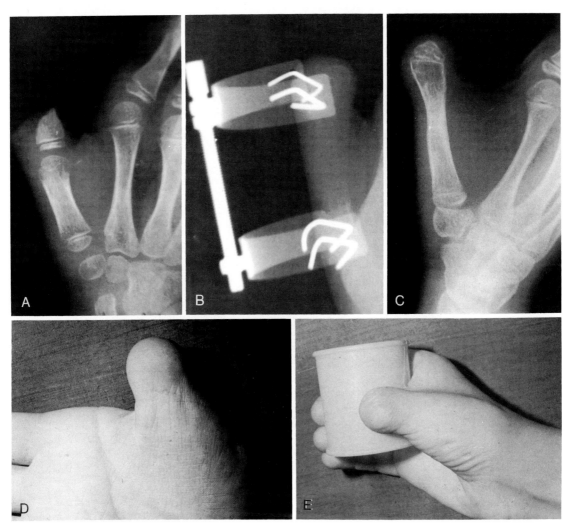

Figure 127–16. In this 11 year old boy a 3.5 cm lengthening of the first metacarpal was accomplished in 30 days. The fragments fused spontaneously 45 days after cessation of the distraction. *A,* Radiograph before the osteotomy. *B,* During the lengthening period. *C to E,* Three years after treatment.

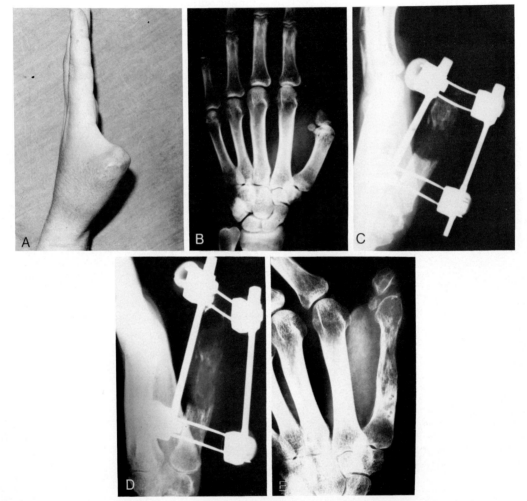

Figure 127–17. A 24 year old female patient before and five years after treatment. *A, B,* Condition before the operation. *C, D,* Note the fast bone growth in the interfragmental space during the lengthening period. *E,* The metacarpal is lengthened by 2.8 cm; the first cleft is deepened by Z-plasty.

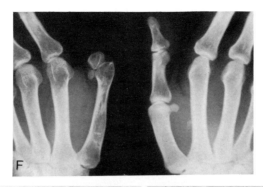

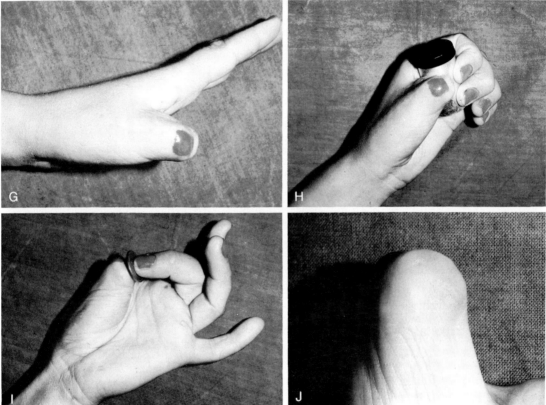

Figure 127–17 *Continued F to I,* Five years after completion of treatment. *J,* Note the sulci cutis of the pulp.

Parents are instructed how to turn the screws of the device at home, so that there is no need for long hospitalization.

The metacarpal lengthening accomplished in children is greater than that in adolescents or adults. One can safely obtain an elongation of even a 110 per cent increase on the initial length of the metacarpal.

The gap between the pulled apart fragments usually fuses in a natural way through spontaneous ossification, owing to the high reactivity of the growing elements of the bone. The author has never carried out a

bone grafting operation for fusion of the lengthened metacarpal in children (Fig. 127–16).

Check-up examinations, including x-ray, are necessary once in seven to ten days during the elongation period to ensure that distraction is proceeding accurately. In the immobilization period examination once every two weeks is sufficient.

Immobilization of the hand and wrist joint with a plaster of Paris splint during the bone fusion period proves to be necessary in children more often than in adults.

LONG-TERM RESULTS

Long-term follow-up studies up to ten years after completion of treatment show a good functional condition of the reconstructed thumb, free of trophic changes and with preserved sensibility on the whole surface. X-ray films do not disclose osteolytic changes in the tip regions of the elongated metacarpal. Beyond any doubt, the lack of trophic disorders in the thumb metacarpal end is attributable to the interposition type of bone lengthening, i.e., the additional bone structure is placed into the bone, and not superimposed on the bone stump end, as practiced in other thumb reconstruction procedures (Fig. 127–17).

REFERENCES

Ben-Hur, N.: Reconstruction of traumatic loss of fingers by a free sensory dorsalis pedis flap and Matev procedure. Proceedings of the First Congress of the International Federation of Societies for Surgery of the Hand, Rotterdam, 1980, p. 121 (abstr.).

Codivilla, A.: On the means of lengthening in the lower limbs the muscles and tissues which are shortened through deformity. Am. J. Orthop. Surg., 2:353, 1904.

Cowen, N. (Ed.): Practical Hand Surgery. Chicago, Year Book Medical Publishers, 1980, pp. 186, 191.

Cugola, L., Colognese, L., and Marcer, M.: L'allungamento del I metacarpo per ricostruire una pinza pollice-digitale. Riv. Chir. della Mano, 12:137, 1974.

Kessler, I.: Transposition lengthening of a digital ray after multiple amputations of fingers. Hand, 8:176, 1976.

Kessler, I., Baruch, A., and Hecht, O.: Experience with distraction lengthening of digital rays in congenital anomalies. J. Hand Surg., 2:394, 1977.

Manninger, J.: Hüvelykujj potlas, ujjcsere, szigetlebeny plasztika serules utan. Proceedings of the Combined Meeting of the Deutschsprachige Arbeitsgemeinschaft für Handchirurgie and the Hungarian Society for Hand Surgery, Budapest, 1980, p. 128 (abstr.).

Matev, I.B.: Reconstruction of the thumb by adjacent skin flaps. Scientific Works of the Institute for Reconstructive Surgery, Prosthetics and Rehabilitation. Sofia, Medicina i Fizkultura, 6:25, 1965 (in Bulgarian).

Matev, I.B.: Gradual elongation of the first metacarpal as a method of thumb reconstruction. Read at the 23rd Meeting, Lausanne and Vienna. In Stack, H.G., and Bolton, H. (Eds.): Proceedings of the Second Hand Club. London, 1967, pp. 431, 495.

Matev, I.B.: Reconstruction of the thumb through gradual lengthening of the first metacarpal with the soft tissues. Ortoped. Travmatol., 6:11, 1969 (in Bulgarian).

Matev, I.B.: Thumb reconstruction after amputation at the metacarpophalangeal joint by bone lengthening. A preliminary report of three cases. J. Bone Joint Surg., 52A:957, 1970.

Matev, I.B.: New thoughts on hand surgery. In Apley, A.G. (Ed.): Modern Trends in Orthopaedics. London, Butterworths, 1972, p. 95.

Matev, I.B.: Thumb reconstruction in children through metacarpal lengthening. Plast. Reconstr. Surg., 64:665, 1979.

Matev, I.B.: Thumb reconstruction through metacarpal bone lengthening. J. Hand Surg., 5:482, 1980.

Matev, I.B.: Reconstructive Surgery of the Thumb. Brentwood, Essex, England, Pilgrims Press, 1983.

Neff, G.: Verlängerung nach Matev bei Handfehlbildungen. Zeitschr. Orthop., 119:14, 1981.

Putti, V.: The operative lengthening of the femur. J.A.M.A., 77:934, 1921.

Ulitzkii, G.I., and Maligin, G.D.: Digital reconstruction by distraction of the metacarpals. Ortoped. Travmatol. Protezirovanie, 11:55, 1971 (in Russian).

Vossman, H., and Zellner, P.R.: Verlängerung des I Mittelhandknochens bei Verlust des Daumens nach Matev. Proceedings of the Combined Meeting of the Deutschsprachige Arbeitsgemeinschaft für Handchirurgie and the Hungarian Society for Hand Surgery, Budapest, 1980, p. 128 (abstr.).

Joseph Upton

Congenital Anomalies of the Hand and Forearm

Hand surgery as a surgical discipline has blossomed since the initial impetus it received from the organization of regional hand centers by Sterling Bunnell during World War II. During the past 40 years, the subject of congenital anomalies has remained a quiet backwater compared with the torrent of information in other subject areas, such as trauma, arthritis, tendon surgery, and microsurgery. Paradoxically, the study of congenital hand deformities was one of the earliest topics to be pursued by medical academia and one of the most noticeable to benefit from recent advances in surgical techniques and bioengineering technology.

Early references to limb anomalies are found in the Old Testament of the Bible:

Goliath was a member of a band of giants with polydactyly (Temtamy and McKusick, 1982). Monsters and pedigrees with limb malformations were documented by Ambroise Paré in 1634, when causes were thought to be related to "bad thoughts or deeds," and when interruption of pregnancy and avoidance of consanguinity were accepted social solutions (Fig. 128–1).

Further, the stigma of a congenital malformation has always been present in varied forms. A six-fingered hand was so common in one Arabian tribe, the Hyabites, that a child with five digits was considered abnormal and subsequently sacrificed (Boinet, 1898)! Extra digits in England were considered a sign of royalty, owing to the frequent appearance of polydactyly in the royal line since Mary Queen of Scots (Flatt, 1977). As early as 1832, St. Hilaire published a detailed classification of congenital deformities of the hand; soon after, Velpeau (1847) and Vrolik (1849) produced thoughtful treatises on the subject. Although most deformities of that time were unapproachable surgically, the treatment of syndactyly was hotly debated when Felizet proposed in 1892 his classic techniques for separation of digits.

The embryology of the upper limb has been studied in great detail for over 100 years; the interested reader is referred to Bardeen and Lewis's (1901–1902) eloquent 40-page disser-

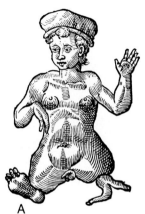

Anno Dom. 1573. I saw at St. *Andrewes* Church in *Paris,* a boy nine yeeres old, borne in the village *Parpavilla,* sixe miles from *Guise;* his fathers name was *Peter Renard,* and his mother, *Marquete* : hee had but two fingers on his right hand, his arm was well proportioned from the top of his shoulder almost to his wrest, but from thence to his two fingers ends it was very deformed, he wanted his legs and thighes, although from the right buttocke a certaine unperfect figure, having onely foure toes, seemed to put it selfe forth; from the midst of the left buttock two toes sprung out, the one of which was not much unlike a mans yard, as you may see by the figure.

A

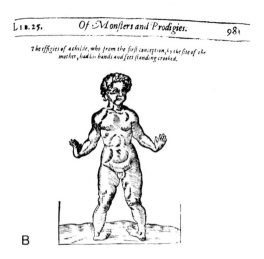

B

C

Figure 128–1. *A,* Woodcut of a boy with phocomelia. This child may also have had the cleft hand-foot syndrome with a positive family history. *B,* Another illustration of an adult with marked deviation of hands and feet, which could have been secondary to a preaxial failure of formation, arthrogryposis, or clubbed feet. *C,* Another robust adult male may have had phocomelia or complete upper limb aplasia. It is unlikely that he had survived post-traumatic bilateral shoulder disarticulations. (From Paré, A.: The Works of That Famous Chirurgion Ambroise Parey. Translated Out of Latin and Compared with the French by Thomas Johnson. London, T. Cotes and R. Young, 1634.)

Ossification Centers

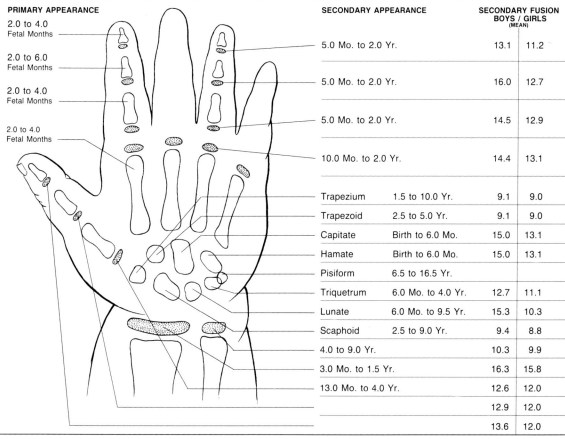

PRIMARY APPEARANCE		SECONDARY APPEARANCE		SECONDARY FUSION BOYS / GIRLS (MEAN)	
2.0 to 4.0 Fetal Months			5.0 Mo. to 2.0 Yr.	13.1	11.2
2.0 to 6.0 Fetal Months			5.0 Mo. to 2.0 Yr.	16.0	12.7
2.0 to 4.0 Fetal Months			5.0 Mo. to 2.0 Yr.	14.5	12.9
2.0 to 4.0 Fetal Months			10.0 Mo. to 2.0 Yr.	14.4	13.1
		Trapezium	1.5 to 10.0 Yr.	9.1	9.0
		Trapezoid	2.5 to 5.0 Yr.	9.1	9.0
		Capitate	Birth to 6.0 Mo.	15.0	13.1
		Hamate	Birth to 6.0 Mo.	15.0	13.1
		Pisiform	6.5 to 16.5 Yr.		
		Triquetrum	6.0 Mo. to 4.0 Yr.	12.7	11.1
		Lunate	6.0 Mo. to 9.5 Yr.	15.3	10.3
		Scaphoid	2.5 to 9.0 Yr.	9.4	8.8
			4.0 to 9.0 Yr.	10.3	9.9
			3.0 Mo. to 1.5 Yr.	16.3	15.8
			13.0 Mo. to 4.0 Yr.	12.6	12.0
				12.9	12.0
				13.6	12.0

Figure 128–2. Ossification centers. The time of appearance of primary and secondary ossification centers in the hand (Caffey, 1978) and the average time of fusion of secondary centers for both boys and girls. There is great variation in these numbers for both ages and individuals. Time of appearance and of fusion can also be altered in the presence of a congenital anomaly (Stuart and associates, 1962). Time for secondary fusion is given in years.

tation. Yet, despite this long history, the classification and treatment of congenital anomalies of the hand have only recently reached a high degree of definition and consensus that has elevated the study of this branch of hand surgery to the level of its kindred subspecialties. The thalidomide tragedy of the 1960's served to focus public awareness on limb anomalies and provided a stimulus for basic research and development of new surgical solutions for difficult problems. Even today, when thalidomide babies are in their 30's, much progress has been achieved.

One cannot always transfer principles of adult hand surgery to that of congenitally deformed children. Surgery on the infantile hand always has been hampered by restrictions imposed by the small size of the anatomic structures that the surgeon is attempting to correct. The child is not merely a miniature adult and presents many problems in both evaluation and treatment. It is difficult to predict how one will respond psychologically and functionally to a deformed limb or to a proposed reconstruction. Valid functional evaluation is most difficult to obtain in the young child, who is unable to cooperate or to articulate his needs precisely (Smith and Lipke, 1979). History is usually obtained from a parent, who may be surprisingly uncertain of the manual dexterity and limitations of the child. Methods for sensory evaluation are most difficult. Radiographic evaluation is of limited value because most of the infant hand is primarily cartilage. Ossification appears at different ages, and knowledge of the ossification centers may be most helpful (Fig. 128–2). Surgical decisions and recommendations will be greatly influenced by the development of hand function, hand-eye coordination, and growth.

Although a small amount of surgery is

performed, particular care and time will be necessary with informed consent. The surgeon who examines and operates upon the baby is actually treating an entire family. The parents may be initially devastated by guilt when an imperfection is seen in their otherwise normal child. They must be counseled honestly and informed clearly about potentials from the time of the initial consultation. When a complex deformity exists, they should not be given unrealistic expectations about the anticipated functional result; every attempt should be made to answer their questions with precision and sincerity. When there are multiple alternative methods of treatment, it is often wise to enlist the help of a knowledgeable colleague for a second opinion.

EMBRYOLOGY

Limb development and differentiation is a rapid process occurring between the third and eighth postovulatory weeks. Until recently, systematic study of upper limb embryogenesis was based on descriptive accounts of limited dissections and histologic study (Lewis, 1901–1902; Streeter, 1930). The development of molecular biology, histochemistry, chromosomal analysis, and genetic engineering with recombinant DNA methods is beginning to shed more light on the mechanisms of malformation. With new technology, classic descriptive embryology is being augmented by experimental techniques for elucidating cell interactions, genetic events, and teratogens (Krey, Dayton, and Goetnick, 1984).

Morphologic Development

Streeter's (1949) staging system for the human divides upper limb development into 23 stages, starting with the fertilized egg and ending with nutrient artery penetration of the humerus. An approximate timetable is summarized in Table 128–1. The beginning of limb development is marked by the migration of paired somatopleure, consisting of surface ectoderm and underlying somatic mesoderm. Swellings on the ventrolateral side of the embryo called limb buds make their appearance between the fourth and fifth intrauterine weeks. This bud, called Wolff's crest, consists of a ventral swelling of mesoderm covered by a thick layer of ectoderm called the apical ectodermal ridge (AER) (O'Rahilly and Gardner, 1975) (Fig. 128–3). This ridge is located opposite the eighth to 12th myotomes, which correspond to the C6, T1, and T2 vertebral bodies. Growth of the upper limb bud is always a few days ahead of the lower limb and progresses in a proximal to distal direction.

During the beginning of the fifth week, this bud straightens and a constriction separates the arm from the forearm; a depression forms,

Table 128–1. Staging of Embryonic Development as Defined by Streeter (1949)*

Stage	Length (mm)	Age (Days)	Limb Developments
I		0—1	Fertilized ovum, single cell
III		4	Free blastocyst
IV	0.1	8	Implantation
V	0.2	9–10	Ovum implanted
IX	1.0	21–22	Neural folds, notochord
X	2.0	24	Early somites appear
XI		24	13–20 paired somites
XII	4.0	30	Arm bud appears
XIII	5.0	32	Leg bud appears
XIV	7.0	34	Marginal vessels within arm bed
XV			Hand segment appears
XVI	11.0	38	Major nerve trunks enter limb
XVII	13.0	41	Digital rays evident
XVIII	17.0	44	Muscle groups form around cartilage
XIX	21.0	48	Joint interzones present
XX	23.0	52	Arm flexed at elbow
XI			
XXII	28.0	55	Periosteal bone around humerus
XXIII		56	Nutrient vessel penetrates humerus

*By 56 days, the upper limb is a well-differentiated part.

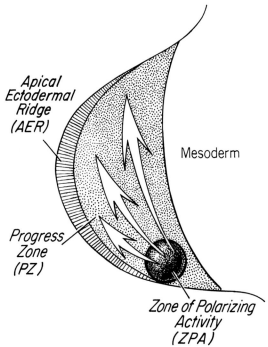

Apical
Ectodermal
Ridge
(AER)

Mesoderm

Progress
Zone
(PZ)

Zone of Polarizing
Activity
(ZPA)

Figure 128–3. The early limb bud, called Wolff's crest, consists of an outer layer called the apical ectodermal ridge (AER), which has a dynamic relationship with underlying mesoderm labeled the progress zone (PZ). The AER expands to cover the entire rim of the hand and eventually breaks up when digits separate. The zone of polarizing activity (ZPA), located on the more posterior aspect of the limb bud, produces morphogens that control anteroposterior relationships. (Adapted from Wolpert, L.: Positional information, pattern formation and morphogenesis. *In* Connelly, T. G. (Ed.): Morphogenesis and Pattern Formation. New York, Raven Press, 1981.)

namic growth and refinement of limbs continue.

Experimental Embryology

The true mechanisms of malformation are poorly understood, but an expanding body of literature by limb developmentalists is helping to elucidate basic principles. Two general approaches to development have been espoused: one holding that the process is programmed from start to finish, and another postulating that development is the result of a sequence of biochemical and physical forces that occur and are influenced by combinations of time and three-dimensional space. Many experiments have demonstrated that the latter approach may be the more reasonable (Zaleski and Holmes, 1985).

In classic amphibian ablation experiments, Harrison (1918) found that limb mesoderm could be differentiating when transferred to heterotopic locations. Others then established the very close relationship between the mesoderm and specialized ectoderm, or apical ectodermal ridge (AER), which is a transient structure appearing at Stage 12 and disappearing at Stage 17 (Zwilling, 1955; Saunders, Gasseling, and Saunders, 1962). The mesoderm elaborates as apical ectodermal maintenance factor (AEMF), a morphogen or inducer that, in turn, communicates commensurate information from one cell to another and influences cytodifferentiation (Wolpert, 1981). Electron microscopy has shown that although the outer layer of the apical ectodermal ridge is sealed from the amnionic fluid, open gap junctions do exist adjacent to underlying mesoderm.

The AER is important in directing longitudinal axes of the limb. Grafting experiments have demonstrated that the mechanisms for other axes (dorsal-ventral; preaxial and postaxial) are complicated and involve communications between the ridge and a 350 micron thick layer called the progress zone (Wolpert, Lewis, and Summerbell, 1975), which can influence proximal-distal relationships (Fig. 128–5). Within the progress zone is a specialized zone of polarizing activity that controls anteroposterior morphology. Wolpert, Lewis, and Summerbell (1975) propose that this region produces another diffusable morphogen that gradually moves across the limb bud. High concentrations of this

which becomes the axillary fossa. By 37 days of intrauterine life, the hand is present in the form of a flattened structure with small swellings representing digits. At the same time, vessels grow into the limb to supply the ectodermal surface (Feinberg and Saunders, 1982). Nerve trunks have entered the arm, and within the next five days, individual digits begin to form. The hand begins to pronate, and elbow flexion takes form (Fig. 128–4). At this point, the size of the hand equals that of the arm and forearm. By Stages 18 and 19, well-defined muscle groups have formed around cartilage, and joint interzones begin to appear. By Stage 23, a well-formed and well-differentiated limb is present, and the crown-rump length of the fetus is 3.0 cm. Shortly after the mother realizes she is pregnant, a well-differentiated upper limb has been completed. Although Stage 23 marks the end of Streeter's embryonic period, dy-

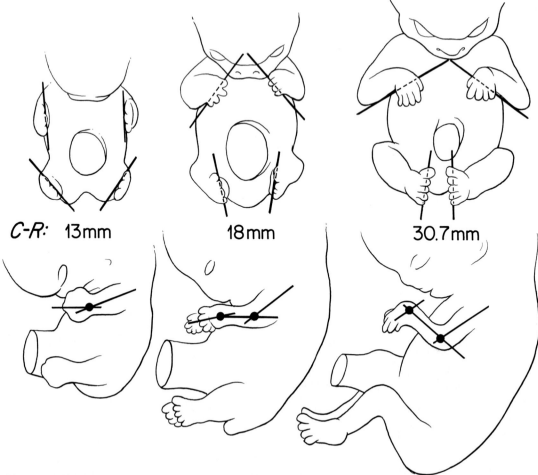

C-R: 13mm   18mm   30.7mm

Figure 128–4. During the embryonic period, the position of the upper limbs changes rapidly. In this series of embryos at five *(left)*, six *(middle)*, and eight *(right)* week's gestation, the hands and arms became pronated from the anterior view *(top)*. With development, the elbow becomes flexed, and the hand-wrist assumes slight ulnar deviation, flexion, and pronation. As the upper limb extends outward or laterally, the lower limb rotates medially. C-R = crown-rump length of embryo in millimeters. (Adapted from O'Rahilly, R., Gray, D. J., and Gardner, E.: Chondrification in the hands and feet of staged human embryos. Contrib. Embryol., *36*:183, 1957.)

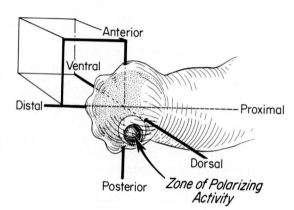

Figure 128–5. Three-dimensional relationships within the growing limb bud are illustrated. The apical ectodermal ridge (AER) and progress zone (PZ) impart proximodistal information to developing cells. The zone of polarizing activity within the PZ controls anteroposterior morphology. The two other axes are proximodistal and dorsoventral. (Adapted from Wolpert, L.: Positional information, pattern formation and morphogenesis. *In* Connelly, T. G. (Ed.): Morphogenesis and Pattern Formation. New York, Raven Press, 1981.)

substance at a critical time may produce a preaxial or postaxial duplication, whereas a deficiency may result in hypoplasia or a complete absence (see Fig. 128–3). Recent work with retinoic acid gradients has shown that limb formation can be chemically directed (Thaller and Eichele, 1987; Tickle, 1987).

With direction from the apical ectodermal ridge, the mesoderm grows and differentiates into distal limb structures. The ectoderm will give rise to skin and its adnexae (hair, sweat and sebaceous glands, and nails), and the mesoderm will develop into muscle-tendon units, skeletal structures, and connective tissues. Dissociated chick embryo mesoderm packed into an ectodermal jacket and grafted to a chick flank will regenerate anomalous limbs, but the inclusion of the specialized zone of polarizing activity within the progress zone will result in a normal limb or wing (Wolpert, Lewis, and Summerbell, 1975; Wolpert, 1981).

This information may help explain the effects of certain teratogens. Klein, Scott, and Wilson (1981) found that aspirin produced both polydactylous and ectrodactylous limbs in rats, predominantly the right hind limb. The ectrodactyly may be related to the asymmetric development of the vascular system, and the polydactyly to the effect of the apical ectodermal ridge upon the mesoderm. These researchers postulate that the amount of mesoderm available, the concentration of circulating morphogens, and the duration of the AER's inductive influence are critical. This concentration gradient produced within the mesoderm "tells the ectoderm just how long it wants to be induced." Aspirin causes preaxial mesodermal abnormalities. If the extent of cell injury or cell death is great, ectrodactyly will result. If the insult causes abnormal release of these morphogens, the action of the AER may be prolonged to produce polydactyly.

The effect of thalidomide has been tested experimentally by Hodgen (1981) in the rhesus monkey. With early administration of this drug, abnormal cells within the progress zone of the limb bud develop. If the cells are excised surgically within a critical period, the gap is filled from its margins by regenerated normal cells and a normal limb differentiates, in contrast to the unoperated control limb, which is deformed ("phocomelia") (Hodgen, 1981) (Fig. 128–6).

These experiments give credence to the

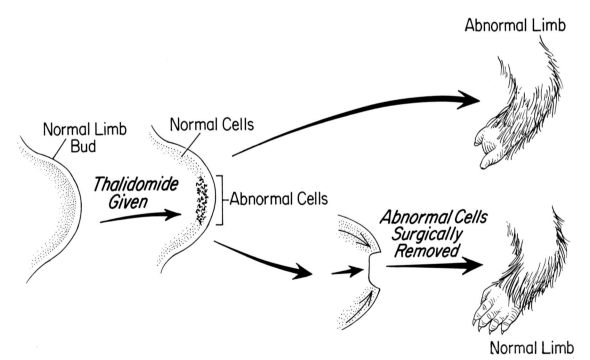

Figure 128–6. The effect of thalidomide on the limb bud of the rhesus monkey has been demonstrated by Hodgen (Hodgen, 1981). If abnormal cells within the limb bud are excised within a critical period, the gap will be filled by bordering normal cells, and a normal limb results. If the abnormal cells remain, severe failure of formation deformities occur, in this case an atypical cleft hand. The time sequence in these experiments is critical. (Adapted from data by Hodgen, 1981.)

idea of condition-generated abnormalities in the explanation of congenital anomalies and point out how the postnatal pathology can vary so tremendously.

Skeletal Development

Once the skeleton begins to develop, progress is rapid. Condensation of mesoderm is quickly followed by chondrification in the fifth postovulatory week. Cartilage cells secrete an extracellular matrix, which pushes mesenchyme peripherally as tubular bones develop from central areas. By the sixth week the humerus begins to ossify, and distal progress occurs, skipping the carpal bones and moving to the distal phalanges (Gray, Gardner, and O'Rahilly, 1957). By the seventh week, the hand takes form and gradually develops a cupped posture in both longitudinal and transverse planes. The arm, well formed and flexed at the elbow, begins to move into a pronated posture (see Fig. 128–4). Continued bone growth and remodeling occur in the prenatal period (O'Rahilly, 1957; O'Rahilly and Gardner, 1975).

Joint development begins during the sixth week, when joint capsules and ligaments are present before separation of joints. A synovial mesenchymal layer with blood vessels forms between the capsule and periosteum, but there are no vessels within the cartilage. By the seventh week, areas of flattened chondrocytes form dense plates within the cartilage called interzones, which are the precursors of articular cartilage (Haines, 1947). At this point motion must occur if cavitation is to result. Embryos paralyzed at this stage will lack proper joint development and will have flat articular surfaces joined by fibrous tissue (Drachman and Sokoloff, 1966). Joints develop as cellular death occurs within the interzone. Lysosomal release and contact play an important role in the process, which can result in either excessive or incomplete joint formation.

Ossification of the phalanges is a prenatal event, but that of the carpals and epiphyses is not and is useful in assessment of skeletal maturity (see Fig. 128–2). Ossification of the congenitally malformed limb is typically *delayed*. The development of the carpus is a fascinating one, well beyond the scope of this chapter. Only the trapezium, trapezoid, and capitate develop in their original form, as the other bones will migrate and fuse during a very complicated process (Cihak, 1972b). The scaphoid and lunate begin to form during the seventh week (20 mm) as separate parts but do not fuse to form their ultimate configuration until the embryo is 50 mm in crown-rump length.

Vascular Development

By the third postovulatory week, thin-walled vessels begin to penetrate the limb mesoderm. A border or marginal vein develops on the postaxial (ulnar) side of the limb bud and remains functional until the apical ectodermal ridge disappears (Milaire, 1965). Myogenic regions of the limb become vascular, and chondrogenic areas avascular, under the influence of metabolic gradients (Caplan and Koutroupas, 1972; Tickle, 1987). Vessels then begin to form adult patterns. Mrazkova (1973) points out that the brachial artery initially gives origin to a large interosseous artery and median artery within the limb bud. By the sixth week, an ulnar artery develops and progresses down the hand plate to form the deep palmar arch. The radial artery develops later on the preaxial side of the limb. The median and interosseous arteries then decrease in size, and the median artery supplies primarily the median nerve, with variable contributions to the hand (Mrazkova, 1973). The same is true for the interosseous artery, which terminates at the carpus (Fig. 128–7).

With this rapid change within a short time, it is not surprising that the arterial supply to the hand has great variation (Edwards, 1960; Coleman and Anson, 1961). The anatomic location of embryologic vessels influences growth and nutrition of developing tissue, and interruption of blood supply is known to cause distal malformations (Hootnick and associates, 1980; Zaleski and Holmes, 1983). What mediates differentiation of primordial cells into arteries, veins, and lymphatics is not known.

Muscle Development

Muscle development in the upper limb parallels, but is less well understood than, skeletal formation. The exact cell of origin is still a matter of some controversy. The somites

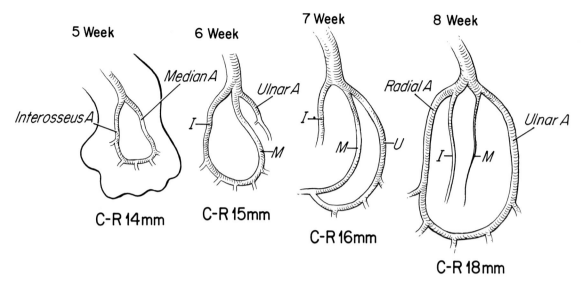

Figure 128–7. This sequence demonstrates the development of the major vessels within the upper extremity from the fifth through the eighth week after ovulation: *Left,* The early blood supply is provided by the median (M) and interosseus (I) arteries. The ulnar artery (U) then sprouts from the median to become the dominant vessel to the hand. *Right,* The radial artery is the last to develop and communicates with the ulnar system within the palm. The interosseus artery persists in the adult on the interosseus membrane and terminates at the wrist, and the median artery persists as the vessel found on the ventral (palmar) surface of the median nerve. In a small number of people, this median artery persists as a major conduit to the hand. C-R = crown-rump embryo length. (Adapted from Mrazkova, O.: Ontogenesis of arterial trunks in the human forearm. Folia Morph. *21:*193, 1973.)

divide into (1) a sclerotome, which forms vertebral bodies and ribs; (2) a dermatome, which forms skin and fascia; and (3) a myotome, which forms segmented muscles. The myoblasts that give rise to limb muscles either arise from limb bud mesenchyme or migrate into the limb from the somite (Zwilling, 1968; Newman, 1977). Two masses of muscle blastoma form: the dorsal, which give origin to the extensor muscles, and the ventral, which give origin to the flexors. As with skeletal structures, proximal muscles differentiate before distal muscles, and by the eighth postovulatory week all major muscle groups have formed (Figs. 128–8 to 128–10).

Muscle blastoma division and differentiation are influenced primarily by local factors, and not by its somite of origin or by any neural influence (Chevallier, Kieny, and Mauger, 1977; Jacob and Christ, 1980). Tendons develop independently of their muscle bellies after the blastomas have split and attach to their skeletal origin (Shellswell and Wolpert, 1977; Bogusch, 1980). If the bone to which they normally attach has not formed, they will adhere to the nearest bone, tendon, or fascial layer, thus accounting for the many bizarre tendon insertions seen in congenital hand malformations. If a tendon does not join its muscle belly, it will degenerate (Kieny and Chevallier, 1979; Graham and associates, 1982). Muscles can survive without tendons,

but they need innervation for growth and development (Jacob and Christ, 1980).

In the forearm, the superficial muscles differentiate before the deeper ones. The blastomas of origin, differentiation, and migration of the extrinsic and intrinsic muscles of the hand are a fascinating subject that has been well described by Cihak (1972a, 1977). The intrinsic muscles, for example, arise from five embryonic muscle layers, which divide and differentiate in a logical but complicated fashion. The interested student of anatomy is referred to the work of Cihak (1972a, 1977).

Nerve Formation

The formation of specific sensory and motor nerve patterns within the limb is a subject of great experimental interest. Unlike caudate amphibians (fish), in which there is specific spinal nerve for each muscle, the human is more complex; all nerves to the limb traverse a cervicobrachial plexus, which is developed by the fourth postovulatory week (Bardeen and Lewis, 1901–1902). The process of guidance and interrelationship between nerve and muscle is not known. Is it random (Horder and Martin, 1982) or specific (Hollyday, 1983)?

Much of the experimentation on nerve formation has been done in eye models and

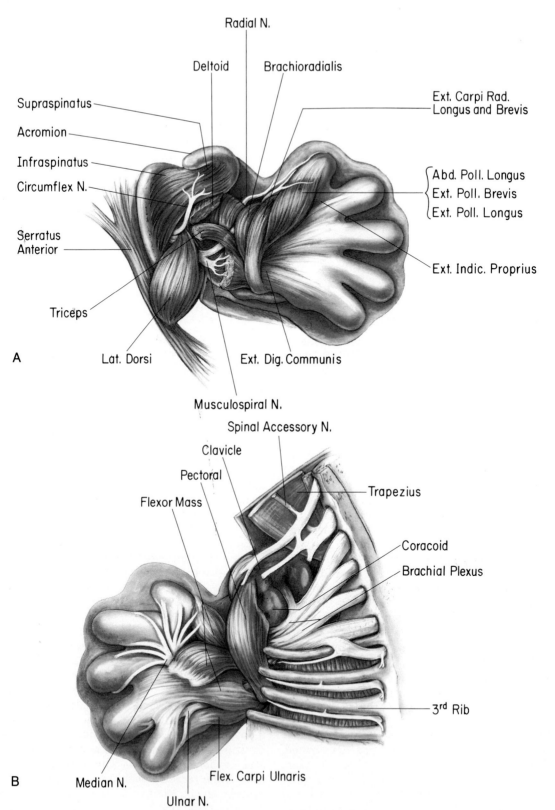

Radial N.

Deltoid   Brachioradialis

Supraspinatus

Acromion

Infraspinatus

Circumflex N.

Ext. Carpi Rad.
Longus and Brevis

Abd. Poll. Longus
Ext. Poll. Brevis
Ext. Poll. Longus

Serratus
Anterior

Ext. Indic. Proprius

Triceps

Lat. Dorsi   Ext. Dig. Communis

A

Musculospiral N.

Spinal Accessory N.

Clavicle

Pectoral

Flexor Mass

Trapezius

Coracoid

Brachial Plexus

3rd Rib

Median N.   Flex. Carpi Ulnaris

Ulnar N.

B

Figure 128–8. *See legend on opposite page*

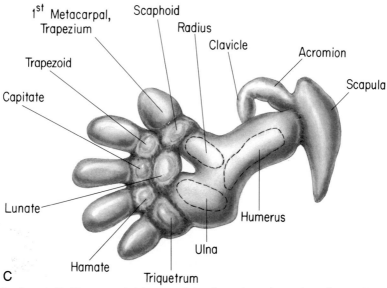

1st Metacarpal, Trapezium — Scaphoid — Radius — Clavicle — Acromion — Scapula

Trapezoid

Capitate

Lunate — Humerus

Hamate — Ulna

C — Triquetrum

Figure 128–8 *Continued C,* The arm skeleton consists of condensations of cartilage with greater degrees of differentiation in the more proximal portions. A poorly defined clavicle is attached to the scapula. The shaft of the humerus is surrounded by very thick perichondrium. There is no evidence of joint cavitation at this stage, nor is there ossification. Radius and ulna are continuous with the humerus as well as the hand plate. Multiple centers of increased condensation correspond to eventual carpal bones. The scaphoid is in line with the radius and the lunate with the ulna. At this stage, the hand and carpus are not in ulnar deviation. (Redrawn, abstracted, and condensed from Lewis, W. H.: The development of the arm in man. Am. J. Anat., *1*:145, 1901–1902.)

avian limbs. Because removal of somatic mesoderm creates muscleless limbs with normal nerves that lack only branches to the missing muscle, muscle may not be the stimulus (Chevallier, Kieny, and Mauger, 1978). Destruction of neural crest results in normal motor nerves but no sensory nerves, an indication that sensory nerves are not important. Removal of the neural tube prevents motor nerve formation, but normal sensory nerve patterns develop. Similarly, it has also been demonstrated that if a whole section of the spinal cord is transferred as a graft, it is still capable of innervating specific nerves if these nerves are allowed to reach the correct limb plexus.

Mixed motor and sensory nerves in chick embryos enter the limb as a pioneer growth cone, which is soon surrounded by mesenchy-mal cells that soon form a perineural sheath. Branches sprout to individual muscles, and these nerves are stretched or pulled distally with the growing limb. In humans, individual muscles can be supplied by more than one nerve root through interconnections within the brachial plexus. In general, the anterior division nerves supply the flexor mass; the posterior, the extensor mass. By the eighth postovulatory week, pronation and internal rotation of the upper limb have changed the inclination and position of the plexus.

Anomalies and Timetables

Embryologic failures are undoubtedly related to malformation of "timetables" upon which the teratogen, chromosomal abnormality, virus, toxic agent, vascular event,

Figure 128–8. Diagrammatic representation of the upper limb of an embryo with a crown-rump length of 11.0 mm at four and one-half five weeks of age. *A,* Dorsal view of the muscles to the limb show the trapezius, latissimus dorsi, and levator scapulae and serratus anterior muscles at a more advanced stage of development. At the forearm level, small triceps and biceps muscle fibers are present, with extrinsic wrist extensors. Window dissection within the triceps demonstrates the radial nerve in its course to the outcropping muscles—extensor pollicis brevis and abductor pollicis longus—of the thumb. The hand plate is well formed. *B,* Ventral view of musculature and its relationship to the chest wall are demonstrated. The pectoralis major and minor muscles exist as a common mass that extends from the second and third ribs to the proximal portion of the humerus. It is not well differentiated into sternal or clavicular portions. The brachial plexus is well formed into lateral (dorsal) and medial (ventral) divisions, and these nerves are quite large in comparison with other structures. Trunks, cords, and major divisions are well formed. With distal progression, the flexor mass within the forearm is less well differentiated, but superficial and deep layers are present (the median nerve lies between these two layers). The flexor carpi ulnaris has attached to the fifth metacarpal base (pisiform region).

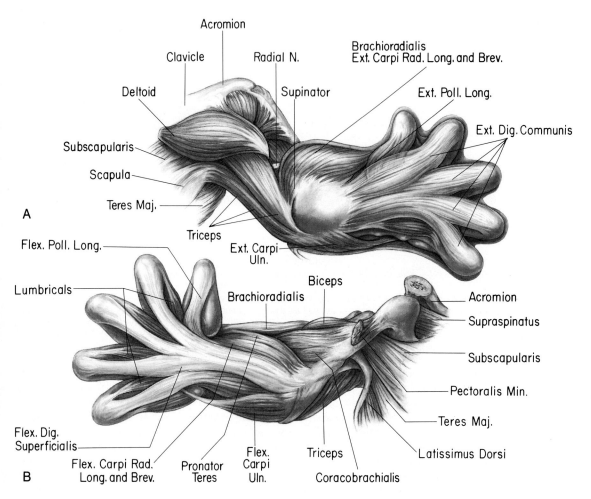

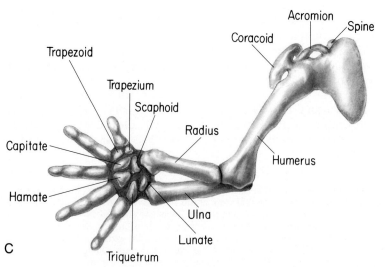

Figure 128–9 *See legend on opposite page*

trauma, or other cause exerts its effect within a very critical time (Triden and Thiret, 1966). The embryologic process is a very coordinated one and can be likened to an orchestra of musical instruments all playing in synchrony. The period of hand differentiation is relatively short, occurring between the 25th and 50th days. Most congenital anomalies occur within this period. For example, failure of breakup of the apical ectodermal ridge by a process of programmed cell death will result in syndactyly (Milaire, 1965). In contrast, prolonged interaction between the AER and mesoderm will result in delayed involution and an extra field of congenital polydactyly (Yasuda, 1975; Klein, Scott, and Wilson, 1981). After the seventh week, any malformations that occur are the result of extrinsic compression upon the uterine wall, local ischemic events, or mechanical influence of local factors, such as seen in the constriction ring (amnionic band) syndromes.

How this complex biologic process works on a cellular, biochemical, and cytogenetic level is complex and the subject of a tremendous amount of current and future experimental work. These fascinating areas of research, aided by recent computer technology, will provide many answers in the future.

INCIDENCE

Congenital anomalies of the hand and upper limb are not uncommon. Analysis of frequency data must be reviewed critically because of the tremendous variation in the genetic make-up of populations being studied, of sampling, and of inconsistencies in precise definitions (Temtamy and McKusick, 1978). The incidence of one in 4000 live births obtained by Birch-Jensen (1949) in his classic study was low because he primarily considered congenital absence deformities in the Danish study population. A more realistic incidence of one in 626 live births was reported by Conway and Bowe (1956), who surveyed all of the births at the New York Hospital between 1932 and 1952.

These and more recent frequency data studies cite camptodactyly, polydactyly (duplication), and syndactyly as the most common deformities in the upper limb (Flatt, 1977; Lamb, Wynne-Davies, and Soto, 1982; Bod, Dzeizel, and Lenz, 1983; Centers for Disease Control, 1984; Kallen, Tamereh, and Winberg, 1984) (Table 128–2).

Flatt's (1977) systematic study of limb anomalies in Iowa, conducted over a 15-year period, reflects the same relative incidence of individual anomalies evaluated and treated by the hand surgeons. Geographic differences highlight the tremendous variation, for example, of polydactyly, which is two to three times more common in Asian countries and in certain well-studied regions within the United States where Negro and American Indian groups predominate (Flatt, 1980; Centers for Disease Control, 1984). Absence deformities including constriction rings occur

Figure 128–9. Diagrammatic presentation of the upper limb of an embryo with a crown-rump length of 16.0 mm at six weeks of age. *A,* Dorsal view of the arm, forearm, and hand shows well differentiated triceps and deltoid muscles. The subscapularis, teres major, and teres minor muscles are now in adult relationships. The triceps muscle has two distinct heads. The extrinsic extensor muscle groups are well differentiated and extend to the wrist and hand, but their development has not been as rapid as their antagonists on the flexor side. The brachioradialis still shares a common muscle origin with the two radial wrist extensors, over which pass the abductor pollicis longus, extensor pollicis brevis, and extensor pollicus longus. Common extensors to the digits are formed and are quite distinct from the extensor indicis proprius and extensor digiti quinti minimi proprius. *B,* Ventral (palmar) view of the same arm shows pectoralis insertion reflected to demonstrate insertions of teres major and latissimus dorsi muscles into the humerus. The triceps has three distinct origins at this stage, and the elongated triceps shows a long head extending to the coracoid process and a short head originating in common with the coracobrachialis muscle. The flexor muscles of the forearm are more advanced than the extensors and show separation into wrist flexors, superficial finger flexors, and deep finger flexors. The pronator teres muscle passes deep along the middle third of the radius. These muscle masses are broad and thin and extend to, but not beyond, the level of the carpals, where they connect to well-formed tendons. The lumbrical muscles have formed, but the other intrinsic muscles are still represented by less well-differentiated masses of tissue adjacent to the metacarpals. *C,* The scapula is composed primarily of cartilage, has grown, and has migrated posteriorly. The coracoid process and acromion are distinct. The humerus is longer and more slender than in the preceding stage and has broadened at either end, but there still is no joint cavity at either end. The radius and ulna are still continuous with the humerus and each other over their proximal third of the forearm. Capsular structures are beginning to form over future joint cavities. The carpals are still a very condensed mass with demarcations between future bones; the distal row is more easily distinguished. Metacarpals are beginning to form and, with distal phalanges attached, are represented by long, slender condensations of cartilage. There are no joint cavities. None of the metacarpal condensations comes in contact with the radius. (Redrawn, abstracted, and condensed from Lewis, W. H.: The development of the arm in man. Am. J. Anat. *1:*145, 1901–1902.)

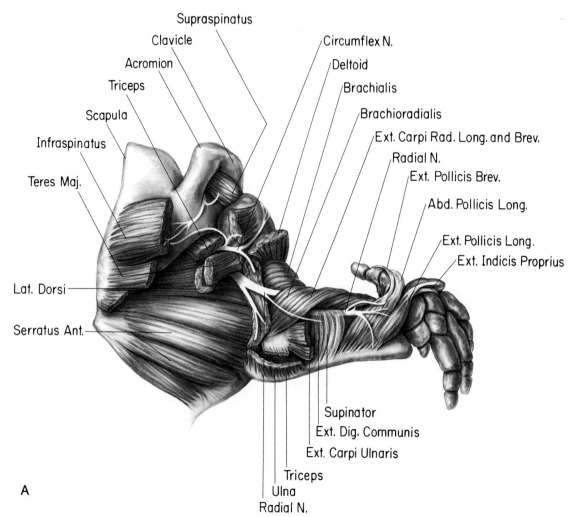

Figure 128–10. Diagrammatic representation of the embryo upper limb with a crown-rump length of 20.0 mm at seven weeks of age. *A,* Within this dissection, many of the proximal limb muscles have been cut to show the very distinct innervation around the shoulder. The deltoid, supraspinatus, infraspinatus, latissimus dorsi, serratus anterior, teres major, and teres minor are all well differentiated. The position of the radial nerve (musculospiral nerve) as it spirals around the humerus to innervate the wrist and finger extensors is demonstrated. The size of the peripheral nerves is still relatively great in comparison with other structures. The brachioradialis and extensor carpi ulnaris longus and brevis are now distinct. The extensor carpi ulnaris has been cut away to show the supinator, through which passes the posterior interosseus nerve, a branch of the radial. In the forearm, the abductor pollicis longus and extensor medius proprius now have distinguishable ulnar portions adjacent to the index extensor digitorum communis. A common extensor muscle mass (not shown) extends to the metacarpal level before tapering into four distinct tendons.

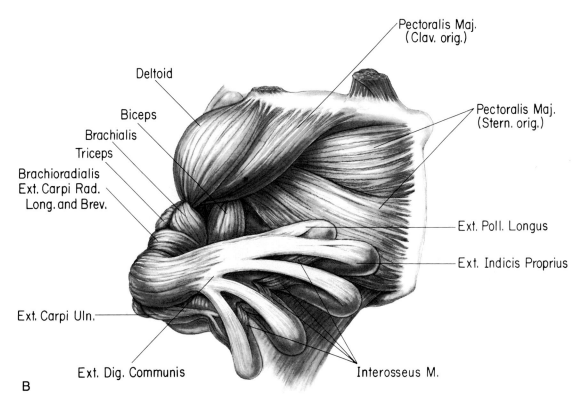

Deltoid

Biceps

Brachialis

Triceps

Brachioradialis
Ext. Carpi Rad.
Long. and Brev.

Pectoralis Maj.
(Clav. orig.)

Pectoralis Maj.
(Stern. orig.)

Ext. Poll. Longus

Ext. Indicis Proprius

Ext. Carpi Uln.

Ext. Dig. Communis

Interosseus M.

B

Figure 128–10 *Continued B,* A dorsal view of the hand from an anterior position shows the arm being pronated from its earlier position. The pectoralis major is distinct from the underlying pectoralis minor and is separated into clavicular and sternal origins. Common extensor tendons extend out along the digital cartilaginous condensations and the intrinsic muscles, both lumbrical, dorsal, and palmar interosseus groups, are forming.

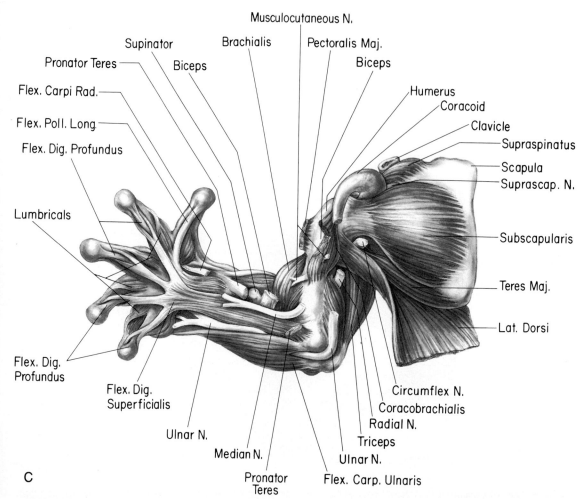

Figure 128–10 *Continued C,* On the ventral surface of the same arm, portions of many superficial flexor muscles have been sectioned to show the relationship of the median and ulnar nerves. The broad latissimus dorsi muscle inserts into the medial border of the humerus distal to the insertion of the subscapularis, which as a muscle group is still relatively large in comparison with the rest of the limb. The biceps muscle belly has been cut away to show its innervation, the musculocutaneous nerve, which also passes through the coracobrachialis muscle. The brachialis muscle has its origin along the humerus and is located deep to the biceps muscle. In the proximal forearm, the median nerve is shown where it passes between the deep and superficial (cut away) heads of the pronator teres muscle. The flexor digitorum superficialis muscle group is a large mass within the forearm tapering to tendons within the hand, which at this stage have split to allow the penetration of the flexor digitorum profundus. The well-formed lumbrical muscles extend to the radial side of their respective digits, where they condense with perichondrium. They are distinct from the palmar interosseus muscles.

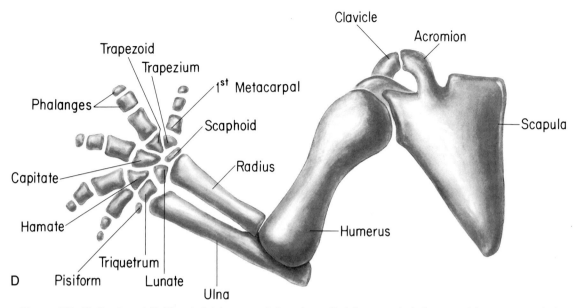

Figure 128–10 *Continued D,* The skeletal representation shows that the scapula is larger and in a more posterior position than in the earlier stage. An acromioclavicular ligament has formed. The cartilaginous humerus is broader and thicker, and a coracohumeral ligament is present. There is still no glenohumeral joint. The radius and ulna are larger, and the olecranon, coracoid, and styloid processes are beginning to form as condensed tissue. No joints are present, and perichondrium between the two bones is still continuous. All carpal bones are still cartilaginous, and ligaments are beginning to form. The carpus has not yet begun to flex and deviate ulnarward. Five metacarpals are distinct, with the first on the preaxial side being the shortest. At the digital level, the first *two* rows of phalanges are evident. (Redrawn, abstracted, and condensed from Lewis, W. H.: The development of the arm in man. Am. J. Anat., *1*:145, 1901–1902.)

much less frequently, with an incidence of one in 2000 to 3000 live births (Goldberg and Bartoshesky, 1985). Between two and four per cent of all children are born with a major or minor hand malformation, and approximately 0.7 per cent have multiple anomalies. The relative incidence of individual anomalies varies with the population being studied. Table 128–3 summarizes frequency data for hand anomalies in four different clinic populations. These are consistent with other collaborative comparative studies (Lamb, Wynne-Davies, and Soto, 1982).

Minor anomalies cannot be fully evaluated by this method. For example, clinodactyly is probably not usually included on birth certificates, one of the sources of information for registries. On examination of 4322 infants with no major anomaly, Marden, Smith, and McDonald (1964) found the incidence of clinodactyly to be 9.9 per 1000 live births, whereas in 90 babies with other major anomalies, the incidence was 122 per 1000 live births. In addition, some anomalies are evident on radiographic study only after a certain amount of maturation has occurred. Triquetrum-lunate synostosis (coalition), for example, cannot be clinically evaluated in

Table 128–2. Relative Frequency of Congenital Upper Limb Anomalies per 1000 Live Births*

Anomaly	Incidence by Location				
	Baltimore	Hungary	Sweden	Atlanta	Nebraska
Polydactyly	3.8			12.2	5.56
Caucasian	0.3			0.2	0.66
Negroes	3.5			12.0	4.9
Syndactyly	0.6		0.65	0.9	
Radial deficiency	0.03	0.09	0.08		
Ulnar deficiency	0.01	0.11	0.02		
Transverse deficiency	0.05	0.14	0.13	0.8	0.4
Camptodactyly (flexion deformity)	4.0				
Constriction ring	0.1	0.11			
Source study	Temtamy and McKusick (1978)	Bod, Dzeizel, and Lenz (1983)	Kallen, Tamerch, and Winberg (1984)	Centers for Disease Control (1984)	Centers for Disease Control (1984)

*Note that in the foreign studies, duplications were not included. (Data summarized from Goldberg, M. J., and Bartoshesky, L. E.: Congenital hand anomaly: Etiology and associated malformations. Hand Clin., *1*:405, 1985.)

Table 128–3. Relative Frequency (Percentage) of Anomalies Seen in Four Hand Clinics*

	Yokohama	Iowa	Hong Kong	Sapporo
Number of patients	227	1,476	326	955
Failure of formation (FOF)				
Transverse (arm, wrist, hand)	7.0	7.1	6.8	2.9
Radial ray	9.6	5.4†	0.5	3.9
Ulnar ray		3.4‡		0.9
Central ray	5.8	3.9	2.5	3.2
Phocomelia (typical, atypical)	0.9	0.8		
Failure of differentiation				
Triphalangeal thumb		0.8		0.6
Clasped thumb		0.7	2.5	5.5
Trigger		2.3	6.3	21.0
Camptodactyly		6.9	2.0	7.2
Syndactyly	10.1	17.5	14.9	4.1
Proximal radioulnar synostosis		1.2	0.7	4.3
Madelung's deformity	0.5	1.7		0.7
Symphalangism		0.5	0.5	0.4
Clinodactyly	1.3	5.6	1.8	1.3
Duplication	28.6	14.3	39.9	18.4
Radial		6.4		16.3
Central		5.2		1.2
Ulnar		2.7		0.8
Ulnar dimelia		0.0		0.1
Overgrowth	1.3	0.8	0.5	0.5
Undergrowth				
Whole hand		0.8	2.0	
Brachydactyly		5.2		4.0
Brachysyndactyly	10.6§			4.5
Ectrosyndactyly	4.4			
Hypoplastic thumb	7.5	3.6	4.5	
Constriction ring	1.3	5.3‖		4.8
Generalized skeletal anomaly				3.2
Poland's syndrome		2.2	11.9	
Apert's syndrome		2.1		

"Top four" anomalies in clinic

Yokohama	Iowa	Hong Kong	Sapporo
Duplication 28.6%	Syndactyly 17.5%	Duplication 39.9%	Trigger Digit 21.0%
Brachysyndactyly 10.6%	Duplication 14.3%	Syndactyly 14.9%	Duplication 18.4%
Syndactyly 10.1%	FOF—transverse 7.1%	Syndromes 11.9%	Camptodactyly 7.2%
Radial Ray defect 9.6%	Radial Ray 5.4%	FOF—transverse 6.8%	Clasped Thumb 5.5%

Source study

Yokohama	Iowa	Hong Kong	Sapporo
Yamaguchi et al. (1973)	Flatt (1980)	Leung, Chan, and Cheng (1982)	Ogino et al. (1986)

*Anomalies chosen for inclusion were those in which data could be expressed in terms of the international classification adapted by all major hand societies.
†Includes radial club hand and radial hyperplasia.
‡Includes ulnar absence, hypoplasia, metacarpal absence.
§Includes microdactyly, brachydactyly.
‖Includes acrosyndactyly.

youngsters. In a study of 7500 Africans, Garn and associates (1971) found the incidence to be 1.6 per 1000, and in 11,663 to be one per 1000 during childhood.

The high associated coincidence of upper and lower limb anomalies is so common in many syndromes that they are almost always expected in entities such as the constriction ring syndrome. In Apert's syndrome (acrocephalosyndactyly), mirror image deformities of the feet are present. In the cleft hand/foot and Goltz's syndromes, the lower limbs are, almost by definition, abnormal.

DYSMORPHOLOGY APPROACH

Although some hand surgeons think geneticists are often speaking a foreign language, it is important to understand their terms, which are actually quite straightforward and simple. Because 0.7 per cent of all babies born have multiple malformations, often involving the upper limb, a clear understanding of the alterations in morphogenesis is necessary in the evaluation of the malformation, formulation of a treatment plan, and counseling for parents.

Initial evaluation by the hand surgeon should consist of: (1) a complete family history; (2) a thorough pregnancy history, including information regarding medical illnesses, medications, alcohol and substance abuse, onset and vigor of fetal movements, gestational timing, any indications of uterine irritability, delivery, and neonatal adaptations; and (3) postnatal growth and development. Minor and major abnormalities should all be recorded. *Major* anomalies are those that have serious medical and surgical implications and characteristically involve the renal, pulmonary, cardiovascular, or central nervous system. Hand anomalies are usually classified as *minor*. When three or more minor anomalies exist in a single patient, there is a 90 per cent chance that a major anomaly will also be found (Holmes, 1980).

The term congenital malformation syndrome may be confusing, as there are problems with all three components of the term. *Congenital* refers to something present at birth, but not all conditions, such as bone dysplasias, are evident at birth. *Malformation* is used to define a gross structural anomaly and, according to some, should not be used for biochemical and nonstructural changes

(Warkeny, 1971). *Syndrome* is even more difficult to define but is generally used to describe a combination of anomalies in a patient, particularly if there is a familial tendency for this combination, a single known biochemical or chromosomal cause for this combination, or a developmental sequence that results in the combination. The distinction between a *syndrome* and the chance *association* of three or more anomalies can be an artificial one (Fig. 128–11).

The interpretation of the patient's anomaly may not be simple. Reference should be made to published stages of prenatal development for an estimate of the time at which the deficiency developed (Smith, 1982). Multiple problems in morphogenesis may be explained in terms of a *sequence,* which is a simple problem leading to a cascade of subsequent problems. Developmentalists have designated three types of sequence: (1) malformation, (2) deformation, and (3) disruption (Smith, 1982). In a *malformation sequence,* poor formation of tissue within the fetus initiates the chain of defects, which may range from minimal to severe. It can occur in all gradations; a good example is radial dysplasia, in which one may see complete absence of the radius with club hand posturing or an isolated loss of thenar muscles. Recurrence rate for malformations is usually in the range of one to five per cent.

In a *deformation sequence,* there is no intrinsic problem with the fetus or embryo, but abnormal external mechanical or structural forces cause secondary distortion or deformation. Leakage of amniotic fluid and bicornuate uterus are common causes for external deformation of the intact fetus in this sequence. In contrast to malformations, recurrence rate in this category is very low, unless the cause is a persistent anatomic defect such as a bicornuate uterus. Tethering or constriction of limb parts by annular bands in the constriction ring syndrome is a prime example. Forearm skin necrosis in cutis aplasia may be caused by impaction of the arm between the pelvis and uterine wall after breech presentation, and a prolonged labor is another cause.

In a *disruption sequence,* the normal fetus or embryo is subjected to tissue breakdown or injury, which may be vascular, infectious, mechanical, or metabolic in origin. The proximal limb deficiencies caused by thalidomide or alcohol are dramatic examples.

It is often important to recognize that not

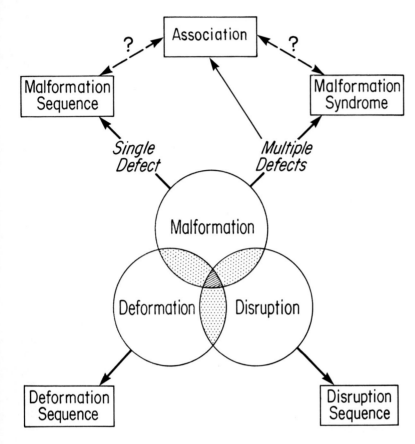

Figure 128–11. The dysmorphology approach to congenital anomalies divides defects into one of three sequences, which are defined as problems that lead to a cascade of events. Overlap between sequences can and does occur. Three types of sequences exist: malformation, disruption, and distortion. When multiple malformation defects exist, they lead to a malformation syndrome. The term association is used when no unifying cause is known and the relationship between an association and malformation sequence is still unclear. (Abstracted from Smith, D. W.: Recognizable Patterns of Human Malformation: Genetic, Embryologic, and Clinical Aspects. 3rd Ed. Philadelphia, W. B. Saunders Company, 1982.)

all of the patient's problems can be explained by a single initiating factor. When the cause of the defect is unknown, *malformation* is usually preferred. Similarly, when the anomalies seen appear to be the result of multiple defects in one or more tissues, *malformation syndrome* is also used. Some known causes for syndromes are chromosomal abnormalities, mutant gene disorders, and teratogens such as thalidomide. The specific etiology of many syndromes is not known. When multiple major and/or minor anomalies exist in combination without any known unifying cause, the term malformation association has been used.

Geneticists use important general principles and terms in their evaluation of multiple anomalies. *Nonspecificity* of an individual defect means that a single anomaly will not necessarily make a specific diagnosis, which is usually based upon the overall pattern of minor and major anomalies. A single defect such as clinodactyly or syndactyly may appear as part of many diagnostic categories, but when considered alone it will not make a

specific diagnosis of a syndrome. *Variance* in the extent or expression of a defect is common among individuals and often within the same individual. *Pleotropism* is another commonly found synonymous term for variance (McKusick, 1969). A good example is the Holt-Oram syndrome, in which hand manifestations may include absence of a thumb, hypoplastic thumb, or even a triphalangeal thumb, all defects involving the radial ray. Similarly, patients with absence of the radius and club hand posturing in one limb may demonstrate only hypothenar muscle absence on the other. The term *heterogeneity* is used often because many deformities with the same phenotype, such as simple syndactyly, or similar physical characteristics may have different etiologies. In the multiply-deformed child, it is important to withhold a diagnosis (and its consequences) until there is a very close resemblance between the overall pattern of anomalies seen in the patient and the syndrome under consideration.

Roughly half of cases with multiple anomalies fall into syndromes; the remaining have not been specifically labelled. In the absence of known genetic information, it is impossible to give accurate information regarding the potential risk for recurrence for future malformations. At this time, Temtany and McKusick's work (1978) is the only comprehensive treatise devoted to this subject. Without very specific knowledge, the hand surgeon should not tell the parents that their child's condition is rare and will not occur in future children. In these situations, geneticists recommend telling parents that the lowest risk is zero and the highest 25 per cent with each pregnancy (Smith, 1982). Referral to a local birth defects service (if available) or a clinical geneticist may be particularly helpful for parents with multiply-deformed children and advisable for the patients when they reach childbearing age. If uncertain about the possible association of upper limb anomalies with other malformations, one should refer to texts by Smith (1982) and Temtamy and McKusick (1978).

GENETICS AND ETIOLOGY

The birth of a child is a long-awaited, often eagerly awaited, event. After parents and family recover from the initial "shock" of a congenital imperfection, the question of etiology is asked. Unfortunately, clear-cut answers are not always available. It is important for the hand surgeon to have a grasp of what little is known.

It is convenient to divide etiologies into three categories: environmental, genetic, and uncertain (Goldberg and Bartoshesky, 1985). At least 40 to 50 per cent of all anomalies belong in the last group.

Genetic Causes

The inherited or genetic disorders depend upon the appropriate gene sequence on chromosomes. They can be classified into three specific groups: single gene, multiple gene, and chromosomal deformities.

The inherited pattern of a *single gene* or Mendelian pattern may be *dominant, recessive,* or *sex-linked.* When the affected gene is *dominant,* only one of the pair of genes on a chromosome must be involved for the deformity to occur. Only one parent needs to be affected. Brachydactyly, camptodactyly, and

central polysyndactylies are common examples of such deformities in the hand. If a heterozygote person who has one affected chromosome mates with someone without the affected gene, there is a 50 per cent chance that the deformity will occur. When a trait is *recessive,* both genes on a given chromosome must be affected for the deformity to occur. The affected person is the homozygote. If both parents are heterozygotes, there is a 25 per cent chance that the deformity will occur (homozygote), a 50 per cent chance that the child will be a carrier (heterozygote), and a 25 per cent chance that the child will be normal. Recessive hand abnormalities are usually more severe than dominant ones. Arthrogryposis and the thrombocytopenia–absent radius (TAR) syndrome are common examples (Temtamy, 1978; Smith, 1982). In the *sex-linked* inheritance pattern, the affected gene is always the X chromosome and can never be passed from father to son. If a mother is a carrier, male children have a 50 per cent chance of having the deformity, and female offspring have a 50 per cent chance of being carriers. Some types of syndactyly, metacarpal synostosis, and Goltz's syndrome are good examples.

Environmental Causes

Changes that occur within the internal environment of the womb may result in a congenital limb anomaly. This internal milieu is known to have been affected by mechanical forces such as intrauterine fibromas and other factors such as drugs, irradiation, hormones, alcohol, and viral infections. The thalidomide tragedy of the 1960's in Europe focused much attention on a large series of helpless children with major reduction limb deformities (usually phocomelia) (Fig. 128–5) as well as anorectal and cardiac malformations (McBride, 1977). Warfarin (Coumadin) (Hall, 1980), heroin, and phenytoin (Dilantin) (Hanson, 1976) have also been directly associated with limb anomalies. Despite a considerable amount of research and exposure in the lay press, Bendectin, synthetic hormones (Holmes, 1983; Schardein, 1980), pesticides (Pearn, 1983), herbicides, particularly Agent Orange, which was used in Vietnam (Friedman, 1984), and x-ray exposure (Soyka, 1979) have not been definitely shown to cause limb defects directly or indirectly. Because limb

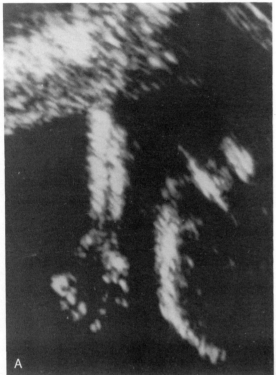

Figure 128–12. An ultrasound examination at 22 weeks of gestation is sensitive enough to diagnose normal from abnormal development. *A,* A normal hand and forearm. *B,* Radial club hand and total absence of the radius seen in comparison with the clinical and radiographic appearance.

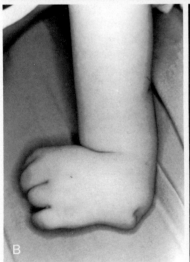
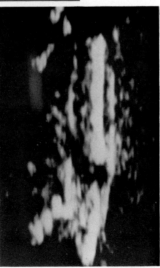
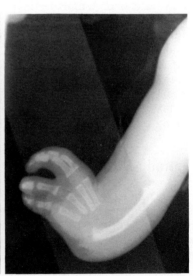

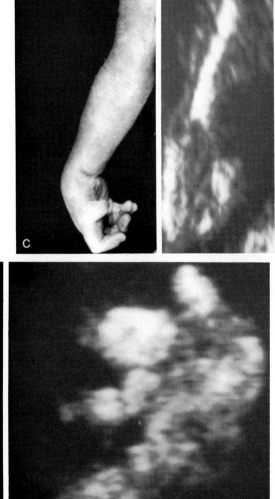

Figure 128–12 *Continued C,* Ulnar deviation and flexion of the wrist associated with total absence of the ulna. *D,* A close-up of the hand in *C* with multiple pterygium syndrome. (*B* courtesy of B. Benacerraf, M.D.; *C* and *D* courtesy of P. Doubilet, M.D.)

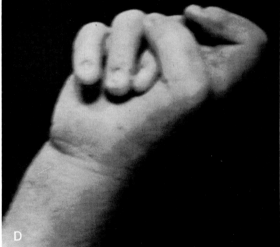

development is complete by seven to eight weeks of gestation, the effect of many of these teratogens after that time will be minimal. The type and configuration of the deformity will depend upon when, in the sequence of proximal to distal development, exposure occurs. Recent and past interest in vascular compromise within the developing limb results in a number of anomalies (Bouwes-Bavinck and Weaver, 1986). Besides the direct compression of a limb with subsequent ischemic arrest of growth (Graham and associates, 1980), more subtle factors such as vasoactive drugs, placental vascular insufficiency, maternal vascular disease such as diabetes, toxemia, and hypertension (Wilson and Fraser, 1978), and emboli (Hoyme and associates, 1982) have all been postulated to influence the development of upper limb defects.

Uncertain Etiology

The impression that most congenital limb malformations have a genetic basis is erroneous. Fraser (1959) emphasized, "A minority of congenital anomalies have a major environmental cause, a minority have a major genetic cause." The cause of most is uncertain and probably involves a complex interaction between genetic predisposition and very subtle factors within the intrauterine environment. Isolated transverse limb anomalies such as below elbow amputations with no identifiable cause fall into this group (Goldberg, Bartoshesky, and O'Toole, 1981).

SYNDROMES

The hand surgeon not only must recognize that a hand anomaly may have the likelihood of future occurrence within a given family or kindred, but also must consider that the deformity may be part of a syndrome. Identification of a syndrome may be difficult because all of the cardinal features may not be present and observations may be limited by the interest of the observer, but as Greenfield states, "A three legged dog is still a dog" (Poznanski, 1984).

Syndromes are difficult to remember, and even though most are related to some chromosomal aberration (single gene, multiple gene, or sex-linked), only five per cent of all upper limb malformations occur as part of a well-recognized syndrome (Lamb, Wynne-Davies, and Soto, 1982). Over the years, geneticists have become fascinated with four particular hand anomalies: syndactyly, which is part of 48 different syndromes; clinodactyly, part of 36 syndromes; camptodactyly, part of 20 syndromes; and brachydactyly, part of 18 syndromes (Goldberg and Bartoshesky, 1985). Many potential associations (with radial ray defects) will be made by the hand surgeon—Fanconi's pancytopenia or syndrome, thrombocytopenia–absent radius (TAR) syndrome, Holt-Oram syndrome, and the VATER association—in which the hand anomaly may be the most obvious malformation in a patient with hematologic, cardiac, genitourinary, or other musculoskeletal anomalies. The hematologic and cardiac lesions may be life threatening. One is referred to appropriate genetics textbooks for a full description of these syndromes (Smith, 1982). Temtamy and McKusick's (1982) work is the only one currently available that specifically deals with genetics of upper limb anomalies. An excellent review of the International Nomenclature of Constitutional Diseases of Bone and the Hand is contained in Poznanski's (1984) book on the radiology of hand syndromes. The glossary of Flatt's (1977) book contains a useful outline of common syndromes and eponyms involving the upper limb.

Radiologic measurements of the hand are the parameters most commonly used for evaluation of maturation, which includes the presence or absence of ossification centers, modeling characteristics, and presence or absence of epiphyseal closure (see Fig. 128–2). Although skeletal maturation and size may be related, they can vary independently. Variations exist in all 28 bones of the hand and wrist in terms of length, width, mineralization (density), relative size, and position; to be clinically useful these features must be compared with normative tables that specifically define sex, race, and nutritional and social background of the group studied (Poznanski, 1984). The simplest method for evaluating maturation to identify congenital defects is to look through the standards and find a radiograph that corresponds to the hand being studied (Greulich and Pyle, 1959) or to compare the onset of ossification centers (Garn, 1964). When uncertainty exists, comparison of individual maturation characteristics of each bone should be made. Comparison of ossification centers in children with unilateral limb anomalies will often show delay on the affected side. No standards are available for common anomalies such as radial dysplasias, cleft hands, and hypoplastic hands.

CLASSIFICATION

During the past 100 years attempts to establish a universal classification of congenital hand anomalies have been frustrated by the confusing array of Greek and Latin terms used to describe similar deformities with the emphasis on different pathologic features. With no systematic approach, there has been confusion, duplication, and overlapping of terms. Some anomalies have seemed too bizarre to fit into any specific category. Isidore St. Hilaire (1832) proposed probably the first classification in 1832, introducing terms such as phocomele (seal limb), hemimele (part of limb missing), and ectromele (complete absence); and numerous authors have championed their own versions at regular intervals since (Kelikian, 1974). There was so much confusion by the midportion of the 20th century that The National Research Council adopted the Frantz and O'Rahilly (1961) classification, which was based on skeletal appearance and still contained terms such as miromelia (partial limb) and amelia (missing limb). The principal underlying difficulty has remained our limited understanding of embryogenesis.

An ideal classification system should contain simple descriptive terms, should permit easy recording of common conditions, but also should allow full categorization of complex cases. While being specific, it should not be so detailed that its use is burdensome. Few systems are likely to hold a surgeon's interest for long, nor has any of the myriad systems advanced the treatment of any specific anomaly. Nonetheless, until surgeons, pediatricians, embryologists, geneticists, and others who deal with these conditions use the same terms, communication and the advancement of knowledge remain difficult, particularly when international boundaries are crossed. The true incidence of a deformity and international comparisons are impossible to establish unless the classification is common to all. Toward this end, the American Society for Surgery of the Hand and the International Federation of Societies for Surgery of the Hand have adopted a classification proposed by Swanson, Barsky, and Entin in 1968, which is based on grouping according to the parts that have been primarily affected by certain embryonic failures (Table 128–4). Within this classification, provisions for the continued use of widely used terms that are easily understood and cause no confusion have been made. They include *melia* (limb), *cheir* (hand), *dactyly* (fingers), *phalangia* (segments of fingers), *brachy* (short), *syn* (together), *poly* (many), and *macro* (large). All authors agree that it is beneficial to avoid confusion and to minimize the use of Latin and Greek derivatives in the description of these anomalies. The author's expanded version of this classification system is shown in Table 128–4. An excellent glossary of terms is provided in Flatt's (1977) textbook and a comprehensive discussion of classifications is found in Kelikian's (1974) classic work.

Classification of congenitally deficient limbs is made more difficult in the infant by the absence or delay of ossification. Any diagnosis in the early years should, therefore, be guarded.

In the light of limited knowledge about the embryologic mechanism(s) of malformations, such a comprehensive classification will be frustrating for the strict constructionist. Many anomalies will fit easily into two or more categories. Some current authors hypothesize that polydactyly, syndactyly, and the typical cleft hand may have a common teratologic mechanism, on the basis of the similarities of osseous fusions; given deformities may be conveniently placed in several categories (Miura, 1978; Ogino, 1979).

The deformity association that has provoked the most recent controversy are hypoplastic hands with central deficiencies. Should these be called "atypical" cleft hands in the failure of formation category, or "symbrachydactyly" in the failure of differentiation category? Blauth and Gekeler (1971) have commented that the predominant feature is a reduction and sometimes a transverse arrest, so the association belongs in the failure of formation of the central rays. Within these hypoplastic hands, the whole spectrum of deformity exists, from short, webbed fingers to no digits at all. According to Blauth and Gekeler (1971) brachysyndactyly, atypical cleft hand, and transverse deficiency should be put in the same category. With expansion of knowledge within developmental embryopathy, this classification may stand the test of time and, one hopes,

Table 128–4. Classification of Congenital Hand Anomalies (Expanded Version)*

I. Failure of Formation
  A. Transverse arrest
    1. Shoulder
      a. Shoulder level (amelia)
      b. Clavicle
    2. Upper arm
      a. Upper arm level
        (1) Long above elbow
        (2) Short above elbow
    3. Elbow
      a. Elbow level
    4. Forearm
      a. Forearm level
        (1) Long below elbow
        (2) Short below elbow
    5. Wrist
      a. Wrist level (acheira)
    6. Carpal
      a. Carpal level (no metacarpals present)
        (1) Proximal carpal row
        (2) Distal carpal row
    7. Metacarpal
      a. Metacarpal level (adactyly)
    8. Phalanx
      a. Phalangeal level
        (1) Proximal level
        (2) Middle level
        (3) Distal level
  B. Longitudinal arrest
    1. Radial ray (preaxial)
      a. Radial ray deficiency
        (1) Normal radius
          (a) Thumb hypoplastic—functional
          (b) Thumb hypoplastic—nonfunctional
          (c) Thumb absent
        (2) Hypoplasia of radius (complete but small)
          (a) Thumb hypoplastic—functional
          (b) Thumb hypoplastic—nonfunctional
          (c) Thumb absent
          (d) Madelung's deformity
          (e) Other
        (3) Partial absence of radius (distal end absent)
          (a) Thumb hypoplastic—functional
          (b) Thumb hypoplastic—nonfunctional
          (c) Thumb absent
        (4) Complete absence of radius
          (a) Thumb hypoplastic—functional
          (b) Thumb hypoplastic—nonfunctional
          (c) Thumb absent
        (5) Absent/hypoplastic thenar muscles
        (6) Absent/hypoplastic extensor muscles
        (7) Absent/hypoplastic flexor muscles
    2. Ulnar ray (postaxial)
      a. Ulnar ray deficiency
        (1) Normal ulna
          (a) Metacarpals, digits hypoplastic
          (b) Metacarpals hypoplastic, digits absent
          (c) Metacarpals, digits absent
        (2) Hypoplasia of ulna (complete but small)
          (a) Metacarpals, digits hypoplastic
          (b) Metacarpals hypoplastic, digits absent
          (c) Metacarpals, digits absent
        (3) Partial absence of ulna (distal end absent)

          (a) Metacarpals, digits hypoplastic
          (b) Metacarpals hypoplastic, digits absent
          (c) Metacarpals, digits absent
        (4) Complete absence of ulna
          (a) Metacarpals, digits hypoplastic
          (b) Metacarpals hypoplastic, digits absent
          (c) Metacarpals, digits absent
        (5) Defect of ulna with humeroradial synostosis
        (6) Absent/hypoplastic hypothenar muscles
        (7) Absent/hypoplastic extensor muscles
        (8) Absent/hypoplastic flexor muscles
    3. Central ray (cleft hand)
      a. Central ray deficiency
        (1) Typical type (deficiency type)
          (a) Metacarpals, digits hypoplastic
          (b) Metacarpals hypoplastic, digits absent
          (c) Metacarpals, digits absent
        (2) Atypical type
          (a) Syndactylous type
          (b) Polydactylous type
          (c) Monodactyly
          (d) Other
    4. Intersegmental (intercalated) type of longitudinal arrest
      a. Phocomelia
        (1) Proximal type (hand-to-forearm-to-trunk)
        (2) Distal type (hand-to-arm-to-trunk)
        (3) Total type (hand-to-trunk)
      b. Other
II. Failure of Differentiation (Separation) of Parts
  A. Soft tissue involvement
    1. Disseminated
      a. Arthrogryposis (including multiplex congenita)
        (1) Severe
        (2) Moderate
        (3) Mild
    2. Shoulder
      a. Undescended shoulder
        (1) Sprengel's shoulder
      b. Absence of thorax muscles (including Poland's syndrome)
        (1) Pectoralis major
        (2) Pectoralis major and minor
        (3) Other
    3. Elbow and forearm
      a. Aberrant muscle
        (1) Aberrant muscles of long extrinsic flexors
        (2) Aberrant muscles of long extrinsic extensors
        (3) Aberrant intrinsics of the hand
        (4) Other
    4. Wrist and hand
      a. Cutaneous syndactyly (complete and incomplete)
        (1) Radial (1st interdigital space)
        (2) Central (2nd/3rd interdigital space)
        (3) Ulnar (3rd interdigital space)
        (4) Combination of (1) ± (2) or (3)
      b. Congenital flexion contracture (camptodactyly)
        (1) Fifth digit
        (2) Others

Table 128–4. Classification of Congenital Hand Anomalies (Expanded Version)* *Continued*

    c. Thumb-in-palm deformity
    d. Deviated finger without bony deformity (laxity secondary to differentiation of muscle ligament or capsule)
      (1) Radial/ulnar
        (a) Isolated digit
        (b) Congenital ulnar drift (including "windblown hand")
      (2) Other
    e. Congenital trigger digit or thumb
    f. Other
  5. Skin and appendages
    a. Pterygium (webbing) of axilla or elbow
    b. Cutis aplasia congenita
    c. Congenital clubbing of nails
    d. Tusk nail deformity, volar nail
    e. Other
B. Skeletal involvement
  1. Shoulder
    a. Congenital humerus varus
    b. Other
  2. Elbow
    a. Elbow synostosis
      (1) Humeroradial
      (2) Humeroulnar
      (3) Total elbow
    b. Elbow ankylosis (joint segmentation present)
  3. Forearm
    a. Proximal radioulnar synostosis
      (1) Without radial head dislocation
      (2) With radial head dislocation
    b. Distal radioulnar synostosis
  4. Wrist and hand
    a. Synostosis of carpal bones
      (1) Lunate-triquetrum synostosis
      (2) Capitate-hamate synostosis
      (3) Scaphoid-lunate synostosis
      (4) Others
    b. Synostosis of metacarpal bones
      (1) Ring-small synostosis
      (2) Others
    c. Synostosis of phalanges (osseous syndactyly, complex syndactyly)
      (1) Radial (1st-2nd rays)
      (2) Central (2nd-3rd, 3rd-4th rays)
      (3) Ulnar (4th-5th rays)
      (4) Mitten hand (including Apert's hand)
      (5) Other
    d. Symphalangia
      (1) Proximal interphalangeal joint
      (2) Other
    e. Congenital deviation (clinodactyly)
      (1) Idiopathic clinodactyly
        (a) Fifth finger (including delta phalanx)
        (b) Thumb (including delta phalanx)
        (c) Others
    f. Hypersegmentation
      (1) Triphalangeal thumb
      (2) Others
C. Congenital tumorous conditions
  1. Vascular system
    a. Hemangioma
    b. Malformations
      (1) Capillary
        (a) Port wine stain
        (b) Others
      (2) Venous

      (3) Venolymphatic
      (4) Arterial (including AV fistulas)
      (5) Lymphatic
      (6) Others
  2. Neurologic
    a. Neurofibromatosis
    b. Neuroblastoma
    c. Others
  3. Connective tissue
    a. Juvenile (aponeurotic) fibroma
    b. Other
  4. Skeletal (not including overgrowth syndromes)
    a. Osteochondromatosis (including multiple hereditary exostosis)
    b. Enchondromatosis
    c. Fibrous dysplasia
    d. Epiphyseal abnormalities
    e. Other
III. Duplication†
  1. Whole limb
  2. Humerus
  3. Radius
  4. Ulna
    a. Mirror hand
    b. Other
  5. Digit
    a. Polydactyly
      (1) Radial (preaxial, 1st ray, including triphalangeal thumb)
      (2) Central
      (3) Ulnar (postaxial, 5th ray)
      (4) Combinations
  6. Epiphyseal (extra)
    a. 1st ray
    b. 2nd ray
    c. Other
IV. Overgrowth†
  1. Whole limb
    a. Hemihypertrophy
    b. Associated with vascular condition
    c. Other
  2. Partial limb
    a. With associated vascular condition
    b. Other
  3. Digit
    a. Macrodactyly
      (1) With associated vascular condition
      (2) With neurofibromatosis
      (3) With bone or cartilage exostoses
      (4) Other
V. Undergrowth†
  1. Whole limb
  2. Forearm and hand
  3. Hand alone
    a. Entire
    b. Partial
  4. Metacarpal
    a. Brachymetacarpia
      (1) Fifth ray
      (2) Other
    b. Other
  5. Digit
    a. Brachysyndactyly
      (1) With associated absence of thorax muscles (Poland's syndrome)
      (2) Without associated absence of thorax muscles

Table continued on following page

Table 128–4. Classification of Congenital Hand Anomalies (Expanded Version)* *Continued*

b. Brachydactyly
  (1) Defect of middle phalanx only (brachy-mesophalangia)
  (2) Defect of two or more phalanges
  (3) Defect of either proximal or distal phalanx
  (4) Other
VI. Constriction ring syndrome ("Streeter's dysplasia," annular band syndrome)†
  1. Focal necrosis
    a. Constriction band (partial or circumferential)
      (1) With lymphedema
      (2) Without lymphedema
    b. Acrosyndactyly
  2. Amputation ("intrauterine")
    a. Wrist
    b. Metacarpal
    c. Digit
    d. Combination a and b or b and c
    e. Other
VII. Generalized abnormalities and syndromes†

*This is an expanded version of the classification adopted by the American Society for Surgery of the Hand and all major international hand societies and associations. Clearly, one anomaly or group of malformations may be included in more than one category. Some malformations, such as tumorous conditions, may not be considered by some to be genuine upper limb anomalies.
  Notation is as follows:
  I. Main category
    A. Subcategory
      1. Level of deformity
        a. Diagnosis
          (1) Subclassification
            (a) Details
†Standard subcategories are not specified in III through VI.

prove to be both flexible enough for the scientist and helpful enough for the clinician.

The two opposing trends in nosology must include traditional "lumpers" and "splitters." The "lumpers" try to find new things in common, an attempt that seems logical because it is easier to find similarities and variance (pleotropism) within many syndromes. "Splitting" a subclassification into smaller subcategories becomes necessary as genetic and biochemical heterogeneity becomes apparent. This is important when prognostication depends on specific biochemical or genetic factors. Splitting congenital hand deformities strictly on morphologic grounds, however, can be an exercise in futility.

TIMING OF SURGERY

The optimal age for surgical correction of various deformities remains controversial. Ideally, one would like to perform all reconstruction within the first few months of life, to provide the infant with everything possible for normal growth and development (Eaton, 1967). Many physical and psychologic factors will critically influence surgical judgment; agreement upon the relative importance of these factors is not widespread, as some surgeons favor early (infancy) surgery, whereas others prefer later (childhood) correction.

Arguments that favor late correction of the congenitally malformed hands are many. Because the hand is larger, a more precise operation can be done on delicate structures. Difficulties with immobilization of skin grafted regions, tenuous flaps, osteotomies, and ligament reconstructions are reduced. The infant may scar more readily than the older child, and precise incisional design may be more difficult in smaller hands. Developmental studies indicate that a primitive grasp mechanism functions early in infancy and that three digit prehension with eye-hand coordination is not fully developed until 2 to 3 years of age (McGraw, 1943). Finally, the functional needs of the child can be evaluated more adequately, particularly in less severe deformities.

Many objective arguments favor early surgery, which is defined as that performed within the first two years of life. Tethering of adjacent structures, such as a complex syndactyly involving digits of unequal length, will result in irreversible angulation, rotation, and deviation of skeletal parts. The infant or young child can begin using the reconstructed part early in development and will develop fewer bad habits. Anatomic adaptation of the reconstructed part will occur with growth and the external forces placed upon it. Examples include the broadening of the distal ulnar following centralization of the radial club hand (Zaricznyj, 1977) or intrinsic muscle hypertrophy and broadening of the metaphysis of the proximal phalanx of a pollicized index finger that has been moved into the metacarpal position (Buck-Gramcko, 1975). Parental anxiety and potential psychologic problems for the child are reduced with earlier surgery. Functionless nubbins and the small floating thumb ("pouce flotant") are best eliminated before the child or parents become psychologically attached. Many have stated that the congenitally malformed hand represents a static situation wherein changes occur only with growth or surgery. Early surgical release of tight deforming structures may unlock potential growth and lessen progressive deformity.

The determination of the optimal time for correction of these varied hands also is guided in great part by the experience, knowledge, and special training of the surgeon (Eaton, 1967). Those who operate primarily upon children and perform microsurgery on a regular basis will feel more confident with smaller structures and will operate within the first year of life. Those who regularly reduce fractures, reconstruct ligaments, and perform osteotomies will be less tentative about early skeletal corrections. Those who work in rural regions or developing countries may need to wait and stage their procedures differently. The general condition of the patient and associated malformations will obviously influence decision-making. Correction of a congenital heart defect or gastrointestinal or genitourinary obstruction will take precedence over a hand anomaly, which is not life threatening. Severe mental retardation associated with impaired neurologic function may obviate any practical need for hand surgery.

There seems no urgency to operate on most congenital hand anomalies until growth has been sufficient to allow exacting surgery. Early release of tethering structures such as the radial club hand, central polysyndactylies, complex syndactylies, transverse phalanges, and cleft hands can be safely performed between six and 18 months. Other soft tissue releases of tight constriction rings and thumb-index web spaces can be done during the same period. Routine syndactyly release, polydactyly correction, and pollicizations are usually reserved for the second year of life. All major reconstructions should be completed by school age so that the deformity is the least source of ridicule by other children and so that maximum function can be achieved during the formative developmental period. Imbalance of major muscle-tendon units should be corrected early so that they will influence growth and proper skeletal alignment. Follow-up of all complex deformity patients is mandatory at least until patients reach skeletal maturity, and preferably into adulthood.

Occasionally, an adult presents for correction of a congenital anomaly to which he or she has adapted comfortably. The prime reason and primary motivation of such patients should be determined (Fig. 128–13A). Often, they have observed a very functional correction in one of their children or have changed to an occupation that requires new functional demands. Just as frequently, however, these adults may be displacing anxieties to their obvious deformity, and referral to a psychiatrist before any surgical recommendations are made may be justified (Fig. 128–13B).

FAILURES OF FORMATION

Transverse Absences

UPPER ARM

Clinical Presentation

Transverse absence at the upper arm level is, fortunately, rare, occurring in one in every 270,000 live births (Birch-Jensen, 1949). It has also been called terminal transverse defect (Frantz and O'Rahilly, 1961) and is occasionally seen in association with the constriction ring syndrome. The deformities are usually bilateral and have an autosomal recessive inheritance pattern with variable expression (Temtamy and McKusick, 1978). Children with these bilateral deformities become amazingly dextrous with their feet but

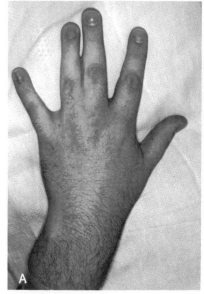
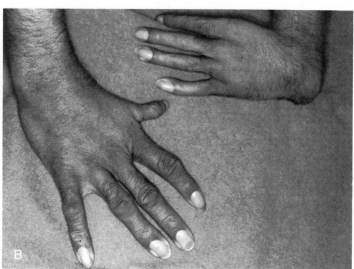

Figure 128–13. *A,* Correction of congenital deformities of the hand and forearm in adults may often be justified, as with the hand of a young man who was ineligible for induction into the Marine Corps unless he had his bilateral simple syndactyly corrected. *B,* In contrast, the motivation for correction was not as clear for the 58 year old man with severe radial dysplasia who had lived and worked as an engineer for many years. It is often helpful to request psychiatric evaluations in these patients.

are often embarrassed to use them in public settings. Although these patients can perform incredible tasks with their toes, other modes of prehension become important in later years, when their hips, knees, and ankles become less mobile. The amputation stump may have a variety of configurations but is usually bulbous and contains some useless rudimentary hand remnants. A deep dimple may be caused by attachment of these elements to what humerus is present. Remaining proximal parts of the limb are always hypoplastic, along with chest wall musculature attaching to the humerus. This arm amputation has the highest incidence of distal bone overgrowth, for which surgery may be necessary.

Treatment

Rarely is surgical intervention necessary. Indications for treatment are covered under "Phocomelia." See also Chapter 94 for a discussion of upper limb prostheses.

INTERCALATED "PHOCOMELIA"

Clinical Presentation

Phocomelia (seal limb) is distinguished from *amelia* (complete absence of the extrem-

ity at the shoulder level) by the presence in phocomelia of hand skeletal structures in which one or more digits may be missing but a functional terminal element is always present. There is always an intercalated loss of upper arm and forearm elements (Frantz, 1961; Smith and Lipke, 1979).

In most series, phocomelias are bilateral and account for 0.8 per cent of congenital limb deformities (Flatt, 1977). These deformities became widespread in Western Europe during the 1960's when the sedative thalidomide was taken (between the 38th and 45th days of gestation) by pregnant women (Taussig, 1962; Sulamaa and Ryoppy, 1964) (see Fig. 128–6).

The three basic types of phocomelia are determined by the intermediate segment (Fig. 128–14). In the most severe type, arm and forearm skeleton is missing, and the hand attaches directly to the shoulder. In the second type, the arm segment is deficient and the forearm-hand segment attaches directly to the shoulder; in the third, the forearm portion of the limb is absent, so that the hand attaches to the humerus (Swanson, 1965; Clippinger, Avery, and Titus, 1974). Arm, forearm, and hand segments are hypoplastic in the last two types, and a longitudinal radial or ulnar deficiency is also usually present (Kay and associates, 1974) (Fig. 128–15). Digital function varies tremendously and is achieved primarily with intrinsic muscles. Strength and function of these digits is rarely normal but is sufficient to manipulate shoulder or elbow locking mechanisms for control of myoelectric prostheses. Half of the West German thalidomide patients studied presented with upper limb deformities, and one-fourth with upper limb involvement; more than 10 per cent had congenital cardiac anomalies (Taussig, 1962; Fletcher, 1980). Some syndromes that the hand surgeon may see are Robert's syndrome, with four deficient limbs plus cleft lip or palate; the Holt-Oram syndrome, with congenital heart disease; and the adactyly-adontia syndrome, in which major proximal limb amputations may be present (Temtamy and McKusick, 1978).

Treatment

Phocomelia presents a problem primarily to the prosthetist and engineer, and the surgeon rarely intervenes (Aitkin and Frantz, 1960). Occasionally, digital function may be enhanced by a web release, rotational osteotomy, or tendon transfer (Kelikian, 1974). Lengthening of whatever humerus is present with and without bone grafts (Dick and Tietjen, 1978), removal of vestigial tags, mobilization of the clavicle (Taussig, 1962; Sulamaa and Ryoppy, 1964), and fibular transfer and

fusion to the glenoid may be beneficial for prosthetic fitting. Associated radial or ulnar deviation of the hand may require centralization. These techniques are discussed in other sections.

Amputation of hand remnants is rarely indicated, as the affected child can often use them to control a prosthetic terminal device. When phocomelic limbs can reach the mouth, prosthetic fitting is rarely indicated (Posner, 1985). The objective of any reconstructive surgery is to gain a motor end organ with sensation that will achieve maximum function. Malformations can be corrected at an early age so function can be optimized, as most of these children will achieve some degree of upper extremity function. When no hand is present (amelia), there is no surgical treatment.

The use of a prosthesis is less than ideal. If prosthetic wear is indicated, it is adviseable to start early in order to integrate the brain and functional development. The prosthesis, chosen from a wide variety of shoulder joints, elbow joints, and terminal devices available, must be individualized to the patient's age, size, opposite limb, and adaptation. Shoulder motion may be used to trigger elbow and finger motion within prostheses. Newer myoelectric devices amplify impulses from muscular contraction to do the same thing (Kadefors and Taylor, 1973). These larger prostheses are readily accepted by patients

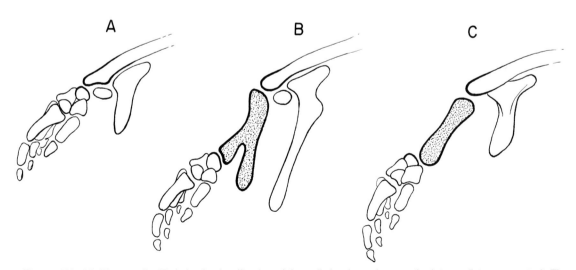

Figure 128–14. Phocomelia. The simple classification of these limbs depends upon the intermediate segment. *A,* The arm and forearm are absent as the hand attaches to the shoulder. *B,* A hypoplastic forearm attaches to the shoulder. *C,* The forearm segment is absent. In all types, the remaining portions of the limb are never normal, and treatment must be carefully individualized to specific functional needs.

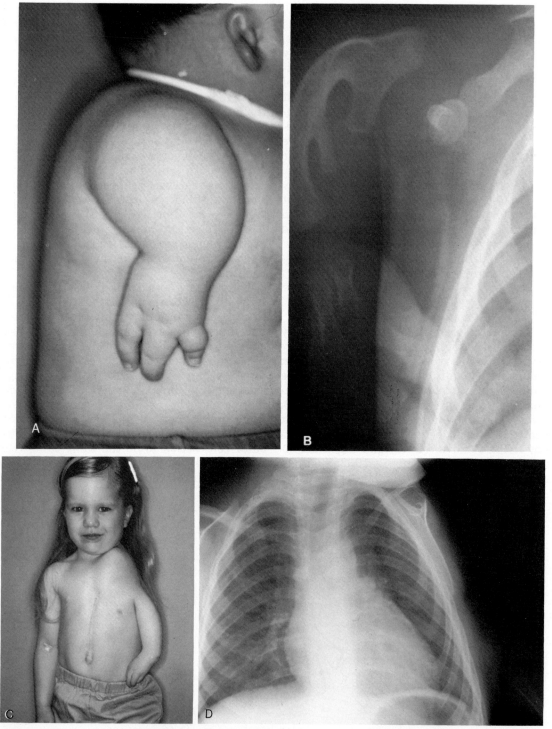

Figure 128–15. *A, B,* Presentation in the most common type of phocomelia is hand and hypoplastic forearm attaching at the shoulder level. Hypoplastic thumb, index, and long fingers are present. A child with this deformity has difficulty getting objects to the mouth because the deformity is bilateral and the profound ulnar failure of formation positions the limb posteriorly. Digital flexion and extension are present. *C and D,* The very unusual intercalated total absence of the humerus is demonstrated. A rudimentary scapula is present. This child has a floating forearm and hand with absence of the radius, thumb, and index fingers. She uses this limb as a helper in balancing, grasping, and hooking maneuvers. No surgery has been performed, but splinting and stretching of the wrist have continued since birth. Recommendations for vascularized bone reconstruction of the humerus will be deferred until she is older. She may ultimately need no surgery.

and playmates as soon as curiosity is overcome. As long as these limbs are painless, functional, durable, and within the "gadget tolerance" of the patient and family, they are tolerated well. The principle of sensory feedback between a terminal device and an implanted electrode within a major nerve has been introduced; though appealing, it is not clinically predictable at this time (Clippinger, Avery, and Titus, 1974).

FOREARM

Clinical Presentation

Transverse absence at the forearm level is more common, having a frequency of one in 20,000 (Birch-Jensen, 1949). It is more frequently found in females than males by a ratio of 3:2, most often involves the left side, and rarely is bilateral. Sex distribution is equal in transverse absence of the forearm associated with the constriction ring syndrome, which does not usually occur bilaterally. Subluxation of the proximal radioulnar joint and radial head dislocation are common, and elbow flexion greater than 100 degrees is usually present with normal shoulder musculature.

The cause of these malformations is unknown. Most are thought to occur sporadically. Growth of the forearm portion of the limb is usually decreased, rarely exceeding 10 cm (Marquardt, 1981). Most malformations occur in the proximal one-third of the forearm. Vestigial bulbous remnants and deep dimples connecting skin to fibrous anlages are often present in the ends of these stumps. Rarely are well-developed hand structures present.

Treatment

Surgery is indicated in less than 10 per cent of patients with transverse absence of the forearm. Stump revision in the form of excision of functionless nubbins, recontouring of bulbous skin folds, and elimination of deep dimples make initial prosthetic fitting easier but are not absolute requisites. Soft tissue deepening of the axillary web may facilitate fixation of the stump socket. Very infrequently, lengthening of a humeral stump using a sliding osteotomy may be indicated (Dick, 1978). In patients with transverse amputations at the elbow level, humeral overgrowth is common. Stump capping with au-

togenous cartilage may be useful to avoid overgrowth (Marquardt, 1981). Angulation osteotomies have been advocated in selected cases to provide a 20 to 45 degree flexion at the elbow (Marquardt, 1981; Pellicore and Lambert, 1981). Stump lengthening with bone grafts and tube pedicle flaps have produced an unpredictable amount of resorption, and vascularized bone transfers have not been described as having been attempted in these patients, primarily because it is much easier to revise a prosthesis than to operate upon a patient. Treatment of the below elbow transverse amputation is a problem for the prosthetist.

One option for the patient with bilateral amputations below the elbow or at the wrist is the Krukenberg (1917) procedure, in which a prehensile pincer is created by separating the radius and the ulna (Sung, 1957; Nathan and Trung, 1977; Chan and associates, 1984). With pronation, the two forearm bones adduct, and an adult with a Krukenberg arm can hold objects weighing up to 10 kg. With supination the two limbs of the pincer abduct as much as 45 degrees. The best candidates for this operation are those with bilateral absence of the hand, particularly in regions of the world where prostheses are not available, and blind patients, who require constant sensory feedback for use of the extremity. Clinical reports on results of the Krukenberg procedure have described very few congenital amputees, focusing primarily upon adults with bilateral traumatic amputations in Southeast Asia and other countries where machete accidents are common. Chan and colleagues' (1984) report of eight procedures for unilateral congenital amputees indicates that there may be a place for this operation, but most children do not have long enough forearm stumps for the procedure. Sighted children with unilateral deformities (and their parents) find the pincer functional but so unattractive and conspicuous that they reject its use in public. The Krukenberg arm is also compatible with prosthetic wear when desired.

Prosthetic Fitting

Early prosthetic fitting is the treatment of choice in patients with congenital absence of the forearm. (Aitken, 1964, 1972; Murray, Shore, and Trefler, 1972). The timing of the initial fitting has changed dramatically in the past ten years (MacDonell, 1958). Most centers now recommend fitting below elbow amputees with a smooth plastic mitten or paddle at 6 months of age so they can crawl, balance, and grasp with both extremities (Fig. 128–16). Early fitting and wear avoid substitution patterns, and sensory stimulation at the stump-prosthesis interface will stimulate visual cues (Pellicore and Lambert, 1981). At 18 to 24 months of age, a hook is added to the terminal device, and the child is taught to control it with a shoulder harness. More sophisticated myoelectric prostheses are now being introduced for children between 3 and 6 years of age (Marquardt, 1965; Sorbye, 1980). Impulses from contracting muscles are amplified by skin electrodes to motor these devices, which provide a basic key pinch between thumb and index fingers. Technologic improvements in the design and function of these prostheses are beginning to increase exponentially (Lamb, 1983; Lamb and Law, 1987).

The child with unilateral arm or forearm amputation is an unpredictable user of a prosthesis, tending instead to use the deficient limb as a helper for support and hook activities. The normal limb, both of necessity and with development, becomes stronger, more dextrous, and adaptable. Prosthetic wear is worthwhile for restoration of bimanual function. It is important to encourage the child to use prosthesis, which may improve function; its continued use is ultimately determined by the patient, however, and not by an enthusiastic surgeon, therapist, or parent.

Continual retraining and refitting is mandatory in these children so that the device will become fully integrated into the child's activities of daily living and body image. Prosthetic acceptance is directly related to parental acceptance and participation in the prosthesis program (Laboriel and Setoguchi, 1981). The prosthetic goals should be restoration of optimal function, cosmetic effect, and comfort. One of the greatest pitfalls has been to "overgadget" these devices in children, who will provide the ultimate test for the most durable biomaterials. The child's prosthetic needs are most concerned with durability and adaptability. The other problems in childhood amputees are prosthetic training and occasional psychologic difficulties.

The psychologic concern about the limb absence deformity becomes a very real problem for most adolescents who have adapted well with or without a prosthesis. Counseling and open discussion with these children should be encouraged.

As a member of a prosthetic team, the surgeon must realize that the patient's acceptance of and willingness to wear a prosthesis may at times be difficult and unpredictable. These children should be fitted only when necessary, and care should be taken not to make patient acceptance a focal point of family life (Murray, Shore, and Trefler, 1972). Those working with such children are referred to the *Atlas of Limb Prosthetics* sponsored by the American Academy of Orthopedic Surgery.

CARPAL AND METACARPAL

Clinical Presentation

Transverse amputation of the hand at the wrist level (*acheira*) or at the metacarpal level (*adactyly*) may be complete or incomplete. There may be motion of the radiocarpal joint through well-formed extrinsic flexor and extensor tendons present in the forearm. Other portions of the limb are often hypoplastic. These deformities may present in a wide variety of clinical patterns: as a true transverse absence, as part of a cleft hand, as localized amputations within the constriction ring syndrome, and as symbrachydactyly (Lister, 1984). Theoretically, the presence of a hypoplastic nubbin with a small nail remnant in symbrachydactyly discounts this anomaly as a true transverse amputation. Most of these incomplete limbs contain vestigial hypoplastic nubbins with or without miniature nail remnants. The dimpling or retraction of this tissue is indicative of present but usually abnormal extrinsic flexor and extensor tendons, which lie in normal position over the carpal and metacarpal portions of the hand and insert into the hypoplastic nubbins. Grasping and pulling on the soft tissue nubbins will give the examiner some indication of the size of the skin envelope and the strength of the tendons. Radiographs are of limited predictive value early in life, because the hypoplastic skeletal parts are not ossified. Congenital carpal and metacarpal amputations are usually unilateral and are not commonly associated with other malformations.

Treatment

Vestigial nubbins without underlying skeletal elements and with no functional poten-

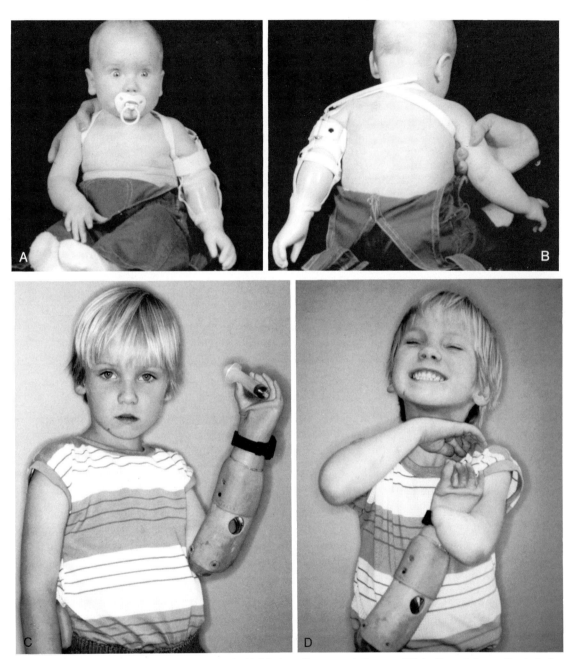

Figure 128–16. *A, B,* The child with a congenital left below elbow amputation was fitted with a static prosthesis before 1 year of age, once he could sit and had good trunk and shoulder control. The primary goal is sensorimotor acceptance of the prosthesis. Parents were very cooperative and encouraged the child to use the prosthesis, which was converted to a myoelectric device when he was 5 years old. *C,* At age 6 years, he wears the prosthesis at least 12 hours per day and functions very well at school. He has learned to wear the device when faced with fine prehension tasks! *D,* Because children are rambunctious, the materials used in construction must be durable and fitting, and readjustment service capabilities must be available.

tial should be excised early in life, before they become bizarre objects of curiosity and of psychologic attachment for both parent and child. Most authors agree that removal of the nubbins "removes the stigma of congenitalism" and makes a more acceptable deformity that appears to be the result of trauma (Flatt, 1977; Hentz and Littler, 1977).

Treatment options for the carpal hand are difficult because the child adaptively uses the flexible wrist as a hook and manages to hold objects against the torso as a paddle. Prosthetic fitting may be not only unnecessary but also contraindicated because the prosthesis may interfere with normal sensory feedback between the sensate stump and the external environment.

When a mobile wrist is present, a palmar plate prosthesis may provide a post against which the child may grasp and pick up and hold objects (Lamb and Kuczynski, 1981). Many children develop two point discrimination that is better than normal on both dorsal and palmar surfaces (Lister, 1984) (Fig. 128–17). After 2 years of age, the CAPP multipositional part may be strapped to the distal forearm and adjusted to various positions for functional purposes. When not in use it can be folded back up against the forearm (Posner, 1985) (Fig. 128–17). The size and length of the carpus can be increased by bone grafts beneath the often redundant soft tissue on the end of the extremity. Distraction techniques and bone grafting at the carpal level to increase the amount of contact surface may be considered.

If metacarpal elements are present distal to the carpals, reconstructive possibilities increase dramatically, and the need for prostheses almost disappears. The goal should be to create a "basic hand" that is more functional than a prosthesis and that contains, by definition, (1) a mobile ray on the radial side, (2) a cleft, and (3) a post or at least one additional mobile ray on the opposite side of the hand (Entin, 1959). This is a realistic approach, because often the first and fifth metacarpals are commonly present in this type of transverse deficiency. The presence of a joint at the base of the thumb metacarpal and of thenar intrinsic muscles is the most critical factor in this reconstruction. Many workers believe that the unilateral deformity does not require reconstruction (Dobyns, 1982). The decision to perform any reconstruction requires careful evaluation, counseling, and planning.

Every deformity is different, and there are many reconstructive possibilities. These should be carefully evaluated and discussed with parents, who should be urged to articulate their desires and questions. In few other areas of congenital hand surgery are the reconstruction options so great.

Web Deepening. Older methods of deepening the cleft to create a pincer mechanism between metacarpal remnants, or "phalangealization," will probably decrease in popularity as newer methods of distraction lengthening become available. Dorsal flaps are used to line the base of the commissure, and skin grafts are usually needed (Kelikian, 1974). The major problem with deepening webs to create a pincer between metacarpals is injury to intrinsic muscles, particularly within the thumb-index web space.

Metacarpal Transposition. Transfer of metacarpal remnants from the central portion of the hand to the border serves to lengthen an existing border ray or to deepen the central cleft. Consideration must be given to this procedure before any hypoplastic metacarpals with potential usefulness are discarded. The soft tissue may be lengthened by distraction techniques or with a combination of local flaps and grafts (Buck-Gramcko, 1981).

Phalangeal Transfer. The nonvascularized transfer of the proximal phalangeal segments of toes may be useful to fill floppy soft tissue masses that have attached extrinsic tendons. The presence of these muscle tendon units can be seen by deep retraction of distal skin dimples at the end of amputation stumps. When toes are used to fill abundant and redundant soft tissue nubbins distal to hypoplastic metacarpals, remarkable improvement in function can be achieved, particularly with the thumb (Fig. 128–18). The reported success of this procedure varies from no growth in 159 phalanges transferred without periosteum (Carroll and Green, 1975) to 90 per cent growth in 20 of 27 phalanges that were transferred with intact periosteum and collateral ligaments, which were then attached to skeletal elements (Goldberg and Watson, 1982). Most authors agree that considerable resorption occurs when the toe segment is transferred as a free floating segment within a soft tissue tube. Even if the epiphysis remains open and growth occurs, the maximal length gained is not great, owing to the disproportionate sizes of the toe and digital phalanges. Others suggest that these free,

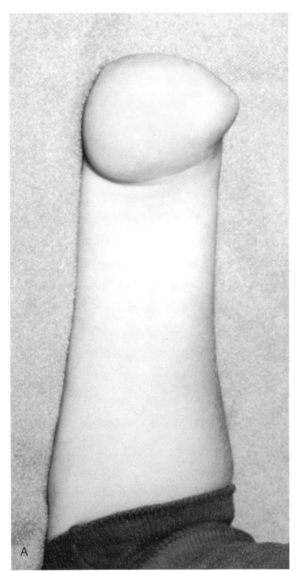

Figure 128–17. The patient with a transverse deficiency at the carpal level with good wrist motion *(A)* usually functions extremely well, but may benefit from a simple palmar plate prosthesis *(B)*, which can be worn and adjusted for specific functional needs. Two-point discrimination in these palms is more acute than in the normal palm. *C,* The CAPP device allows positioning of the palmar plate.

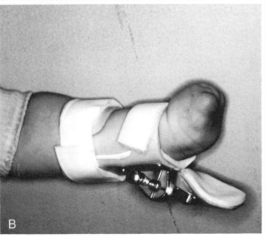

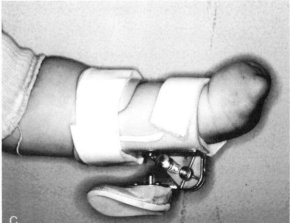

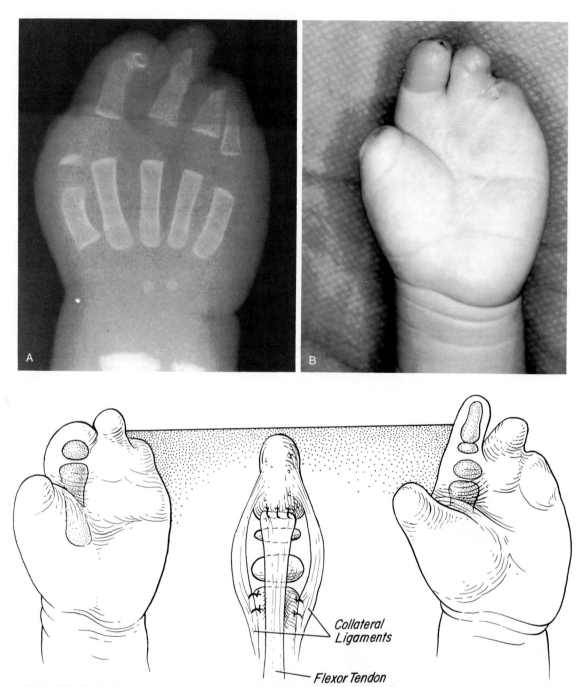

Figure 128–18. *A, B,* Appearance of the hand and radiograph of a child born with the constriction ring syndrome. Distal soft tissue bands (acrosyndactyly) between the hypoplastic index and long fingers were released in the newborn nursery. Both thumbs and index tips were unstable. *C,* Schematic drawing of the phalangeal transfer "on top" of the existing proximal phalanx with attachment of extrinsic flexor and extensor tendons and collateral ligament segments into periosteum.

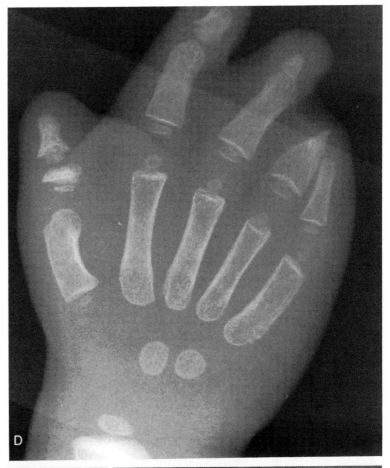

Figure 128–18 *Continued D, E, and F,* Eighteen months later, the child retains stability and has developed a strong grasp on this (her best) hand. Nonvascularized toe phalanges have been placed upon the thumb and index fingers. Radiograph shows that the epiphysis is open. The total growth over the next 15 years is not predictable.

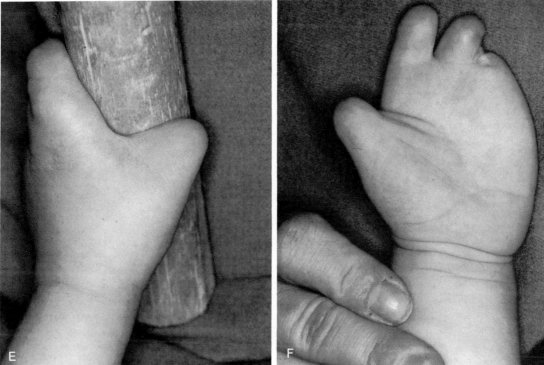

nonvascularized transfers both stimulate adjacent bone growth and are incorporated more effectively when they are attached to bone or used as interpositional grafts (Rank, 1978) (Fig. 128–18C). In the future these phalangeal transfers will be used in conjunction with skeletal distraction methods.

The technique most authors prefer involves removal of the third and fourth toe proximal phalanges through zigzag dorsal incisions. Other surgeons prefer the second toe phalanx because of its size. The collateral ligaments, capsule, and volar (palmar) plate may be retained with periosteum and attached to the hypoplastic metacarpal head. The articular cartilage may be shaved on opposing surfaces if no pseudojoint function is desired. Flexor and extensor tendons may be attached to the transferred segment. Internal fixation of the phalanx may result in a premature closure of the central portion of the transferred physis (Rank, 1978), and stabilization can be maintained with extraosseous pins. The donor toe will predictably retract and will not have as much stability as its neighbors, but gait will not be altered. This issue is of prime importance to parents and must be explained thoroughly (Lipton, May, and Simon, 1987).

Metacarpal Distraction Lengthening. If enough metacarpal bone is present, satisfactory length can be achieved using distraction methods (see Fig. 128–20). The initial application of this technique was described by Codvilla (1905) for use in the lower limb, and much later, Matev (1975, 1985) introduced it to the upper extremity for the correction of post-traumatic thumb deformities. Matev and others have subsequently applied this method to congenital hand malformations (Kessler, Baruch, and Hecht, 1977; Cowen and Loftus, 1978; Smith and Gumley, 1985). The procedure is quite useful in clinical situations where increased length of a border ray is required, or when an opposition post should be created in a hand with no digits and a hypoplastic thumb. Most authors wait until the patient is 5 years of age to perform these staged procedures. Distraction can be done earlier if enough bone stock is present to avoid damage to growth centers.

Technique of Distraction. The distraction apparatuses that are available commercially consist of metal blocks that attach to a longitudinal screw mechanism on either side of the bone to be lengthened. Turning the screw knobs clockwise will increase or decrease the interval distance 0.5 to 0.6 mm for each complete 360 degree turn (Fig. 128–19). In the first stage of this reconstruction, the site of metacarpal osteotomy is selected, in the widest portion of the bone at a sufficient distance from the growth plate. Two or three small (0.28 or 0.35 mm) wires are passed transversely through the bone on either side of the planned osteotomy site. The holes within the metal blocks can be used as a drill guide. A dorsal incision is made, the extensor mechanism retracted, the periosteum *incised* transversely, and the osteotomy completed. Direct observation of pin placement will prevent penetration of digital nerves or flexor tendons. The complete apparatus is assembled and stabilized with malleable struts connecting the block on either side of the hand or digit. In Matev's (1975) original work on the thumb, the periosteum was not incised, and bone formation by creeping substitution occurred as the distractor was left on for several months. Owing to the unpredictable quality of this bone (Ulitsky and Malygin, 1974; Mulliken and Curtis, 1980), most authors prefer to insert a bone graft once satisfactory length has been achieved. The skin is closed and a protective splint is applied.

The lengthening is started several days later and proceeds at about one and one-half to two complete revolutions per day. Distraction is stopped temporarily if there is any sign of vascular compromise or skin irritation, or significant pain. The hand in a young child should be protected with a splint or bulky dressing. Parents can do the distracting at home by turning the screw knobs, which should all be marked with a reference point. At weekly intervals the amount of distraction is measured radiographically. Most metacarpal distractions are completed within 4 to 5 weeks and the child is admitted to the hospital for the second stage, a bone graft procedure.

Although autogenous donor sites from iliac crest or fibula are preferred, allografts (Smith and Gumley, 1985) and demineralized bone implants (Upton and associates, 1983) have been useful. Nonfunctional skeletal segments within the hand may serve as bone graft donor sites, particularly at the metacarpal level in the cleft hand/foot and the constriction ring syndromes. Grafts are fixed with either interosseous wires or, preferably, longitudinal C wires. In selected cases, the lengthened segment may be transposed onto

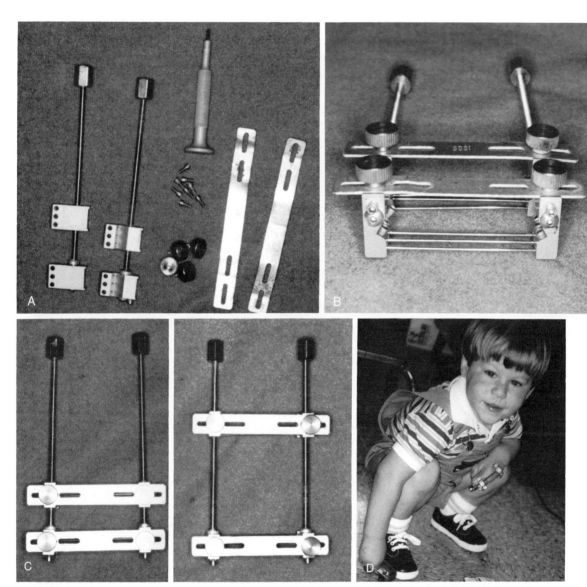

Figure 128–19. Distraction. *A,* The basic components of most commercially available distraction apparatuses include two side pieces and crossbars with screws. The small screws for fixation of the transverse wires and especially the special hexagonal wrench are the items that are most commonly "lost." *B,* The assembled apparatus. Some designs contain a lock screw that will secure position when not being turned. If lock screws are positioned inside during distraction, the child will be less likely to play with them. *C,* The device in shortened and lengthened positions. One-and-one-half turns in a clockwise direction will lengthen the device by approximately 1.0 mm. *D,* Children tolerate and protect the attached distractors quite well, but their siblings and playmates do not and usually are the cause of breakage problems.

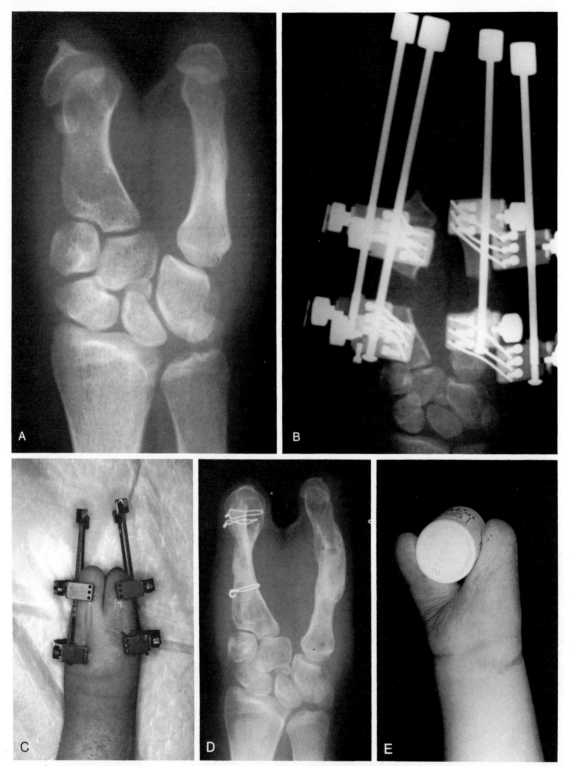

Figure 128–20. *A,* Radiograph of a metacarpal hand in a young teenaged girl with the constriction ring syndrome. A below elbow amputation was present on the other arm, and all toes were absent from both feet. *B,* Osteotomies have been performed and distraction apparatuses attached to both metacarpals. A 1.0 cm gap is present four days after operation. *C,* Appearance of the hand several weeks later shows an area of skin tightness between the pins. *D,* Four weeks later, autogenous iliac crest bone grafts have been used to fill the intercalated gaps. Interosseus wire fixation incorporated C wire holes. *E,* Following web deepening, the patient developed excellent pincer function, and she now works as a microbiology technician.

an adjacent ray (Dobyns, 1982). In appropriate cases, adjacent metacarpals may also be inserted into the distracted segment as vascularized bone grafts. The transverse pins and apparatus are removed, and the extremity is immobilized in a cast.

Significant amounts of lengthening can be achieved within short periods. Usually only 30 to 40 mm of length is required at the metacarpal level, but up to 80 mm has been reported. Intrinsic muscles cannot be rapidly stretched more than 75 per cent of their resting length (Matev, 1985). Skin and neurovascular bundles tolerate the 1.0 to 1.5 mm daily expansion quite well. In patients with previous surgery and scar formation adjacent to the bone to be distracted, especially in the first web space, the contracture should be released before distraction is performed.

Complications can occur early and late; careful vigilance over these children is required. Active children will invariably bump and break a portion of the apparatus if they discard the protective splints. An inventory of spare parts is, therefore, necessary. Pin tract irritation, skin blanching, a tight ridge between pins across the distraction site, and neurovascular compromise are best treated by stopping the distraction for a few days. Skin maceration can occur if the metal blocks of the apparatus are too close to adjacent skin surfaces. Possible late problems include contracture of joints distal to the distracted segment, intrinsic muscle fibrosis, and nonunion of the bone graft to the distal distracted segment. Infections are often related to soft tissue loss and skeletal extrusion associated with too rapid distraction.

Bone Grafting. Often an abundant amount of soft tissue is present beyond the hypoplastic metacarpal remnants. Insertion of autogenous bone grafts will transform the floppy palm or digital remnant into a rigid functional post with sensation. At a later date this post either can be augmented with distraction methods or can serve as the foundation for a phalangeal reconstruction. Primary autogenous bone grafting to increase length at the digital level often results in significant graft resorption (Fig. 128–21). Occasionally, a local flap can be combined with a bone graft to create functional border rays in the hypoplastic hand (Reid, 1980; Lister, 1984).

Vascularized Toe to Hand Transfer. The most elaborate reconstruction for the missing digit would be the toe to hand transfer. As with distraction methods, these techniques were initially developed for post-traumatic defects, and many have applied them to the hypoplastic hand with no digits or thumb (O'Brien and associates, 1978; May, Smith, and Peimer, 1981; Gilbert, 1982). The prime indication would be the thumb that has a carpometacarpal joint but no phalangeal segments. The technique and results of toe transfer are discussed in Chapter 125. The major disadvantages of toe transfers are limitation of flexion arc and motion, and appearance. Gait alterations in the donor site have not been reported as being significant (Lipton, 1987), but some authors with extensive experience have raised doubts about such functions as running and walking on upwardly inclined surfaces (Leung, 1982, 1985).

Transfer of the great or second toe is often more difficult in young children, and the predictability of function is much less than with a post-traumatic deformity because of the underdevelopment of necessary muscle tendon units in the forearm. Typically, broad sheets of tendon attached to a common muscle mass are found in the dorsal and palmar forearm. Median and ulnar nerves are often so rudimentary that toe digital nerves must be joined to cutaneous branches at the carpal level (Gilbert, 1982). The major exception to the rule is the constriction ring syndrome, in which most of the normal anatomic structures are present and well differentiated in the forearm and up to the level of constriction. The results of these transfers at the proximal phalangeal level can be esthetically quite natural looking.

PHALANGEAL

Clinical Presentation

Transverse arrest in development at the digital level runs the whole gamut of variations. These amputations are not as common as the hypoplastic digit and are often classified as variants of the longitudinal deficiencies: radial, central, or ulnar. The greatest number of isolated or multiple digit amputations is seen in the constriction ring syndrome, in which all fingers and thumb may be involved alone or in combination at any phalangeal level. Often the hand and occasionally the forearm are hypoplastic.

Length and bulk are usually the presenting problems, although abnormalities in align-

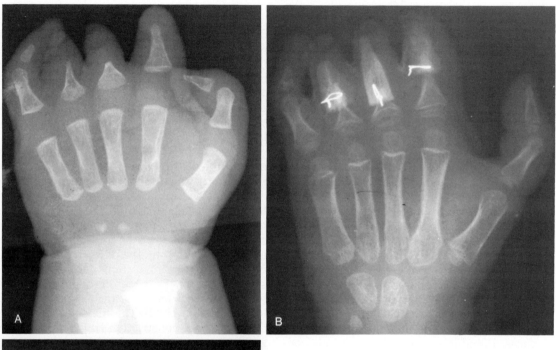

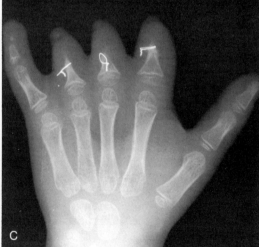

Figure 128–21. Nonvascularized autogenous bone grafting for augmentation of phalangeal length is disappointing, as illustrated by this hand with the constriction ring syndrome. The preoperative condition *(A)* and immediate postoperative result *(B)* is contracted, with total absorption of the grafts seen four years later *(C)*. Direct toe phalangeal transfers, metacarpal distraction, or later microvascular toe transfers are more satisfactory considerations for treatment.

ment, mobility, and stability may also be present. Bulbous lymphedematous soft tissue masses may be present in the constriction ring syndrome (see later discussion). The radiographic and clinical evaluations are good indicators of what structures are anatomically present. Terminal phalanges in this syndrome characteristically show a trumpet appearance, broad at the base and narrow at the distal tip. Extrinsic and intrinsic muscle tendon units usually accompany a well-formed proximal phalanx. Often, all normal structures are present up to the level of the transverse arrest. This is in contrast to the severely hypoplastic digit, in which many structures may be present but abnormal.

Treatment

Reconstruction is often beneficial and must always be considered in the context of the existing hand malformations. When the level of arrest is in the proximal half of the proximal phalangeal segment, nonvascularized phalangeal transfers or metacarpal distraction may be considered, especially if multiple digits and/or the thumb is abnormal. Microvascular toe transfers may be a reasonable functional and esthetic option but are often unacceptable to young parents. In selected cases, complete and partial toe transfer may be indicated (Gilbert, 1985). Enthusiasm for such an operation will be much less with congenital than with post-traumatic deformities. The functional gain with excessive web deepening or phalangization of the thumb is usually limited. Pollicization of a finger, partial ray ablation to create a web space, or the shifting of bone segments from one ray to another may be indicated. When the majority of the proximal phalanx is present, function is usually excellent and lengthening rarely required.

Distraction methods have been used at this level with a lesser degree of predictability, particularly when hypoplastic phalanges are being manipulated. Pin tract infections and nonunion of the distal distracted fragment are the primary complications of digital distraction, which, although restoring length to the finger, does not provide normal circumferential width or, of course, interphalangeal joint motion.

Partial or total finger prostheses are available commercially but are not consistently used by children, who prefer the shorter working surface with sensation. Protheses are also easily lost, damaged, and discolored by active children. Adolescents will wear them for social occasions. In contrast, a partial hand prosthesis may be advisable for the older child or adolescent with multiple digit amputations and a normal thumb.

Longitudinal Absences

PREAXIAL (RADIAL)

Partial or complete absence of structures on the preaxial side of the limb constitutes the deformities often referred to as the radial deficiencies. Deficiencies may vary from minor abnormalities of the thenar muscles to complete absence of all preaxial structures as well as anomalies involving the upper arm and brachial plexus. Although this is considered a preaxial affliction, the ulna on the postaxial side is never normal in severe cases, as neurovascular and skeletal deficiencies are more pronounced with severity of the deformities. The most common presentation is a present but short radius, absence of scaphoid and trapezium, and total absence or hypoplasia of the thumb, all of which combine to give the appearance of the deviated "radial club hand" (Flatt, 1977). Because of lack of radial support, the hand and wrist deviate toward the side of the deficiency. Elbow stiffness, which is marked within the first few years of life, may improve with time and is an important consideration in the planning of later surgical treatment (Lamb, 1977).

There is no clear etiology—genetic, environmental, or other—for these deformities. Associated malformations are common, and many patients have recognizable malformation syndromes. Autosomal dominant genetic association has been recognized (Forbes, 1938; Goldenberg, 1948). Most cases do not have recognizable genetic causes; other factors such as environment, irradiation, viral infections, and drugs, including thalidomide, have been implicated. The deformity has been produced in chick embryos by Duraiswami (1952), who cauterized preaxial portions of the limb bud.

The incidence of radial deficiencies is approximately one in every 100,000 live births, and the "club hand" posture occurs bilaterally about as frequently as unilaterally. If one looks carefully in unilateral cases, some form of hypoplasia can usually be found in the opposite extremity (Forbes, 1938; Lamb, 1977; Bayne and Klug, 1987). The severity of the hand abnormality may not be related to the amount of radial absence, which directly determines the degree of radial deviation and the extent of soft tissue deficiencies (Skerik and Flatt, 1969; Flatt, 1977).

Associated defects are particularly common with bilateral radial deficiencies. The limb anomaly may be considered by the hand surgeon to be a symptom of another underlying defect, which occurs in 40 per cent of unilateral and 77 per cent of bilateral cases; possible defects are congenital heart disease (approximately 25 per cent); pulmonary hypoplasia; and genitourinary, gastrointestinal, hematologic, and other musculoskeletal anomalies (Goldberg and Bartoshesky, 1985; Lin and Perloff, 1985). Of these, only the anemias are not present at birth, occurring later in childhood. Syndromes most commonly associated with radial defects include: the VATERR association (vertebral anomalies, anal atresia, tracheoesophageal fistula, renal and radial abnormalities) (Quan and Smith, 1973), the Holt-Oram syndrome (Holt and Oram, 1960; Lin, 1985), the ventriculoradial dysplasia syndrome (Carroll and Louis, 1974), thrombocytopenia–absent radius (TAR) syndrome (Hall and associates, 1969; Sheppard, 1982; Hays, Bartoshesky, and Feingold, 1982), Fanconi's pancytopenia or syndrome (Gmyrek and Sullum-Rapopoa, 1964; Fanconi, 1967), and the Najar–acrofacial dysostoses syndrome (Smith, 1982). The most common cardiac defects seen are atrial septal defect (ASD) and ventriculoseptal defects (VSD), but more severe anomalies, such as tetralogy of Fallot, aortic coarctation, transposition of the great vessels, and valvular anomalies, can also occur.

Clinical Presentation

The clinical picture of a child with severe deficiencies consists of a youngster who uses both hands to perform a single task. Many two-handed activities cannot be done, and individually handed tasks are very difficult with severe thumb deficiencies. The unsupported hand and carpus are deviated, and the wrist is often unstable.

Passive motion is markedly reduced in severe deformities in both palmar flexion and dorsiflexion. The power of the deforming forces is often reflected by the amount of passive correction with manipulation. With ulnar deviation, there is a paucity of soft tissue on the radial side and a redundancy on the ulnar side. The bump in the distal forearm is the ulna. The tightest soft tissue structures on the radial side are flexor carpi radialis (if present), median nerve, and a fibrous anlage in the place of the deficient radius (see Fig. 128–25).

The thumb may be absent, hypoplastic, or rudimentary and connected by a soft tissue bridge with no skeletal support (often called "pouce flotant" by the French and "floating thumb" by the English). Digital hypoplasia with stiffness is more common in the index and long fingers than in the ring and small fingers. Poor range of motion is often heralded by the lack of flexion and extension creases. The primary cause of this stiffness is not known to be intrinsic to the joint or muscle tendon units. Instead of being well differentiated, flexor and extensor muscles and tendons are often found in large sheets or bands in the forearm (Skerik and Flatt, 1969). Tendon excursion and power vary in direct relation to the severity of the deformity and the amount of wrist instability (Riordan, 1963).

Classification

Skeletal size of the radius offers a practical method for classifying these deformities (O'Rahilly, 1951; Heikel, 1959; Bayne and Klug, 1987) (Fig. 128–22). There is a direct relationship between the radial deficiency and the clinical deformity. Because the hand deformities associated with radial dysplasia are covered in Chapter 123, they are not discussed here in detail. Early correction or adjustment of arm, elbow, and wrist deformities must be carefully evaluated before thumb construction is undertaken. Carpal abnormalities, particularly of the trapezium, scaphoid, and lunate, parallel the thumb, index, and long finger deficiencies.

Type I: Short Radius. Support of the hand and wrist is adequate, but there is a growth deficiency of the proximal or distal radial epiphyses. There is no radial bowing and little deviation of the hand and wrist; the elbow is normal. No treatment is necessary for the forearm. Function is good, and surgical procedures are confined to the aplastic or hypoplastic thumb (see Chapter 123).

Type II: Hypoplastic Radius. In this unusual variant, the radius is short owing to

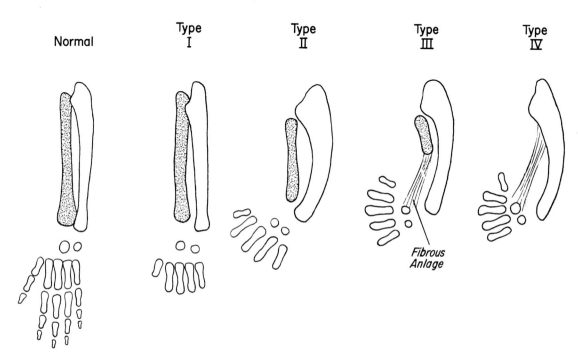

Figure 128–22. The classification of longitudinal preaxial radial deficiencies parallel the skeletal abnormalities. In Type I, there is a growth deficiency in the proximal or distal radius, no bowing, and little deviation of the hand and wrist. In the more unusual Type II variant, the radius is short owing to a more profound growth disturbance; the hand is deviated at the distal ulna, which may be thickened and bowed. In Type III, the most common type, a portion of the radius is present, the hand and carpus are deviated, and the ulna is thickened and bowed as it is pulled "like a fiber glass fishing pole" in a radial deviation by the tight fibrous anlage. The amount of radius absent varies, as do the carpal and thumb deficiencies. In the most severe Type IV abnormalities, the radius is completely absent, the wrist and hand are usually subluxed and deviated over the distal ulna, the ulna is bowed, and the elbow joint is usually deficient.

abnormal growth in both proximal and distal epiphyses and presents as a radius "in miniature" (Bayne, 1982). The hand is deviated, and the ulna is thick and often bowed toward the radial side. The thumb ray and its carpals are usually deficient. Hand deviation can be controlled with splinting, and later, radial shortness can be corrected with distraction and bone grafting.

Type III: Partial Absence of the Radius. Absence or hypoplasia of the middle and distal thirds of the radius is the most common deformity in most series. The ulna is bowed, and deviation of the hand varies from moderate to extreme, depending on the length of the radius. The hand usually lies in a pronated, flexed, and radially deviated position. The thumb ray and carpals are usually deficient. The ulnar two digits are the most normal. A fibrous band or anlage is usually found in place of the deficient distal radius and contributes to bowing of the ulna (see Fig. 128–22). Abnormalities in muscles, tendons, nerves, and major arteries vary tremendously but usually correspond closely to the degree of skeletal deficiency. Blauth and Schmidt (1969) and Heikel (1959) have noted that deficient but present structures tend to course radially at the distal end of the ulna. The radial nerve usually ends at the elbow, and the median nerve substitute supplies the radial side of the existing hand. At surgery this latter nerve is often thickened and may provide an unyielding obstacle to total passive correction of the wrist and hand. The ulnar nerve and artery are in their normal locations.

In severe cases, preaxial flexor and extensor muscles and tendons are deficient; abnormalities in muscle, skeleton, nerves, and vessels may extend up to the shoulder level. The radial artery is usually absent. Review of excellent descriptions of abnormal anatomy by Flatt (1977) and others is recommended and is almost mandatory before one contemplates approaching these deformities surgically (Stoffel and Stempel, 1909; Skerik and Flatt, 1969). Some type of centralization procedure is needed to improve hand function in affected patients.

Type IV: Total Absence of the Radius. The second most common presentation in the author's patients, total absence of the radius, demonstrates all the anatomic characteristics of the severe form of partial absence. The wrist is deviated and subluxed over the distal ulna. If it is left alone, a pseudoarthrosis develops with the distal ulna (Fig. 128–23). The radial structures of the hand are deficient but may not *all* be severely deformed. Elbow motion is restricted. The ulna is bowed and will never achieve its normal growth (Lamb, 1977). Aggressive soft tissue release with centralization is the most common form of treatment. Hand anomalies increase from the ulnar to the radial side. Index and long fingers rarely have normal range of motion and intrinsic tendons.

Treatment

Treatment depends upon the severity of the deformity, associated malformations, and functional deficits (Bayne, 1982). Surgical correction often presents the conflict between the need for cosmetic acceptance versus the risk of functional loss. Patients who should not be treated include older persons who have adapted well, patients with minimal deformities, patients with malformations incompatible with a long life, patients who lack adequate elbow flexion, and patients with severe tightness of neurovascular structures, which would prevent centralization of the hand and wrist. Surgical correction for the aplastic and hypoplastic thumb is covered in Chapter 123.

Timing of procedures varies, and more than one is usually needed for these deficient limbs. All clinicians ideally start *splinting* and *passive stretching* of all severe deformities in the newborn nursery. The use of serial casts or Aquaplast splints can aid a remarkable correction if started early but must be considered secondary in importance to passive manipulation of both wrist and elbow by the parents. Passive maneuvers of the carpus and hand should include stretching the hand out of a flexed-pronated position while maintaining axial traction. Static orthoplast splints or a ratchet-type device may be used with appropriate passive stretching exercises (Lamb, 1977). If serial casts are used, they must extend proximal to the flexed elbow to be effective and to maintain position. Riordan (1963) prefers to centralize the carpus at age 2 to 3 months, but most others wait until 6 to 8 months of age (Bayne, 1982), at which time anatomic identification of all structures is much easier. Early soft tissue release may be necessary in some patients with tight

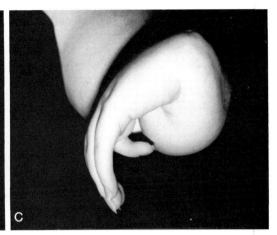

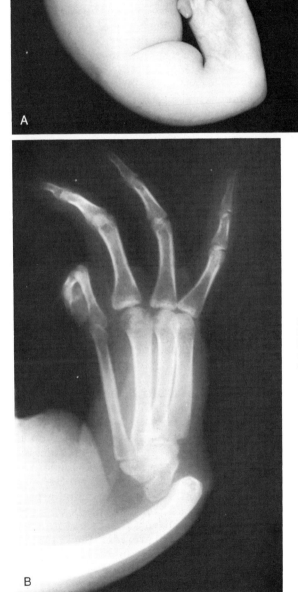

Figure 128–23. *A,* In severe Type IV deficiencies, growth may occur with the carpus subluxed radial to the distal ulna. The condition of the digits and range of motion of interphalangeal joints improve toward the ulnar side of the hand, because the ring and small fingers are always more functional. A pseudojoint and indentation have developed in the ulna. *B* and *C,* Despite significant radial deviation and rotation, this adult patient worked as a bookkeeper and could type 25 words per minute. (Courtesy of R. G. Eaton, M.D., 1976.)

contractures in Type III and IV deformities prior to formal centralization, but if splinting is started early, this maneuver may be avoided.

Four general types of surgical procedures have been performed alone or in combination to correct absence of the radius: soft tissue releases, replacement or lengthening of the missing radius, centralization of the hand over the distal ulna, and tendon transfers and arthrodeses. Soft tissue releases consist of excision of the fibrous anlage, tenotomies of tight radial structures, and Z-plasties. Most are performed prior to a formal centralization in Type III and IV deformities.

Centralization can be delayed in patients when deviation is passively correctable by a splint, but the results of centralization done prior to 3 years of age are superior. *Pollicization* procedures for the absent thumb are usually completed by age 2 years. *Tendon transfers,* such as the abductor digiti quinti muscle transfer (Huber procedure) to provide palmar abduction for the thumb, are usually completed by school age (Huber, 1921; Manske and McCarroll, 1978). Toe transfers are not regarded as the treatment of choice in congenital absence of the thumb. This general timetable is not absolute, particularly in children with very slow development or other severe associated anomalies.

Replacement of the deficient radius with a nonvascularized bone graft has a long historical precedence but is no longer used because of the lack of growth potential and ultimate recurrence of the deformity (Albee, 1928; Riordan, 1963; Bora, Nicholson, and Cheema, 1970). Recent success with vascular fibular grafts has not yielded sufficient long-term results and is a very difficult procedure because a separate pedicle to the proximal epiphysis of the fibula must be isolated and revascularized to ensure growth (Weiland and associates, 1978; Tsai, Ludwig, and Tonkin, 1987). Distraction lengthening of the ulna with interdigital bone grafts for Type II and III deformities is beneficial but has not been performed in sufficient numbers of patients to warrant general conclusions about its efficacy (Dick and associates, 1977).

Centralization of the hand and wrist over the distal ulna is recommended for all severe deformities if elbow flexion has been achieved (Sayer, 1893). If the elbow remains stiff after adequate manipulation and splinting, the centralized hand cannot reach the face. Elbow capsular release and anterior transfer of the triceps will produce a forearm that can flex dynamically and extend by gravity (Bunnell, 1951; Manelaus, 1976). The centralization technique of Lidge (1969) and Lamb (1977) has become standard (Fig. 128–24*A*). Bayne and Klug (1987) have preserved some wrist motion in most patients by avoiding carpal resections (Fig. 128–24*B*) (Watson, Beebe, and Cruz, 1984). Recently, Buck-Gramcko's (1985) radialization method positions the ulna beneath the most radial portion of the carpus, avoids the making of a carpal notch and removal of the lunate, and results in more motion (Fig. 128–24*C*). The relocated hand and wrist are held with a substantial Kirschner wire, which is left in for at least six to 12 months. Muscular balance can be achieved by releasing or lengthening tight motors on the radial side and shortening lax motors on the ulnar side, usually the flexor and extensor carpi ulnaris tendons. Some have recommended rerouting the superficial flexors to the ring and long fingers to maintain both position and balance (Bora, Nicholson, and Cheema, 1970), and others transfer a tight flexion carpi radialis to the ulnar side of the hand if the muscle is long enough (Buck-Gramko, 1985).

Arthrodesis of the wrist is usually reserved as a definitive posturing procedure after full growth has been achieved. The procedure should not be done in patients with bilateral deformities because of sacrifice of motion (Lamb, 1977) or in patients with no elbow motion.

Technique of Centralization. The goal of this procedure is a stable wrist, centralized over the distal ulna with its motion preserved. The operation is performed under general anesthesia and with pneumatic tourniquet. A transverse incision is made over the distal ulna and carpus with an S-shaped extension down the dorsal and radial aspects of the forearm as needed. The flexor carpi ulnaris tendon and dorsal sensory branches of the ulnar nerve are identified and retracted. The extensor retinaculum is incised in a ulnar to radial direction after all extensor tendons, particularly the fourth dorsal compartment, have been identified. In most cases, the radial extrinsic flexors and extensors have a common muscle mass and need to be detached from the radial carpal bones. In a

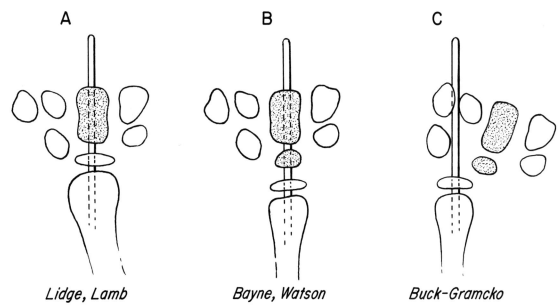

A   *Lidge, Lamb*

B   *Bayne, Watson*

C   *Buck-Gramcko*

Figure 128–24. Three basic types of centralization techniques have been used during the past 15 years. *A,* In the classic Lidge (1969) and Lamb (1977) procedure, the rudimentary lunate is excised, and a notch is created at the base of the capitate to receive the distal ulna. The distal ulna should not be traumatized. *B,* Watson and Bayne modified this approach by preserving the carpals despite their deficiencies and also by centralizing the ulna beneath the capitate. The opposing articular surfaces are shaved to accept each other. A pseudoarthrosis develops, and some motion is preserved (Bayne, 1982; Watson and associates, 1984). *C,* Buck-Gramcko (1981) also performs an aggressive capsular release, but centralizes the ulna in a more radial position beneath the existing carpal bones.

few cases, separate tendons with metacarpal insertions are present. The distal ulna is exposed, and the interval between it and the carpus located. The dorsal and then palmar joint capsule is incised transversely to mobilize the distal ulna, and the important ulnar collateral ligament is preserved as a distally based capsular flap is created (Fig. 128–25).

Fibrosed and contracted muscle or scar on the radial side may require release for mobilization of the carpus and hand. Although this may often be visualized through the dorsal incision, an additional incision over the forearm may be necessary. A Z-plasty may be used for closure if length is needed (Bayne and Klug, 1987). Tendons and median nerve should be carefully identified before any structures are incised. If present, a tight fibrocartilaginous "anlage" should be excised; this is usually found in partial and complete radial absence deformities (Types III and IV). With mobilization of the joint capsule, care must be taken not to injure the periosteum and blood supply growth plate of the distal ulna. The median nerve often becomes the structure most limiting to immobilization on

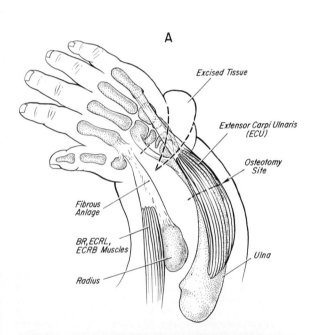

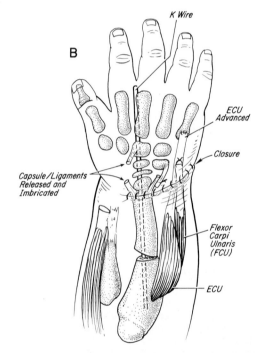

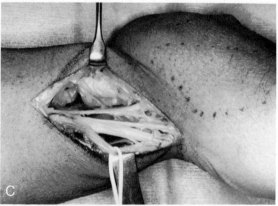

Figure 128–25. A, The abnormal structures that require alteration in a centralization procedure are the fibrous anlage and hypoplastic brachioradialis (BR), extensor carpi radialis longus (ERCL) and extensor carpi radialis brevis (ECRB), tight joint capsules, elongated ulnar wrist flexors and extensors, and a bowed ulna. B, Through a dorsal ulnar approach, the tight capsular ligaments are released, the fibrous anlage is incised at the carpal level, and the hand is centralized over the distal ulna. Separate palmar and radial forearm incisions may be required to provide better exposure of tight radial structures. Dynamic rebalancing is often achieved by shortening and/or advancing the extensor carpi ulnaris (ECU) and then transferring the flexor carpi ulnaris (FCU) into it to eliminate the major flexion deforming force. The dorsal and palmar joint capsule and ligament are imbricated and sutured. Significant ulnar bowing is corrected with a transverse osteotomy at the site of maximum angulation through a more proximal forearm incision. C, Following an aggressive release in a severe "club hand," the median nerve (in a more radial position) often becomes the limiting structure in the correction.

the radial side of the wrist. The hand is now ready for repositioning over the distal ulna.

Centralization (Lidge, 1969; Lamb, 1977; Bayne, 1982; Watson, Beebe, and Cruz, 1984). The distal radius is exposed and shaved slightly to flatten its surface (Watson, Beebe, and Cruz, 1984; Bayne and Klug, 1987). A Kirschner wire is then predrilled into the distal ulnar articular surface and passed down its shaft. A separate wire is then passed retrograde through the lunate and capitate, and into the base of the third metacarpal. Lamb (1977) chooses to prepare a notch for reception of the distal ulna with partial or complete excision of the lunate. The capitate and the metacarpal are then centered directly over the distal ulna, and the second pin is advanced in a retrograde fashion down the ulnar shaft. The hand and carpus are in neutral position between dorsiflexion and palmar flexion. Opening or closing wedge osteotomies may be performed to correct radial bowing greater than 30 degrees. Healing of these osteotomies is better if done in the distal third of the ulna. Radiographs are then obtained intraoperatively to confirm position.

Radialization (Buck-Gramcko, 1985). Following aggressive mobilization of the hand and carpus with preservation of the ulnar collateral ligament, the distal ulna is predrilled. The distal Kirschner wire is then passed through the radial carpal bones and obliquely through the base of the second (index) metacarpal. After the articular surface of the ulna has been shaved to match the radial side of the carpus, the hand is positioned in an ulnar direction with the second (index) metacarpal and trapezium centered directly over the distal ulna. Wedge osteotomies are also incorporated within the distal third of the ulna to correct bowing.

In both techniques the capsular structures are trimmed, and tight closure is performed with nonabsorbable sutures. Dynamic rebalancing is achieved by imbrication or advancement of the extensor carpi ulnaris, transfer of the flexor carpi ulnaris to become an extensor, and lengthening or tenotomy of wellformed radial tendons, if present. The flexor carpi radialis, extensor carpi radialis longus and brevis, and brachioradialis, often indistinguishable from one another, are transferred as a mass dorsally into the extensor carpi ulnaris insertion to become dorsiflexors and ulnar deviators (Buck-Gramcko, 1985). Bora and associates (1981) have advocated

using some superficial flexors for the same purpose. Before transfers are made absolute, the muscle and tendon to be moved must be identified, as both extrinsic flexors and extensors are often undifferentiated from one another. The dorsal retinaculum is then transposed between the extensor tendons and wrist capsule to prevent adhesions. Excess skin on the ulnar side of the hand is then excised during closure with preservation of the dorsal sensory branch of the ulnar nerve. A wellpadded, long arm cast extending well above the flexed elbow is applied. Active stretching of the fingers is started in the early postoperative period. The Kirschner wire is left in place for at least eight weeks; after it is removed, active motion is begun (Bayne and Klug, 1987). Use of night splints that leave the fingers and elbows free is recommended until skeletal maturity has been reached.

Complications. Recurrence of deformity is a common complication of centralization procedures with the exception of arthrodeses. This may be due to poor pin fixation, inadequate tendon balance, tight soft tissues, pin fractures, or progressive bowing of the ulna with growth. The last can be the result of damage to one side of the ulnar epiphysis, excessive pull of radial muscles, or an internal growth deficiency within the ulna. Noncompliant patients who do not wear splints or do exercises will achieve poor correction. Recentralization and correction of deforming forces is indicated when recurrence affects function. The same is true for osteotomy of the bowed ulna, which most prefer to delay until after skeletal maturity.

A well-supported hand located on the distal ulna is a functional and esthetic hand. Wrist motion following most centralization procedures measures 30 to 40 degrees in Type III and IV cases. With functional use and growth, the distal ulna broadens and becomes less bowed if it supports a well-balanced hand and wrist (Fig. 128–26D). The most predictable results are obtained in young patients (less than 3 years of age) with ulnar bowing less than 30 degrees and no significant preoperative soft tissue tightness.

Preservation of wrist motion is recommended by most authors (Buck-Gramcko, 1985; Bayne and Klug, 1987). Surgical stabilization produces a happier patient with a more acceptable appearance and as much dexterity as the unoperated patient has despite some obligatory loss of wrist motion.

In evaluating adults with untreated Type

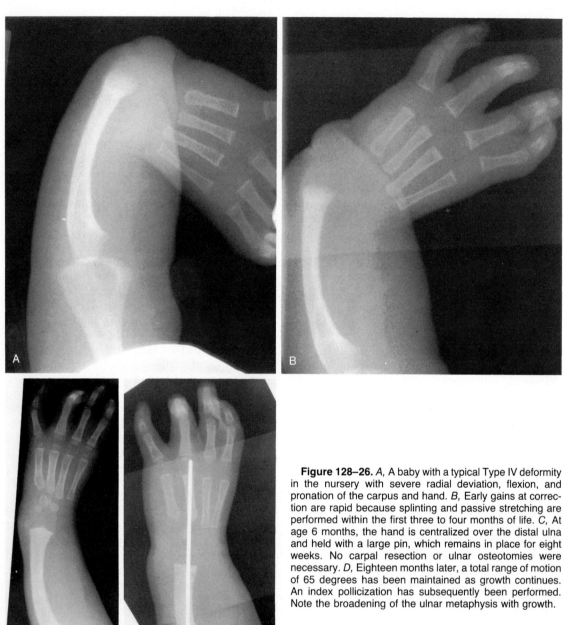

Figure 128–26. *A,* A baby with a typical Type IV deformity in the nursery with severe radial deviation, flexion, and pronation of the carpus and hand. *B,* Early gains at correction are rapid because splinting and passive stretching are performed within the first three to four months of life. *C,* At age 6 months, the hand is centralized over the distal ulna and held with a large pin, which remains in place for eight weeks. No carpal resection or ulnar osteotomies were necessary. *D,* Eighteen months later, a total range of motion of 65 degrees has been maintained as growth continues. An index pollicization has subsequently been performed. Note the broadening of the ulnar metaphysis with growth.

II, III, or IV deformities, most authors have found that all had adjusted adequately but would have preferred centralization at an early age for cosmetic reasons.

CENTRAL

The absence of digits or metacarpals within the central portion of the hand constitutes the cleft hand. Radius and ulna are present. More extensive involvement may result in complete absence of the index, long, and, occasionally, ring rays. In his comprehensive review, Barsky (1964) proposed a classification of two types, "typical" and "atypical." These terms have raised considerable nosologic controversy, because many German and Japanese authors hold that the atypical type should be in another category (Ogino, 1979; Buck-Gramcko, 1985). Atypical cleft hands have historically been called "ectrodactyly" or "symbrachydactyly."

Clinical Presentation

"Typical" Type. The classic type of cleft hand has a defect of variable depth within the central portion of the hand. In severe forms, syndactyly between the thumb-index and ring-small rays may be present, and the long ray may be completely absent. More extensive involvement may result in complete absence of the index and long rays. Involvement of the hand and foot is bilateral (Fig. 128–27). Many pedigrees have demonstrated dominant or recessive inheritance patterns (David, 1974; Flatt, 1977). Associated malformations include ectodermal deficiencies such as cleft lip and palate, cataracts, dislocating lens, tibial defects, and genitourinary and cardiovascular abnormalities (Barsky, 1964; Watari and Tsuge, 1979; Nutt and Flatt, 1981).

These hand anomalies are unusual, accounting for between 2.3 per cent (Flatt, 1977) and 5.8 per cent (Birch-Jensen, 1949) of large series studied and occurring once in approximately every 90,000 live births. The etiology is unknown. Maisels (1970) has proposed a centripedal suppression theory, in which the apical ectrodermal ridge does not develop normally but creates a central wedge of varying size. At about the seventh week of fetal development, a central defect occurs in the hand plate. In minimal cases, a soft tissue cleft exists between the long and ring rays

but no bone is missing. In more severe cases, the soft tissue deficiency pushes skeletal elements laterally and accounts for skeletal malalignment and syndactyly on the other side of the central cleft. Manske (1983) has suggested that a developmental relationship may exist between cleft hands and central polydactyly. The ultimate forms of this suppression are a monodactylous hand and a hand with no digits (Maisels, 1970). Many of these concepts may correlate well with basic research by Klein, Scott, and Wilson (1981), Thaller and Eichele (1987), and others, described under Embryology.

Although hand function is usually quite satisfactory, the cosmetic appearance is poor, creating "functional triumphs and social disasters" (Flatt, 1977). In severe forms, syndactyly on one or the other side of the cleft varies, but soft tissue is always deficient. A tight thumb-index web space severely limits key pinch between these two rays. The degree of adduction depends on the varying deficiencies of the thumb intrinsic muscles. A hypoplastic thumb supinated in the same plane as the digits may be seen in severe cases with syndactyly. Often the distal portion of the thumb is hypoplastic. The patient often neglects the deficient index ray, accomplishing pinch between the thumb and ring fingers. Bizarre appearing, contracted digits often bordering the central cleft are commonly used in ingenious hooking maneuvers by these children. Transverse oriented phalanges are often present at the metacarpal level. Reduced interphalangeal joint motion and symphalangism are common in the digits.

Hand formation is severely impaired in many of these children despite their adaptations. Grasp is usually achieved either within the central cleft or between the thumb and best remaining digit on the hand. Often, a hypoplastic index finger obstructs effective thumb–ring finger prehension. Digital proximal and distal interphalangeal flexion contractures may be present and are characteristically worse in digits adjacent to the cleft. Abnormal rotation of the ulnar digits usually in supination may affect prehension, and reduced interphalangeal joint motion and symphalangism lessen grasp. Fortunately, wrist motion and anatomy are usually normal.

"Atypical" Type. In this form of cleft hand, the central rays either are missing or have deficient components. Phalanges are commonly absent, but a portion of metacar-

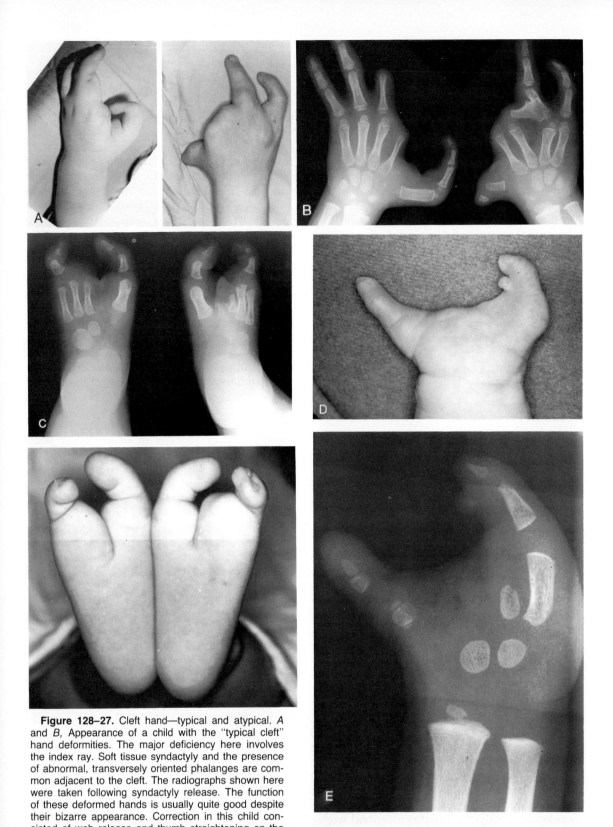

Figure 128–27. Cleft hand—typical and atypical. *A* and *B,* Appearance of a child with the "typical cleft" hand deformities. The major deficiency here involves the index ray. Soft tissue syndactyly and the presence of abnormal, transversely oriented phalanges are common adjacent to the cleft. The radiographs shown here were taken following syndactyly release. The function of these deformed hands is usually quite good despite their bizarre appearance. Correction in this child consisted of web release and thumb straightening on the right and thumb lengthening on the left. The parents did not want a toe-to-thumb transfer. Despite the appearance, function of these hands has been excellent. *C,* Symmetric involvement of both feet. The major deficiency involving the second ray is demonstrated. *D* and *E,* The "atypical cleft," in contrast, is usually unilateral and has a U-shaped defect involving more than one central ray. Fingers are often represented by small nubbins, and the border rays (thumb, fifth) are usually hypoplastic. Feet are normal.

pals is present. The hand is occasionally hypoplastic, and the thumb and fifth (small) rays are the best-developed digits in the entire hand. Soft tissue nubbins often represent the hypoplastic central three digits. Unlike in the typical cleft hand, the proximal phalanx and metacarpals on either side of the cleft are smaller than on the unaffected hand (Maisels, 1970) (Fig. 128–27D) (Table 128–5). Most authors prefer to classify this anomaly as symbrachydactyly, which belongs in the failure of differentiation category (Tada, Yonenobu, and Swanson, 1981; Miura and Suzuki, 1984; Buck-Gramcko, 1985). In contrast to "typical" clefts, the deformity is unilateral and is not accompanied by foot and musculoskeletal deformities or a positive family history. The incidence is difficult to determine, because this entity has often been placed in other diagnostic categories, such as the constriction ring syndrome and ectrodactyly.

Muller (1937) has proposed a progression of severity in the condition, starting with short middle phalanges (brachymesophalangia) and continuing to total absence of metacarpals with digits represented by small soft tissue remnants, frequently bearing miniature nails (Muller, 1937; Buck-Gramcko, 1985). *Lobster claw hand* has been used to describe an atypical cleft hand with border rays (thumb and small), a large intervening cleft, and, often, nubbins representing hypoplastic digits to the missing index, long, and ring fingers.

Table 128–5. Comparison of Types of Cleft Hand

Feature	Typical Cleft Hand	Atypical Cleft Hand
Laterality	Bilateral	Unilateral
Inheritance	Familial	Nonfamilial
Shape of defect	V shape	U shape
Foot involvement	Present	Absent
Syndactyly	Common	Less likely
Absence/deficiencies of finger rays	Middle ray absent (sometimes index, rarely ring)	Several rays deficient
Eponyms	Cleft hand	Lobster claw hand, symbrachydactyly, ectrodactyly

Treatment

Typical Cleft. Surgical treatment of the typical cleft hand varies with the severity of the deformity. The surgeon must carefully weigh the merits of surgical correction for these deformities because a supple, unscarred, but functional hand will usually be much more acceptable than a stiff, scarred hand with digits in closer alignment (Lister, 1985).

The central cleft can be narrowed in mild cases. This is more than a simple closure, and a local flap should be used to provide the normal breadth and dorsal slope for the new commissure (Kelikian and Doumanian, 1957; Barsky, 1964). Zigzag incisions on the palmar surface will reduce contracture with growth. In deeper clefts, a new transverse metacarpal ligament should be reconstructed with a tendon graft or by connecting the index and ring finger extensor mechanism (Ueba, 1981) or with a bone peg as an arthrodesis (Snow and Littler, 1969). Syndactyly releases should be done initially to release the border rays. Obstructing transverse bone segments, usually proximal phalanges, often require removal (Fig. 128–27B). Flexion contractures of the interphalangeal joints often require aggressive soft tissue release and closure with Z-plasty or grafts, if necessary. Recurrent contracture with growth should be carefully monitored so that re-release can be accomplished before permanent joint deformities develop, particularly in the fifth finger. Persistent proximal interphalangeal joint flexion contractures may be seen adjacent to either the central cleft or an incomplete digit. This may be caused by a dynamic imbalance caused by insertion of the intrinsic and/or extrinsic tendons from the incomplete ray into its neighbor.

Wide clefts often have an associated adduction contracture between the thumb and index rays and an index finger situated in a functional "no man's land" between the thumb and ring fingers. These cases are best treated by transposition of the index to the long metacarpal (if present) and release of the muscular attachments between the thumb and index metacarpals. Excellent techniques are described by Snow and Littler (1969), who prefer to correct this deformity as a one stage procedure (Fig. 128–28), and by Miura and Komada (1979), who prefer to first close the cleft and second release the thumb-index adduction contracture. Release

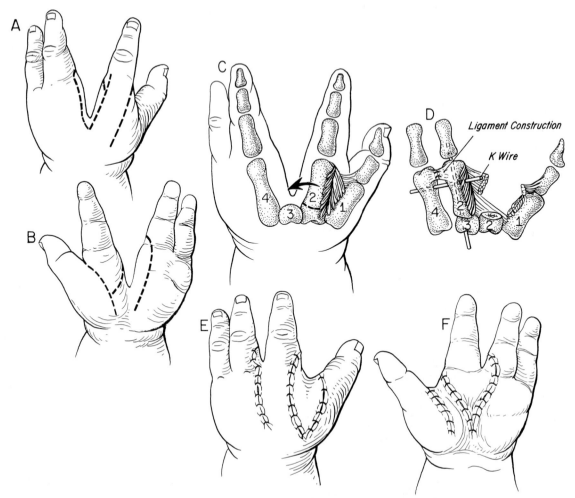

Figure 128–28. Cleft hand correction. *A* and *B,* Outline of complex incisions used for a one-stage cleft hand correction that will close the cleft and transpose the index metacarpal into the third (long) metacarpal position. Dorsal skin continuity is designed to preserve draining veins. *C* and *D,* The metacarpal osteotomy and transfer are shown. Most of the first dorsal interosseus muscle must be released, and a new transverse metacarpal ligament is constructed between metacarpals 2 and 4. Anomalous anatomy is frequently found in these hands. *E* and *F,* Skin closure. Metacarpal 1 = thumb; 2 = index finger; 3 = long finger; 4 = ring finger; 5 = small finger.

of these tight contractures often involves excision of fibrous bands, incision of fascia, and, occasionally, total release of first dorsal interosseous muscular origin from the thumb metacarpal. Transposition procedures are difficult because the transferred ray is moved as a neurovascular island to provide better functional and aesthetic results and to maintain skeletal alignment (Ahstrom, 1977; Wood, 1982) (Fig. 128–28). Vascular compromise of the transferred ray or skin flaps is a feared complication. Extensor imbalance may be improved with tendon transfers using the flexor digitorum superficialis of the ring finger. Anomalous anatomy is frequently encountered and can result in partial loss of the

index digit, which is rarely normal (Buck-Gramcko, 1985). Review of well-illustrated summaries of these procedures, particularly incisions, is suggested before one attempts to perform these operations (Snow and Littler, 1969; Wood, 1982; Sandzen, 1985).

Transfers of toes to augment initial aplastic digits will often jeopardize much of the function of these well-adapted hands. Transfer of a toe from a cleft foot is beneficial for thumb deficiencies, in which the metacarpal and thenar intrinsic muscles are present (May, Smith, and Peimer, 1981).

The timing of these individualized procedures should be arranged so that releases and skeletal realignment are finished before school age to achieve optimal results. Hand function should be very carefully assessed preoperatively because, as stated, these children often function remarkably well. Although correction and reduction of the central cleft is beneficial to all, other procedures such as metacarpal transposition, rotational osteotomies, athrodeses, and release of flexion contractures may jeopardize function. Syndactyly releases are recommended within the first year of life because, when present, they involve digits of unequal length. Cleft closure and release of the first web space can be safely done together, but one must exercise caution in performing rotational osteotomies before the rest of the hand is in a set position. Conservative judgment should also prevail when the thumb is hypoplastic and is in the same plane as the digits. Syndactyly is invariably present in these hands and should be released prior to definitive repositioning of the thumb with a pollicization. Preoperative angiograms are quite helpful. Metacarpals should be aligned as anatomically as possible and may require capsulotomies, osteotomies, or actual transposition.

Atypical Cleft. The management of the atypical cleft hand does not follow as logical a sequence as that for the typical cleft. Treatment is individualized to the particular functional or aesthetic problem. Rudimentary nubbins are best excised early in life, before they become the focus of peer group or parental concern.

Creation of a "basic hand" with a mobile thumb, central cleft, and at least one digit or post for opposition is often a very realistic goal. Unlike in the typical cleft, the central cleft may be deepened with Z-plasty techniques to improve the gripping capacity of the border rays. Hypoplastic digits may be transposed on top of adjacent digits for lengthening (Dobyns, 1985). Useless central metacarpals may be used to lengthen the more functional border digits after a gap has been created by means of distraction techniques. Rotational osteotomies may improve the opposition of the functional digits on either side of the cleft, particularly if all metacarpals lie in the same plane. Flail finger joints may be fused with arthrodeses in older children and chondrodeses in the young.

Flexor tendon grafts may improve flexor power to the thumb and small fingers, which are usually hypoplastic and have passively mobile interphalangeal joints (Fig. 128–29).

Small but functional motors are usually present in the forearm. Retraction of soft tissue nubbins or skin dimples within the central cleft is a good clinical indication that muscles are present in the forearm.

In the severe suppression deformities, in which there is one digit or none, distraction lengthening techniques or toe transfers should be considered in lieu of older, staged osteoplastic reconstructions with tubed pedicle flaps and bone grafts (Lister, 1985). For any free toe transfer, preoperative angiographic evaluation of the hand and foot are necessary. Although prostheses are often recommended, these patients usually do not persist in using them because of adaptation made since the time of birth.

Because the spectrum of the atypical or lobster claw cleft hand is so widespread, the possibilities for surgical reconstruction vary tremendously. Many options for reconstruction are covered in sections on transverse amputations—metacarpal and digital level, hypoplasia, and syndactyly. Procedures for the one digit hand and the no digit hand are also covered in other sections of this chapter.

ULNAR

Absences along the ulnar or postaxial portion of the upper limb are characterized by a much greater degree of variation than those that occur along the radial side and do not represent the mirror image of radial deficiencies. They may be as subtle as carpal or metacarpal hypoplasia, but most are expressed as shortening of the ulna with slight ulnar deviation of the hand. Usually, one will see complete absence of the ulnar two digits, a shortened ulna, bowing of the radius, and, in the most severe forms, a fused elbow and shortening of the humerus. These deformities are not common. Birch-Jensen (1949) found an incidence of one in 100,000 live births, and most authors find one ulnar absence for every five to 10 radial deficiencies (Carroll and Bowel, 1977; Broudy and Smith, 1979; Swanson, Tada, and Yonenobu, 1984). The etiology is unknown, but familial inheritance has been described (Temtamy and McKusick, 1978). No teratogens have been identified in reported cases. Ulnar deficiencies may occur as part of syndromes that demonstrate great variation in Mendelian inheritance patterns, but most cases show autosomal dominant patterns, which are well summarized in re-

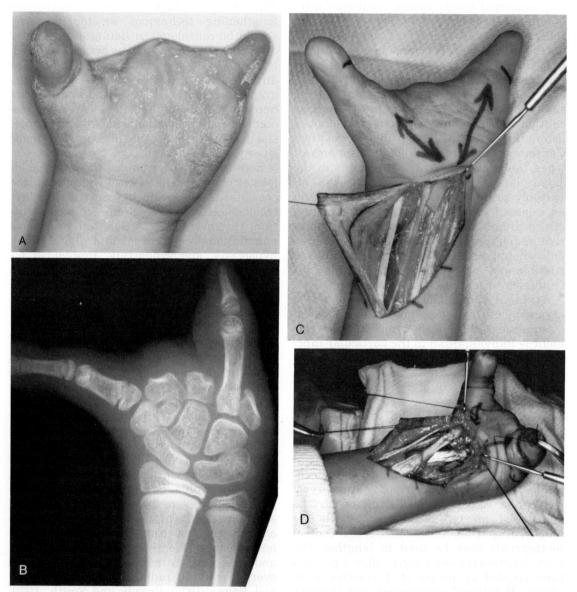

Figure 128–29. *A* and *B,* Treatment in this "atypical" cleft hand consisted of excision of hypoplastic nubbins within the first year of life, followed by deepening of the soft tissue cleft. Radiograph shows central metacarpals following shortening. *C* and *D,* Flexor tendon grafts to the border rays enabled basic pincer function. In the forearm, sheets of flexor tendons were present but poorly differentiated. Grafts were criss-crossed in order to provide a direct pull with adduction.

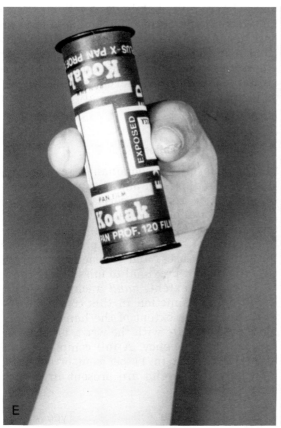

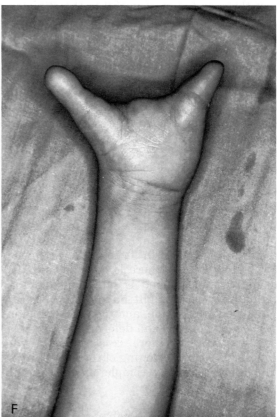

Figure 128–29 *Continued E* and *F,* Flexion and extension five years later.

cent texts (Temtamy and McKusick, 1978; Johnson and Omer, 1985).

Almost half of affected patients have associated defects, all of which are musculoskeletal; they include femoral focal deficiency, fibular defects, scoliosis, club feet, and congenital dislocation of the hip. In contrast to radial defects, ulnar deficiencies are not associated with abnormalities in the hematopoietic, gastrointestinal, genitourinary, and cardiopulmonary organ systems (Table 128–6). Only one-fourth of these patients have defects on the opposite upper extremity (Ogden, Watson, and Bohne, 1976).

Classification

Classification systems have been proposed by Kummel (1895), Riordan, Mills, and Aldredge (1961), Swanson, Tada, and Yonenobu (1984), Ogden, Watson, and Bone (1976), and more recently by Miller, Wenner, and Kruger (1986). Bayne's (1982) system combines the

Table 128–6. Comparison of Radial and Ulnar Longitudinal Absence Deformities

Feature	Ulnar	Radial
Inheritance	Sporadic	Sometimes genetic
Associated anomalies	Musculoskeletal	GI, GU, cardiac, hematopoetic
Syndromic associations	Rare	Common
Involved digits	Any	Predominantly radial
Elbow involvement	Frequent	Less frequent
Joint stability	Wrist stable, elbow unstable	Wrist unstable, elbow stable
Common presentation	Partial absence	Total absence
Presence of opposite limb anomaly	25%	100%

last three and is most useful to the clinician (Fig. 128–30).

In Type I deformities, the distal ulnar epiphysis is present but deficient. There is minimal shortening or clinical deviation of the hand. The proximal ulna is normal. In Type II deformity, the most common type, the distal or middle one-third of the ulna is deficient. A fibrous anlage is present, and there may be bowing of the radius. The radial head may be dislocated, and the distal radial epiphysis may be slanted in an ulnar direction. A proximal ulna is present and articulates with the humerus. The hand and wrist may be deviated and may exhibit deformities unrelated to the severity of the forearm abnormality. Some postaxial hand deficiency is invariably present. In Type III, the ulna is completely absent, there is no ulnar anlage, deviation of the hand is minimal, and the radius may be straight but is often bowed. The elbow is unstable, and the radial head is dislocated. Severe hand deformities are present. In Type IV there is a radiohumeral synostosis with shortening of the entire limb. The ulna is usually completely absent but

may be represented by a small olecranon fused to the humerus. The hand and forearm are usually supinated away from the body and held in a posterior posture or "hand on flank" position. A fibrous ulnar anlage is usually present with severe radial bowing, and hand anomalies are always present (Bayne, 1982).

Clinical Presentations

This deformity predominantly involves the hand, wrist, forearm and elbow. In a review of all major reported series, Johnson and Omer (1985) tabulated that (1) in only 11 per cent of cases is there a normal complement of digits, (2) syndactyly is present in over one-third of cases, and (3) metacarpals are usually absent proximal to missing digits.

To a great extent, *hand* anomalies determine patient function in this condition. Interestingly, the extent of the hand anomaly does not correlate with the wrist, forearm, or upper arm deficiency. A full complement of digits is present in 11 per cent of patients, and only four digits are present in 12 per

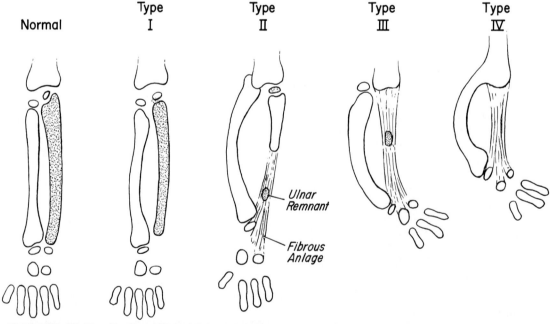

Figure 128–30. Classification of ulnar deficiencies. In Type I, the ulnar epiphysis is present, there is no fibrous anlage, and minimal deformity occurs. In Type II, the proximal two-thirds of the ulna is present, the fibrous anlage acts as a tethering for creation of some radial bowing, and the radial articular surface is often slanted. The radial head may or may not be dislocated. In Type III, there is complete absence of the ulna; the radius is usually bowed but may be straight. An anlage may be present, and the elbow is usually unstable with or without radial head dislocation. Significant postaxial ray deficiencies are usually present. In the most severe, Type IV deformity, the radius is fused to the humerus, and the ulna is completely absent. An anlage is present with significant radial bowing, which positions the hand and carpus posteriorly and severely limits upper limb function.

cent. More than half of these patients have a thumb deficiency, ranging from complete absence to hypoplasia to duplication (Broudy and Smith, 1979; Blair, Shurr, and Buckwalter, 1983; Johnson and Omer, 1985).

At the *wrist level,* one-fourth of the patients have carpal coalitions. In contrast to radial ray defects, in which deformity is common, only 30 per cent of patients demonstrate any ulnar deviation, and most of these have an ulnar slant to the radial articular surface. Carpal bones are frequently missing, and ossification centers appear delayed, in descending frequency, in the pisiform, hamate, triquetrum, capitate, and trapezoid (Ogden and associates, 1976). Often carpal bones fail to differentiate, manifesting as coalitions that articulate well with the radius (Swanson, Tada, and Yonenobu, 1984). The degree of ulnar deviation is less than 30 degrees in most cases (Broudy and Smith, 1977). There has been a lack of agreement regarding the initial treatment of the ulnar deviation. Some believe it is secondary to an intrinsic mesenchymal defect during development (Broudy and Smith, 1979), whereas others hold that the bowing is secondary to the tethering effect of the fibrous anlage, which has been compared to a fiber glass fishing pole that will bend but not lengthen (Southwood, 1926–1927; Riordan, Mills, and Aldredge, 1961). Combined data indicate that in a minority of cases the deviation is severe, measuring more than 30 degrees and significantly affecting growth and formation.

Abnormalities of the *forearm* are variable. Type II deformities predominate in almost two-thirds of all cases. In these patients there is partial hypoplasia of the forearm, and a distal ulnar epiphysis does appear, but growth is delayed. Although some patients demonstrate "catch-up" growth, in most the forearm grows proportionately with the rest of the limb (Johnson and Omer, 1985). Variable degrees of bowing of the radius and ulnar deviation of the hand exist.

The existence of an "anlage" in Type II and III deformities has aroused considerable interest (Straub, 1965). Some believe that with growth this "fibrous cord" acts as a check rein and contributes to bowing of the radius, dislocation of the radial head, which is often present at birth, and the ulnar slant of the distal radius (Fig. 128–31). They recommend excision of the cord early in life to avoid progressive radial bowing, ulnar tilt of the distal radius, impaired growth, ulnar deviation of the hand, and dislocation of the radial head (Riordan, Mills, and Aldredge, 1961; Ogden, Watson, and Bohne, 1976; Carroll and Bowel, 1977). Others hold that severe ulnar deviation occurs so infrequently that routine resection of the anlage is warranted only for those cases showing progressive deviation with growth (Broudy and Smith, 1979; Johnson and Omer, 1985). Absence of extrinsic flexor and extensor muscles within the forearm parallels the degree of the deformity. Although the ulnar artery is noted to be absent, the ulnar nerve is usually present in Type II cases, lying directly beneath the fibrous anlage.

In the minimal and moderate deformities, the distal radial epiphysis is present but demonstrates delayed growth in 60 per cent of cases. Growth does occur and provides adequate support for the wrist and hand. The radius is almost always short. There appears to be no correlation between the ulnar tilt of the distal radius and the degree of radial bowing in severe deformities.

Although the hand is usually stable at the wrist, the *elbow* is frequently unstable or fused. Elbow abnormalities occur in all severe cases. A radial head dislocation is usually present at birth and may or may not improve with growth but frequently affects motion. These patients may have functional but limited pronation and supination. A humeroradial synostosis is present in the most severe deficiencies. In such cases the humerus is hypoplastic and the hand and forearm are usually not positioned optimally, lying in a supinated position in the posterior axillary line. Children with bilateral deformities are unable to reach their mouths.

Despite significant anatomic deformities, these patients function quite well. "The deformed limb is much more useful than its anatomical condition would lead one to expect" (Southwood, 1926–1927). Total active motion of the wrist averages 70 per cent of normal and is not severely affected by radial head dislocation or bowing. Grip is significantly reduced and prehension difficult, especially in children with limited numbers of digits (Blair, Shurr, and Buckwalter, 1983; Johnson and Omer, 1985). Functional testing by Flatt (1977), Johnson and Omer (1985), and Blair, Shurr, and Buckwalter (1983) has documented that the hand deformity provides the greatest functional limitation and that

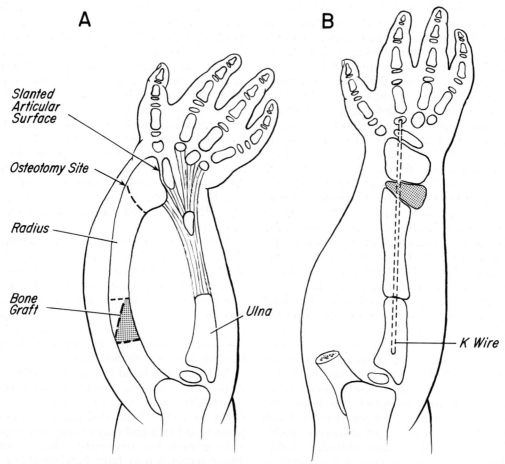

A

Slanted
Articular
Surface

Osteotomy Site

Radius

Bone
Graft

Ulna

B

K Wire

Figure 128–31. Ulnar deficiency. *A,* The anatomic abnormalities in the common Types II and III include a short or absent ulna, bowed radius, ulnar slant of the radial articular surface, and a fibrous anlage in place of the missing ulna. *B,* Treatment may include conversion to a one bone forearm and use of a portion of the radius as an opening wedge bone graft if needed. In severe cases, the radial head may be dislocated, creating a cosmetic deformity. The one bone forearm will provide increased length and alignment at the expense of some limitation of pronation and supination. There is usually, but not always, a hand and carpal deficiency.

patients adapt to and use these limbs much better than expected.

Treatment

Infants with ulnar deviation should receive manipulation or splinting as early as possible to achieve passive correction. Splinting should be done continuously during the first year of life and at night only thereafter in an effort to gain maximum correction early. Some recommend resection of the fibrous anlage early in life for patients with severe radial bowing, an ulnar slant to the radial articular surface, and radial head dislocation, before growth accentuates the deformities (Ogden, Watson, and Bohne, 1976). Resection of the cord should start as far distally as

possible in Type II and III deformities, and care must be taken to avoid injury to the ulnar nerve, which is located directly beneath the fibrous anlage, and to the posterior interosseous nerve in the proximal forearm. At the same time, the forearm can be straightened with an opening wedge osteotomy and bone graft (see Fig. 128–31).

Resection of the anlage remains controversial; many authors prefer to wait because (1) the natural history of the more severe deformities indicates that some radial bowing may improve spontaneously, (2) the ulnar tilt of the epiphysis is rarely extensive, (3) radial head dislocation is not progressive, and (4) the functional results without anlage resection are usually excellent (Broudy and Smith, 1979; Johnson and Omer, 1985). Most authors

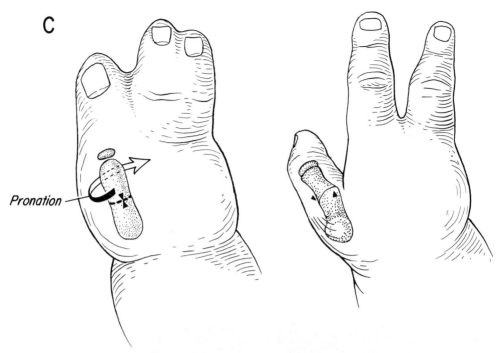

Figure 128–31 *Continued C,* Common procedures required in the hand of a child with severe ulnar deficiencies include separation of soft tissue syndactyly and pronation/angulation osteotomies of the thumb metacarpal to position this ray in more palmar abduction. For the two digit hand, formal rotation and recession or full pollicization of the radial digit is beneficial.

agree that this procedure does improve ulnar deviation and that resection should be considered for angulation greater than 30 per cent that occurs over a period of 6 months.

Creating a one bone forearm by fusing the proximal ulna to the distal radius has been recommended for moderate and severe deformities (Straub, 1956; Riordan, Mills, and Aldredge, 1961). Advantages include increased length, removal of the obstruction to full extension caused by the radial head, a stable forearm, and better appearance. All this is gained at the expense of pronation and some supination (see Fig. 128–31*B*). Other forearm procedures of value when growth is complete are wedge osteotomies for correction of excessive bowing and derotational osteotomies for correction of excessive pronation or supination. Resection of the dislocated radial head is not often done and must be combined with creation of a one bone forearm (Bayne, 1982). This procedure is reserved for patients with a demonstrable decrease in elbow motion and greater proximal migration of the radial head (Tachdian, 1972).

Distraction devices can be used to maximize potential length lost by overriding of the proximal radius. It should be emphasized that patients with Type II, III and IV deform-

ities have extremely good function. Although ranges of motion at the elbow and wrist as well as grip strength are markedly reduced, these youngsters, including those with bilateral deformities, manage quite well.

Hand deformities vary, and absence of rays on the ulnar side are common. Complete syndactylies between the thumb-index and index-long webs should be released early to avoid discrepant growth problems. When ectrodactyly type deformities exist, rotational osteotomy at the metacarpal level is often necessary for opposition of what mobile digits are present (Fig. 128–32). A rotational flap that is a form of Z-plasty is helpful (Broudy and Smith, 1985). For the two digit hand or hand with no thumb, a formal pollicization of the radial digit is recommended. Short metacarpals with functional digits are easily lengthened with distraction techniques and bone grafts.

Frequently, surgery on the upper arm and forearm precedes refinement procedures on the hand. Derotational osteotomies of the humerus are necessary in most Type IV patients if the hand is to be of functional value. Osteotomy is most effectively performed at the humeroradial synostosis, with direct observation of the abnormal neurovascular

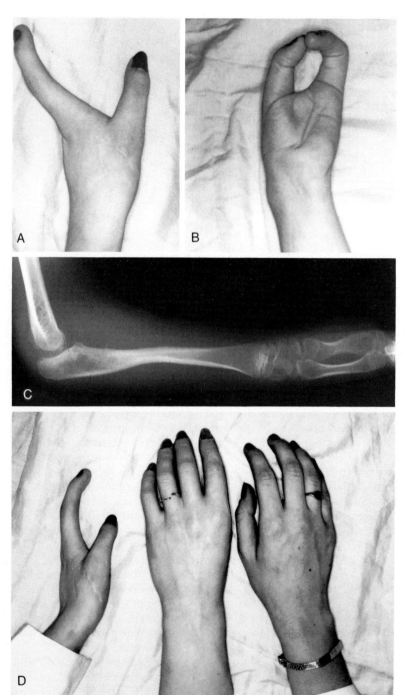

Figure 128–32. A and B, Postoperative appearance and radiograph of a teenager's hand following rotation recession osteotomy (performed by Richard Smith, M.D.). C, Radiographic appearance of one bone forearm. D, Despite excellent function, the patient still wears a cosmetic prosthetic glove (middle) for social functions.

structures to avoid kinking and entrapment. The goal of the procedure is to place the hand in front of the body and in mid-forearm rotation with approximately 60 degrees of elbow flexion. Removal of a segment of bone often releases tension on neurovascular structures. Arthroplasty of these congenital elbow synostoses does not produce predictable stability or motion, and total joint replacement utilizing alloplastic materials or free vascularized joint transfers have not been reported.

FAILURES OF DIFFERENTIATION

Syndactyly

Syndactyly is consistently one of the two most common congenital anomalies of the hand seen in different cultures (see "Incidence"). Although digital webbing usually is an isolated deformity, it is also frequently seen in association with other malformations (Goldberg and Bartoshesky, 1985). Failure of digital rays to separate from one another by a process of programmed cell death during the seventh to eighth week of intrauterine life has been classified as a failure of differentiation (Swanson, 1976). The major exception to this rule is acrosyndactyly, which is associated with the constriction ring syndrome and represents a refusion of adjacent digits following separation and a local ischemic insult.

The true incidence of syndactyly varies from one part of the world to another but is seen in approximately one of every 2000 live births (Kelikian, 1974; Flatt, 1977). Half of the cases are bilateral, and males are more commonly affected. Familial syndactyly is seen in 15 to 40 per cent of more series and, when present, commonly is one of the more complex and complicated forms of polysyndactyly. All types of genetic inheritance patterns have been documented with syndactyly; the most common is sporadic with incomplete penetrance (Temtamy and McKusick, 1978). In familial cases the dominant genes show reduced penetrance and variable expression, meaning that there is little consistency from one generation to another (Woolf and Woolf, 1973). The third web space in the hand and the second web space in the foot are the most commonly affected areas. The first web space in the hand is the least frequently affected

because the thumb separates from the rest of the hand at a much earlier stage. The incidence of ray involvement varies from one series to another but is generally thumb–index 5 per cent, index-long 15 per cent, middle-ring 50 per cent, and ring-small 30 per cent (Flatt, 1977; Posch and associates, 1981).

Associated anomalies are common and occur with defects in all other organ systems. Syndactyly is part of at least 28 syndromes, of which the most common are Apert's (acrocephalosyndactyly), Poland's, constriction ring, and multiple facial syndromes. Often syndactyly is one of the most treatable defects in the multiply-deformed child (Kelikian, 1974; Poznanski, 1984; Goldberg and Bartoshesky, 1985).

Classification

Syndactyly is clinically classified according to (1) the degree of webbing along the length of the digit (complete versus incomplete) and (2) the presence or absence of a bone union or other skeletal abnormality (simple versus complex) (Flatt, 1977). First the degree of webbing is determined. A *complete* syndactyly extends out to the tip of the terminal phalanx of the involved digit. An *incomplete* syndactyly may end anywhere between the level of the normal commissure and the fingertip but does not extend to the most distal point of the finger. In a *simple* syndactyly, the interdigital connection consists of only skin and abnormal fibrous connections; and in a *complex* syndactyly, abnormal osseous and/or cartilaginous unions are present between adjacent fingers (Fig. 128–33). Growth deformities and joint abnormalities will occur, as these fingers grow disproportionately while fused at or near the tip. Dorsal buckling or lateral angulation of the proximal interphalangeal joint of a long finger fused at the tip of a ring finger will, for example, progress unless the distal fusion is released. The useful term *complicated* syndactyly may be reserved for those cases involving more than simple side-to-side bone fusions (Dobyns, 1982). Examples of such cases are Apert's syndrome, central polysyndactyly, and typical cleft hand, in which an array of abnormal bones, joints, tendons, muscles, and nerves may be present. The degree of abnormality of skeletal elements within a web space is often a good indicator of other abnormal anatomical relationships.

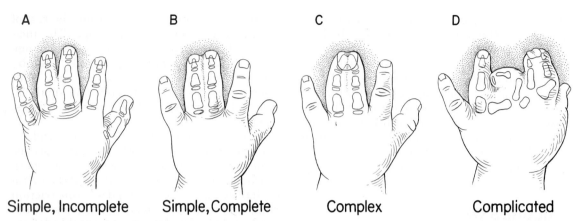

A — Simple, Incomplete B — Simple, Complete C — Complex D — Complicated

Figure 128–33. Classification of syndactyly. *A,* A simple, incomplete syndactyly involves soft tissue and does not extend to the tip of the terminal phalanx. *B,* A simple, complete form extends to the tip of involved digits. *C,* Skeletal union, usually at the distal phalangeal level, is present in complex varieties. Here, distal bone excision will result in progressive proximal buckling or angulation owing to discrepant growth of digits. *D,* Bone union, duplications, delta phalanges, and bizarre disorganization of normal skeletal ray alignment is common in the complicated forms.

Abnormal Anatomy

Almost all permutations and combinations of abnormal anatomy can be present in syndactyly. Skin is invariably deficient, especially in the region of the normal commissure (Fig. 128–34). This can easily be demonstrated to curious parents by measuring the circumference of two digits held together and comparing it with the sum of the circumferences of the individual digits (Flatt, 1974). Although infrequently webbed, the thumb-

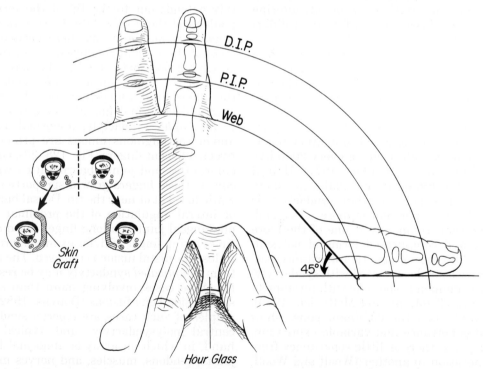

Figure 128–34. The normal anatomy of an interdigital web space (IDS) demonstrates an hourglass configuration of non–hair-bearing skin that subtends at 45 degrees dorsal to palmar angulation. The base of the web commissure is located at the midportion of the proximal phalanx on a lateral view. The transverse width of the second and fourth webspaces is greater than that of the central (third) web space. *Inset left,* A relative deficiency of skin always exists in syndactyly, particularly at the base of the digit adjacent to the commissure. With release, additional skin is necessary to cover the raw area created. D.I.P. = distal interphalangeal joint; P.I.P. = proximal interphalangeal joint.

index web space is usually deficient in the hypoplastic hand, where webbing of the digits is commonly present.

Broad or short fascial interconnections are present in all webbed digits and extend across the interdigital space at the level of the proximal and middle phalanges in the midaxial line. These bands do not have names but incorporate Clelland's ligaments of either digit. Their size varies, and when seen in the first web space, they may appear to be a band above the adductor pollicis muscle and connecting the first and second metacarpals. The transverse metacarpal ligaments, retinacular sheaths, investing fascia of intrinsic muscles, and palmar aponeurosis may be hypertrophied and tight in the small hypoplastic hand or Apert's hand and provide static check-rein forces to growth and mobility. These tight, unyielding fascial interconnections are some of the most statically deforming structures with growth (Dobyns, 1982).

Bones and joints may present bizarre and erratic configurations. Central duplications within the web (polysyndactylies) often demonstrate interconnections of phalanges and metacarpals articulating with one another at any level. Occasionally, alignment of skeletal elements into digital rays is impossible. Transversely oriented phalanges and symphalangism are encountered in the complex central problems as well as the typical cleft hand deformities. Joints in patients with syndactyly may be incompletely developed, angulated, ankylosed or even fused in a wide range of variations. What appears to be a well-segmented joint with no motion at birth may rapidly fuse to form a symphalangism. Phalanges may be crooked, broad, short, long, or fused. These abnormal patterns occur with the highest incidence in the hereditary forms of syndactyly. The thumb proximal phalanx may often present as a triangular ("delta") instead of rectangular bone, placing the distal portion of the thumb in radial or ulnar (uncommon) deviation. The middle phalanx of the fifth finger, the last to ossify in the hand, is abnormal, creating the familiar radial deviation known as clinodactyly (Kelikian, 1974). Missing or hypoplastic phalanges and/or metacarpals are as common as duplicated skeletal structures and are often accompanied by tendon, nerve, and ligament deficiencies.

Digital nerves and arteries often have a wide variety of branching patterns within a web space. Distal branching is most common

for both. An artery may form loops around a digital nerve, and vice versa. Nerves can easily be teased apart under the microscope, but arterial loops present a much more complex problem if they represent the primary or only arterial conduit to a digit or thumb. In complex and complicated syndactylies, there is often incomplete or missing neurovascular structures on one or both sides of a digital ray. Flexor and extensor tendons may have similar distal branching patterns and interconnections within a web. Distal insertions may be abnormal in complex and complicated cases. Often, the radiographic appearance of the skeletal structures and degree of hypoplasia are good indicators of associated tendon, nerve, arterial, or ligamentous abnormalities. The precise configuration must be individualized to each case, as few broad generalizations can be made.

Treatment

Principles of Correction. The history of the surgical correction of syndactyly is fascinating, and refinements made over the past 170 years have established many important principles. The well-known early surgical operations date back to the early nineteenth century, when lead beads, glass setons, rubber tubes, and ligatures were used to create epithelium-lined commissures and to separate the webbing segmentally. Often, large raw surfaces were left to heal secondarily, resulting in contractures that accentuated growth deformities (Davis and German, 1930; Hentz and Littler, 1977) (Fig. 128–35). The goals of surgery should be the separation of independent digits, provision of a lined commissure, and avoidance of scars that might cause constricting deformities with growth. Syndactyly separation is a simple soft tissue problem and should not be made complicated.

Current principles of a syndactyly correction are: (1) creation of dorsal and/or palmar flap tissue to create and line the commissure, (2) zigzag incisions to lessen contracture, (3) skin grafts to cover raw areas, (4) meticulous surgical technique, (5) operations on one side of a digit at a time, (6) emphasis upon the creation of normal nails, and (7) correction of skeletal deformities (Fig. 128–36). Generations of surgeons have designed many types of flaps to line the commissure, all of which utilize the flap principle of Zeller (Zeller, 1810). The most popular techniques today

Text continued on page 5288

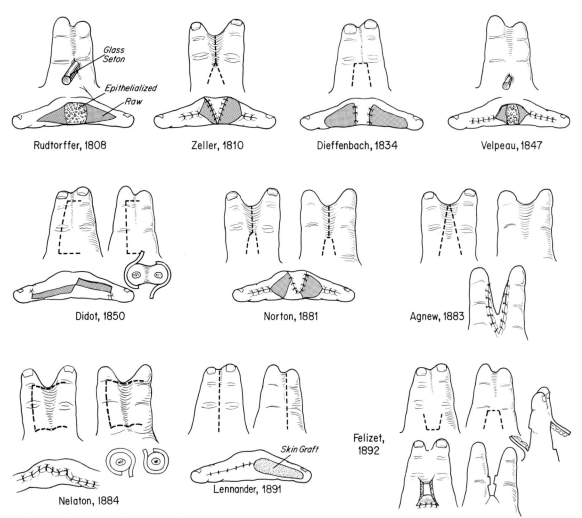

Figure 128–35. The evolution of methods for correction of interdigital webbing has varied tremendously. Although early attempts at simple division were probably made prior to the 19th century, the literature documents methods beginning at the turn of that century. Earlier methods included the use of glass rods or setons, which created epithelialized traits serving as the commissure base. Skin grafts were first employed by Lennander. Although primary closure of many of these incisions seems impractical, review of original source articles indicates that many of these cases were simple, incomplete syndactylies with wide interdigital webbing. Raw areas are indicated by dense stripping, epithelialized areas by pebbling, and skin grafted areas by fine stippling.

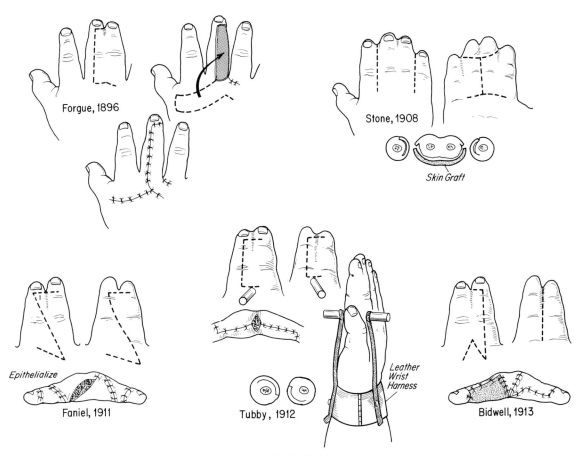

Forgue, 1896

Stone, 1908

Skin Graft

Epithelialize

Faniel, 1911

Tubby, 1912

Leather Wrist Harness

Bidwell, 1913

Figure 128–35 Continued

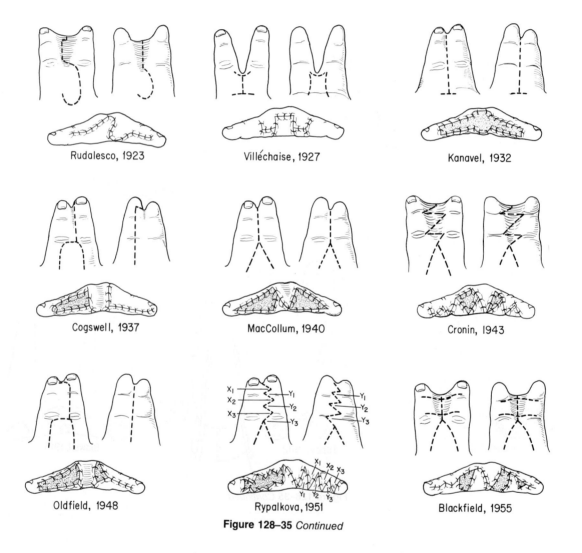

Rudalesco, 1923

Villéchaise, 1927

Kanavel, 1932

Cogswell, 1937

MacCollum, 1940

Cronin, 1943

Oldfield, 1948

Rypalkova, 1951

Blackfield, 1955

Figure 128–35 *Continued*

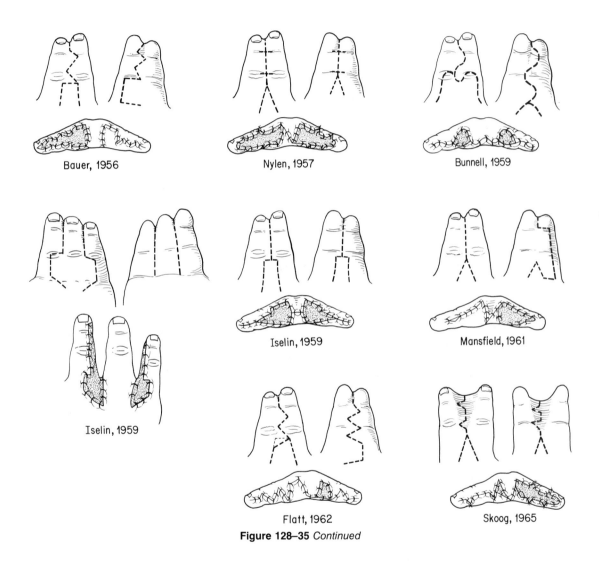

Bauer, 1956

Nylen, 1957

Bunnell, 1959

Iselin, 1959

Iselin, 1959

Mansfield, 1961

Flatt, 1962

Skoog, 1965

Figure 128–35 *Continued*

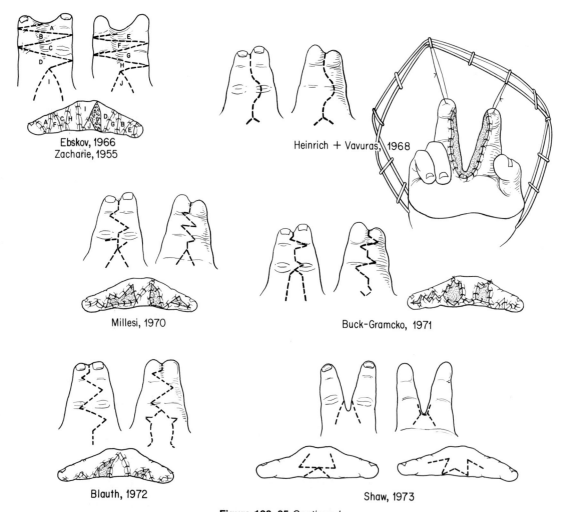

Ebskov, 1966
Zacharie, 1955

Heinrich + Vavuras, 1968

Millesi, 1970

Buck-Gramcko, 1971

Blauth, 1972

Shaw, 1973

Figure 128–35 *Continued*

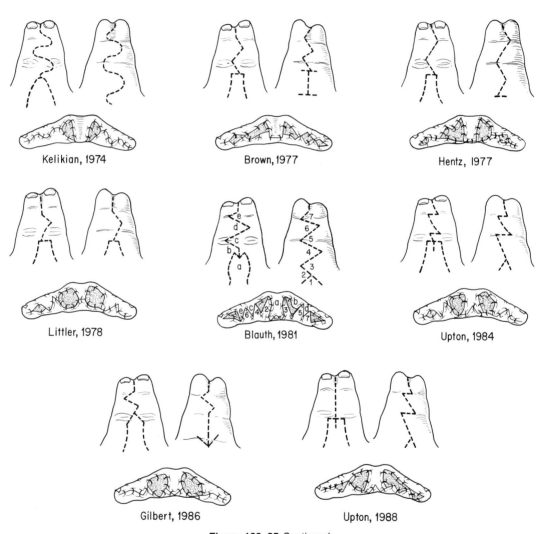

Kelikian, 1974

Brown, 1977

Hentz, 1977

Littler, 1978

Blauth, 1981

Upton, 1984

Gilbert, 1986

Upton, 1988

Figure 128–35 *Continued*

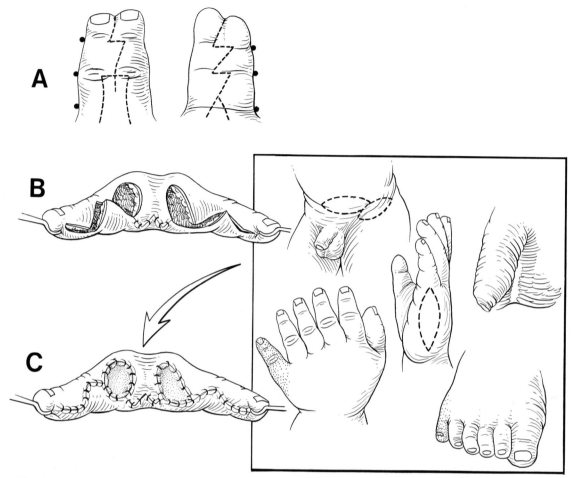

Figure 128–36. Principles and techniques of syndactyly release. *A,* Dorsal and palmar markings create zigzag incisions in order to minimize straight-line scar contractures with growth. A large dorsal flap is used to line the depth of the commissure. Reference points made on the side of the digit are helpful in obtaining correct alignment in the distal half of the digit, where flaps often interdigitate. *B,* After flaps have been sutured, templates are made for skin grafts, which may be obtained from a variety of sources. *Inset,* "Like tissues" from a similar part such as a finger or toe are preferred but are usually not available. The inguinal crease is most commonly used, and lower abdominal crease utilized when large amounts of skin are required during sequential release of multiple web spaces in the same hand, such as the Apert hand. The use of preputial skin, although practical, often results in partial graft loss owing to infection and a dark pigmentation often develops. The hypothenar eminence is very useful when small amounts of graft are required. *C,* Following meticulous graft application, the released web space is ready for a dressing.

employ either interdigitating dorsal-palmar flaps (MacCollum, 1940) or a single large dorsal flap (Dieffenbach, 1834; Norton, 1881; Bauer, Tondra, and Trusler, 1956). All combinations of dorsal and palmar flaps have been described as having good results, indicating that the surgeon's technical proficiency and experience with a given method is a strong determinant of a good functional result.

Constricting palmar scars are minimized with the use of zigzag incisions (Pieri, 1949; Cronin, 1956). Historically, raw edges were left to epithelialize (Rudtorffer, 1808; Zeller,

1810) and tremendous contractures developed. Many ingenious patterns of incision have been developed through the decades to avoid this specific problem (see Fig. 128–35). The most problematic region following release is still the palmar edge of the commissure; several helpful modifications have been made here either to overcorrect the commissure depth or to interdigitate flaps to break up a straight line scar (Blauth and Schneider-Sickert, 1981; Upton, 1986). Because skin is deficient in all but the most incomplete simple syndactyly or the thin newborn infant, skin grafts are necessary (Lennander, 1891).

Full-thickness grafts are preferred because they are less likely to result in contracture (Kanavel, 1932). The inguinal crease donor site is still preferred over other regions such as the palmar wrist flexion crease, antecubital fossa, upper arm, thigh, and instep of foot. A lower abdominal crease is often useful in patients who require large amounts of skin for multiple web releases. Occasionally, portions of amputated duplicate (supernumerary) toes or fingers are available; skin grafts from such sites have ideal consistency and color match (Rowsell and Godfrey, 1984). Our experience with the use of the elastic penile skin following simultaneous circumcision has not been as good because of postoperative infection (see Fig. 128–36).

Timing of Surgery. Timing of surgical correction varies with the complexity of the deformity and the web space involved. Although there is no consensus, most hand surgeons agree that complicated complex webbing involving adjacent digits with different growth potential warrants early release by 1 year of age. Patterns of prehensile function are established by 24 months, which should be the upper age limit for correction (Gesell and associates, 1940). There has been recent interest in correction within the first two weeks of life in infants with an abundance of mobile skin and less complex deformities (Raus, 1984) (Fig. 128–37). Restoration of maximum functional potential and liberation of all digits should be completed by school age.

Our preference has been not to routinely release simple syndactylies at birth, although several trials of such treatment have been reported (Fig. 128–37A to D). Complete webbing involving the important first (thumb-index) and fourth (ring-small) web spaces are released by 6 to 12 months of age. Surgery before 1 year of age is often necessary in patients with complex syndactylies in order to avoid skeletal deformities, which once established may not correct with growth. The urgency for correction increases with greater discrepancy between the webbed digits; thus, one should not wait as long with the thumb-index web space as with the middle-ring web space. The majority of simple and complex syndactylies are corrected between 12 and 36 months of age. Whenever possible, bilateral procedures should be performed on patients with deformities in both hands. This is conveniently done in children less than 14 months of age, because youngsters between 2 and 3 years of age are most active and difficult to manage. In the older child, bilateral procedures should be avoided (Flatt, 1977).

Alterations in this timetable are, of course, dictated by associated anomalies, size of the hand, medical problems of higher priority, and concerns about anesthesia exposures. Several authors of long-term review series cite a higher incidence for complications and resultant contractures with early surgery and recommend delay of initial procedures (Brown, 1977; Posch and associates, 1981). Although infants and children of any age can be safely anesthesized during a long operation, elective syndactyly releases may need to be postponed in the multiply-deformed child with cardiopulmonary, hematologic, and severe musculoskeletal problems.

Technique of Release

Interdigital Web Space. Syndactyly release is a simple but meticulous operation that should not be made complicated. General anesthesia is preferred. Following routine preparation and draping, incisions are planned with the pediatric tourniquet deflated. The dorsal and palmar levels of the cleft are marked, and a large dorsal, slightly truncated rectangular flap is outlined. Dorsal skin dimples in chubby hands denote the metacarpal phalangeal joint level. Measurements of adjacent web spaces and of the opposite hand are often useful. The normal web space has a palmar inclination of 40 to 45 degrees and an "hourglass" configuration (see Fig. 128–34). The size of the dorsal flap varies; it is often 18 mm long and 9 mm wide in the normal 12 month old child and extends almost to the proximal interphalangeal joint extension crease. The palmar inset flap is marked so that there is always slight overcorrection. The third web space extends more distal than the second and fourth. Distal zigzag incisions are measured so that mirror images are created on the two sides of each finger. Sharp, acute angles are preferable to gentle, obtuse angles, which often become straight with growth. Marked reference points along the sides of the digits (Flatt, 1974), bent dental wires (Cronin, 1956), or 25 gauge needles passed through the webbing may help align this precision marking (see Fig. 128–36A). The flaps are equally distributed between the two digits. Techniques designed to totally resurface one side of the release with flap tissue and the other with a

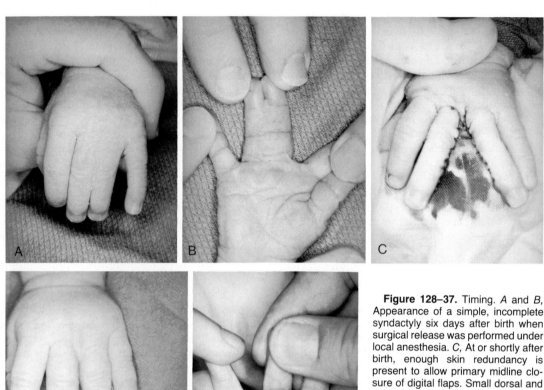

Figure 128–37. Timing. *A* and *B*, Appearance of a simple, incomplete syndactyly six days after birth when surgical release was performed under local anesthesia. *C*, At or shortly after birth, enough skin redundancy is present to allow primary midline closure of digital flaps. Small dorsal and palmar triangular flaps were used here to line the commissure (see Norton, 1881). Skin flaps were tight with the digits held in abduction. *D* and *E*, Excellent primary healing is present six months later. Slight constriction at the base of the commissure can be released at a later date with Z-plasties. Surgical release during infancy has limited application at this time.

skin graft (Bauer, Tondra, and Trusler, 1956) often yield inconsistent results.

Following limb exsanguination and tourniquet inflation, the web is released beginning distally and progressing proximally. A knife or small osteotome is often sufficient to release distal bone or cartilaginous coalitions beneath conjoined nails. Palmar pulp can often be defatted and advanced dorsally to create a new paronychial fold. In some cases, a portion of the lateral nail matrix and underlying bone may provide enough space for advancement. Composite grafts from the lateral portion of the great toe may also provide a smooth rounded fold (Hentz, 1985). For complex syndactylies with a conjoined nail, some authors have advocated separation of the nail and application of a thenar flap as a

preliminary procedure to web separation (Johannsen, 1982). This procedure is not routinely performed.

Neurovascular structures are identified, and the interdigital separation is performed in the midline toward the proximal interphalangeal joint. The fascial interconnecting fibers between Clelland's ligaments on either digit are incised, and excised if thick and fibrous. Magnification is essential in the dissection of this tissue from the underlying neurovascular structures on either side of the web. The dorsal flap is next raised with careful preservation of large dorsal veins. Nerves are identified and can easily be teased proximally if a distal bifurcation is found. The arborization of the common digital artery to the adjacent sides of the cleft will often be

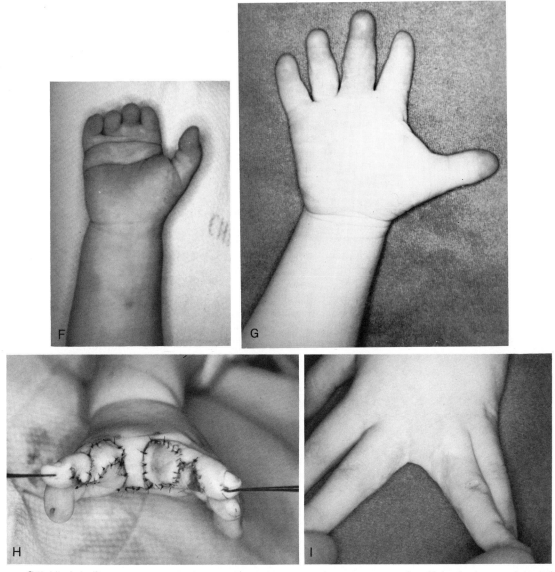

Figure 128–37 *Continued F* and *G,* Preoperative and postoperative appearance of multiple simple, complete web releases which were performed at two stages at 24 and 32 months of age. *H* and *I,* The large dorsal flap has provided excellent lining to the commissure.

the structure limiting the depth of the commissure release. At least one digital artery per digit should be preserved. If an artery is injured or cut in a digit with known absence of an artery on the opposite side, revascularization utilizing the operating microscope is recommended.

The transverse metacarpal ligament is identified and is incised if greater metacarpal mobility is desired, as in the hypoplastic hand or Apert's hand. Abnormal osseous structures may require rearrangement at this point, but most surgeons prefer to delay definitive skeletal correction until the patient is older.

Damage to growth centers and periosteum must be avoided. The dorsal flap is rotated into the depth of the release, and the palmar flap is interdigitated and secured with 5-0 or 6-0 absorbable sutures tied under no tension. The distal flaps along the sides of the digits are closed. Excessive defatting in order to gain mobilization and close these flaps is not recommended but may be helpful along the borders. Exact templates are made of all areas to be grafted. The tourniquet is released, flap circulation checked, and hemostasis controlled.

A pressure dressing is applied after tourniquet release, while full-thickness skin grafts are harvested from the inguinal crease, well lateral to the future hair-bearing eschutcheon (see Fig. 128–36, *inset*). The donor site is closed using buried absorbable sutures and external Steri-Strips. The skin grafts are defatted and sutured into position with 6-0 chromic sutures.

The dressing is important! All grafts and incisions are covered with one layer of a medicated gauze followed by a compressible synthetic foam or moistened cotton placed as a stent within the interdigital web space. The fingers are positioned in abduction to avoid kinking of the commissure flaps. A bulky fluff dressing is then applied and secured with a circumferential Kling wrap. The extremity is then immobilized with a well-padded long arm cast or splint extending well above the flexed elbow. Because the forearm of a 2 year old child is bulky in its midportion and tapers distally, casts easily slip off unless elbow flexion is maintained. The thumb or at least one other finger is left exposed distally to act as a monitor of hand position within the cast. A stockinette-sling is then passed around the cast and tied behind the child's back. The other end can also be tied to a line strapped above the child's bed for elevation. At night the second end is looped around a line strung above the crib. Proper dressings and immobilization of an active child's arm are the single most important factors in obtaining a satisfactory skin graft take. The cast is left in place for two to three weeks, depending upon the amount of bone or soft tissue reconstruction performed (Fig. 128–38).

Problematic grafts or flaps may require earlier inspection. Cast removal is usually most efficiently accomplished in the ambulatory surgery room under sedation or light general anesthesia for the uncooperative child or equally anxious parent. When healing has been incomplete and small areas of scar are present at the base of the commissure, small splints and molded inserts are made for the child to wear at night.

Thumb-Index Web Space. The first web space has the configuration of a diamond-shaped tetrahedron (Littler, 1977). Complete syndactyly of this web space occurs in less than 10 per cent of all cases, but very frequently this region is deficient in the congenitally deformed hand, limiting abduction and independent motion of the thumb. Often, thenar muscles are deficient; their reconstruction is covered in Chapter 123.

Correction of the thumb-index deficiency varies with the severity of the contracture. For small defects, commonly seen in the hypoplastic hand with a small thumb, or broad defects with loose mobile skin, variations of Z-plasties may be used. A single large Z-plasty is often sufficient to provide a greater release than multiple small flaps (Fig. 128–39A). In many cases the four-flap Z-plasty

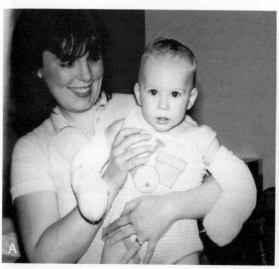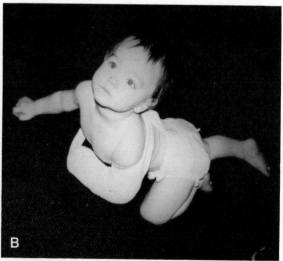

Figure 128–38. *A,* Immobilization of the youngster, one of the single most important variables in syndactyly surgery, can be achieved with a good compression dressing secured with a long arm cast (fiber glass or plaster), extending well proximal to the flexed elbow. Fingertips can be covered, but the thumb is left exposed and is a good indicator of hand position within the cast. *B,* A stockinette tied around the back provides a "Chinese handcuff," which permits crawling but restricts use.

provides excellent length and contour within the depth of the web space (Furnas and Fischer, 1971; Woolf and Broadbent, 1972) (Fig. 128–39B and C). In a similar procedure, a complex central V-Y, lateral Z-plasty approach may also accomplish the same result and is more useful within interdigital web space (Hirschowitz, Karev, and Rousso, 1975). Techniques for providing dynamic muscle balance following soft tissue release are covered in other sections.

In patients with mild or moderate webbing, more than skin is tight. The investing fascia of the adductor pollicis and first dorsal interosseous muscles and, occasionally, the capsule of the carpometacarpal joint, particularly in complex syndactyly, require release. Ideally, the surgeon would like to gain maximal thumb-index span and close with local glabrous skin. In moderately severe defects, skin flaps should be used following web release to line the depth of the commissure and the ulnar border of the thumb, and a full-thickness skin graft should be placed over the dorsal interosseous muscle. A large diamond-shaped graft can be used to cover the entire defect. Releases are effectively maintained with temporary internal Kirschner wire fixation traversing the midportion of the first and second metacarpals.

When the defect is severe, types of dorsal rotation flaps are used to resurface the ulnar side of the thumb and the depth of the commissure (Fig. 128–39D). Rarely are pedicle flaps or free tissue transfers practical considerations in the small child. Newer methods of distraction and skin expansion have not yet been applied to the congenitally deficient first web space. In the most severe restriction of the first web space, ray resection of the index finger should be considered. The tight investing fascia of the first dorsal interosseous and abductor pollicis muscles must be released to gain maximum space. Occasionally the tight capsule of the carpometacarpal joint must be released to improve mobility. A skin graft is used to cover the donor defect. The sliding flap from the radial side of the index finger may be used in the same fashion. A large diamond-shaped, split-thickness skin graft may be sufficient cover.

Complications. Fortunately, complications following a carefully planned and executed procedure are unusual, but when present, they greatly affect the long-term functional result. The most dramatic early complication is *vascular compromise* due to tight dressings, suturing of skin flaps under tension, or injury to digital vessels. Before a dressing is applied the optimal position of the commissure flaps must be checked with the tourniquet deflated, because placing adjacent digits in too much adduction may kink the flap(s). Five or six days postoperatively, *infection* or *maceration* may occur beneath the bulky dressings and may be difficult to detect. Temperature elevation, erythema, extreme irritability, and odiferous dressings are important clues.

The most significant late complication of any web release is scar contracture resulting in a distal migration of the reconstructed commissure. Contracture can be secondary to an initial graft or flap loss, but can also simply be due to a growth discrepancy between scar and normal tissue. A 1.0 mm loss of tissue or graft in an infant translates into a 1.0 cm distraction in the adult (Fig. 128–40). Compression garments, with or without malleable inserts, Coban wrapping, and interdigital splints are of limited value in these young patients, who are known to develop hypertrophic scars or keloids, particularly Oriental and black patients. Early release with Z-plasties or skin grafts is recommended for these difficult problems, but each case must be carefully individualized.

Syndactyly-Related Syndromes

APERT'S SYNDROME

Clinical Presentation

Apert's syndrome is the most common of six acrocephalosyndactyly (ACS) syndromes seen by the hand surgeon. It may affect persons of all races and has an autosomal dominant inheritance pattern and an incidence higher than one in 100,000 live births (Blank, 1960). The physical findings are striking. Facial features consist of a wide variety of skull deformities due to premature closure of the basal portions of the coronal and, frequently, the lambdoidal sutures. The orbits are shallow, with exorbitism. There is a failure of forward growth of the maxilla, with a parrot-beaked nose, a high-arched palate, and crowding of maxillary teeth and tongue, which can frequently cause upper airway difficulty. The forehead is deeply furrowed (Fig. 128–41).

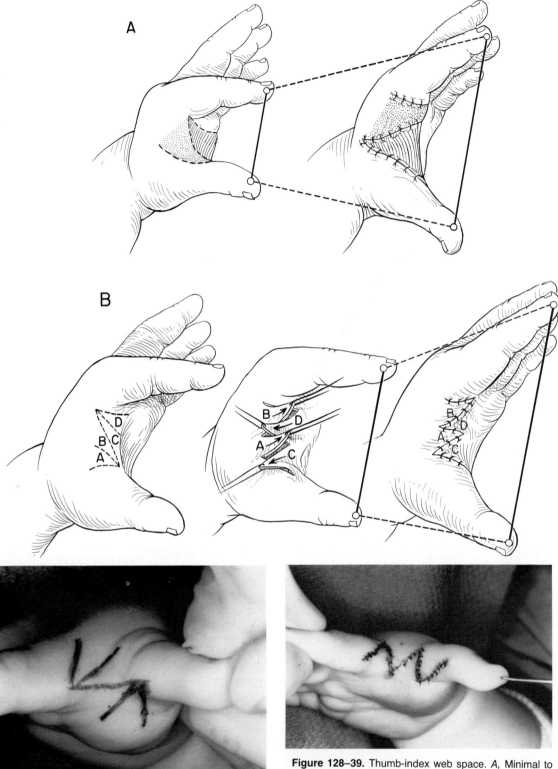

Figure 128–39. Thumb-index web space. *A,* Minimal to moderate contractures within this web space best corrected with simple Z-plasties. The central incision is made over the area of maximal tightness between the bases of the thumb and index finger (*left*). The palmar transposition flap (stippled) is incised first and matched. The dorsal flap of more mobile skin is then raised and can be made asymmetrical, depending upon the geometry of the defect. After transposition and closure, the thumb-index span is greatly increased (*right*). *B,* A greater release and excellent contour are obtained with a four flap Z-plasty; *left,* incisions; *middle,* flaps transposed; *right,* after closure. *C,* A clinical case illustration demonstrates the incisions and the significant increase in web span that can be obtained.

D

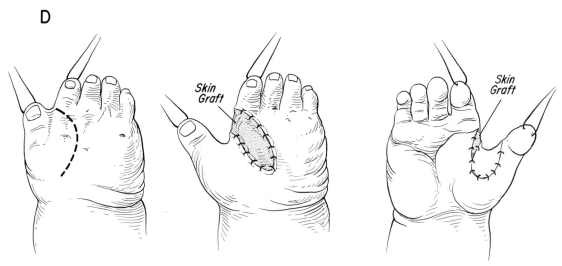

Figure 128–39 *Continued D,* A dorsal rotation flap of full-thickness skin graft is often necessary for the tight web space with hypoplastic hands. This web can then be subsequently broadened with Z-plasties if necessary with growth.

Figure 128–40. Complications can and do occur following routine syndactyly release when graft "take" has been incomplete or partial flap loss has occurred at the base of the commissure. The hand of this child demonstrates linear contractures and distal migration of the commissure with growth. Z-plasty correction was possible without additional skin grafts.

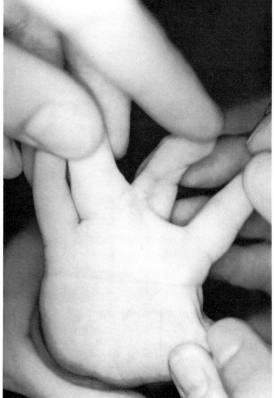

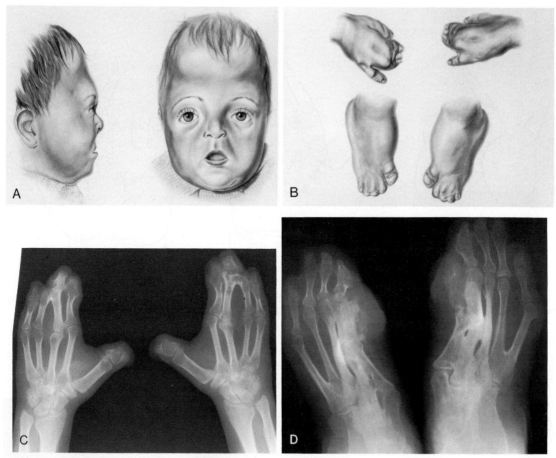

Figure 128–41. Apert's syndrome. *A,* Common features in Apert's syndrome include a midface hypoplasia resulting in exorbitism, a "parrot-beaked" nose, and retruded maxilla with a high arched palate. Upper airway obstruction is common, and the tongue often contains a central furrow. Skull deformities may vary but are usually accompanied by a deep forehead furrow. *B,* Mirror image hand (*top*) and foot (*bottom*) anomalies are always present. *C* and *D,* The first ray on all extremities is always deficient. In the hand, a short thumb with radial clinodactyly is present, and in the foot, the great toe is so short and medially displaced that partial amputation is occasionally necessary to accommodate the wearing of conventional shoes.

There are no commonly associated malformations besides those of the musculoskeletal and central nervous systems. Although mental retardation is *not* part of this syndrome, at least half of affected children require special assistance in school, but many are normal if intracranial pressure problems are aggressively treated in infancy. Historically, many of these individuals have been institutionalized, and their intellectual potentials never developed.

Symmetric complex and complicated syndactylies of both hands and feet are present (Hoover, Flatt, and Weiss, 1970). Usually there is skeletal dysplasia of the glenohu-

meral joint (Fig. 128–42), and occasionally the elbow joint, which limits proximal limb function (Mah and associates, in press). Two basic types of hand patterns are seen, the flat, spade-like hand and the constricted, cupped, mitten hand (Fig. 128–43A and B). Common to both are (1) a short, radially deviated thumb with an abnormal, delta-shaped proximal phalanx; (2) a complex side-to-side fusion involving phalanges of the index, long, and ring fingers; (3) symphalangism within the four digits; and (4) a simple syndactyly involving the fourth web space. Less than half of these patients have syndactyly of the first web space (Upton, 1986).

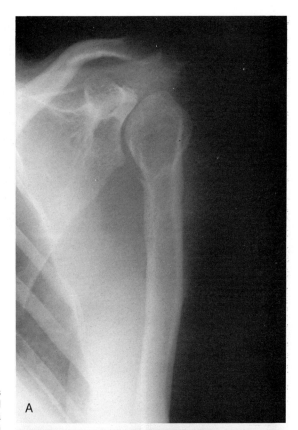

Figure 128–42. Proximal upper limb anomalies of Apert's syndrome will greatly affect hand function. Seen in internal (*A*) and external (*B*) rotation, the abnormal shoulder with a dysplastic glenoid cavity and abnormal humeral head often gives the clinical appearance of an anterior dislocation. Elbow ankylosis and proximal radioulnar synostosis may also restrict proximal limb motion.

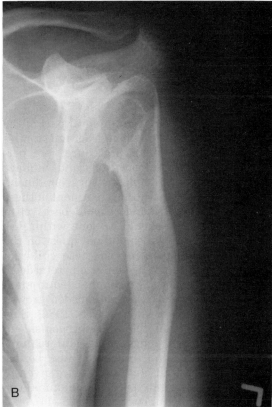

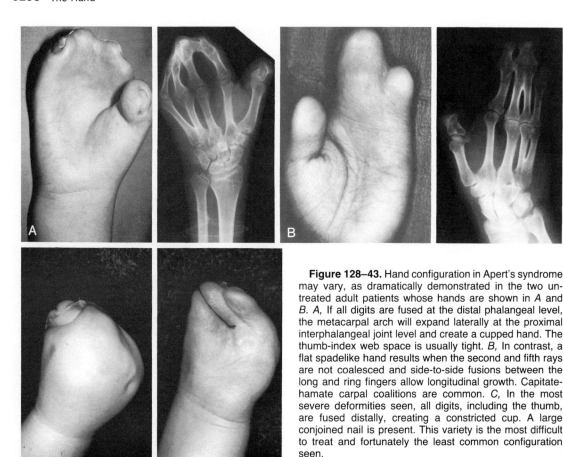

Figure 128–43. Hand configuration in Apert's syndrome may vary, as dramatically demonstrated in the two untreated adult patients whose hands are shown in *A* and *B*. *A*, If all digits are fused at the distal phalangeal level, the metacarpal arch will expand laterally at the proximal interphalangeal joint level and create a cupped hand. The thumb-index web space is usually tight. *B*, In contrast, a flat spadelike hand results when the second and fifth rays are not coalesced and side-to-side fusions between the long and ring fingers allow longitudinal growth. Capitate-hamate carpal coalitions are common. *C*, In the most severe deformities seen, all digits, including the thumb, are fused distally, creating a constricted cup. A large conjoined nail is present. This variety is the most difficult to treat and fortunately the least common configuration seen.

Treatment

The hand surgeon is an integral part of the craniofacial team. Although craniectomies and intracranial shunt procedures are performed by the neurosurgeon, and midface advancements by the plastic surgeon, during the first few months of life, treatment of these severely deformed hands should be given a high priority and should be done within the first 24 months. One should not question the advisability of operating on these children, because they are not by definition "retarded." Early hand surgery is recommended to maximize function and allow unimpeded growth (Barot and Caplan, 1986; Upton, 1986). Surgical treatment has the following goals: separation of digits, lengthening and realignment of the thumb, release of the border digits first, with absolute preference given to the thumb-index web space, and maximal use of potential joint function (Fig. 128–44).

In mild cases, Z-plasty techniques are sufficient in the first web space, but large dorsal rotation flaps and skin grafts are necessary when this web space is tight or completely webbed, particularly in the spoon-shaped hand configuration, which is the most difficult to treat. Abnormal extensions of palmar fascia and tight bands over the adductor pollicis should be released. Because well over 50 per cent of hand function is achieved with the thumb and index finger pinch or grasp in these patients, careful preservation of all thumb intrinsic tendons is mandatory. The adductor pollicis is universally hypertrophied. Index metacarpal ray resection to create an adequate first web space may be advisable, and the creation of a three-fingered hand may often be both more functional and more esthetic. The central index-long-ring coalition is then released before 3 years of age to allow unrestricted growth of adjacent digits. Skeletal alignment of interphalangeal

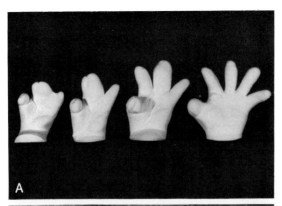

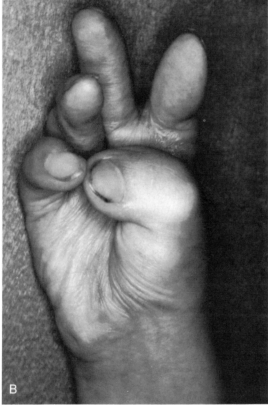

Figure 128–44. Apert's syndrome. *A,* Hand casts of the same patient show the results of sequential web releases, which started at 8 months of age. The released digits often show a sunburst appearance. At age 6 years the radial clinodactyly of the thumb will be corrected. *B,* Although most prehension in these patients exists between the thumb and index finger, mobilization of the fifth ray with excision of the fourth-fifth metacarpal synostosis can be beneficial for creation of thumb–fifth finger pinch grasp.

bifurcations of neurovascular and tendinous structures, abnormal intrinsic muscles, distal and crossed insertions of extrinsic flexor and extensor tendons, and all variations of abnormal phalanges and interphalangeal joints. The site for distal osteotomy or ostectomy with separation of the index-long-ring complex is the most difficult region to resurface and is treated with dorsal advancement of palmar pulp, dorsal flaps (Buck-Gramcko, 1986), skin grafts, or a combination of these techniques. Careful attention to reconstruct the normal size and contour of the nail bed and construct paronychial fold can be rewarding. Before or shortly after 5 years of age, the radially deviated thumb should be lengthened with an opening wedge osteotomy, bone graft, and soft tissue lengthening with a Z-plasty or a skin graft (see "Clinodactyly" and Fig. 128–82).

Ironically, the fifth ray is often anatomically the most normal digit in the hand but is furthest from the mobile thumb. Its distal interphalangeal joint is commonly the only functional interphalangeal joint in the hand. Mobility of this finger can be improved with excision of the ring-small metacarpal synostosis that is often present and release of the transverse metacarpal ligament. Interpositional material such as fascia, tendon, or silicone must be placed to prevent refusion in children (Fig. 128–44). After the child reaches skeletal maturity, implant arthroplasty at the metacarpophalangeal joint may improve motion. Implants at the interphalangeal joint level are not recommended, because long-term follow-up indicates that these digits possess very little motion (Upton, 1986).

Refinement procedures such as arthrodeses, osteotomies, and soft tissue and nail revisions are necessary at later ages, but the surgeon should make every effort to combine multiple procedures during single operations in an effort to reduce the total number of hospitalizations, anesthesia episodes, cost, etc., for these children and their families. The author's current experience with over 50 children with Apert's syndrome is that by the time they are 20 years of age they will have had undergone general anesthesia at least 15 times. All major reconstruction should be completed by school age. Hyperhidrosis often creates wound and graft maceration and healing problems during warm weather in these children, in whom the indications for cast and dressing changes is much lower. As teenagers, these children will have many skin prob-

joints is recommended, because these three rays have very poor, if any, motion beyond the metacarpophalangeal joint level.

Only one side of a digit should be released at a time in this central area, where abnormal anatomy is the rule and consists of very distal lems on the face, chest, and arms secondary to acne. Their hands will never look normal but can be extremely functional.

Serial psychologic evaluations in these patients indicate that their sense of mastery, self-esteem, and competence is very much a part of upper limb and hand function. The earlier they are able to increase hand function, the more likely these children, on whatever cognitive level, will demonstrate important psychologic development (Belfer, Harrison, and Murray, 1979).

POLAND'S SYNDROME

Clinical Presentation

This common syndactyly-related syndrome seen by the hand surgeon classically consists of (1) the absence of the sternocostal portion of the pectoralis major muscles, (2) hypoplasia of the hand and, to a lesser degree, of the forearm and upper arm, (3) simple, complete, or incomplete syndactyly, and (4) short fingers (brachysymphalangism) (Clarkson, 1962; Ireland, Takayama, and Flatt, 1976; Sugiura, 1976) (Figs. 128–45 and 128–46). The etiology of the condition is unknown, and there is no inheritance pattern or predisposition. There also are no commonly associated anomalies (Bouvet and associates, 1976; Goldberg and Mazzei, 1977).

A wide variety of hand presentations are found, as the central index, long, and ring fingers are more commonly affected than the thumb and fifth rays. The first web space is invariably restricted, and all degrees of skeletal hypoplasia are present within the digits, which are joined by simple syndactylies. In the most severe form of Poland's syndrome, hypoplastic thumb and fifth fingers are present and the remaining digits are represented by hypoplastic nubbins. The ipsilateral pectoralis major muscle deficit may also be associated with absence or hypoplasia of the serratus anterior, latissimus dorsi, and deltoid muscles, breast hypoplasia (33 per cent of females), rib cage deficiencies, scoliosis, and rarely, dextrocardia.

Associated chest wall skeletal and soft tissue deformities often require treatment, particularly in the adolescent female with a hypoplastic breast. Restoration of contour to ipsilateral chest wall deformities is seldom required. Alloplastic materials rarely remain in place for a lifetime, but more recently, local latissimus dorsi muscle pedicle transfers and custom-made silicone implants have gained popularity (Ohmori and Takada, 1980).

Treatment

The lack of skeletal fusions and complicated syndactylies makes treatment of Poland's syndrome more straightforward. The optimal age for correction depends upon the age and the extent of the deformity, but major functional reconstruction should be completed by school age. Nonadjacent webs are released before 2 to 3 years of age. If a Z-plasty technique is not sufficient for release of the first web space, a dorsal rotational flap and skin graft will provide adequate release (see Fig. 128–39D). Exaggeration of web deepening will often add relative length to the short digit but if overdone creates a bizarre appearance. Distraction techniques and bone grafts have been used to lengthen these hypoplastic digits but should be performed with caution, because complications secondary to rapid overstretching are common at this level. Broad commissure release within the second and fourth web spaces will effectively increase mobility and abduction of index and fifth fingers. Rotational osteotomy of the thumb metacarpal and tendon transfers are occasionally indicated to improve thumb position and strength. Tendon transfers are not needed in less severe cases. The mitten hand with the thumb in the same plane as the digits is treated by early release of the first web with a generous dorsal flap and release of a tight carpometacarpal joint. With time and growth, functioning thenar intrinsic muscles will position the thumb in sufficient palmar abduction and avoid the necessity for rotational osteotomy (Fig. 128–46C).

Follow-up evaluation in these children is very important, because soft tissue and skeletal deformities may be accentuated by growth. Correction of the symphalangism with insertion of implants seen at the interphalangeal level is not helpful; this technique is discussed in more detail in another section (Flatt, 1977). Occasionally, a patient may request augmentation of a severely hypoplastic forearm. This can be accomplished with skin expansion followed by insertion of custom-made soft gel silicone implants (Fig. 128–47).

In the most severe form of Poland's syndrome, the hand deformity resembles either

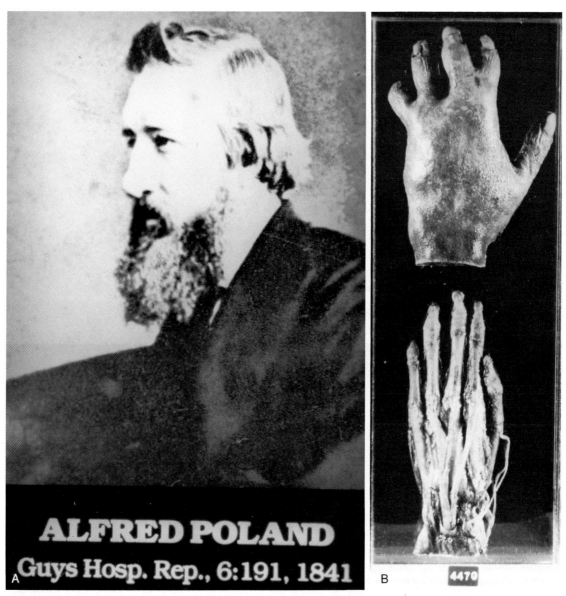

Figure 128–45. Poland's syndrome. Photographs of Alfred Poland, M.D. (*A*), and the dried preparation of the hand (specimen 4470) that he dissected in 1840 (*B*). Although not described in detail in his article published in the Guy's Hospital Report, the hand has short digits with incomplete simple syndactylies primarily involving the central three rays. (Courtesy of Joe Dawes, curator of Guy's Hospital Museum, London, England.)

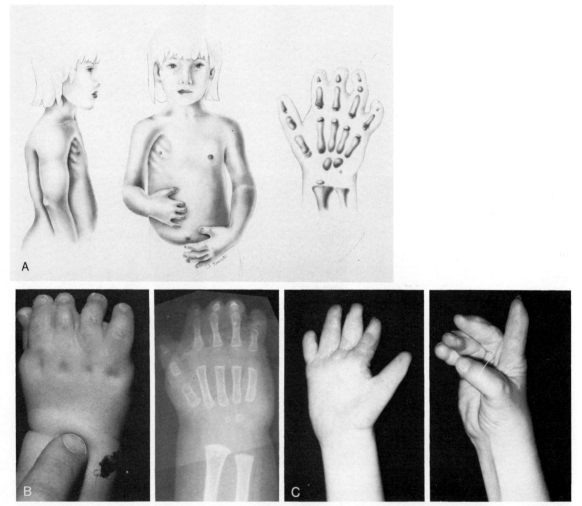

Figure 128–46. Poland's syndrome. *A,* Features commonly seen by the hand surgeon are an ipsilateral deficiency of the pectoralis major and occasionally the pectoralis minor muscle, hypoplasia of the hand, short digits often with missing phalanges, and incomplete simple syndactyly. *B,* Clinical and radiographic appearances of typical hand before web separation. *C,* The thumb commonly rotates into more palmar abduction when a flap hand is initially present. Appearance five years after interdigital web releases and four flap Z-plasty of the thumb-index web space.

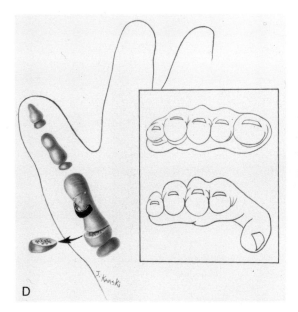

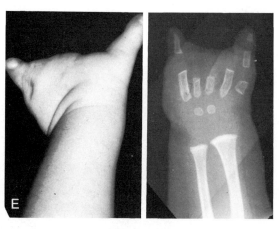

Figure 128–46 *Continued D,* When thumb abduction does not occur, rotational angulation osteotomy may be indicated. *E,* In severe cases, the three central rays are represented by nubbins, yielding a two-finger ("lobster claw") hand.

"symbrachydactyly" or "ectrodactyly," with only hypoplastic first and fifth rays, or consists of a hand with no digits at all (adactyly). The first two forms are best treated with functional alignment of the two digits to add opposable pinch and tendon grafts to provide power (see Fig. 128–46*E*). Extrinsic muscle-tendon units are present in the forearm, frequently with abnormal distal tendon insertions within the proximal palm. Staged flexor or extensor tendon grafts with pulley reconstruction can be done to provide pincer grasp. Adactylous patients should be considered for (1) no treatment, (2) toe transfers, or (3) partial hand prostheses, depending on needs and bimanual function. Distraction at the metacarpal level may be helpful to increase the length of functioning border digits (i.e., thumb and fifth finger).

ACROSYNDACTYLY

Clinical Presentation

The term *acrosyndactyly* denotes digits (Gr., *dactylos*) formed together (Gr., *syn*) in a peak (Gr., *acro*) and is generally considered part of the constriction ring syndrome. There is always a proximal dorsal to palmar epithelium-lined space or sinus. Dissections by Lösch and Duncker (1971) and extensive studies by Patterson (1961) and Torpin and Faulkner (1966) indicate that some type of disruption sequence initiated by an ischemic insult occurs after the digits have been sep-

arated and that the resulting scar tissue draws adjacent soft tissue and bone together. Patterson (1961) has also noted the possibility that there is a more fundamental tissue problem because of the high number of associated anomalies, including facial clefts, congenital heart defects, and clubbed feet. Frequently, upper and lower limbs are involved. The author's series of 175 patients with the constriction ring syndrome has an associated anomaly rate of 13 per cent. It is quite possible that a combination of malformations, disruption, and deformation sequences may be involved in this syndrome (Granick and associates, 1987) (see also "Dysmorphology").

Walsh (1970) has documented a very wide range of hand presentations and categorized them as mild, moderate, and severe, depending on skeletal structure. In mild cases, three phalanges with two segmental joints are present with well-formed proximal clefts. In moderately involved hands, there are two phalanges and a single interphalangeal joint. In severe cases, only hypoplastic nubbins with small phalanges are present. Of the 68 cases Walsh (1970) studied, four were mild, 44 moderate, and 20 severe. There is no standard pattern of involvement in a single hand or in opposite limbs of the same child (Walsh, 1970). A typical pattern of syndactyly is present in all of these hands. Large and small epithelium-lined spaces or sinuses are present, denoting web commissures that are characteristically more distal to their normal lo-

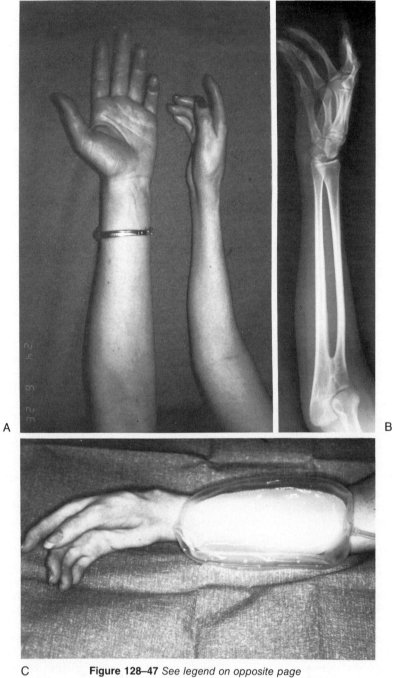

A

B

C   **Figure 128–47** *See legend on opposite page*

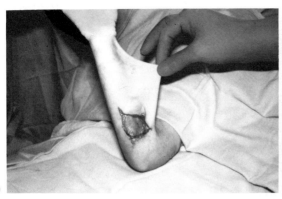

D

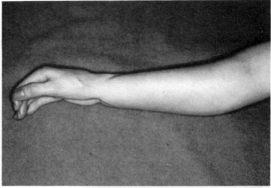

E

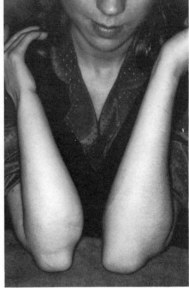

F

Figure 128–47. *A* and *B,* Preoperative appearance of an adult female with rightsided Poland's syndrome seeking esthetic improvement of her hand. A preaxial radioulnar synostosis prevented forearm rotation. *C,* Skin expansion was used to create room within a subcutaneous pocket for a custom-made implant. *D,* Eight years later, this implant is still in place. The syndactyly was corrected in two stages, with a four flap Z-plasty for the first interdigital web and dorsal flaps, and skin flaps for the remaining webs. *E* and *F,* Appearance eight years after operation.

cation (Lösch and Duncker, 1972). Congenital transverse amputation of one or more digits is common, and soft tissue at and distal to the level of digital coalescence is always deficient. Digits are short and osseous involvement is different from that in other forms of syndactyly. Extra skeletal parts are never found, and fusion is between common scars in a side-to-side or on-top position.

Treatment

The size of the clefts, extent of fusion, and relative deformities of adjacent digits all play a role in surgical decision making. Generally, doing many smaller procedures in lieu of a large one is recommended, because of the precarious blood supply to these digits (Blauth, 1972). Digits joined at the tips in mild and moderate cases should be released early to allow unrestricted longitudinal

growth. Incising a small band in the newborn in the nursery will often liberate one or more border digits being held to the central scar mass (Fig. 128–48*B*). Walsh (1970) did not find any correlation between the method of tip release and ultimate function. Often, bizarre nubbins with and without nails are saved initially only to become the focus of peer group curiosity a few years later. The epithelium-lined clefts should be deepened at a later date and often overcorrected in order to provide additional relative length for the hypoplastic digits (Fig. 128–49).

Incision planning may be quite difficult because of these lined clefts or sinuses. The level of the existing sinus is usually distal and should not necessarily become the level of commissure. When available, dorsal skin should be used to line the depth of the ultimate commissure, and full-thickness skin grafts should be used to line the sides of the

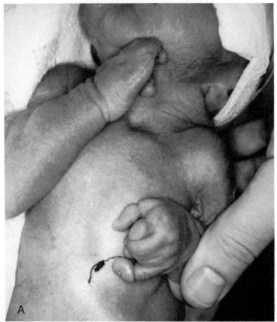

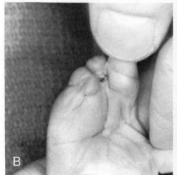

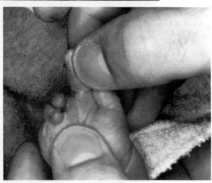

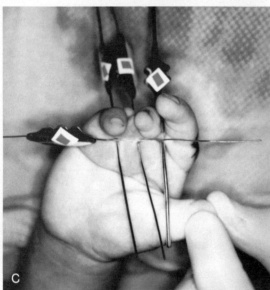

Figure 128–48. Acrosyndactyly. *A,* Occasionally at birth, the tight band may still be attached to the patient. Histology of this strand is consistent with the inner layer of chorion. Soft tissue swelling distal to these bands may be marked. *B,* Simple release of small soft tissue bridges in the newborn nursery will liberate constricted digits. *C,* Dorsal to palmar communicating sinuses lined with epithelium are characteristically present. These represent the depth of commissures that had formed prior to the ischemic necrosis precipitated by the constriction band.

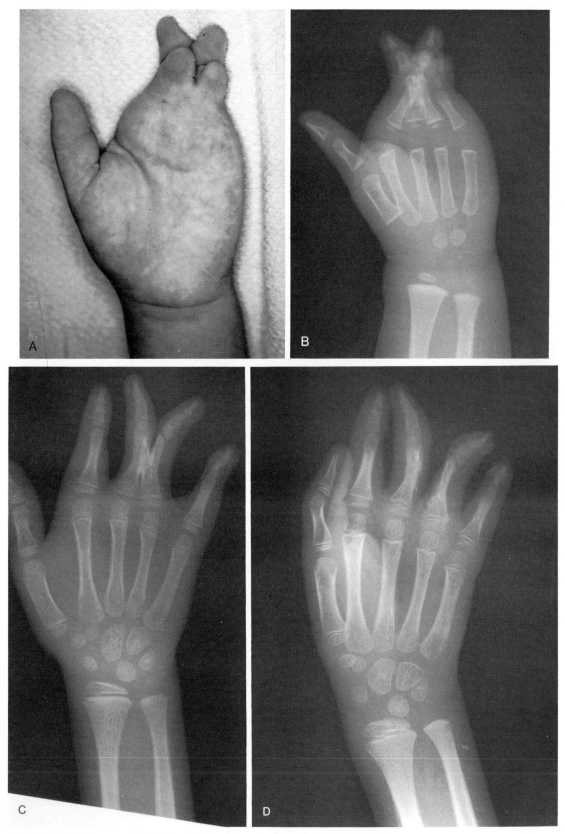

Figure 128–49. Acrosyndactyly. *A* and *B,* Appearance and x-ray of a baby with all digits stacked in side-to-side fashion. *C* and *D,* Treatment consisted of separation of the index and fifth fingers in separate procedures followed by separation and osteotomy of the long-ring coalition at one year intervals. The two central fingers will be straightened when the child is older.

digits, which in most cases will have limited joint motion. Coalesced scar tissue will be found at the point of common union between adjacent digits or finger and thumb, but normal anatomy is characteristically found proximal to these areas. In severe cases, early separation is recommended. Often a functionless nubbin can be sacrificed and its skin used as a full-thickness skin graft. The most difficult problems occur when there is not enough proximal finger skeletal remnant to accommodate its distal partner beyond the point of common scar.

No generalities can be given for the management of hypoplastic nails and fingertip nubbins, which are usually preserved initially and excised later if they create functional or esthetic problems. The management of the individual constriction ring or annular band and distal lymphedematous tissue is covered in another section (see "Constriction Rings Syndrome").

Symphalangism

Clinical Presentation

Cushing (1916) noted that one of his patients with an intracranial glioma was unable to bend her proximal interphalangeal joints, and after 10 years of studying her kindred, he published a classic paper, in which he introduced the term "symphalangism" in the description of a family with 84 involved persons from a kindred of 313 examined. This pedigree was later updated by Strasburger and associates (1965). The largest pedigree in the genetic literature involves the Talbot family of England, from the mid 1450's through the twentieth century (Drinkwater, 1917; Elkington and Huntsman, 1967).

Failure of segmentation or incomplete segmentation with cavitation has for generations been of great interest to geneticists, who have classified at least 15 conditions with stiff fingers. Inheritance in most conditions follows an autosomal dominant pattern, but isolated cases do occur frequently. The true incidence of symphalangism has never been determined, because this is rarely a primary diagnosis, usually seen in conjunction with another condition (see "Etiology and Genetics") (Goldberg and Bartoshesky, 1985). Flatt and Wood (1975) classify the conditions as (1) true symphalangism, in which digits have normal length, (2) symbrachydactyly, in which digits are short as well as stiff, or (3) symphalangism with associated anomalies (Flatt and Wood, 1975). The majority of cases in the third group include syndactyly, and most are diagnosed as either Apert's or Poland's syndrome (Fig. 128–50). Many other conditions that demonstrate this deformity, such as gargoylism, are not frequently seen by the hand surgeon.

The proximal interphalangeal joint is the most common site of involvement. In contrast, congenital fusion at the metacarpophalangeal

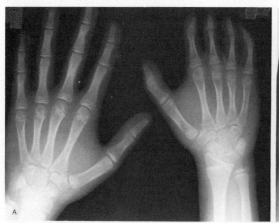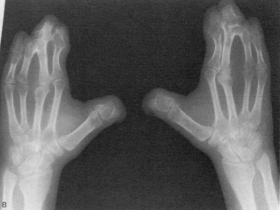

Figure 128–50. Symphalangism. *A,* The proximal interphalangeal joint fusion in Poland's syndrome is common and is usually associated with thin, short digits and an incomplete simple syndactyly. A radial clinodactyly of the fifth finger is common. Comparison with the other hand shows diminished size. A complete coalition of the proximal and middle phalangeal segments is seen in the long and ring rays. *B,* Much more extensive symphalangism exists in Apert's syndrome, in which there is very little, if any, proximal and distal interphalangeal joint motion at skeletal maturity. Only the distal interphalangeal joint of the fifth finger is consistently segmented and has good clinical motion. Proximal fourth-fifth metacarpal synostosis and capitate to hamate carpal coalitions are also present.

joint is extremely rare; fusion of the distal interphalangeal joint is seen with symbrachydactyly in which other abnormalities of the digit exist. In very young children, physical findings may range from a well-segmented but stiff joint space to a minimal space seen on radiograph that is represented on gross examination by a solid cartilaginous bar joining articular surfaces. Initial radiographs of the infant's hand will appear normal because the cartilage representing the epiphysis and joint space is radiolucent. Early radiographic evaluations in these children may be confusing, because the middle phalangeal epiphysis may be mistaken for a joint space. The middle phalanx is usually deficient. When the proximal interphalangeal joint is primarily involved, a tremendous amount of compensatory motion in flexion is often present at the distal level, whereas metacarpophalangeal motion in flexion is usually normal. Affected digits are more slender and lack normal flexion creases in the involved regions. Skin is often atrophic but sensation is normal. One or more digits may be involved, but the thumb is rarely affected. Although the patient cannot make a full fist and power grip is deficient, use of the ulnar three digits may be quite effective despite the loss of normal flexion (Fig. 128–51).

Treatment

Treatment of symphalangism is usually conservative. Attempts to create functional motion with interpositional arthroplasties with silicone caps (Flatt, 1977) and silicone implant arthroplasties (Palmieri, 1980; Dobyns and associates, 1982) have produced unstable joints, despite attempts at collateral ligament construction. Perichondral arthroplasties have been successful at the metacarpophalangeal joint level for post-traumatic conditions but have performed poorly at the interphalangeal joint level (Upton, Sohn, and Glowacki, 1981). Repositioning the flexion position of the three ulnar fingers with angulation osteotomy and arthrodesis improves functional pinch and grip; however, such procedures are usually deferred until skeletal maturity has been reached. Recommended angles for arthrodesis at the proximal interphalangeal joint level are index, 20 degrees; middle, 30 degrees; ring, 40 degrees, and small, 50 degrees (Lister, 1984).

In children less than 2 or 3 years old, exploration of a well-segmented joint space may be useful, because in some cases a solid cartilaginous bar is not present and functional motion may be achieved by release of tight collateral ligaments and the dorsal capsule. After soft tissue release and early passive motion, function may be maintained, although long-term results are less predictable. When a segmented joint is visible on radiograph, early release may be worthwhile (Fig. 128–52). Excision of the cartilaginous bar, with creation of concave/convex surfaces, and early postoperative motion can be frustrating, as these joints rapidly fuse. Methods of maintaining periodic distraction to these digits after release have not been reported.

Radioulnar Synostosis

Clinical Presentation

This condition occurs more commonly than is perceived by most hand surgeons and is often part of syndromes that may have skeletal coalitions at other levels, such as Crouzon's, Apert's, and Poland's varieties. Although etiology is unknown, there appears to be some genetic basis for this failure of differentiation between the radius and ulna (Robinson and associates, 1964). The elbow joint is discernible at 34 days, at which time the cartilaginous anlage representing the humerus, radius, and ulna is present (see Fig. 128–10D). Longitudinal segmentation between the radius and ulna starts distally and progresses proximally. If proper cavitation and segmentation between these forearm anlagen does not occur, the proximal radioulnar joint will not develop, and all degrees of synostosis may result (Fig. 128–53). During this embryologic period the forearm is in pronation, the position found with almost all radioulnar synostoses (Lewis, 1901; Wilkie, 1914).

The proximal one-third of the forearm is the most common site of involvement. About 40 per cent are unilateral, and 60 per cent bilateral. Males and females are equally affected (Mital, 1976). Although these anomalies are not usually noted during infancy, most children present to the surgeon or pediatrician before the age of 3 years with functional problems including difficulty holding objects two-handed and problems with dressing or feeding, and they are often seen holding objects such as coins with a backhanded posture. They will compensate by positioning their shoulders in hyperabduction. These difficulties are most accentuated with bilateral involvement or in children

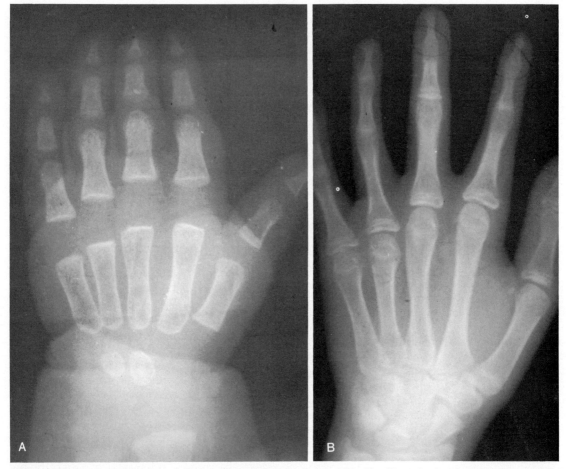

Figure 128–51. Symphalangism. *A,* Early radiographs of this young child with stiff proximal and distal interphalangeal joints show segmentation, even though no more than 15 degrees of passive motion was present. The ring finger appears no different than the adjacent digits. *B,* A solid fusion develops at skeletal maturity in all interphalangeal joints except the ring proximal interphalangeal joint.

with more proximal limb anomalies at the elbow or shoulder level. Adaptive rotational hypermobility at the wrist occurs commonly in most of these patients, who interestingly do not have a higher incidence of internal derangements of the wrist as adults, despite the ligamentous laxity (Simmons, Southmayd, and Riseborough, 1983). With a pronation angle increased beyond 40 degrees, these children also compensate with abduction-elevation of the shoulder.

Approximately one-third of patients with radioulnar synostosis have associated anomalies involving the cardiovascular, genitourinary, gastrointestinal, central nervous, and musculoskeletal systems. Many have hand duplication or absence deformities. No common patterns of association are seen, but proximal radioulnar synostosis frequently occurs in Poland's syndrome and many of the

acrocephalysyndactyly syndromes, particularly the Crouzon, Apert and Carpenter variations (Wynne-Davies, 1973).

All degrees of fixed pronation deformities occur, with approximately 40 per cent of cases having less than 30 degrees, 20 per cent between 31 and 59 degrees, and 40 per cent more than 60 degrees of pronation. The radiologic analysis of these patients spans a wide spectrum from a complete fusion of the entire radius and ulna to a very localized proximal synostosis, which is the most common type (Fig. 128–53). Localized proximal synostosis has been further subdivided into the *primary* type, in which the radial head is absent and the synostosis is extensive, and the *secondary* type, in which the radial head is normal but often dislocated and the synostosis is not as great. The most common presentation is a diminutive radial head and a well-formed

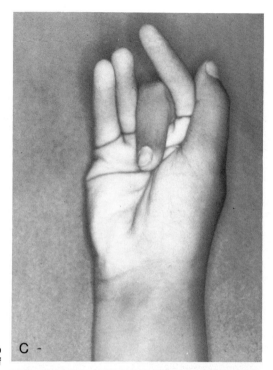

Figure 128–51 *Continued C* and *D,* Despite loss of grip strength, the patient has had few functional deficits. Lack of skin creases and the narrow width of these digits is characteristic.

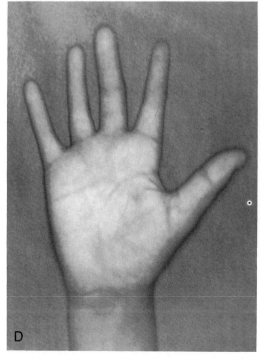

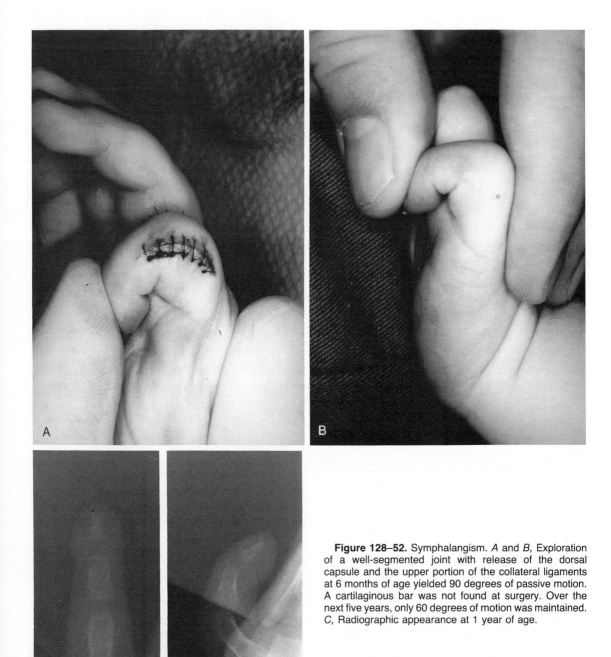

Figure 128–52. Symphalangism. *A* and *B,* Exploration of a well-segmented joint with release of the dorsal capsule and the upper portion of the collateral ligaments at 6 months of age yielded 90 degrees of passive motion. A cartilaginous bar was not found at surgery. Over the next five years, only 60 degrees of motion was maintained. *C,* Radiographic appearance at 1 year of age.

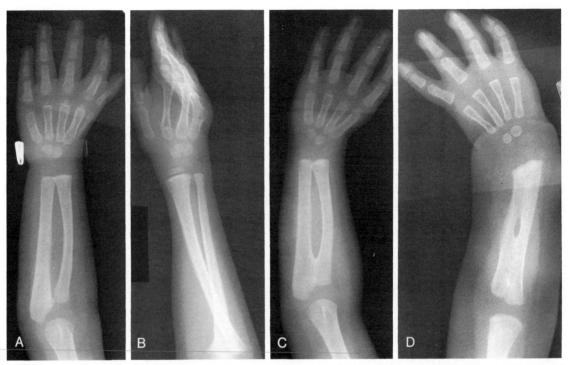

Figure 128–53. Radioulnar synostosis. The degree of involvement varies, as shown in these illustrations. *A,* A localized fibrous union with segmentation on x-ray, but no active pronation and supination. *B,* Absence of bone fusion with radial head subluxation or dislocation with bowing of the radius. *C,* Partial proximal fusion. *D,* Almost complete coalition of both bones in the forearm. The forearm is hypoplastic in the most severe forms. Elbow flexion and extension will be normal in the absence of radial head mechanical obstruction or severe bowing. Hand anomalies frequently coexist but are not always present.

proximal bone coalition. In the evaluation of any radiographs, it is important to differentiate, by means of history, congenital synostosis from post-traumatic cross union in children after forearm fracture, which usually occurs at the distal or middle third of the forearm.

Treatment

Treatment is usually not initiated for unilateral involvement unless fixed pronation is sufficiently great, but it may be quite helpful with bilateral synostosis. Operations to restore motion with resection of the synostosis (Wilkie, 1914), insertion of "swivel apparatuses" (Kelikian, 1974), and reconstruction with interpositional materials (Brady, 1960) are of historical interest only. These innovative procedures have been inconsistent over time because of bone overgrowth around implant materials, angulation of the forearm distal to the osteotomy, and ineffective strength of tendon transfers designed to provide pronation or supination and preexisting contractures of soft tissue (Mital, 1976). The only encouraging results with resection and interposition procedures have been obtained in patients with post-traumatic deformities. The pervading pessimism and surgical nihilism expressed in the literature (Feidt, 1917; Hansen and Anderson, 1970) is not, however, warranted.

Patients with unilateral or bilateral deformities with less than 30 degrees of pronation generally do not need surgery (Dawson, 1912), because they easily compensate. With 60 degrees or more of fixed pronation, there is obvious functional impairment in children with both unilateral and bilateral radioulnar synostosis. The dominant extremity should be given preference. For those with between 30 and 60 degrees of pronation, one must carefully individualize functional limitations, esthetic needs, and degree of involvement. The most common clinical situation in which surgery is recommended is the child with bilateral involvement greater than 40 to 50 degrees of fixed pronation. Derotational osteotomy through the area of synostosis is the treatment of choice, and the ideal time to complete the surgery is before school age (Fig. 128–54).

Technique of Osteotomy. The osteotomy described by Green and Mital (1979) is predictable and reliable. A longitudinal pin is used to stabilize the osteotomy, and a transverse wire to control the amount of rotation. In most cases, 50 to 70 degrees of rotation, from a very pronated position to neutral or slight pronation, is required.

The synostosis is explored through a longitudinal incision over the ulna and subperiosteal elevation dorsally and palmarly. The osteotomy is made through the midportion of the synostosis, and the longitudinal pin is placed through the olecranon across the osteotomy site. The exact amount of derotation accomplished with the transverse pin can be measured by marking the ulna (Fig. 128–54).

It is often difficult to obtain more than 45 degrees of derotation, as tight soft tissue is the limiting factor. If a correction of more than 80 degrees is needed, properly spaced, staged procedures may provide the safest means for total correction. The final position is then stabilized with an additional Kirschner wire. Some prefer to incorporate a single transverse pin into a plaster cast so that potential vascular compromise, the most feared complication of this operation, can be easily relieved with a cast change. The tourniquet should be released and vascular status assessed before final fixation and position are confirmed.

Additional distal radial osteotomies or hand procedures should be done at other times. Besides vascular compromise and compartment syndromes, other reported complications include loss of position when only one

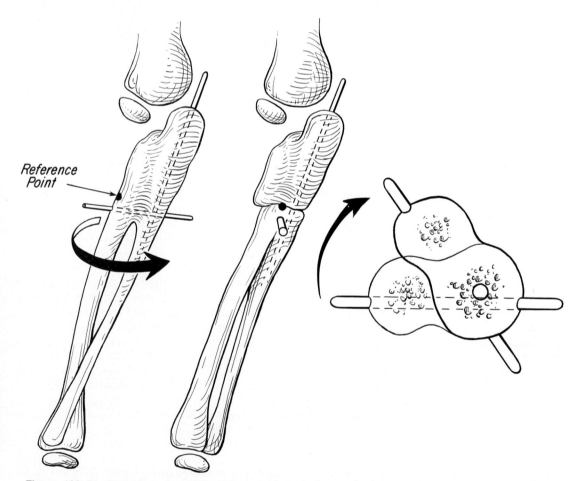

Figure 128–54. Radioulnar synostosis. Osteotomy through the proximal synostosis, the treatment of choice, is demonstrated. The longitudinal pin placed after the osteotomy will control angulation, and the transverse pin can be used to guide the amount of correction. A neutral position of slight pronation is preferred.

transverse pin is used, infection, and transient posterior interosseous nerve palsies.

What is the most functional position? Most authors agree that the corrected position of a unilateral synostosis should be slight, 10 to 20 degrees of, pronation. For bilateral cases, older reports recommended that one arm be placed in 20 to 30 degrees of pronation and the other in slight supination in order to provide a more complete spectrum of function. Because this supinated forearm is often both cosmetically and functionally unpleasant, causing compensatory shoulder hyperabduction, most authors now recommend placing the dominant extremity in 10 to 20 degrees of pronation and the other in neutral position (Green and Mital, 1979; Bayne, 1982). Good to excellent results are achieved in the majority of these patients, who are often surprised by the improved function and by less musculoskeletal discomfort at other levels, such as back, neck, and shoulders.

Vascular Malformations

Although less than 10 per cent of all large vascular tumors involve the upper extremity, those encountered may be extensive and very difficult to treat (Watson and McCarthy, 1940). These lesions represent a failure of differentiation of the primitive vascular elements within the limb bud and may have many forms: arterial, venous, and lymphatic. The literature and management have been hampered by a confusing nomenclature, in which most classification systems present anomalies with differing natural histories and etiologies, so that applying reported treatments to solutions for individual patients is difficult (Table 128–7).

Classification

The suffix -oma should be reserved for lesions that increase in size and grow by cellular proliferation. *Hemangioma* is used for those lesions that demonstrate endothelial activity. Hemangiomas grow shortly after birth, and then undergo a slow spontaneous involution by the third or fourth year of life (Mulliken and Glowacki, 1982). Affected females outnumber males five to one. Not all lesions are noticeable at birth, but all are characterized by rapid growth in the first year, and during this proliferative phase, larger numbers of mast cells are present (Glowacki and Mulliken, 1982).

In contrast, those congenital vascular lesions that show normal endothelial growth characteristics throughout their natural history and normal mast cell counts are *malformations*. Spontaneous involution does not occur, and the lesions grow at the same rate as the rest of the child's body. They may expand with trauma, hemodynamic alterations, or endocrine modulation, especially during menarche, pregnancies, and the adolescent growth spurt, and with antiovulatory medication. Vascular malformations are the result of defective differentiation of vascular elements and may contain one or a combination of arterial, capillary, venous, or lymphatic structures (Mulliken and Glowacki, 1982). For this reason, these vascular anomalies have been included in the failure of differentiation category. Hypertrophy of bone and soft tissue may accompany malformations, which may be further subdivided according to flow dynamics into low flow and high flow lesions. Capillary, lymphatic, and venous elements predominate in low flow lesions, and arterial or "arterialized" vessels with fistulization are more common in the high flow malformations.

Although malformations can be differentiated from hemangiomas by radiography, only clinical examination and natural history are necessary to classify them (Finn, Glowacki, and Mulliken, 1983). The presence of a vascular malformation does not necessarily dictate the need for invasive diagnostic techniques (Table 128–7).

HEMANGIOMA

Clinical Presentation

A hemangioma is usually first noted within the first few weeks of life, beginning as a macular red spot. By 1 to 2 months of age, these vascular lesions are obvious and rapidly growing faster than the child. If the superficial dermis is involved, the epidermal surface has a bulging red appearance similar to that of a strawberry, and if the lesion involves the subcutaneous fat or muscle, the overlying skin often displays a faint bluish hue. Frequently, a large lesion may ulcerate, bleed, and be associated with secondary infection, as its rapid growth ironically exceeds the blood supply. By 8 to 12 months of age, small gray areas called "herald spots" develop, and the hemangioma begins to soften. By 4 to 5 years of age this involution is usually complete.

Table 128–7. Comparison of Hemangiomas and Vascular Malformations in the Upper Limb*

Feature	Hemangiomas	Malformations
Sexual predominance	Females: 5:1	Equal
Endothelium	Endothelial cell proliferation	Normal endothelial cell and turnover cell cycle
Growth	Rapid postnatal growth	Grow proportionate to that of rest of body
Involution	Present	Absent
Percentage present (recognized) at birth	40%	90%
Histology	Mast cells present Thickened basement membrane	No mast cells Normal endothelial cell characteristics

*The clinical and biologic cell-oriented characteristics of hemangiomas and malformations in the upper limb parallel those in the rest of the body. The major distinction is that hemangiomas involute and malformations do not (Mulliken and Glowacki, 1982).

Although within Mulliken and Glowacki's (1982) classification the term hemangioma does not nosologically represent a true failure of differentiation, it has been included here to make this group of vascular anomalies distinct from malformations.

Treatment

Treatment is conservative. Watchful waiting and continued support and reassurance for the parents are required. Ulceration should be treated with appropriate dressings. Central scarred areas will contract when the child is older (Fig. 128–55). In time, when involution is complete, the redundant fibrofatty tissue may be excised. Removal is usually requested by the patients during the adolescent years, more for esthetic reasons than because of functional problems. Low dose irradiation (Watson and McCarthy, 1940), laser therapy (Noe and associates, 1980), sodium morrhuate injections (Owens and Stephenson, 1948), and cryosurgery (Jarzab, 1975) should not be used routinely. In rare instances, when large lesions are associated with congestive heart failure or sys-

temic clotting disorders, oral or intravenous steroid therapy may accelerate involution (Zarem and Edgerton, 1967). Large ipsilateral chest, head, and neck involvement is usually present. Compression garments have been recommended to reduce the size and bulk of these lesions and to relieve symptoms, if present (Miller, Smith, and Sochat, 1976).

CAPILLARY MALFORMATIONS

Clinical Presentation

This congenital ectasia of the dermal vasculature is the familiar "port wine stain," "nevus flammeus," or capillary malformation. Capillary malformations may be well localized or more diffuse, involving an entire extremity or possibly the hemithorax. They are characteristically pink in childhood, becoming purple by adulthood as the channels enlarge and eventually form pedunculated excresences. They are frequently associated with deeper malformations containing lymphatic, arterial, or venous elements.

Treatment

In capillary malformations of the upper extremity, the treatment is conservative. Local cosmetics can be used to cover up the lesions and make them less conspicuous. Laser therapy and local tattooing may be helpful but will invariably leave a nonhomogeneous region of hypopigmentation or scarring (Hall and associates, 1971; Noe and associates, 1980). Replacement of involved skin with flaps or grafts for esthetic reasons has usually been reserved for the facial regions and has not routinely been applied in the upper limb and hand.

Symptoms in these patients are indicative of a deeper malformation and associated physiologic problems. A capillary malformation alone is not associated with local changes in sudomotor function or sensation.

VENOUS MALFORMATIONS

Clinical Presentation

Although present at birth, venous vascular anomalies may not become noticeable until about the first year of life, because they grow proportionately with the rest of the child's body (Mulliken and Glowacki, 1982). Small localized spots or blue marks within the palm, a web space, or the antecubital fossa may

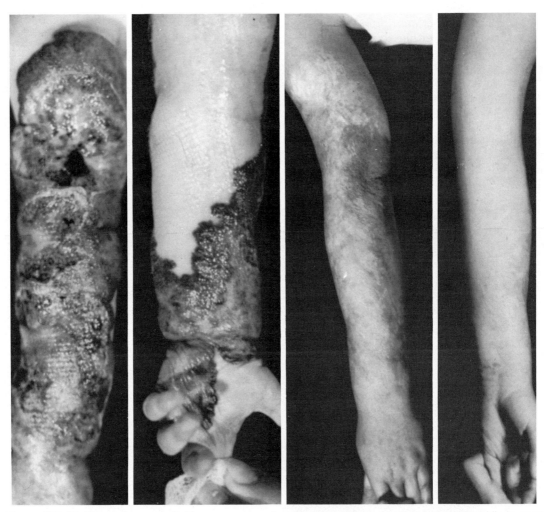

Figure 128–55. Hemangiomas. *Left,* The appearance of a diffuse vascular lesion that increased rapidly in growth shortly after birth and at age 24 months shows areas of involution and central gray areas (Herald spots). Areas of maceration and skin breakdown were treated with local wound care. *Right,* Ten years later. The patient has had no surgery, although some areas of redundant fibrofatty tissue remain. Soft tissue contour is good, and regions of hypopigmentation and hyperpigmentation constitute the primary deformity. (Courtesy of Joseph E. Murray, M.D.)

remain unnoticed. Large lesions are obvious and become engorged when the limb is held in a dependent position and completely decompress with elevation (Fig. 128–56). Enlargement can occur after trauma, during puberty and pregnancies, and with birth control medication. Skin ulceration rarely occurs. Subcutaneous thrombi or calcifications may be accompanied by pain. Any or all of the tissues within the limb may be involved, including bone. Functional problems are predominantly related either to pain or to limitation of motion by size and bulk (Fig. 128–57). Patients with massively enlarged upper arms and forearms occasionally develop intertriginous macerations and infections. Hypertrophy of any or all portions of the skeleton may occur; the degree of enlargement is not predictable from the primary vascular element or flow characteristics of the lesion (Boyd and associates, 1984).

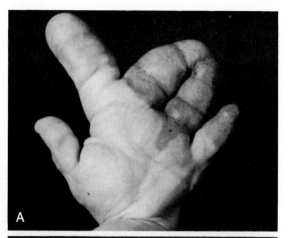

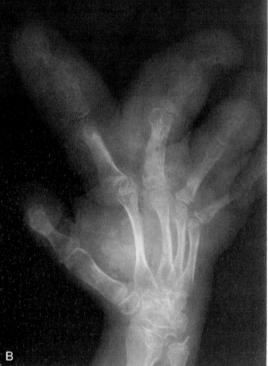

Figure 128–57. Venous malformation. *A* and *B,* Diffuse enlargement and skeletal hypertrophy may occur. The mechanisms of overgrowth in this low flow lesion are not known. Note the associated capillary malformation ("port wine stain"). Hand surgery was deferred owing to associated medical problems in other organ systems. The size and weight of the digits in this patient provided the primary functional deterrents.

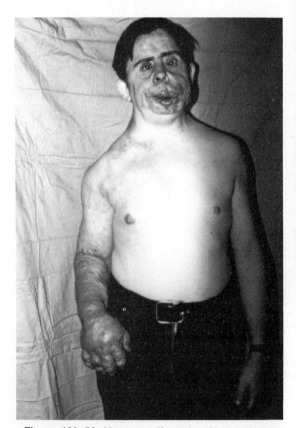

Figure 128–56. Venous malformation. Venous lesions may be massive, extending beyond the extremity to the head and neck region and hemithorax. Hand size here is controlled with a compression garment, and function is quite good when the hand is not engorged because of being held in a dependent position. (Courtesy of J. B. Mulliken, M.D.)

Many eponyms have been used to describe the presence of malformations with associated overgrowth. The Klippel-Trenaunay syndrome is primarily reserved for lesions with venous varicosities and dysplasia, capillary malformations (port-wine stain), and overgrowth (Klippel and Trenaunay, 1900) (Fig. 128–57). Overgrowth, the mechanisms of which are poorly understood, may occur with both high flow and low flow lesions (Boyd and associates, 1984). Involvement of multiple internal organs is common in the patients with Klippel-Trenaunay syndrome, whose upper limb is often not the most significant medical problem.

Treatment

Occurrence of a venous malformation beyond the upper extremity is not predictable and does not justify an extensive diagnostic evaluation of the gastrointestinal, gastrourinary, cardiovascular, and central nervous systems. The treatment of these low flow venous lesions varies with both size and symptoms. When localized pain occurs, treatment with aspirin, elevation, and elastic support is beneficial. Excision may be chosen for small, well-defined malformations on the dorsum of the hand or a digit. Deeper and often insidious lesions may often be found within the metacarpal and forearm regions. These lesions are always more extensive than they initially appear. Large, diffuse masses cannot be completely excised but can usually be debulked safely.

The decision to operate on diffuse lesions is difficult and should not be made without the aid of arterial and sometimes venous angiography, which precisely defines the anatomic size, extent, and caliber of abnormal vessels (McNeil and associates, 1974; Burrows and associates, 1983). Although closed venous angiography has been of demonstrated value in these low flow lesions, which often contain diffuse, interconnecting, large saccular dilatations, arterial studies are still preferred (Upton, Mulliken, and Murray, 1985; Upton, 1988). Radiography is still more helpful than less invasive studies, including computerized tomography, nuclear magnetic resonance imaging, xeroradiography, and thermography. Compression garments are quite satisfactory for large, asymptomatic malformations, which can be cumbersome in dependent positions. Surgery is reserved primarily for *persistently symptomatic* lesions.

Staged debulking procedures are beneficial with venous lesions and can be safely done. Planning should require only one surgical dissection in any anatomic region, so that surgical reentry into a scarred portion of the forearm, palm, or digit will not be necessary. Microscopic dissection and preservation of normal neurovascular structures are essential (Fig. 128–58). Simple ligation of feeding "afferent" vessels is not effective, as flow will rapidly be shunted into adjacent interconnecting channels. Intraneural dissections should be avoided. Tendons should not be sacrificed, and intra-articular dissection and synovectomies often result in stiff, immobile joints, a condition often much worse than the original presenting symptoms. Proper postoperative drainage must be used to avoid hematoma, the most common complication. Delay of primary closure may be necessary. Complications occurring with surgery are related to operative damage to nerves, extensive scar formation around gliding tendons, sacrifice of supporting ligaments, and ischemic necrosis of the skin. Debulking large regions is a procedure with considerable risk that must be planned and executed meticulously (Szilagyi and associates, 1976; Newmeyer, 1982; Upton, 1988).

LYMPHATIC MALFORMATIONS

Clinical Presentation

These malformations are often mislabelled as *lymphangioma* and may involve a single digit, the dorsum of the hand, or the forearm, or may be extensive, often encompassing the entire hand or arm with extension to the ipsilateral chest wall and neck regions. Skeletal hypertrophy is often present at an early age. Lymphatic channels vary tremendously from large cystic cavities, usually found in the axilla and upper arm, to smaller catacomb-like channels that do not freely communicate and therefore trap fluid. Lesions in the lower neck, supraclavicular fossa, and axilla characteristically encompass the brachial plexus and are rarely symptomatic (Fig. 128–59C). Arterial and skeletal architecture is often distorted by the lymphatic malformation. Drainage from small skin blebs that look like vesicles is common. Functional impairment of the extremity or hand is directly related to the malformation's size and location.

Treatment

The most commonly required treatment is for recurrent episodic beta-hemolytic strep-

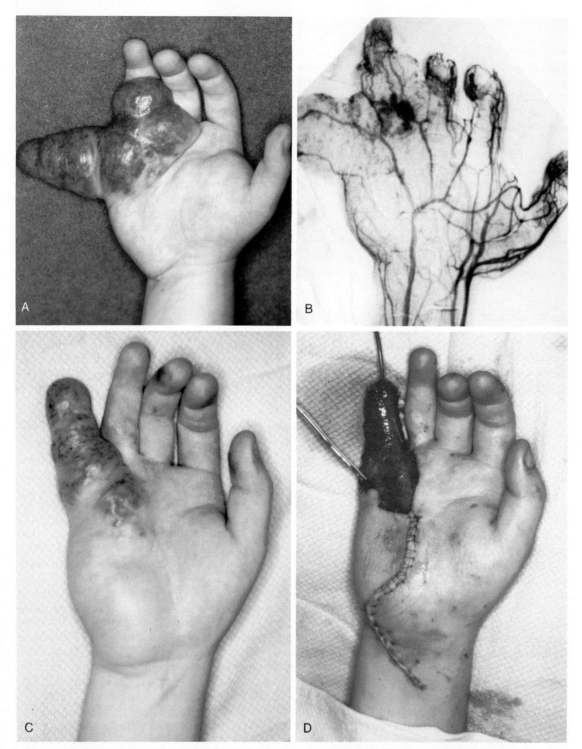

Figure 128–58. Venous malformation. *A* and *B*, Preoperative appearance and angiogram of a low flow, predominantly venous lesion involving the hand in a 3 year old boy. Contrast dye study showed normal arterial anatomy with a diffuse venous anomaly. Large saccular varicosities are located dorsally and within the intermetacarpal regions, and a more plexiform pattern involves all layers of skin and subcutaneous fat. Sensation, joint, and tendon function are normal. Note the capillary ("port wine stain") malformation associated with underlying varicosities. Not shown on the angiogram is a subtle but diffuse extension into the radial half of the palm. *C*, Staged reconstructions were planned. First, the midpalm and thenar eminence radial to the fourth ray were thoroughly dissected, debulked, and closed with redundant skin from the dorsum of the finger. *D*, One year later, all abnormal soft tissue was excised from the palmar aspect of the fifth finger and palm, and resurfaced with a free vascularized temporoparietal flap obtained from the head. The ulnar and radial digital nerves were splayed out in their normal position beneath the fascia, which was then covered with a thick, split-thickness skin graft.

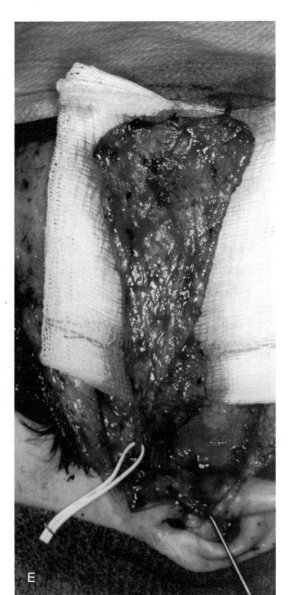

Figure 128–58 *Continued E,* The fascia isolated as a vascular island on the superficial temporal artery and vein. *F,* Guyon's canal (ulnar tunnel) has been dissected with preservation of the ulnar artery (above double background) and flexor tendons (beneath). A subcutaneous vein from the radial side of the wrist (beneath background) was rotated as a pedicle to receive the flap vein. The ulnar nerves, including the deep motor branch, have been dissected and preserved under the operating microscope.

Illustration continued on following page

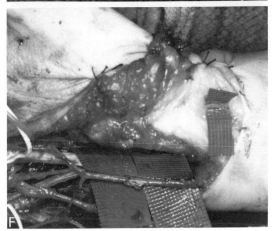

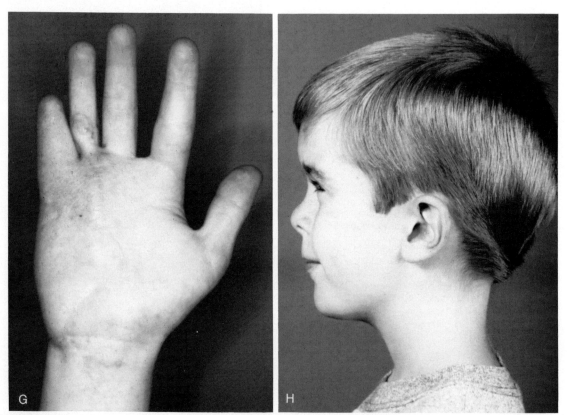

Figure 128–58 *Continued G,* Appearance three years later. Two-point discrimination in the 8 mm range is present. There have been no breakdowns or ulcerations of the skin graft overlying the fascia. *H,* Appearance of donor site. (From Upton, J., Mulliken, J. B., and Murray, J. E.: Classification and rationale for management of vascular anomalies in the upper extremity. J. Hand Surg., *10A*:970, 1985.)

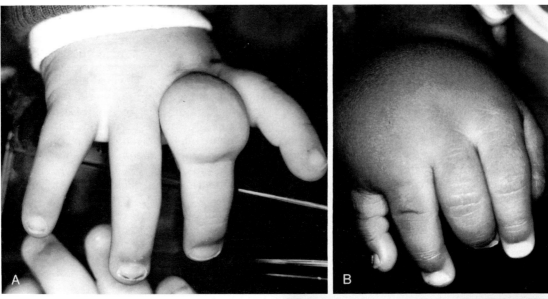

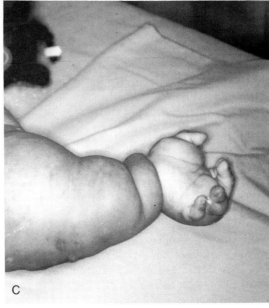

Figure 128–59. The site and extent of lymphatic malformation may be localized to a digit (*A*), or to the dorsum of the hand (*B*), or occasionally to an entire arm (*C*). When the last is seen, extension into the neck and mediastinum is common, with complex, diffuse involvement of the brachial plexus. Surgery in this patient is possible, and bulk and symptoms can be controlled following carefully planned, staged excisions. Functional improvement is not predictable preoperatively.

tococcus infections and consists of elevation, immobilization, warmth, and an antibiotic, usually penicillin. Patients must be careful about small cuts, abrasions, nail infections, and infected bursae. Conservative, nonsurgical therapy is the rule unless size and weight of the lymphatic malformation interfere with function. Compression garments are most useful with lesions that have large intercommunicating cavities, but their effect is not as dramatic as with venous lesions (Miller, 1975).

Surgical debulking of lymphatic malformations can be safe and predictable. The best results are achieved with individual digits or the dorsum of the hand or well-localized lesions elsewhere in the extremity. Removal of all involved tissue is often not possible. The initial dissection is the most opportune time to remove as much malformation as possible, because repeated dissection within the same anatomic region has a very low functional yield and a high incidence of nerve injury, tendon adherence, and stiff joints. Strip excisions with or without excision of underlying muscle or fascia have variable success (Fonkalsrud and Coulson, 1973; Miller, 1975).

In order to avoid vascular compression,

surgical dissections during a single operation should not extend further than 180 degrees circumferentially around an involved digit or arm. Compression garments are useful postoperatively. Postoperative complications include persistent leaking from incisions or blebs, bubbling or serous fluid from involved tissue, and necrosis of excessively thinned flaps. Total excision and skin graft replacement, called the Charles procedure (Charles, 1912), is often complicated by late scarring, persistent ulceration, chronic dermatitis, and contracture, frequently making the end result worse than the initial lymphatic malformation. Historically, this procedure has been performed more frequently in the lower extremity. Massive, diffuse, bulky malformations that are heavy and severely limit function may be best treated by amputation. Although there are anecdotal reports of improvement with suction lipectomy for the treatment of these lesions on the dorsum of the hand or foot, no well-substantiated studies have been published.

COMBINED VENOUS-LYMPHATIC MALFORMATIONS

Clinical Presentation

Combined venous-lymphatic malformation may be clinically indistinguishable from purely venous or lymphatic lesions. Large, easily compressible masses and a bluish discoloration denote venous components; hard, immobile, and often indurated masses with or without cutaneous vesicles are more characteristic of abnormal lymphatic channels. Because veins and lymphatic channels are probably derived from the same embryologic origin, they commonly occur together in malformations.

Treatment

This combination of vascular elements commonly occurs as a low flow malformation in the upper limb. Associated skeletal hypertrophy or gigantism is seen with the larger lesions. Reduction of bulk with compression garments is not as impressive as with purely venous lesions, because of the noncompressible characteristic of many lymphatic lesions. Treatment of smaller lesions is the same as for individual venous and lymphatic malformations, and staged excisions can be safely done for the large and often diffuse anoma-

lies. Resections should be as thorough as possible. Large venous lakes should be obliterated to avoid postoperative bleeding, particularly in the forearm and intermetacarpal regions. Epiphysiodeses of overgrown fingers are not commonly performed but, when done, should completely obliterate the growth plate through a midlateral incision. Return of tendon function in the digit and palm is often dependent upon the reduction or elimination of postoperative edema. Despite use of compression gloves, postoperative edema is very difficult to control in digits, web spaces, and the metacarpal region of the hand. The major complications are the same as with individual venous or lymphatic malformations. The "recurrence" of a lesion after what was thought to have been a thorough dissection represents scarring and redirection of flow into other adjacent, previously existing but empty vascular channels.

HIGH FLOW ARTERIAL MALFORMATIONS

Clinical Presentation

Less than 10 per cent of all malformations involving the upper limb consist of high flow (arteriovenous) channels. When present, these lesions are of significant size to create tremendous problems for the hand surgeon (Malan and Puglionisi, 1965). Symptoms correlate with the size of abnormal arteriovenous fistulous tracts and hemodynamic alterations. The skin may be warm to touch, and a palpable thrill or bruit is usually present (Szilagyi and associates, 1965, 1976). Although most patients seem to accept the increased warmth and hyperhidrosis, the pulsating masses and thrills are most disturbing to them (Fig. 128–60). There may be a previous history of trauma or rapid enlargement during puberty or a pregnancy. Ischemic pain, swelling, or paresthesias secondary to a compression neuropathy often lead the patient to seek medical attention. Associated vascular lesions having both high flow and low flow characteristics may be found in other organ systems and areas, particularly the central nervous system, gastrointestinal tract, and head and neck region. Large shunts not only cause a significant steal phenomenon from the distal portion of the extremity but also may lead to cardiopulmonary overload and congestive heart failure. Shunting does not usually occur with lesions located distal to the mid-forearm. Consumption coagulopa-

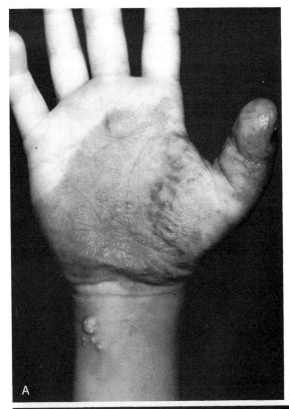

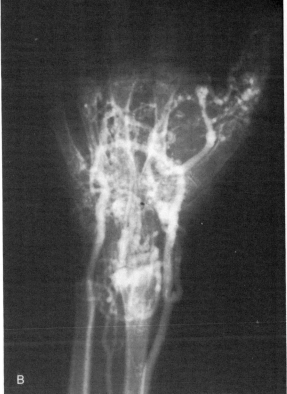

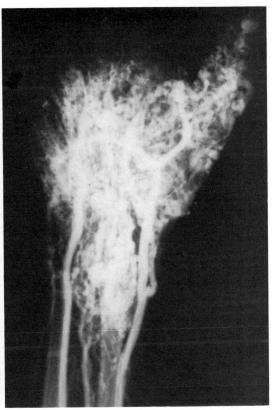

Figure 128–60. Arteriovenous malformation. *A,* The hand of this 5 year old has always been warm with a pulsatile thrill. The associated capillary malformation is common. *B,* Early angiogram views show diffuse high flow shunts that are not approachable surgically in any predictable fashion. No surgery has been done, and the dynamic characteristics of the lesions have not changed during the 12 years of follow-up, during which time the patient has worn a compressive garment. In contrast to low flow venous anomalies, these high flow lesions are not predictably amenable to surgery.

thies may develop in extensive lesions (Rodriguez-Erdman and associates, 1971).

A reduction of the pulse with tourniquet application at the upper arm constitutes the Branham-Nicoladoni sign (Nicoladoni, 1875; Branham, 1890). Distal skin mottling and trophic fingertip ulcerations frequently occur with the paradoxic proximal steal through microfistulous or macrofistulous shunts (Wakim and Janes, 1958). The presence of intraosseus destructive changes carries an unfavorable prognosis but is not an absolute contraindication to subtotal surgical excision. Massive limb hypertrophy and skeletal overgrowth are common in this group of patients. Common eponyms used are the Parkes Weber syndrome (skeletal hypertrophy), extremity arterial malformation with fistulas (Weber, 1918), and Klippel-Trenaunay syndrome (combined capillary lymphaticovenous malformation with skeletal hypertrophy of hypoplasia) (Klippel and Trenaunay, 1900). The last does not classically have high flow characteristics but is often applied to any limb with overgrowth.

Diagnostic Studies

Diagnostic studies such as roentgenography, xeroradiography, computerized axial tomography, thermography, Doppler flow studies, radionucleotide scanning, blood gas determinations, nuclear magnetic resonance scanning, and thermography tend to be confirmatory studies rather than primary diagnostic tools. They are very useful in determining various characteristics of these difficult lesions. Selective angiography is still the single most important study to perform prior to making any surgical approach to any high flow arterial malformation of significant size. This study demonstrates best the anatomic configuration, caliber, and flow characteristics of all major shunts. Even such an invasive study may not, however, define the extent of the malformation adequately.

Treatment

The initial treatment of symptomatic high flow arterial lesions is conservative, consisting of use of compression garments. As patients grow, microfistulous tracts enlarge, pain increases, and distal ischemic ulcers due to the proximal steal phenomenon become more painful. Irradiation and systemic steroid therapy are not indicated and often aggravate symptoms. Surgery is performed with varying predictability, depending on the region of the extremity and the flow dynamics of the lesion; it is palliative in all but the most localized malformations (Curtis, 1953; Malan and Puglionisi, 1965; Szilagyi and associates, 1976; Newmeyer, 1982). Attempts to control high flow malformations by proximal ligation have been unsuccessful and often result in a redirection of flow into other anomalous channels of least resistance, with worsening of symptoms. Partial, staged excisions and, preferably, complete excision of the malformation with revascularization, if needed, via intercalated vein grafts may be more successful.

At least one major artery to a hand or digit should be preserved or reconstructed using microvascular techniques to ensure viability. Soft tissue replacement may often be required after massive excisions. These are all major procedures performed with the understanding that amputation may be the end result. Even amputation may not alleviate all problems, as redirection of flow into adjacent abnormal tissues may result in a chronically ulcerating would or new symptoms (Fig. 128–61). Surgery is palliative in all but the most localized lesions. Selective embolization, used frequently for such malformations in the head and neck location, is not routinely employed in the upper limb, where the risk for distal gangrene is great. In the only reported case, embolization was performed prior to a planned amputation (Moore and Weiland, 1985).

The incidence of early and late complications is great. Incomplete excision may often enhance proximal extension of the lesion. Persistent leaking, wound breakdown, chronic ulceration, uncontrollable pain, injury to peripheral nerves, late scarring of tendons, and formation of new macrofistulous or microfistulous tracts may all occur. Recurrence does not represent a regrowth of new channels but is a redirection of flow into unexcised abnormal vessels.

Although high flow arterial malformations constitute one of the major unsolved problems in upper limb surgery, carefully planned and executed operations can succeed. The surgeon planning such an operation should be cautious but not disheartened about its potential success, because this group of very symptomatic patients may be helped (Fig. 128–62).

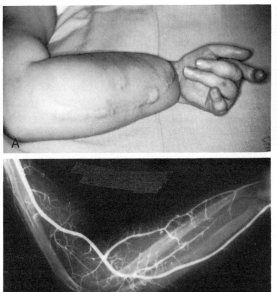

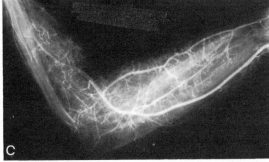

Figure 128–61. Arterial malformation. *A,* Appearance of forearm and hand of a teenage boy whose high flow arterial malformation had been followed since birth. All extrinsic flexors are tight, and he has lost sensation in the median nerve distribution, as he presents with a Volkmann's ischemic contracture secondary to a large, diffuse hematoma within the flexor pronator compartment. Two previous attempts at partial resection and ligation of afferent vessels years earlier had been unrewarding. *B* and *C,* Two angiographic views taken within two seconds of injection show an extensive, diffuse, high flow malformation. The brachial artery and ulnar arteries are twice normal size, and Branham's sign was positive. A below elbow amputation was performed as a salvage procedure to control pain and bleeding.

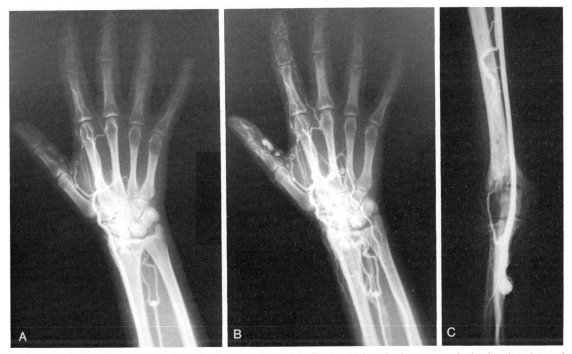

Figure 128–62. Arterial malformation. Angiograpic views (*A* to *C*) of multiple pulsating masses in the thumb, wrist, and forearm of a 12 year old girl. Excision of symptomatic aneurysm in the wrist and thumb relieved local symptoms. Note the large brachial artery and twice normal size persistent median artery, which are commonly seen in vascular malformations. At age 28, the patient's symptoms revolved around the distal humerus, where no surgery has been done or fractures have occurred. The localized bone involvement has not changed over two decades. There have been no neurologic symptoms, and the patient has functioned well as a marine biologist.

Flexion Deformities

The newborn infant will normally keep the thumb in a flexed-adducted position overlapped by the fingers until 3 to 4 months of age. The developmental reason for this is not well understood but may relate to early flexor forces' overpowering the extensor muscle masses, innervation of which occurs later. Lack of independent extension after this period may be due to a number of conditions that, if not corrected, may result in secondary fixed flexion contractures. The majority of these patients have either (1) a trigger thumb, (2) congenital absence of thumb or finger extrinsic extensors, or (3) camptodactyly (Flatt, 1977). Flexion deformities as a part of syndromes such as arthrogryposis, the Freeman-Sheldon syndrome, congenital ulnar drift, and cerebral palsy occur with much less frequency and are easily distinguished by other hand anomalies or associated problems.

Congenital trigger thumb and the "clasped thumb" due to absence or hypoplasia of extensors are discussed in Chapter 123.

FLEXION DEFORMITY OF DIGITS SECONDARY TO EXTENSOR HYPOPLASIA

Clinical Presentation

Flexion deformity of the digits is rare and can occur as an isolated extensor loss to a single digit or as a common loss of extensors to two or more fingers. Patients with an isolated loss demonstrate good metacarpophalangeal extension but lack adequate proximal interphalangeal joint extension. These anomalies are much less common than thumb extensor loss, which creates the "clasped thumb" posture (Loomis, 1958; McCarroll, 1985). The extensor mechanism and often a lumbrical muscle can be deficient at the proximal interphalangeal joint level, and no functional central slip is present. The long and ring fingers are most commonly involved. Patients with deficient thumb extensors commonly have weakness or absence of common extensors to the index and occasionally long rays. In contrast, patients with multiple extensor deficiencies lack metacarpophalangeal extension (with the wrist held in a dorsiflexed position) but do have good proximal and distal interphalangeal joint extension through intact intrinsic muscles. Radiographic evaluation is not very helpful.

Treatment

Treatment is difficult in both isolated and multiple flexion deformities of the digit(s). At a young age, splinting and passive exercises should be used to maintain passive correction and to avoid contractures. When flexion contractures have occurred, soft tissue releases of skin, palmar plate, and collateral ligaments may be necessary prior to tendon transfers. Patients with isolated extensor losses can undergo reconstruction either by transfer of a lateral band from an adjacent normal digit (Snow, 1976) (see Fig. 128–70) or by transfer of the flexor digitorum superficialis to the same finger (Kelikian, 1974) (Figure 128–64A and B). In either case, incomplete palmar release will result in a residual flexion contracture. Multiple finger extensor loss can be corrected by transfer of the extensor carpi radialis longus plus a many-tailed graft (Flatt, 1977) or by rerouting one or two of the superficial finger flexors around the ulnar border of the hand beneath the dorsal retinaculum and transfer into the common extensors to the individual digits (Figs. 128–63 and 128–64). The deficient extensor tendons are usually present distally, the major abnormality existing in the proximal muscles (Crawford, Horton, and Adamson, 1966). Most surgeons prefer the latter procedure because these tendons have sufficient length, more excursion, and independence of motion. The major prerequisite to all these transfers is full passive extension and adequate release of tight palmar skin and other contractures.

CAMPTODACTYLY

Clinical Presentation

The term *camptodactyly*, introduced by Tamplin (Tamplin, 1846) comes from Greek derivatives meaning "bent finger" and is used to describe a flexion deformity of the proximal interphalangeal joint in an anteroposterior direction. This deformity should be clearly distinguished from clinodactyly, in which there is a deviation in the radioulnar plane (Welch, 1966). Camptodactyly accounts for at least 5 per cent of congenital hand anomalies in most studies and may occur in up to 1 per cent of the general population, almost exclusively Caucasian (Littman, Yates, and Treger, 1968). A true incidence is difficult to establish, because contractures of 20 degrees or less are rarely symptomatic and not recorded. Most reported cases are sporadic in

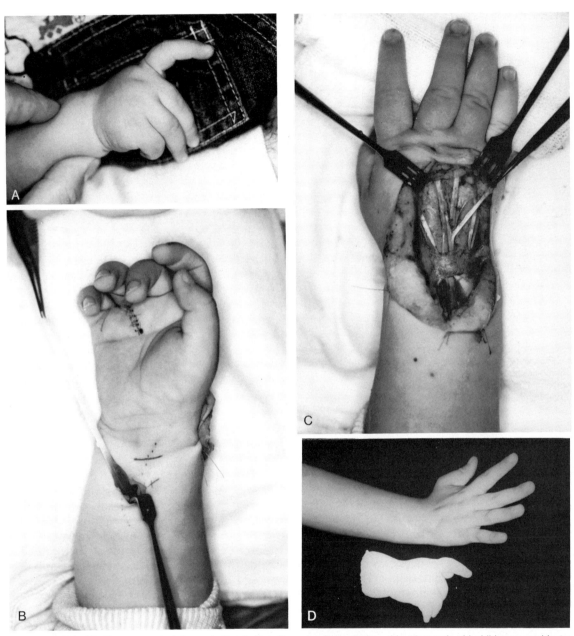

Figure 128–63. Extensor aplasia/hypoplasia. *A,* Despite extensive splinting, this 18 month old child was unable to extend the metacarpophalangeal joints of his ulnar three fingers actively. At surgical exploration, hypoplastic extensor tendons were found to be causing deficient forearm muscles. *B* and *C,* The ring finger superficial flexor was harvested at the level of the distal palmar flexion crease, brought out through the wrist, and split into several tails, which were transferred around the ulnar border of the forearm and placed beneath the extensor retinaculum before being attached to the deficient common extensor tendons. One tail has been attached to the long extensor, and the other to the ring and small extensors at the level of the juncturae tendinei. *D,* Six years later, excellent function has been achieved in comparison with the preoperative hand mold.

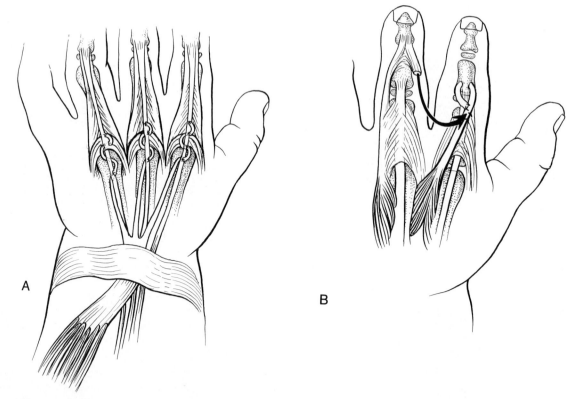

Figure 128–64. Extensor aplasia/hypoplasia. *A,* The most popular method of restoration of extrinsic metacarpophalangeal joint extension is with the transfer of a superficial flexor tendon *around* the ulnar border of the forearm. The extensor mechanism may be rudimentary, but tendons are usually present. *B,* The isolated extensor deficiency in a single digit may be treated with an intrinsic transfer with insertion into either the extensor mechanism or bone, as illustrated.

distribution, but when a familial pattern is noted, it is autosomal dominant. Camptodactyly is not a disease, but rather an individual defect with tremendous nonspecificity that frequently occurs with associated anomalies and as part of many syndromes (Murphy, 1926; Welch and Temtany, 1966; Smith and Kaplan, 1968; Poznanski, 1974; Baraitser, Burn, and Fixsen, 1983).

Camptodactyly is seen in two distinct age groups, infants and adolescents. The majority of cases (84 per cent) are noted within the first year of life and form the "congenital" group, which affects males and females equally. The remainder manifest after 10 years of age and affect primarily females (Engber and Flatt, 1977) (Fig. 128–65). In both groups, the flexion deformity may become dramatically worse during the adolescent growth spurt and does not resolve spontaneously. The deformity is usually bilateral and is most commonly seen in the small (fifth) finger but can occur, in decreasing order of frequency, in the ring, long, and, rarely, the index finger (Fig. 128–66). This finding paralleles the incidence of anomalous intrinsic muscles in the hand (Wilhelm and Kleinschmidt, 1968; Millesi, 1974; McFarlane, Curry, and Evans, 1983). Only 20 per cent of patients show involvement of more than one digit. The degree of contracture in the other hand is not necessarily symmetric. The severity and incidence of contractures are greater on the the ulnar side of the hand.

Most flexion deformities are slight and are ignored by parents as the child compensates by hyperextending the metacarpophalangeal joint. Contractures range from 20 to 100 degrees, and surprisingly little functional impairment is seen in the most marked deformities. Function is rarely affected with bilateral fifth finger involvement, and the appearance is what prompts many affected teenagers to see the hand surgeon. Only in severe cases will these children complain of functional problems, such as with putting on gloves, gripping large objects, playing musical instruments, and typing, and the annoyance of the finger getting in the way.

Long-standing or well-established cases

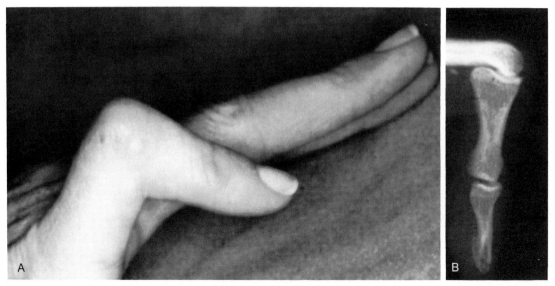

Figure 128–65. Camptodactyly. Clinical (*A*) and radiographic (*B*) appearance of one hand of an adult female with a 90 degree fixed flexion contracture of both fifth fingers. Her deformity started to progress during the adolescent growth spurt and did not respond to splinting. She compensated by hyperextending the metacarpophalangeal joint and as an adult was treated with arthrodesis in 45 degrees of flexion. The radiograph demonstrates flattened condyles, narrowing of the joint space, and a boadened metaphysis of the middle phalanx.

show subtle radiologic changes on *true lateral* view. Careful scrutiny reveals a dorsal and palmar flattening of the normal circular surface of the condyle of the proximal phalanx, narrowing of the joint space, and an indentation in the neck of the proximal phalanx corresponding to the anterior (palmar) lip of the middle phalanx. In addition, the base of the middle phalanx may be broad in teenag-

ers or adults with fixed contractures (Smith and Kaplan, 1968; Lister, 1984) and may show greater subchondral bone density. These changes are thought to be the result and not cause of the contractures (Fig. 128–67).

Diagnosis can be confusing. Camptodactyly is differentiated from a traumatic boutonnière deformity by the lack of distal inter-

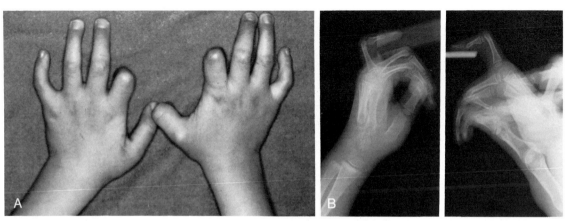

Figure 128–66. Clinical (*A*) and radiographic (*B*) appearance of the much rarer bilateral index finger flexion contractures present since birth.

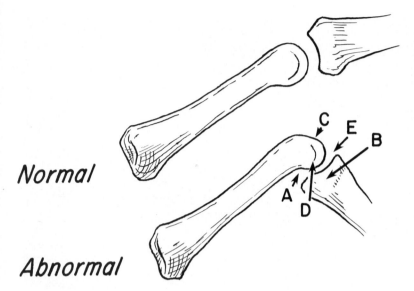

Normal

Abnormal

Figure 128–67. Diagrammatic representation of radiographic changes that will occur with time and growth; indentation of the neck of the proximal phalanx (*A*), broad base of the middle phalanx (*B*), dorsal flattening of the condyle (*C*), flattening of the palmar surface of the condyle (*D*), and narrowed joint space (*E*).

phalangeal joint hyperextension and an appropriate history, from trigger finger by the constant nature of the contracture, and from Dupuytren's contracture by the absence of palmar nodules and subcutaneous bands (Welch and Temtamy, 1966). Rarely, Dupuytren's contracture involves just the palmar aspect of the proximal interphalangeal joint, and in the young patient this distinction can be confusing (Hueston, 1963). In congenital absence of central extensor tendons, there is a lack of extension at the metacarpophalangeal joint and normal passive proximal interphalangeal joint motion with the metacarpophalangeal joint held in flexion or extension.

Normal Intrinsic Muscle Anatomy

The lumbricals originate from the flexor digitorum profundus and insert into another tendon, the extensor aponeurosis. All four pass radial to the metacarpophalangeal joint. Innervation, origins, and insertions are variable in the third and fourth lumbricals, as the first (index) lumbrical is most consistent (Eyler and Markee, 1954; Mehta and Gardner, 1961; Faher, 1975).

Each finger has two interossei, with the exception of the fifth (small), which has an abductor digiti quinti minimi. Three palmar interosseous muscles adduct the long, ring, and small fingers toward the index, and four dorsal interosseous muscles abduct the digits. Distal insertions can be classified either as superficial (into the extensor aponeurosis) or deep (into bone) (Montant and Baumann,

1937) or as proximal (into bone) or distal (into extensor aponeurosis) (Stack, 1963). The first dorsal interosseous inserts into bone (i.e., proximal, or deep). The third inserts primarily into the extensor, whereas the second and fourth have mixed insertions. The palmar interosseous muscles have predominant superficial insertions into the extensor apneurosis on the ulnar side of the index finger and the radial sides of the ring and small fingers (Fig. 128–68).

Abnormal Anatomy

The etiology of camptodactyly is confusing, and virtually every structure surrounding the proximal interphalangeal joint has been implicated in its pathogenesis (Smith and Kaplan, 1968). Most authors emphasize the dynamic imbalance caused by abnormal intrinsic muscle anatomy as the primary cause of these flexion contractures. Currently, the most culpable factor is thought to be an abnormal lumbrical insertion into either (1) the superficialis tendon just distal to the metacarpophalangeal joint (Courtemanche, 1969) or (2) into the fibrous flexor sheath or the capsule of the metacarpophalangeal joint instead of into the lateral band (McFarlane, Curry, and Evans, 1983). Abnormal lumbrical and interosseous anatomy is common, more so in the radial side of the hand. The high frequency of anomalies between the fourth lumbrical and fourth palmar interosseous insertions have consistently been implicated (McFarlane, Curry, and Evans, 1983) (Fig. 128–69).

Other abnormal anatomic findings are a tight superficialis muscle-tendon unit (Stoddard, 1939) (Fig. 128–75), contracture of collateral ligaments and palmar plate (Todd, 1929), tight palmar skin (Steindler, 1920), a slow retracting flexor tendon (O'Brien and Hodgson, 1974), deficient extensor tendons over the proximal interphalangeal joint (Millesi, 1974), including palmar interossei, and a "fibrous substrata" beneath the skin (McCash and Backhouse, 1966; Welch and Temtamy, 1966). When the deformity can be relieved by flexing the wrist and metacarpophalangeal joint and there is active proximal interphalangeal joint extension against resistance, the primary cause probably lies on the palmar aspect (Engber and Flatt, 1977). Miura (1983) postulated that the flexion-extension imbalance is the result of malposition of the extensor lateral slips due to anchoring of the middle phalanx in the flexed position by fibrous substrata, abnormal shortening of the superficialis tendon, or abnormal insertion of the lumbrical muscle into the superficialis tendon. Ochi and associates (1983) reported two cases of camptodactyly, which they attributed to intrauterine tenosynovitis. It is very difficult to separate the primary from the secondary deformities, but most authors agree that capsular, ligamentous, and skeletal changes are secondary and that the dynamic muscular imbalance precipitates these changes (Fig. 128–70).

Treatment

The correct treatment is as difficult to establish as the pathogenesis. For mild cases, the best advice is to encourage the patient and parents to accept the deformity for as long as possible, with the knowledge that it may worsen during the adolescent growth spurt and that aggressive surgery may worsen the function of the finger. Splinting and passive stretching exercises are instituted in the very young and may obviate the need for surgery entirely if maintained religiously (Hori and associates, 1987). This approach is much less successful in adolescents. Approximately 50 per cent of cases improve with conservative treatment, and 50 per cent progress with growth. When the deformity has progressed or has stabilized, some form of surgical correction is generally advised.

Who are good candidates for surgery? Splinting should be used first in children with progressive contractures and a strong family history and adolescents with symptomatic, progressive contractures. Older children and adults with contractures 50 to 70 degrees or greater may benefit from surgical correction. If the joint can be actively extended with the metacarpophalangeal and wrist flexed, release of the flexor superficialis alone is indicated (Smith and Kaplan, 1968).

The operation for significant contractures involves four logical steps: (1) the incision, (2) examination of abnormal lumbrical, interosseous, and superficial flexor tendon anatomy, (3) release of secondary contractures, and (4) rebalance with tendon transfer, if necessary. A longitudinal palmar approach in the distal palm with extension to the digit provides access to abnormal muscles and allows Z-plasty closure at several levels. More aggressive soft tissue release, Z-plasties, and skin grafts may be necessary with contractures greater than 40 degrees. In patients with established skeletal changes, the results of shaving of the joint articular surface are remarkably poor and this is not recommended.

If an anomalous lumbrical can be released (McFarlane, Curry, and Evans, 1983) or a tight superficialis lengthened (Stack, 1963) or released (Smith and Kaplan, 1968), correction may be achieved. The chances of success may be improved if the tight flexor can be converted into a proximal interphalangeal joint extensor by transferring the two slips of the sublimis to the lateral band and the central slip via the lumbrical canal (Lankford, 1975) (Fig. 128–71). This may be quite effective if the metacarpophalangeal joint has been held in hyperextension for a long time. In long-standing cases, it is generally necessary to correct secondary deformities such as palmar plate and collateral ligament shortening. McFarlane, Curry, and Evans (1983) suggest that results are never as good when capsular or palmar plate release is necessary. They further suggest using the ring finger sublimis tendon rather than the little finger tendon, which may lack independence.

Permanent correction of severe camptodactyly is unlikely without tendon transfer. For the best long-term results, small C-wires are used to hold the proximal interphalangeal joint extended for three weeks, and night splints are worn for three to six months postoperatively. The distal phalanx should not be used as a pivot point in these splints,

NORMAL

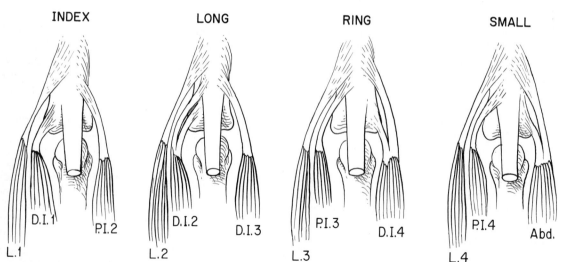

INDEX   LONG   RING   SMALL

D.I.1   D.I.2   P.I.3   P.I.4
      P.I.2   D.I.3   D.I.4   Abd.
L.1   L.2   L.3   L.4

Figure 128–68. Camptodactyly. Normal distal insertions of intrinsic muscles of the hand. Variations in distal insertion are common and more frequently seen with the ulnar digits. (Adapted from Landsmeer, 1976.) L = lumbrical; D.I. = dorsal interosseus; P.I. = palmar interosseus; Abd. = abductor digiti quinti minimi.

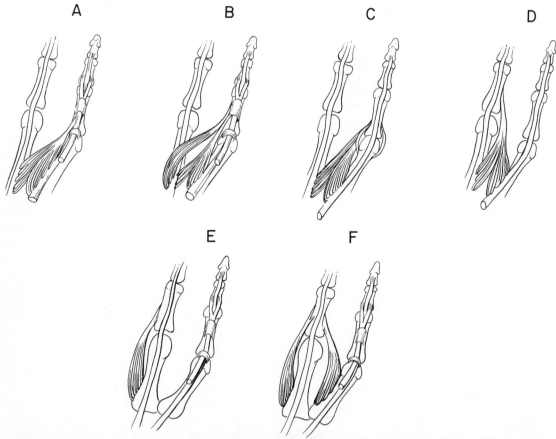

A   B   C   D

E   F

Figure 128–69. A lack of equilibrium between flexion and extension forces due to variations in intrinsic muscle origin and insertion may be the primary cause of camptodactyly. The classic patterns of origin and insertion are present in 40 per cent of all patients. Lumbrical origins may be single or double, and their insertions are more variable, particularly with ulnar digits. *A,* Abnormal lumbrical (4) attaching to flexor digitorum superficialis of 5. *B,* Abnormal lumbrical of 4 attaching to flexor sheath of 5. *C,* Lumbrical of 5 (usually with double origin) inserting into joint capsule, collateral ligament, and a flexor sheath. This is the most common reported anomaly. *D,* Lumbrical of 5 inserting into extensor mechanism of 4. Common interosseus variations include total absence of palmar interosseus 4 to the fifth finger (*E*) and palmar interosseus 4 insertion into the ring instead of the fifth finger (*F*).

5334

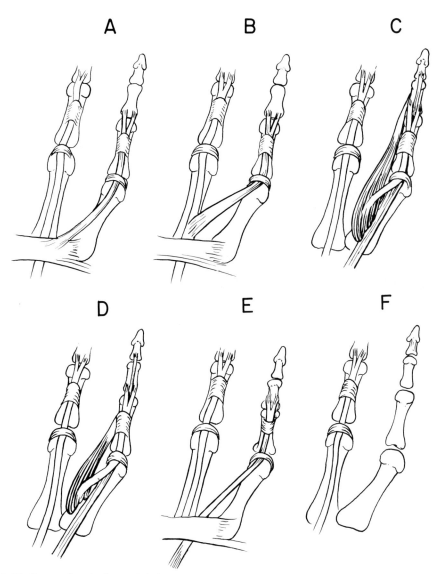

Figure 128–70. Camptodactyly. Dynamic imbalance at the proximal interphalangeal joint may be caused by anomalous extrinsic superficial flexor tendons. *A,* An origin of the flexor superficialis (5) from the transverse carpal ligament. *B,* An origin of the flexor superficialis (5) from the flexor superficialis (4). *C,* An origin from the lumbrical (4). *D,* An origin from the palmar interosseus. *E,* An intact, but very tight, flexor superficialis (5) muscle tendon unit. *F,* Total absence or marked hypoplasia. This last abnormality is reported to be the most common.

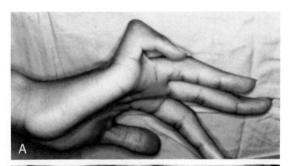

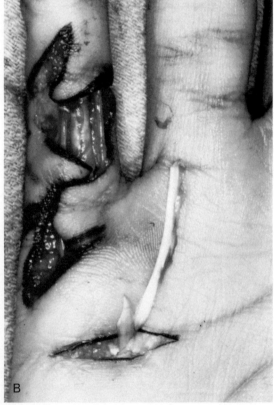

Figure 128–71. Camptodactyly. *A*, Appearance of a significant flexion contracture in a 10 year old boy who compensated by hyperextending the metacarpophalangeal joint. *B*, Surgical release was performed by sequentially incising skin, then flexor sheath, then "fibrous substrata," then palmar plate, then accessory collateral ligaments. The superficial flexor tendon was then transferred palmar to the transverse metacarpal ligament into the extensor mechanism, to act as a metacarpophalangeal joint flexor and an interohalangeal extensor. The midpalmar incision was converted to a Z-plasty and then closed.

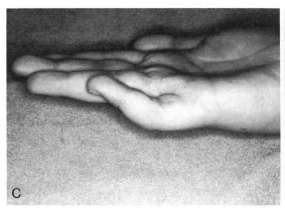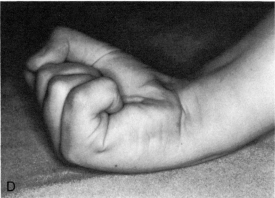

Figure 128–71 *Continued C and D,* Improved flexion and extension eight years later. Flexion and extension following surgery in these patients is rarely normal.

because hyperextension may result. The three pressure points should be the dorsum of the proximal interphalangeal joint and the palmar aspects of the proximal and middle phalanges. These are very difficult splints to maintain in children.

In older patients with significant bony changes and proximal interphalangeal contractures of 90 degrees that severely compromise function, a corrective osteotomy at the neck of the proximal phalanx may achieve proximal interphalangeal extension without losing flexion (Oldfield, 1956) (see Fig. 128–65). If the severe contracture is fixed, arthrodesis and shortening in a more functional position should be considered. Established skeletal deformities are a contraindication to performing only soft tissue procedures.

CLINODACTYLY

Clinical Presentation

Clinodactyly denotes a deviation of a finger or thumb in a radioulnar or mediolateral direction, but when used initially by Fort (1869) meant deviation in any direction. The deviation is the end product of an abnormally shaped bone, which may be triangular or trapezoidal instead of rectangular (see Fig. 128–81). Progressive deviation of the distal phalanx at the distal interphalangeal joint is inevitable when the middle phalanx is shorter on one side than the other. Middle phalanges are the most commonly involved because they are the last bones of the hand to ossify (Kelikian, 1974). Inward inclination of the border digits, particularly the fifth, is probably the most common congenital anom-

aly of the hand and has been noted to occur in up to 19.5 per cent of non-Caucasian populations (Flatt, 1977) (see Fig. 128–73). Clinodactyly has been reported to occur in up to one per cent of normal newborns and up to ten per cent of abnormal newborns (Hersch, DeMarinis, and Stecher, 1953). The proximal phalanx of the thumb is the second most common site of occurrence.

Not all types of clinodactyly are caused by bone abnormalities; some involve soft tissue deficiencies. With large amounts of angulation, certain amounts of joint rotation and flexion will occur, making this a three-dimensional deformity. In such cases, the terms clinodactyly and camptodactyly are as related as hand and glove.

Clinodactyly is often an important symptom or indicator of an underlying malformation, because it has been described in association with over 30 syndromes (Poznanski and associates, 1969). It is frequently associated with syndactyly, polydactyly, cleft hand, triphalangeal thumb, and symphalangism. Because of its ubiquitous appearance in congenital hand anomalies, clinodactyly is often perceived as "background noise" or as a descriptive term that can be applied to identical deformities with different causes. The degree of deformity correlates directly with associated malformations, i.e., a small amount of deviation is more likely to be an isolated anomaly. In most cases there is a positive family history with an autosomal dominant pattern with variable penetrance (Hersch, DeMarinis, and Stecher, 1953), but it can appear in a random occurrence. There can be a very high correlation with mental retardation when clinodactyly is part of a syndrome;

up to 79 per cent of children with Down syndrome have clinodactyly. Males outnumber females, and bilateral involvement is most commonly seen.

Up to 10 degrees of deviation is considered normal in the thumb and fifth digit (Ashley, 1947; Burke and Flatt, 1979). Abnormal deviation rarely exceeds 20 degrees in the finger or thumb and presents no functional problems. In cases of the rectangular middle phalanx, the phalanx can vary from being to having normal length (Pol, 1921) (Fig. 128–72). Shortening of the phalangeal segment (brachyphalangia) is common and should be distinguished from the "delta" phalanx (which is discussed in the next section) and from an additional bone (triangular ossile) that is creating induration, as seen in the triphalangeal thumb deformities.

Treatment

Although some authors have recommended splinting, clinodactyly usually does not correct itself with growth. Patient complaints are usually cosmetic rather than functional. Surgery should be postponed until the child is older than 6 years and cooperative (Wood, 1982).

In cases of marked deviation, there are generally three surgical options: a closing wedge osteotomy, a reversed wedge osteotomy, and an opening wedge osteotomy plus bone graft (Fig. 128–74). A closing wedge osteotomy is usually performed for simple clinodactylies during late childhood or adolescence for functional and occasionally esthetic reasons (Figs. 128–75, 128–76) (Flatt, 1977). A reversed wedge osteotomy is technically demanding, requires precise judgment regarding the width of the wedge, and must be performed with osteotomes instead of electric saw blades, which remove small amounts of cortical bone. An opening wedge osteotomy plus bone graft has the advantage of increasing length, leaving the longer cortical surface intact, and avoiding possible malrotation. Results are generally excellent. In the latter

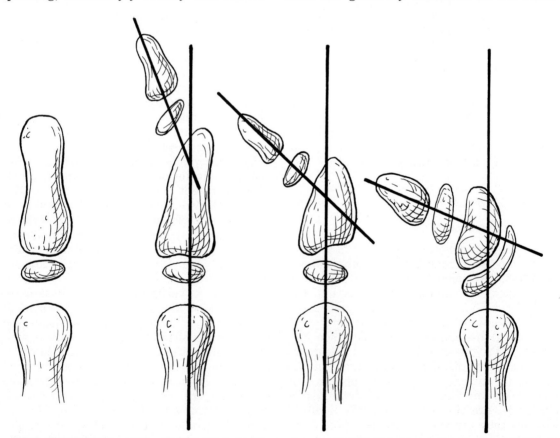

Figure 128–72. Many varieties of abnormal phalanges are seen in congenital hand anomalies. A normal phalanx is shaped like a rectangle (*left*). An abnormal tilt of the distal articular surface results with various trapezoid-shaped phalanges (*center*). The classic "delta" phalanx is smaller and triangular with an abnormal epiphysis extending up along one side of the phalanx (*right*).

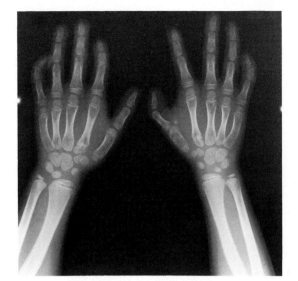

Figure 128–73. Clinodactyly. Radiographic appearance of the most common bilateral fifth finger clinodactyly, which usually does not require correction. This patient had bilateral corrected thumb duplications and demonstrates pseudoepiphyses at the base of both index metacarpals.

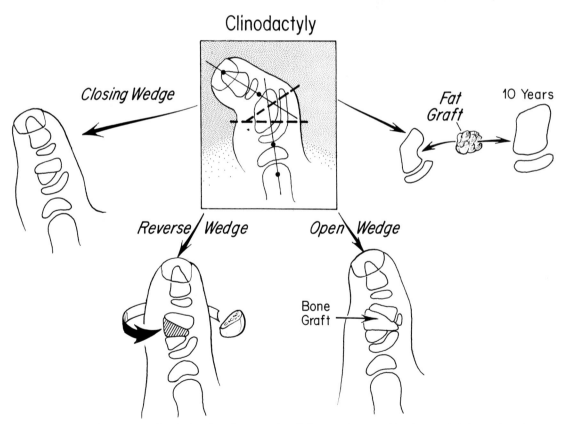

Figure 128–74. Clinodactyly. Surgical options for correction of clinodactyly caused by abnormal phalangeal configuration (*top center*) include a closing wedge osteotomy, an opening wedge osteotomy plus bone graft, the technically demanding reverse wedge osteotomy, and a resection of the mid-zone of the continuous epiphysis along with underlying physis and its replacement by a free, nonvascularized fat graft (physiolysis) (*top right*).

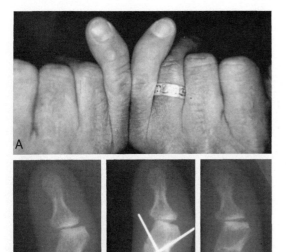

Figure 128–75. Clinodactyly. *A,* Marked radial deviation of both fifth fingers in this adult electrician who complained of extreme scissoring with finger flexion. *B,* He was treated with a closing wedge osteotomy with K wire fixation. Result two years postoperatively is seen on right.

two techniques, soft tissue releases (skin, fibrous tissue, extensor tendon) are occasionally required for simple clinodactyly but are more commonly employed for complex cases such as a delta phalanx. A fourth option for correction, infrequently used for the more severe deviation, consists of excision of the midportion of the continuous epiphysis and underlying physis and replacement with a free fat graft (Vickers, 1987).

Splinting does have a role in postoperative maintenance of correction for at least three to six months. The major problem with an aggressive closing wedge osteotomy is secondary mallet deformity of the distal interphalangeal joint if shortening of the phalanx occurs. The extensor mechanism must be appropriately shortened in this case. Problems that can occur with the other techniques include malrotation, skin tightness and neurosis, and epiphyseal damage.

DELTA PHALANX

Clinical Presentation

When first introduced, the term *delta phalanx* was used to describe a triangular bone with a C-shaped epiphysis running continuously along the shortened side of a phalanx (Jones, 1964). It is an inaccurate term, however, because the bone may be either a metacarpal or a phalanx, and it is usually shaped more like a trapezoid than a delta or triangle (Wood, 1982). Some authors have recommended instead *congenital triangular bone* (Jaeger and Refior, 1971). These bones in any case should be distinguished from those that do have a continuous epiphysis along one entire side (see Fig. 128–72). Theander and Carstam have described a C-shaped epiphysis extending along the short side of the diaphysis that accounts for the abnormal growth of this bone, and have used the term *longitudinally bracketed diaphysis* (LBD) to describe the phalanx (Theander and Carstam, 1974; Carstam and Theander, 1975). Histologically, the osseous bracket consists of trabecular bone with no periosteum that is entirely enclosed in hyaline cartilage in which there is active enchondral ossification. The long side of the bracketed diaphysis is the only part of the phalanx that has a cortex and periosteum (Ogden, Light, and Conlogue, 1981; Theander, Carstam, and Rausing, 1982). Some authors believe that it represents a form of duplication (Watson and Boyes, 1967).

The distal phalanx is never involved. When delta phalanx is present in the small finger, angulation of 10 to 50 degrees will present more cosmetic than functional problems. It is thought that this deformity may be an autosomal dominant trait with incomplete penetrance (Jaeger and Refior, 1971). In most published series, the most common site of occurrence is the middle phalanx of the fifth finger, the next most common being the proximal phalanx of the thumb, followed by the ring finger (Wood, 1976); most reports indicate that it is not inherited. The characteristic radial deviation of the thumb in Apert's syndrome and the Rubenstein-Taybi syndrome, ulnar deviation of the triphalangeal thumb, and the bizarre deviation deformities seen in the central duplications (polysyndactylies) and cleft hand all include delta phalanges. Common to all is the abnormal epiph-

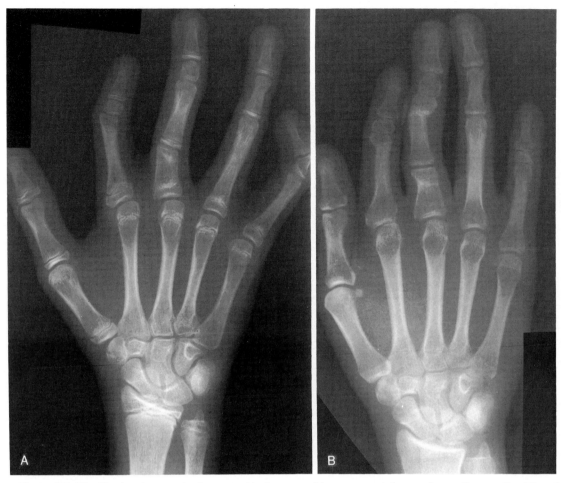

Figure 128-76. Clinodactyly may also be present in the unusual hypersegmentation syndrome. Preoperative (*A*) and postoperative (*B*) radiographs here demonstrate treatment with multiple closing wedge osteotomies in the index, long, and small fingers, which corrected a marked deviation and rotational deformities.

ysis that surrounds one side of the bone like a staple. In delta phalanx of the central digits, the flexion or rotational component of these three-dimensional deformities is often overlooked.

Treatment

Treatment is dictated by the deformity. When it is part of a complicated central polysyndactyly, the pathologic bone is often excised with other duplicated parts, as every effort is made to maintain the longitudinal orientation of a digital ray. A similar approach applies to the care of the triphalangeal thumb, in which the terminal phalanx is deviated because of the interposed delta phalanx. In the small child, this bone should be excised and the collateral ligament reattached. Chondrodesis in the child and arthrodesis in the adult are other alternatives. Osteotomy of the abnormal bone is used for correction of deviation greater than 20 degrees or of any significant rotational deformity. This can be done as an opening wedge osteotomy (Jones, 1964; Wood, 1976; Smith, 1977), as a closing wedge osteotomy (Wood, 1982), or as a reverse wedge osteotomy, in which the central portion is excised as a triangle, turned 180 degrees, and reinserted on the opposite side of the osteotomy site (Carstam and Theander, 1975) (see Fig. 128-74). An H-shaped graft may provide more secure fixation than a simple wedge (Burgess, 1988). When delta phalanx is associated with polydactyly, excised bone is usually the best source for a bone graft. These osteotomies are

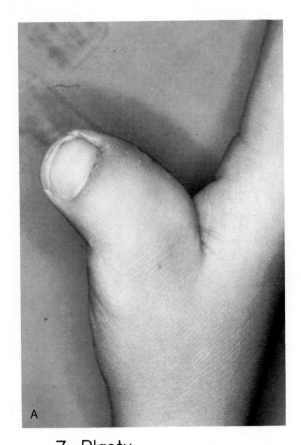

Figure 128–77. Delta phalanx. *A,* Clinical appearance of the common radial deviation of the thumb seen in the acrocephalosyndactyly (ACS) syndromes. *B,* Treatment consists of an opening wedge osteotomy, bone graft, centralization of flexor and extensor tendons (if necessary), and reattachment of the thenar intrinsic muscles. *Inset,* A Z-plasty should be designed so that the dorsal flap is based proximally.

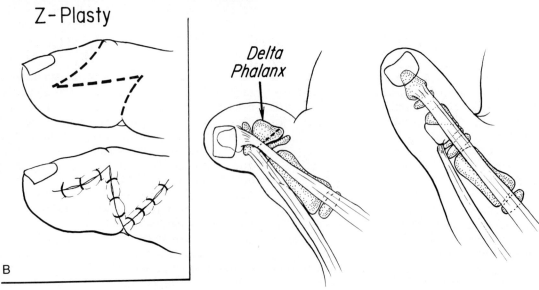

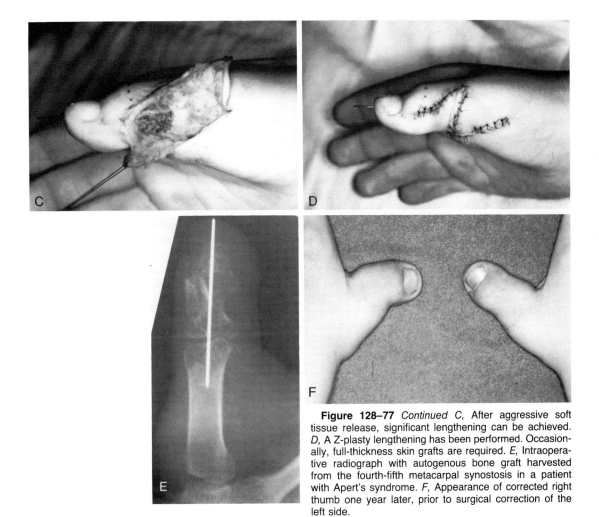

Figure 128–77 *Continued C,* After aggressive soft tissue release, significant lengthening can be achieved. *D,* A Z-plasty lengthening has been performed. Occasionally, full-thickness skin grafts are required. *E,* Intraoperative radiograph with autogenous bone graft harvested from the fourth-fifth metacarpal synostosis in a patient with Apert's syndrome. *F,* Appearance of corrected right thumb one year later, prior to surgical correction of the left side.

quite difficult and will challenge the most gifted surgical technician.

Flatt (1977) emphasizes the brittle nature of the delta phalanx. For cutting the bone, power instruments are less preferable than a sharp osteotome manipulated by hand. If the bone is primarily cartilaginous, a No. 63 Beaver blade will be more delicate. Simple resection of the longitudinal bracket and opening wedge osteotomy are prone to recurrence of deviation.

A different procedure, called "physolysis," involves resection of an abnormal portion of the epiphysis with fat interposition (Vickers, 1980 and 1987). It has had more application in the long bones than in the hand. When angulation is great, an opening wedge osteotomy not only lengthens the digit but also breaks the continuity of the abnormal epiphysis. The radial deviation of the thumb in conditions such as the Rubenstein-Taybi syndrome and Apert's syndrome is best treated with an opening wedge osteotomy, bone graft, and soft tissue release. A carefully planned Z-plasty is usually sufficient for closure but often requires augmentation with a full-thickness skin graft over the abductor pollicis brevis muscle. Eccentric distal insertions of both flexor and extensor tendons should be included to rebalance dynamic forces across the joint space (Fig. 128–77).

In contrast, the common ulnar deviation of the fifth finger is most appropriately treated with a closing wedge osteotomy through the abnormal middle phalangeal segment. In infants, simple resection of the bracket can easily be done while the bone is cartilaginous, with the understanding that the deformity may recur during the adolescent growth spurt. Following growth, arthrodesis may be considered for correction of the clinodactyly deformities.

No generalizations can be made about results because the clinical conditions are so varied. In isolated thumb and fifth finger deformities, functional and cosmetic results are good; but in complex central polysyndactylies, the digits never have normal motion or appearance and often require multiple procedures.

Complications of surgical procedures for clinodactyly correction are nonunion, recurrence of angulation and tendon adhesions (primarily on the extensor side), and malrotation. Corrections performed early in life often require repeat osteotomies after the adolescent growth spurt.

DUPLICATION (POLYDACTYLY)

Duplication of digits and thumbs is the most common congenital anomaly of the upper limb (Mellin, 1963; Flatt, 1977; Goldberg and Bartoshesky, 1985); in most series, the second most common is syndactyly (see "Incidence"). All portions of the hand may be involved. Total duplication of the hand and forearm, or "ulnar dimelia," is so rare that it almost constitutes a medical curiosity. On the preaxial side of the limb bud, thumb duplication occurs in great variation. Central duplications of the index, long, and ring fingers are much less common; usually present with syndactyly, they are reported in the literature as such. Postaxial polydactyly is the most common variety and the single most common congenital anomaly seen in most cultures.

Duplicated digits have been well documented in all races throughout recorded time. The Bible describes polydactylous giants in the eleventh century B.C. (The Holy Bible; Nicolai and Schoch, 1986). The trait was so common in some inbred tribes of Hyamites that a child born without a hexadactylous hand was thought to be illegitimate (Kelikian, 1974). In England, polydactyly was thought to be a sign of royalty because Henry VIII's queen, Anne Boleyn, had an extra finger (Strickland, 1840–1848). In other societies this anomaly was thought to bear a sign of inferiority, and the affected infants were killed. In our society there is both a social and a functional justification to possess a normal number of digits on both hands.

Polydactyly is thought to be the result of an excess longitudinal segmentation that probably represents an increased folding of the apical ectodermal ridge (Zwilling, 1968) (see "Embryology"). The degree of development of extra portions varies enormously, from a small, loosely attached soft tissue anlage to a fully developed functional finger. On this basis, Stelling (1963) and Turek (1967) have classified polydactyly as follows. *Type I* consists of a soft tissue remnant that has no formal skeletal attachment and is devoid of ossified bone. In *Type II,* the most common, there is duplication of a digit or a portion thereof with articulation with an enlarged or bifid metacarpal or phalanx. *Type III* is complete duplication with normal components, including a metacarpal (Fig. 128–78). Hand surgeons have further subclassified these categories of duplications in various

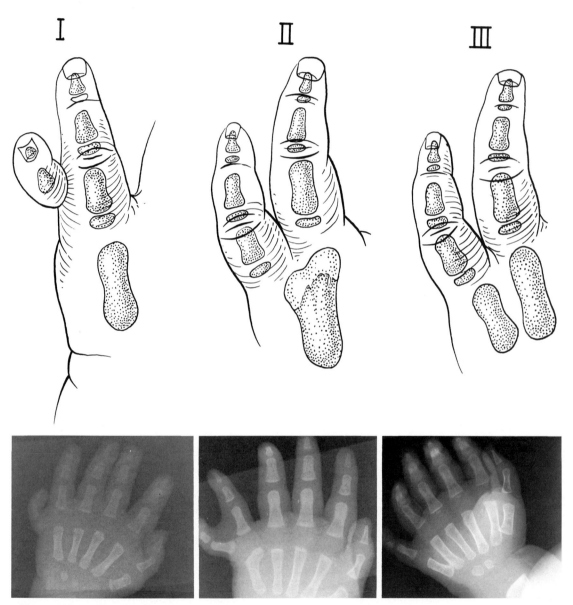

Figure 128–78. The classification of duplication deformities falls into three general types. In Type I, there is a soft tissue remnant, with no bone connections. In Type II, a more complete duplication with a skeletal connection is present. In Type III, there is a complete duplication of the entire ray. Types II and III are more common.

portions of the hand for practical purposes; the subclassifications will be presented in the appropriate sections. Very detailed systems have been described for thumb duplication in particular (see Chapter 123).

Incidence

Polydactyly can occur in isolation or as part of a syndrome. The incidence is as high as one in 300 in American Negroes and American Indians and as low as one in 3000 in Caucasians (Woolf and Myrianthopoulos, 1973; Nathan and Keniston, 1975; Temtamy and McKusick, 1978). The presence of an extra digit may represent an isolated anomaly or a symptom of other significant malformations. Preaxial polydactyly is more common in Caucasians and Orientals and may be an isolated event or part one of eight syndromes that carry either autosomal recessive or dominant inheritance patterns (Leung, Chan, and Cheung, 1982; Goldberg and Bartoshesky, 1985). When it occurs in isolation, postaxial polydactyly has a very positive autosomal dominant pattern, particularly in the Negro population. The true incidence of polydactyly is very difficult to determine because so many Type I deformities are treated by obstetricians and pediatricians in the newborn nursery. Although most patients with postaxial or ulnar duplications have no associated malformations, more than 40 syndromes that include ulnar polydactyly have been described (Goldberg and Bartoshesky, 1985). They involve virtually every organ system. Children born to individuals with Type I accessory digits can produce offspring with both Type I and II duplications. It has been suggested, however, that persons with the better-formed Type II and III duplications usually produce progeny with Type II and III duplications. Preaxial polydactyly associated with or in the form of a triphalangeal thumb carries an autosomal dominant inheritance pattern, in contrast to isolated preaxial polydactyly (Swanson and Brown, 1962; Wood, 1978).

Treatment

The management of polydactyly is surgical and, like the entity itself, varies from the simple to the complex. Removal of a soft tissue anlage may be a simple outpatient or nursery procedure, whereas surgical treatment of a complex preaxial duplication with associated triphalangeal thumb requires well-planned, meticulous skeletal and soft tissue reconstructions.

The timing of the procedure also depends on the complexity of the condition. Most Type I deformities, either preaxial or postaxial, can be corrected as soon as either the anesthesia risks of infancy have receded or associated malformations permit. In contrast, the timing of the complex reconstruction required for Type II duplications becomes a compromise between delay on technical grounds and early operation for functional reasons. If the duplication is distorting normal tissue or restricting the growth of adjacent skeletal structures, early operation, within the first year of life, is advised. Strong clinical evidence for the development of specific cortical patterns after early operations, improvements in instrumentation, and refinements in loupe magnification have all influenced us to advise early performance of complex reconstructions, between 1 and 2 years of age. Some authors prefer to wait until at least 3 years of age or later because the hand is larger and surgery technically easier and because the patient can follow instructions better in the postoperative period (Marks and Bayne, 1978).

Principles of Correction. The major principle of surgical correction is to ablate the least useful digit or parts thereof and to reconstruct its partner. Little reconstruction is necessary for Type I duplications because there usually is no distortion of the normal digit or thumb. Simple excision is followed by primary closure and, occasionally, a Z-plasty closure if the skin incision is in a palmar location.

In Type II polydactylies, a careful assessment of normal and abnormal anatomy should be made with three-dimensional visualization. The less well developed or less functional digit must be removed carefully, with retention of those structures needed for the reconstruction of the retained digit. Functional demands dictate improvement in length, contour, joint stability, position, and adequacy of the web space. Such a goal usually involves collateral ligaments, intrinsic muscles, tendons, periosteum, and skin. Occasionally, nail matrix with paronychial fold and skeletal segments may be preserved. Reconstruction of the retained digit or thumb is often complex, entailing correction of deviation by a combination of soft tissue and skeletal procedures, reconstruction or reinforcement of distorted collateral ligaments, reattachment or advancement of tendons, and reduction of enlarged bones without damage to growth centers. Parents should be reminded that, with growth, a certain amount of deformity may recur despite the elegance of the reconstruction.

Correction of Type III polydactyly is, paradoxically, more straightforward than Type II, because the duplications are more complete, and amputation or ray resection is relatively simple. As in Type I deformities, the extra digit tends not to distort the adjacent digit or thumb, so little or no reconstruction is necessary. Parents should be reminded that the limited joint motion or size of the retained partner will remain the same.

The central duplication, often called complex or complicated polydactyly, is often quite bizarre and requires individualized treatment. Usually enough skeletal elements for three fingers are found in the place of two. Abnormal and often transversely located phalangeal segments require major rearrangement within soft tissue, where abnormal anatomy is more the rule than the exception. The longitudinal orientation of skeletal segments does, however, provide important clues about underlying neurovascular structures. Occasionally, the optimal aesthetic and functional result is conversion to a three-fingered hand.

Duplication: Preaxial (Thumb)

The classification, management, and complications of thumb duplications, including the phalangeal thumb, are covered in Chapter 123.

Duplication: Central (Index, Long, and Ring Fingers)

Clinical Presentation

Because central duplications are so often associated with syndactyly, the terms *central polydactyly* and *polysyndactyly* have often been substituted. The presentation of index finger duplications is much different from those involving the long and ring fingers, which are much more commonly involved in these duplications. Both types have a strong

autosomal dominant inheritance pattern (Goodman, 1965; Temtamy and McKusick, 1969; Flatt, 1977).

Most polysyndactyly cases are bilateral, and the incidence of duplication increases toward the ulnar side of the hand, where the ring ray is most frequently duplicated. Associated anomalies, including toe syndactyly and duplication, are common. There are no major associated anomalies of internal organ systems.

Index duplication is rare, accounting for about three per cent of all central duplications. Wood (1970) has reported five patients with seven index duplications, which were equally divided among Types I to III in terms of complexity. A normal thumb is present, but frequently the first web space may be deficient. Often, when the entire ray is duplicated, the interpretation regarding which of the central rays are duplicated is difficult (Fig. 128–79).

Long and ring finger duplications are much more common; more than half involve the ring ray. Complex and complicated syndactylies are usually present, and the particular anatomic abnormalities range from the simple to the bizarre. In the simplest form, small hypoplastic skeletal remnants will be found between what appears to be a complete simple syndactyly. These cartilaginous skeletal remnants may not be well ossified in infancy and are often missed.

In contrast, a whole array of skeletal elements oriented in longitudinal, oblique, and transverse directions may occur with some frequency. Metacarpals are usually longitudinal but may bifurcate and then articulate with two or more proximal phalanges. Transversely oriented phalanges are typically located at the proximal phalangeal level and often greatly distort the transverse metacarpal arch. Delta-shaped phalanges with longitudinally bracketed diaphyses (LBD) (Carstam and Theander, 1975) are characteristically found within the center of a coalesced mass of phalanges. Marked deviation may occur at all levels. The particular type of soft tissue anatomic abnormalities cannot be absolutely predicted from correlation with the radiographic appearance. Abnormality is the rule distal to the level of duplication. Very distal bifurcations of flexor tendons, digital nerves, and arteries should be expected. If a well-segmented normal ray is adjacent to a central duplication, it is safe to assume that

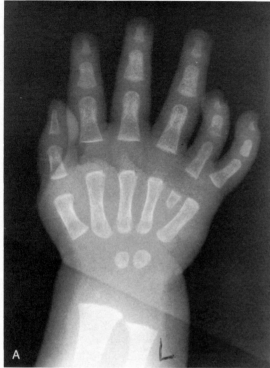

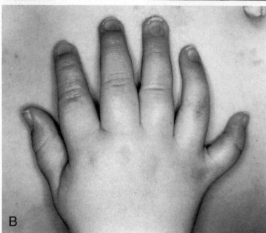

Figure 128–79. Duplication. Radiographic evaluation prior to surgical ablation is very important. *A* and *B*, The radiographs in this patient show a duplication with the more abnormal partner position on the ring finger side.

normal bifurcations of neurovascular structures will contribute to that side of the central duplication (Fig. 128–80).

Treatment

Index duplication is rare and is corrected in much the same fashion as thumb polydactylies, i.e., ablation of accessory parts, collateral ligament reconstruction, realignment of extensor and flexor tendons, and correction of angular deformities. In the more complex Types II and III duplications, early surgery is recommended to prevent excessive angulation deformities. Great care must be taken not to damage the epiphyses of retained skeletal elements as a single longitudinal ray is established and collateral ligaments created. Correction of the complicated Type III deformity is easier in most cases, because the bizarre elements can often be excised and the most normal ray retained as part of a three-fingered hand.

The very bizarre skeletal arrangements in long and ring duplications present difficult and unique reconstructive problems. As with index duplications, it is wise to establish definite, longitudinally oriented skeletal rays before growth further distorts abnormal fingers, as well as to ensure good web spaces (Wood, 1971).

In one series of 16 patients, 91 operations were performed for correction of syndactyly, duplications, angulation, and rotational deformities and for treatment of complications (Wood, 1971). The reported results are typical and document straight digits with deficient interphalangeal joint motion and variable metacarpophalangeal joint mobility. Early operation is recommended, often starting before 1 year of age. In Type III complicated cases the decision regarding the number of digits to be retained on the hand should be discussed with parents and made early in the child's life. When initial web releases are done, excision of extra transverse or obliquely oriented phalanges at the proximal phalangeal level are often necessary to maintain commissure depth and to avoid recurrence (Fig. 128–81B). If a phalanx has deviated, simple excision of the abnormal bone or digit may not correct the problem, and osteotomy may be required. Fusion in complicated hands is currently the best way to maintain normal alignment where the possibility for motion is limited or nonexistent because of incongruence of joint surfaces, absence or abnormality of intrinsic muscles, absence of collateral ligaments, or abnormality of flexor and/or extensor tendons. Every effort should be made to establish proper metacarpal orientation and metacarpophalangeal motion, because most of these digits lack full interphalangeal joint motion. Many women do not care whether their ring fingers are stiff but are

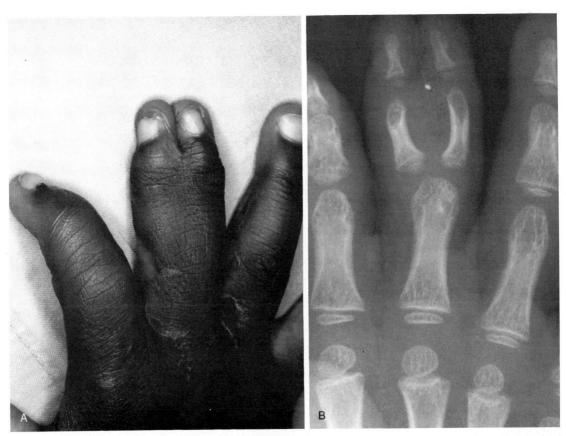

Figure 128–80. Clinical (*A*) and radiographic (*B*) appearance of an unusual central distal duplication at the proximal interphalangeal joint level. Patient had incomplete webbing to both adjacent fingers. A Bilhaut-Cloquet procedure was used for correction of the duplication.

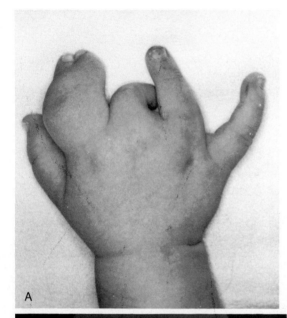

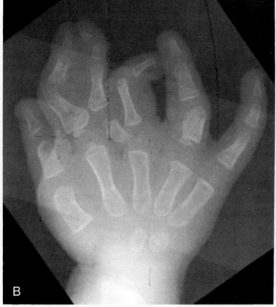

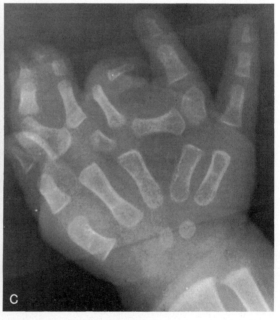

Figure 128–81. Central duplication. Radiographic (*A*) and clinical (*B*) appearance of a very complex duplication involving the central three rays. Staged reconstruction consisted of, first, separation of long-ring web with excision of obstructing transverse phalanx (*C*).

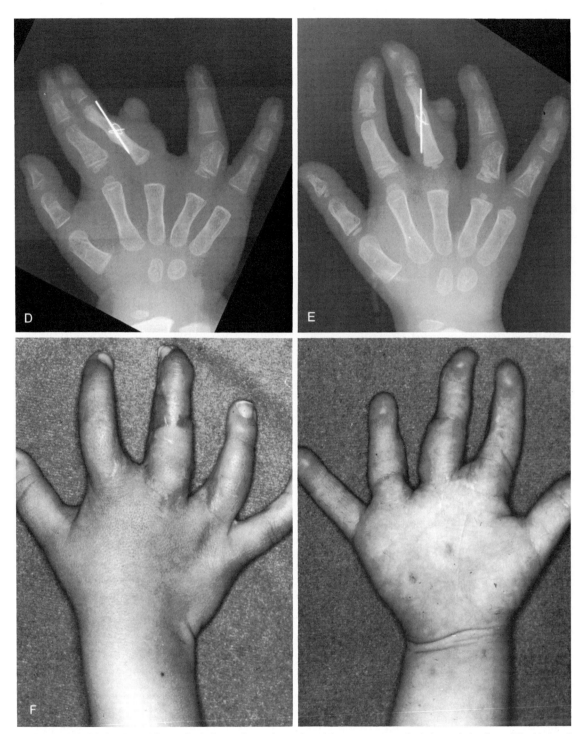

Figure 128–81 *Continued* Second, phalangeal transfer and excision to create a single long skeletal ray (*D*); third, soft tissue separation of the index and long fingers (*E*); and fourth, additional soft tissue debulking. *F,* Four years later, there is very little interphalangeal joint motion in the index and long fingers. Straight digits have been erected with motion at the metacarpophalangeal joint. Excess length and nail angulation will be corrected when the patient reaches skeletal maturity.

quite particular about having a straight digit with satisfactory commissure depth.

Complications of these reconstructions include skin loss, failed skin grafts, and inadequate growth of the central segments. Transversely oriented phalanges invariably block functional motion and should be removed early. Accessory slips, splits, and insertions of intrinsic and extrinsic tendons should be completely removed to avoid a checkrein effect (Wood, 1971). Parents should be advised that children with central duplications require many secondary procedures and that normal rotation, length, and joint mobility are rarely achieved. Distraction techniques and bone grafts with or without joint fusions are useful to gain normal length in adults or adolescents. Conversion to a three finger hand may often be a wise option despite previous efforts to save an extra ray (Flatt, 1977).

Duplication: Postaxial (Small Finger)

The extent of duplication varies from a completely formed digit to a single phalanx or a skin tag. The classification system of Temtamy and McKusick (1969) is quite similar to that outlined previously by Stelling (1963) and Turek (Turek, 1967). In the Type I, a small, poorly formed digit is attached to the ulnar ray of the hand by a skin bridge of variable width. There is no skeletal articulation, and in most cases the rudimentary digit is devoid of bone (Fig. 128–82). Type II involves a duplicated digit with normal components that usually articulates with a bifid metacarpal condyle. The metacarpal may be thickened, and carpal coalition or duplication may occur. Type III, a complete duplication of the entire ray, is rare but does occur (see Fig. 128–79).

Duplication deformities are the most common of all congenital hand anomalies, and postaxial polydactyly is by far the most common duplication. In the United States, it is seen about ten times more frequently in Negroes than Caucasians (Frazier, 1960), with an incidence of one in 300 for the former and one in 3000 for the latter (Woolf, 1978; Nathan and Keniston, 1975; Temtamy and McKusick, 1978). Inheritance in the Type I deformities, which represent rudimentary nubbins with a soft tissue bridge duplicated at the proximal phalangeal level, is dominant with incomplete penetrance, but the whole spectrum exists (Sverdrup, 1922; Odiorne, 1943). In contrast, the more completely formed Types II and III deformities carry a very dominant inheritance pattern (Barsky, 1958). Children born to parents with Types II and III completely formed digits can have progeny with all types of duplication, but children born to parents with Type I duplications can produce only progeny with the same duplications.

Syndromic associations with postaxial polydactyly are common in Caucasians and uncommon in Negroes. Rarely will a Negro with a Type I deformity show any signs of associated anomalies, but a Caucasian with a like deformity should be evaluated for them, as over 40 syndromes have been chronicled by geneticists (Hanson and associates, 1976). They include chromosome syndromes (trisomy 13 and 18), bone dysplasias (Ellis–van Creveld syndrome, achrondroplasia), syndromes involving eyes (Laurence-Moon-Biedl), syndromes involving skin (Goltz's, Bloom's), orofacial syndromes (cleft lip, Meckel's), and syndromes with mental retardation (Cornelia de Lange's, Smith-Lemli-Opitz).

Anatomic abnormalities parallel to those seen with preaxial duplications are present in postaxial duplications. Absence and hypoplasia predominate. In Type I and II deformities, subtle malformations in the extensor mechanism, articular surfaces, and hypothenar intrinsic muscles should be noted in the normal fifth digit. Failure to correctly balance forces and correct angulation will be magnified as the child grows. Subtle differences in the hypothenar muscles, joint surfaces, and potential skeletal growth may not be appreciated until the patient goes through the adolescent growth spurt.

Treatment

The treatment of the accessory digits is straightforward. For Type I deformities, early excision of the digit at the base of the soft tissue bridge is easily done. Although suture ligation at the base of the pedicle may provide satisfactory results, this method often leaves small nubbins with retained cartilage, which grow and often require removal during childhood or adolescence (Fig. 128–82A). Commonly, the mother will bring her 2 to 4 week old infant to the surgeon because a gangrenous duplicated digit has not separated (Fig.

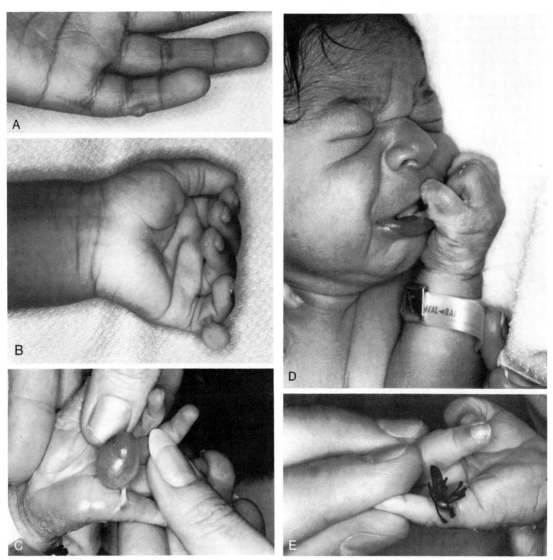

Figure 128–82. A wide variety of Type I duplications may be seen. *A,* Often a small nubbin misdiagnosed as a wart may present the proximal stalk of an in utero amputation. *B,* The most typical form manifests as duplication at the level of the proximal phalanx and a larger soft tissue nubbin. *C* and *D,* Occasionally, a newborn will be found sucking this rudimentary "lollipop" with a long stalk. *E,* Because suture ligation in the nursery is not always initially successful, direct amputation at the skin level and cauterization of the vascular pedicle is recommended. Despite four silk ligatures, this accessory nubbin failed to fall off at four weeks.

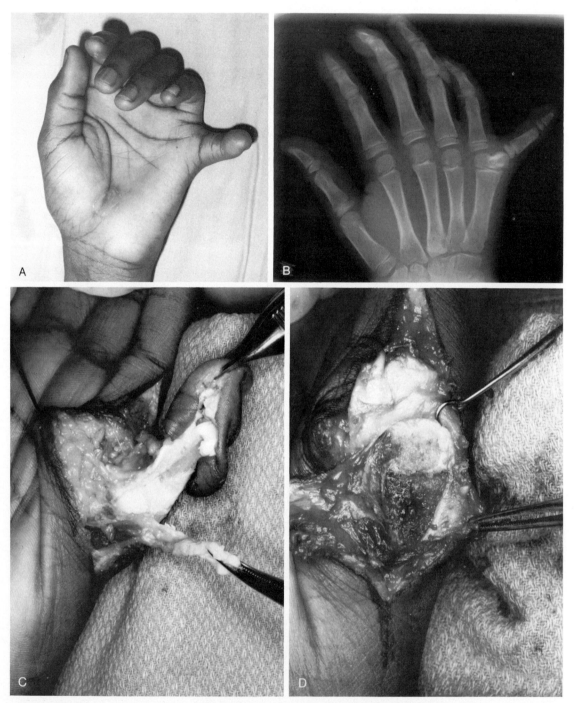

Figure 128–83. Postaxial duplication. Clinical (*A*) and radiographic (*B*) appearance of a right-handed boy unable to get his left hand into a baseball glove. *C,* The hypothenar muscles were detached from the partner to be discarded and transferred to the proximal phalanx of the retained digit. *D,* A generous resection of the bifid metacarpal head was performed as the collateral ligament was retained on the proximal periosteum.

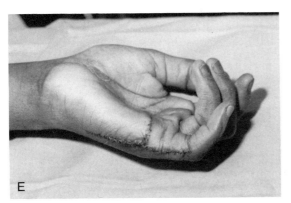

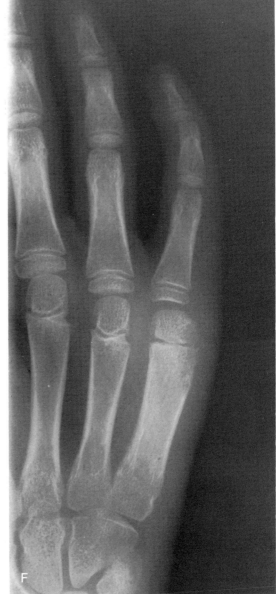

Figure 128–83 *Continued E,* Closure incorporated normal skin creases and incision at the normal line of pigment change. This patient's metacarpophalangeal joint motion was the same after as before operation, but still diminished. *F,* Radiographic appearance five years later.

128–82E). Flatt (1977) has cited one case of death from exsanguination from a ligated pedicle. Suture ligation for the broad pedicle is not recommended. Incisions and closures for broad soft tissue bridges should be made high in the midaxial line of the digit, because with growth, many of these incisions migrate palmarly and create contractures. The pedicle should be electively incised in the newborn nursery or operating room, and the neurovascular pedicle cauterized or ligated directly (Flatt, 1977). Secondary scar contractures, especially in darkly pigmented patients, may need correction with Z-plasties, whose transverse limbs should be designed to fall into transverse flexion creases.

Management of Types II and III ulnar polydactylies is more complex and should be completed by age 2 to 3 years. Surgery on these anomalies does not support earlier statements that these corrections "require no ingenuity and create no problems" (Kelikian, 1974). Some of these corrections may, indeed, be difficult. At operation, incisions should again be kept in the midaxial line, collateral ligaments reconstructed, broad metacarpal heads trimmed, hypothenar intrinsic muscles transferred, and dorsal capsules reconstructed to avoid postoperative problems (Fig. 128–83). Occasionally, the more deformed of the two digits may perform better than its partner. In this case it is often better to reconstruct one good digit using the better structures of both, usually the flexor of the better functional digit and the extensor of its neighbor. It is difficult to transfer a common flexor tendon from one digit to another without creating tendon adherence. The digit with the best flexor power should be preserved. In Type III duplication, the more abnormal partner is occasionally the most functional. In these cases, the more functional digit should be retained, combined with parts of the ablated partner, and placed in a more satisfactory position (Kelikian, 1974). Rarely will the extensor mechanism be normal or metacarpophalangeal joint motion full in these rare types of duplications.

Secondary problems following reconstructions for Type II and III deformities include protuberant metacarpal heads, retained bone or cartilage fragments with collateral ligament reconstructions, extensor tendon imbalance, and rotational deformities. Most are the result of incomplete initial surgery. Waiting longer than 2 to 3 years to correct the more

severe deformities will accentuate associated growth deformities, including flexion contractures, skeletal angulation and rotation, and tight hypothenar intrinsic muscles, collateral ligaments, and joint capsules, all of which may require correction. Commonly, metacarpophalangeal joint motion is deficient after correction of deformities at the joint level or distal metacarpal.

Mirror Hand (Ulnar Dimelia)

Clinical Presentation

The patient with the classic ulnar dimelia will have duplication of the ulna with no radius bones, a hand with seven or eight fingers, and no thumbs, giving a bizarre appearance that is often called "mirror hand." This rare entity is the most complete form of duplication seen in the upper extremity, and slightly more than 60 cases exist in the reported literature (Kelikian, 1974). One of the first clinical descriptions with illustrations appeared in 1587, but the first well-documented case was presented by Jackson (1853), who had the opportunity to describe a mirror hand with duplicated ulnae at necropsy. His patient was a German machinist who found his extra digits and wide span useful while at work and playing the piano; the patient died in Boston in 1852. The dissection by Ainsworth and subsequent description by Jackson labelled the digits properly as little, ring, middle, index, accessory index, accessory middle, accessory ring, and accessory little (Jackson, 1853). The specimen is now in the Warren Museum at the Harvard Medical School (Fig. 128–84).

This abnormality is not inherited but may occur with fibular dimelia of the lower extremity and absence of the tibia. There are no known associated malformations. Geneticists have described the cause as a spontaneous genetic mutation that can be transmitted as an autosomal dominant trait (Sandrow, Sullivan, and Steel, 1970). The embryology of this condition is unknown, but the mechanisms of duplication have great biologic significance. Several interesting theories relating to the inductive specificity of the apical ectrodermal rings have been proposed.

Experimental embryologic studies correlate well with the varied soft tissue abnormalities observed by clinical hand surgeons

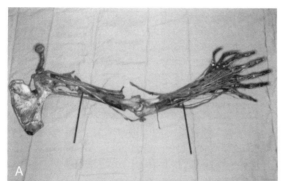

Figure 128–84. Mirror hand. *A*, Dorsal view of entire limb, dissected by Ainsworth and reported by Jackson in 1853, of a German machinist from Boston (see text). *B*, Seven digits are seen from the palmar surface, where very inconsistent anatomy is evident from one digit to another. *C*, Close-up of the elbow demonstrates the two ulnae articulating with the distal humerus. (Specimen photographed in the Warren Museum, Harvard Medical School.)

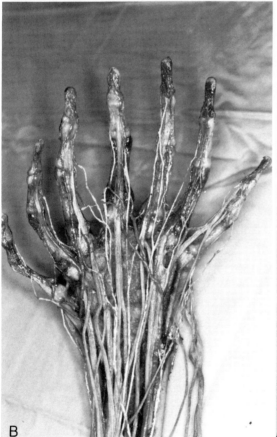

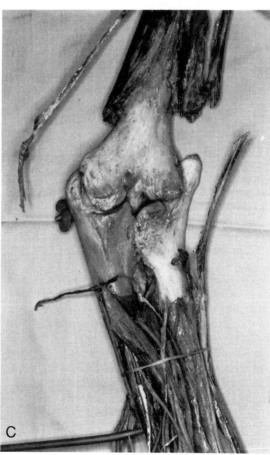

(Barton, Buck-Gramcko, and Evans, 1986). Work with polarizing region grafts within the avian limb buds has shown that there are three planes of growth in the developing limb (Wolpert and Hornbruch, 1981). Cells that spend little time in the progress zone (PZ) of the limb bud form proximal structures such as the upper arm. The second plane is organized as a dorsoventral axis, which correlates with the flexor-extensor components of the arm. Seldom does orientation of this axis go awry. The third plane, radioulnar or preaxial-postaxial, is relevant to the "mirror hand." Saunders and Gasseling in 1968 found that there is a zone of polarizing activity along the postaxial margin of the developing limb bud. Grafting experiments showed that these cells do not form parts but produce substances ("myofibrogens") that diffuse in gradients across the limb bud (Summerbell, 1979). Wolpert (1971) has produced "mirror hands" by grafting polarizing zones to different positions along the anteroposterior axis of the limb bud at specifically appropriate times. He speculates that mirror hand may result from an additional polarizing region in the anterior margins of the limb (Barton, Buck-Gramcko, and Evans, 1986) (Fig. 128–85).

The clinical appearance varies between seven- and eight-fingered hands. All elements are duplicated except those of the radial ray, including scaphoid, trapezoid, trapezium, metacarpal, and thumb phalanges. The hand is flexed at the wrist and may be deviated to one side, depending upon the symmetry of existing carpal bones and length of the two ulnae. There are a central axis and a very exaggerated transverse metacarpal arch, as the border digits oppose one another. Eight digits are usually present; the accessory index ray is often absent, hypoplastic, or webbed to its other index partner. Most digits are held in a flexed position because extensor muscles are often absent or hypoplastic (Barton, Buck-Gramcko, and Evans, 1986). The ulnar (postaxial) set of digits is usually more functional. A duplicated index ray on the radial side of the central hand axis may have either the scaphoid or trapezium missing. The distal articular surface of the preaxial ulna will usually broaden with growth. At the elbow level, the articular surface of each ulna is rotated so that the olecranon fossa face each other (Fig. 128–84C). The humerus lacks a normal capitellum and has two poorly developed trochleae (Tsuyuguchi, Tada, and Yonenobu, 1982).

Function of mirror hands may be quite limited, especially when the forearm and elbow are severely affected. Elbow motion is often limited, and the joint is held in an extended position. Poorly developed upper arm flexors (biceps and brachialis) frequently attach to the distal humerus and do not cross the elbow joint. Pronation and supination are limited, and muscles often are absent. There are weak extensors in a foreshortened forearm, as the wrist is held in a flexed and, usually, ulnarly deviated posture. Most digit function is achieved by the ulnar component of digits, and the radial three or four digits often obstruct the more functional ulnar digits in flexion. As expected, older patients with uncorrected deformities develop ingenious adaptive patterns (Jackson, 1853).

Treatment

Because ulnar dimelia usually involves the entire extremity, surgical management must start proximally. Limited shoulder motion, deficient elbow extension, poor forearm pronation and supination, wrist flexion contractures, extra digits, no thumb, and syndactyly all conspire to make the mirror hand a helping extremity. Elbow motion is achieved by limited excision of one of the ulnae, usually the preaxial. Through a lateral incision, excision of as much of the bulbous bone, including portions of the olecranon, lateral humeral condyle, and trochlea, as will allow flexion/extension and pronation/supination, is advocated (Santero, 1936; Tsuyuguchi, Tada, and Yonenobu, 1982). The articulation of the ulna with the humerus is preserved by resecting ulna proximal to the trochlear notch. The humeral epiphysis must remain unaltered if normal growth is desired. Instability of the elbow may require reconstruction of the collateral ligaments. Elbow motion becomes the next problem, which can be achieved with an anterior transposition of the triceps, transfer of the biceps to the flexor carpi radialis (Tsuyuguchi, Tada, and Yonenobu, 1982), or other transfers such as a Steindler flexorsplasty. Improved active or passive motion of the elbow joint may not last, however (Barton, Buck-Gramcko, and Evans, 1986).

When the forearm and wrist are held in excessive pronation, derotational osteotomy of one or both ulnae may be helpful. Partial excision of one of the olecrena will improve this motion. Wrist flexion contractures present difficult problems and, when combined

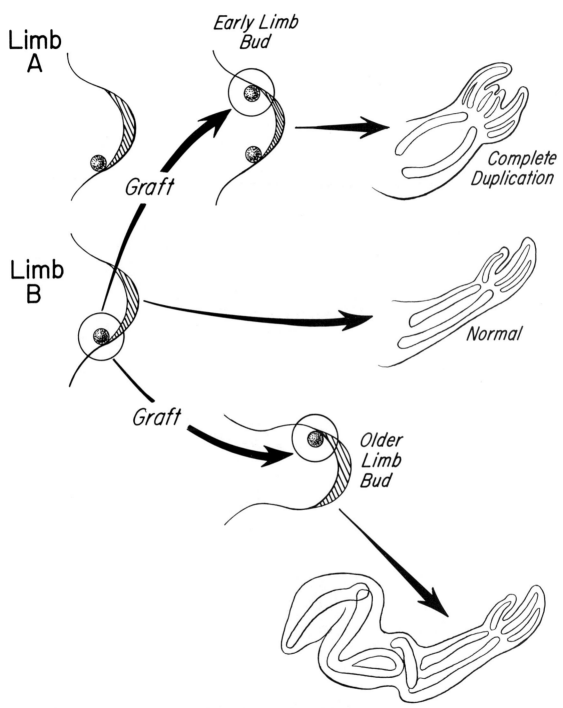

Figure 128–85. Schematic representation of Wolpert's grafting experiments, which created mirror wings in avian limb buds. If cells composing the zone of polarizing activity (PZ) are grafted from one limb (*B*) to the opposite side of another limb (*A*), a complete duplication will result (*top*). If the graft is placed on an older developing limb bud, another distal limb will form on top (*bottom*). (Adapted from Wolpert, L.: Position and pattern formation. Dev. Biol., *6*:183, 1971.)

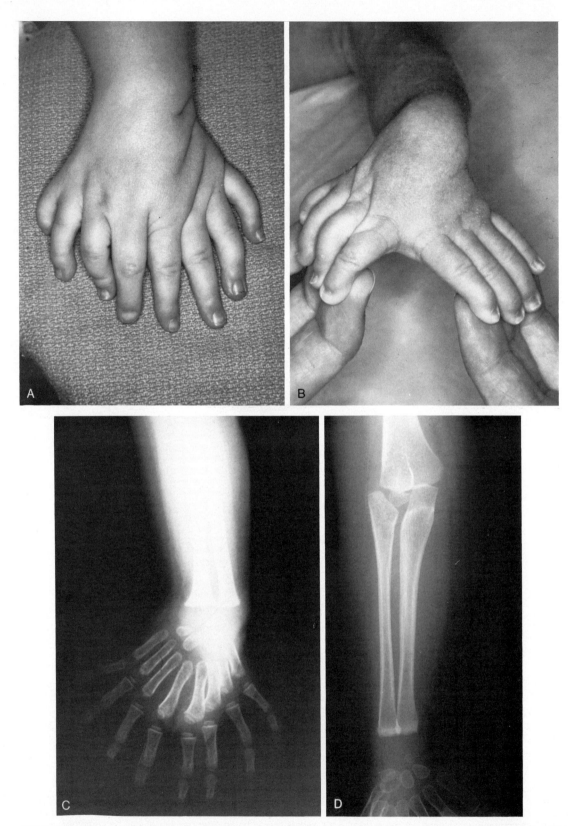

Figure 128–86. *A, B,* and *C,* Preoperative appearance of an 8 year old child with a true mirror hand containing eight rays and duplication of all skeletal elements except the thumb metacarpal, scaphoid, trapezium, trapezoid, and thumb phalanges. A wrist flexion contracture is present. *D,* Two ulnae articulate with a humerus with two poorly developed trochleae.

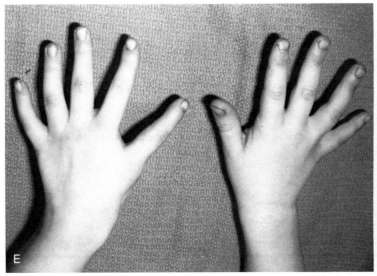

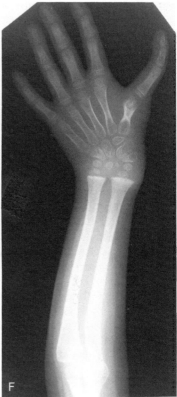

Figure 128–86 *Continued E,* Treatment consisted of excision of the radial three digits of the preaxial set of fingers and rotation-recession repositioning of the index ray into a thumb position. *F,* Postoperative appearance. (Courtesy of V. R. Hentz, M.D.)

with a stiff elbow and pronated forearm, can severely limit function. Skin Z-plasty, capsulotomy, and division of contracted tendons may be required to centralize the hand on the ends of the forearm bones. Osteotomy of distal ulnae has been advocated. Maintaining wrist extension, the next serious problem, can be accomplished with tendon transfers from the amputated digits (Harrison, Pearson, and Roaf, 1960; Pintilie and associates, 1964; Barton, Buck-Gramcko, and Evans, 1986) or of the flexor carpi ulnaris (Tsuyuguchi, Tada, and Yonenobu, 1982). The alternative approach is wrist arthrodesis (Mukerji, 1957; Entin, 1959; Gorriz, 1982). All procedures designed to extend the wrist will be ineffective if the elbow remains in a stiff, extended position.

The last problem becomes the hand with no thumb or thumb index web space. Entin's (1959) procedure has been most widely used; it consists of removing the accessory long and little digits and retaining the accessory ring ray that is in the best position to function as a thumb. A rotation osteotomy and bone block are then used to maintain opposition. Some have attempted to combined two accessory

digits to make a single thumb (Davis and Farmer, 1958). More recently, those experienced in pollicization techniques have advocated repositioning the best of the accessory digits, usually the accessory index (if present) or long finger into a thumb position (Fig. 128–86). Intrinsic muscle transfers convert the interossei of the amputated digits into thumb adductors and the hypothenar mass into the thenar intrinsic muscle mass. The new thumb is then shortened with either a rotation-recession metacarpal osteotomy or subtotal excision with preservation of the metacarpal head (Beasley, 1969).

Despite these sophisticated reconstructions, thumb function is still limited, and additional procedures are required to restore adequate extension. Some have considered complete ablation of all accessory digits and pollicization of the index ray as a more functional solution. Most advocate retaining the most normal accessory digit to create a thumb. Preoperative evaluation, possibly including an angiogram, is critical to this decision and often requires prolonged observation of the child during play activities. No tissues from accessory digits should be discarded until their possible use in web space construction or for tendon transfers for wrist or thumb stabilization dynamics balance has been ruled out.

Long-term follow-ups of mirror hand reconstructions, presented primarily in single case reports or short series, document far from normal thumb function and appearance in just about all cases. In addition, parents should be told that function of the original postaxial hand digits is not completely normal. Multiple operations are invariably required to achieve a maximal functional position and result.

HYPOPLASIA

Limitation in growth commonly occurs in anomalies in all categories except overgrowth. Hypoplasia has not been discussed in detail here by itself but can be found in the sections on failure of formation and of differentiation in this chapter. Difficulties with classification have been presented and common options for treatment covered in discussions of the constriction ring syndrome and distraction lengthening.

OVERGROWTH (GIGANTISM)

Depending upon the location and degree of enlargement, overgrowth has been called many names. The term macrodactyly (Gr., *makros* = large; *dactylos* = digit) has been used most frequently, although the malformation is not restricted solely to digits (Flatt, 1977). The term digital gigantism is preferred by some because it encompasses enlargement of all tissue elements, including the skeleton (Edgerton and Tuerk, 1974). *Gigantism* has simply been defined as "congenital pathologic enlargement of soft tissue parts with associated enlargement of the skeleton" (El Shami, 1969). Many of these conditions have been called hamartomas (Gr., *hamartia* = to sin), as malformed tissue that grow locally. This term is very nonspecific and confusing. In actuality, there is a wide spectrum of overlapping clinical presentations, which will be presented here. These are to be distinguished from other conditions that probably are related to failure of differentiation of certain elements: vascular malformations (arterial, venous, and lymphatic alone or in combination), enchondromatoses (Maffucci's and Ol-

lier's syndromes) (Temtamy and Rogers, 1976), osteoid osteoma (Flatt, 1977), fibrous dysplasia (Flatt, 1977), and lipomatoses.

As a group, overgrowth or gigantism problems occupy a very small portion of congenital hand deformities, but when present, they challenge even the most accomplished hand surgeon. Common to all types is overgrowth of one or more cell types, including the skeleton. It is not known whether enlargement is secondary to actual neoplasia or enlargement of existing cells within the hand. Four entities are presented here, with the common characteristic being skeletal overgrowth of part or all of the hand. Clinical presentation, mode of inheritance, and treatment differ with each entity. Gigantism related to vascular anomalies is covered in the section on vascular malformations.

Types

Gigantism Associated with Nerve-Oriented Lipofibromatosis. This most common type of gigantism is usually unilateral, has no familial inheritance pattern, and is not frequently associated with other malformations (Dell, 1985). The normal stigmata of neurofibromatosis are not present. Males outnumber females by a 3:2 ratio. Kelikian (1974) has introduced the term nerve territory oriented macrodactyly (NTOM), which is useful because it emphasizes the relationship between enlargement and nerve distribution as part of a regional growth disturbance. The median nerve region is most frequently involved, with the second web space predominantly affected. With severe enlargement, the involved digits deviate away from the involved interspace, which is webbed in 10 per cent of patients and may restrict joint motion (Frykman and Wood, 1978) (Fig. 128–87). Multiple digit involvement is three times more likely to occur than single digit enlargement. In 90 per cent of the cases, involvement is unilateral (Wood, 1969). Overgrowth of all digits and the thumb is usually associated with gross overgrowth of the entire limb. Affected thumbs have a characteristic extended, abducted posture (Barsky, 1967). The palm and wrist regions may primarily be involved, with large soft tissue masses but without significant digital gigantism. Carpal tunnel syndromes are common in older patients (Hueston and Millray, 1968; Ranawat, Arora, and Singh, 1968; Tsuge and Ikuta, 1973), but normally, two-point discrimination

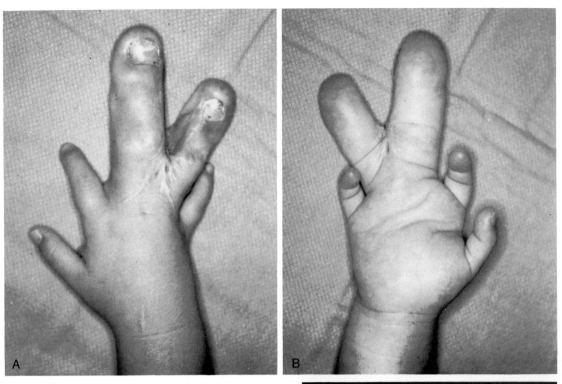

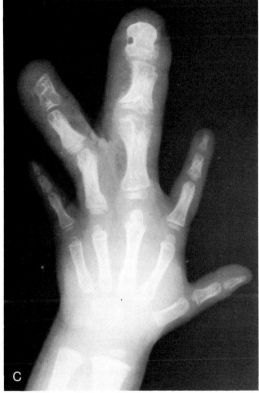

Figure 128–87. Gigantism—lipomatous type. *A* and *B*, Clinical appearance of the hand in a 3 year old child born with grotesque enlargement of the long and ring digits. A third web release had been performed at age one year. *C*, Radiographs show skeletal enlargement from the metacarpal level distal. Note that the bone is increased in length as well as width. Surgical therapy consisted of ablation of the entire long ray and a portion of the ring finger.

and light touch are not impaired with extensive enlargement (Rudolph and Jaffee, 1975).

Two types of growth patterns have been described by Barsky (1967) and DeLaurenzi (1962). In the *static type,* enlargement is present at birth and growth of the limb is proportionate with that of the rest of the child. These patients tend to present for treatment with reasonably good function later in life, usually during adolescence (DeLaurenzi, 1962). In the *progressive type,* very little is obvious at birth, but around age 2 years there is often slow but unrestricted digital and/or hand enlargement (Fig. 128–87). Aggressive overgrowth in both length and circumferential width occurs, ceasing only after epiphyses have closed. Three-dimensional increases in palmar bulk and metacarpal enlargement with a progressive syndactyly between the involved digits characteristically extend into the palm (Barsky, 1967). Early in life it is difficult to differentiate static from progressive growth patterns.

The histology of involved nerves has been well-documented and includes the presence of excessive fat (Edgerton and Turek, 1964; Thorne, Posch, and Mladick, 1968) and distortion by a significant amount of epineural and perineural fibrosis (Ben-Bassat and associates, 1966; Appenzeller and Kornfeld, 1974). These greatly distorted axons are, however, of normal size and caliber. The most impressive finding in these enlarged digits and palms is the markedly excessive fat infiltrating normal-appearing neural structures. Bone contains large numbers of osteoclasts and osteoblasts, and accelerated remodeling of bone at the periosteal level has been noted as the bone grows in length, width, and circumference (Minkowitz and Minkowitz, 1965; Ben-Bassat and associates, 1966). In the immature skeleton, bone remodeling is normal but proceeds at an accelerated rate. Although there is no direct involvement of vascular structures, poor circulation and diminished temperature is common. Symptoms of vascular insufficiency are present in all patients with grotesquely enlarged hands or digits. In every case, comparison radiographs of both the patient's hands should be obtained periodically to document the growth.

The etiology of this condition is not known. An abundance of speculation as to cause ranges from localized neurofibromatosis (Brooks and Lehman, 1964; Edgerton and Tuerk, 1974), to impairment of peripheral nerves (Moore, 1944), to local growth factor (Inglis, 1950; Hueston and Millray, 1968), to defective germ plasm (Streeter, 1930). Tsuge and Ikuta (1973) and others suggest that growth control is mediated through the nerve because incision or resection of the involved nerve in isolated cases has altered progressive growth.

Gigantism and Neurofibromatosis. Digital, hand, and entire extremity gigantism are well-known sequelae of neurofibromatosis (von Recklinghausen's disease), which has an autosomal dominant inheritance pattern and must contain following the clinical hallmarks: (1) six or more areas of cutaneous pigmentation (café au lait spots), (2) pedunculated cutaneous tumors (molluscum fibrosum), and (3) multiple tumors of peripheral nerves. This is a systemic disorder characterized by hyperplasia and neoplasia throughout the connective tissue of the nervous system. Incidence is estimated to be one in every 3000 live births. Neurofibromatosis has also been reported to be one of the most common spontaneously occurring mutations in humans. Digital enlargement and curvature are similar to those seen in gigantism associated with nerve-oriented lipofibromatosis, except that osteochondral masses may be present around the epiphyses of phalanges and metacarpals (Dell, 1985), which cause mechanical obstacles to joint motion and flexor tendon function. When large cartilaginous masses arise within the volar plate, digital flexion can be completely blocked, and nerves, arteries, and flexor tendons significantly displaced (Heiple and Elmer, 1972). Although Dell (1985) includes gigantism in the neurofibromatosis group, it probably represents a completely different process and may fall into the hyperostosis group. The affected nerve may have the same size and tortuosity as those described. Digital enlargement is frequently bilateral and seldom unilateral (Fig. 128–88).

Histologically, the same amount of epineural and perineural fibrosis and tortuosity is present, but there is no marked fatty infiltration of the involved nerves (Johnson and Bonfiglio, 1969). Edgerton and Tuerk (1974) have noted strong clinical similarities between the gigantism seen in lipofibromatosis and that seen in neurofibromatosis and believe that they may be part of the same disease process, neurofibromatosis (Edgerton and Tuerk, 1974). Fat infiltration is not predominant, as one sees an unorganized proliferation of epineurium, perineurium, and endoneurium (Johnson and Bonfiglio, 1969).

Associated features of neurofibromatosis make this entity easier to diagnose and categorize. Bone involvement may result in scoliosis, kyphoscoliosis, pseudoarthrosis of the tibia, seizures disorders, mental retardation, and nerve-related tumors such as astrocytomas, gliomas, and pheochromocytomas. Bone may show either overgrowth or undergrowth patterns, as growth disturbances are common (Holt and Wright, 1948). Peripheral nerve tumors are plentiful and are usually interpreted by pathologists as "plexiform neurofibromas" (Johnson and Bonfiglio, 1969). These neurofibromas arise from both connective tissue and Schwann cells, because both collagen and reticulin are seen with special stains. Multiple nodular thickenings may be seen along the course of an involved nerve.

Gigantism and Hyperostosis. This unusual type of gigantism is associated with local overgrowth of skeletal structures and symmetric enlargement of digits or hand without gross hypertrophy of nerves. The most remarkable findings are large osteochondral and osseous masses or growths adjacent to epiphyses and to the palmar plates of phalanges and metacarpals. Histology shows hypertrophic cartilage in normal-appearing bone. Ironically, these lesions have often been mislabeled enchondromatoses (Hensinger and Rhyne, 1974; Heiple and Elmer, 1972) or hyperostotic lesions (Kelikian, 1974) and multiple hereditary exostosis. The latter term is confusing because there is little evidence to suggest that the lesions have a positive inheritance or represent true exostosis, although they are multiple.

Gross enlargement of metacarpal heads and phalanges may occur without any obvious internal tumor such as an enchondroma. Bilateral and asymmetric involvement is common, and associated problems and other musculoskeletal structures are present. Although there are no cutaneous manifestations of neurofibromatoses, linear nevi and plantar fibromatoses and hemihypertrophy have been noted in some patients with this unusual entity. Digital configuration may be bizarre and unpredictable, in contrast to that seen the first two types of gigantism discussed. The median nerve distribution and the radial three digits and thumb are most commonly involved. Whole hands and digits

may become grotesquely enlarged and small joint motion all but obliterated by the slowly expanding osteochondral masses, particularly within palmar plates at the metacarpophalangeal and interphalangeal joints (Fig. 128–89). Other symptoms are associated with the relative vascular insufficiency. There is no hereditary association in these patients. Approximately 17 patients with this syndrome have been reported in the literature. The author's recent personal experience with five additional patients indicates that this entity is more common than has been assumed, and that it has been classified in other categories. The etiology is unknown.

On histologic examination, nerves are enlarged with all other structures in the involved digit or hand but do not contain fat infiltration, connective tissue, or Schwann cell proliferation.

Gigantism and Hemihypertrophy. This last category of gigantism is rare, difficult to describe, and impossible to find properly categorized in the hand literature. Affected patients usually present soon after birth with an enlargement of one extremity and it is noted that half of their body is enlarged. They do not have vascular malformations, and the gigantism is not necessarily limited to a digit, hand, or single extremity, although certain areas may be more affected than others. The palm and hand are less massive than in the types discussed previously, and there is commensurate enlargement of digits, which do not have the potential of reaching the grotesque proportions seen in other types of gigantism (Fig. 128–90). Early adduction thumb contractures and ulnar deviation of the digits may or may not be present during infancy. Etiology is unknown. Involvement is unilateral. There is no known inheritance pattern. The association of hemihypertrophy with renal, adrenal, and brain tumors is well known (Bjorklund, 1955; Fraumeni and Miller, 1967).

At birth, all joints are supple, but severe flexion contractures and ulnar deviation of digits may occur during adolescence. Early surgery is performed to release individual contractures, and at surgery it is common to find multiple abnormal atavistic intrinsic muscles and abnormal origins and insertions of both intrinsic and extrinsic muscles, which contribute to the contractures. Massive hypertrophy of thenar and hypothenar muscles is common. Forearms and upper arms may

Text continued on page 5371

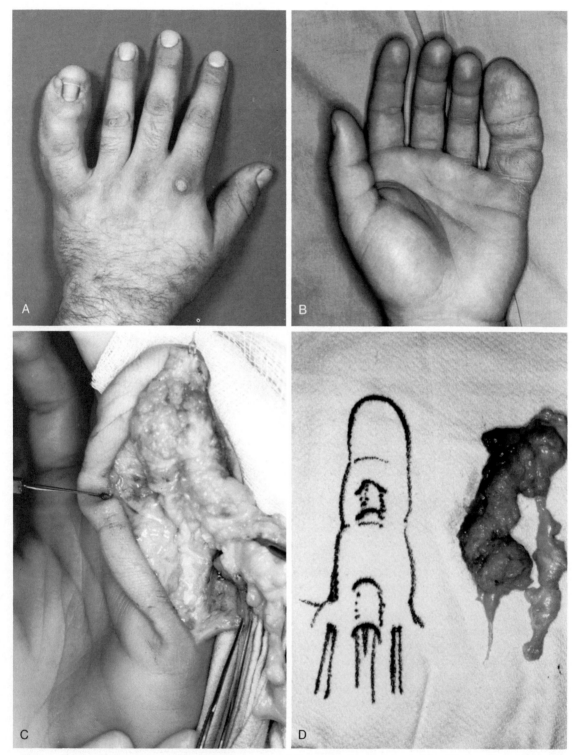

Figure 128–88. Gigantism—neurofibromatosis type. *A* and *B,* Localized enlargement of the fifth finger in a young man with neurofibromatosis. *C* and *D,* Extensive debulking of the ulnar two-thirds of the digit included section of the involved digital nerve, which had multiple segmental enlargements along its course.

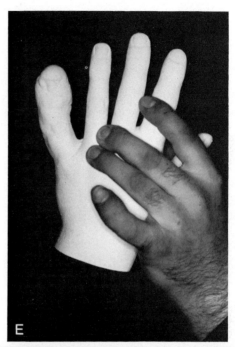

Figure 128–88 *Continued E,* The patient holding his preoperative hand mold four years later. *F,* Flexion of the digit was possible following removal of obstructing soft tissue.

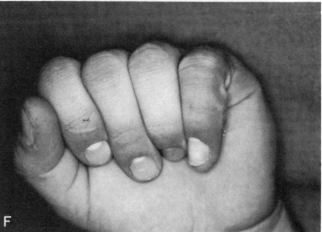

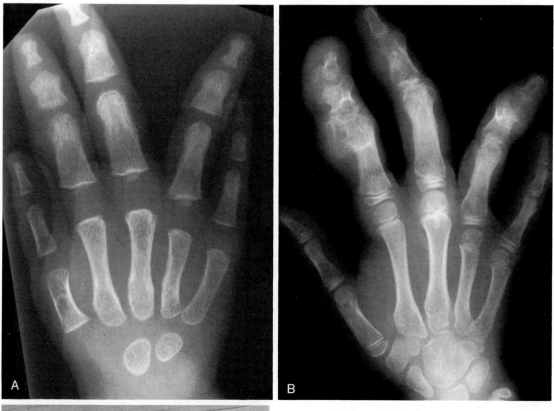

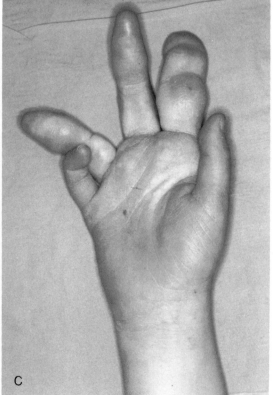

Figure 128–89. Gigantism—hyperostotic type. *A,* At age 3 years, enlargement of the left index, long, and ring fingers was evident in this young boy. *B* and *C,* By age 13 years, marked distortion and limitation of motion were present.

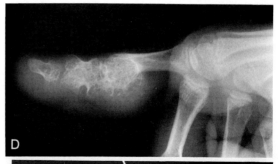

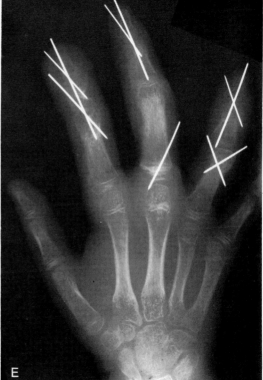

Figure 128–89 *Continued D,* Lateral radiograph of the index finger shows narrowing and distortion of the joint spaces by osseous masses that mechanically block flexion. *E,* Treatment consisted of bone reduction, soft tissue debulking, and interphalangeal joint fusions. When the patient reached skeletal maturity, large masses at the metacarpophalangeal joint were also excised and replaced with implant arthroplasties. *F,* Appearance five years later.

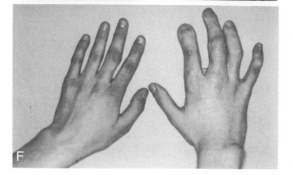

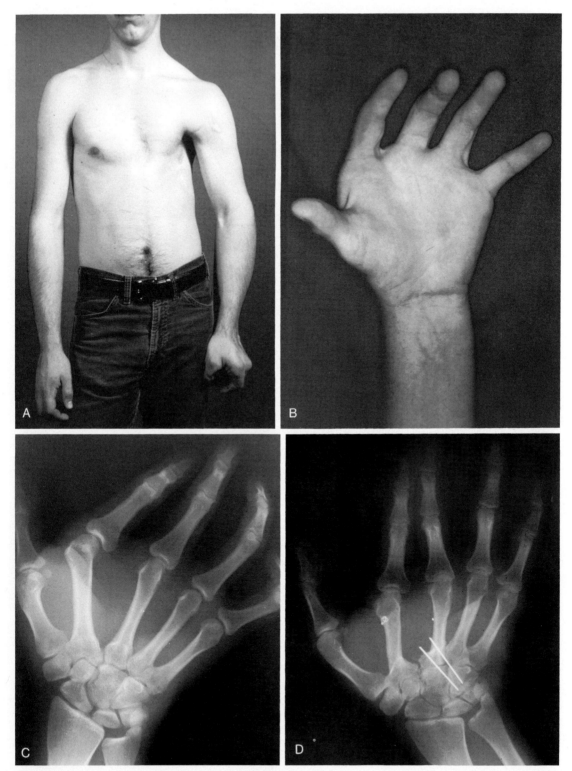

Figure 128–90. Gigantism—hemihypertrophy. *A,* Appearance of a young man born with enlargement of both upper and lower limbs on the left side of his body. A lymphatic malformation was excised from his axilla during infancy. Upper arm and forearm enlargement is due to muscle hypertrophy and not a vascular anomaly. *B,* Typical spadelike appearance of a broad hand with ulnar drift and severe flexion contractures of the digits. Preoperative (*C*) and postoperative (*D*) radiographs show correction of the metacarpal widening with closing wedge osteotomies of the index and long metacarpals.

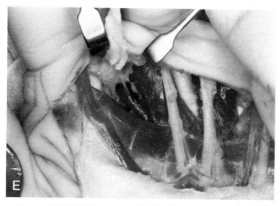

Figure 128–90 *Continued E,* Flexion contractures of the metacarpophalangeal joint were secondary to abnormal sets of atavistic intrinsic muscles inserting into the flexion sheath as well as proximal phalanges. These were released and the flexor tendons were lengthened as a separate procedure following the osteotomies.

be circumferentially massive. Patients' symptoms relate to the progressive adduction contractures of the thumb, flexion contractures at the metacarpophalangeal joint, and ulnar deviation of digits. Vascular insufficiency is not seen.

Treatment

In addition to the obvious functional limitations of these various types of gigantism, the psychologic effect upon a small child and family can be devastating (Edgerton and Tuerk, 1974). There are no predictable ways to inhibit local growth, and surgery tends to be repetitive and ablative. Multiple procedures are often done during a single operation. The patient should be followed very carefully during infancy and early childhood, and a disproportionately large digit(s) should *not* be allowed to go untreated through school ages. Digits with progressive types of gigantism are of primary concern.

Individualization of treatment is more important than in any other area of congenital limb surgery. Patient age, digit involved, type of gigantism, progression, and rehabilitation potential must all be considered both individually and collectively. The major objectives should be to reduce length and circumferential bulk, to maintain sensation and circulation, and to preserve as much motion as possible. Carpal tunnel release will relieve symptoms, but debulking of an enlarged nerve may result in a sensory deficit. Despite the grotesque size of the nerves in the first

two types described, sensation is normal before treatment. Epiphyseal arrest will control longitudinal growth if all growth centers are completely destroyed with a burr. Frykman and Wood (1982) emphasized that total excision of the epiphysis is an easier alternative and pointed out that this does not control circumferential growth or width, which can be reduced by a variety of maneuvers, all resulting in joint stiffness. Staged debulking procedures at three-month intervals have been recommended. They are quite effective but run the risk of injury to neurovascular structures. Incisions made in the high mid to lateral line of the finger grow better and produce less hypertrophy and contractures than palmar zigzag approaches. One side of the digit or hand should be treated at a time. Patients with hyperostotic lesions often form hypertrophic scars in incisions made in glabrous palmar surfaces. Excess bone is usually removed at the same time as soft tissue is debulked. Tsuge and Ikuta (1973) have recommended stripping the digital nerves and attempting to preserve the main nerve trunk in order to avoid major sensory deficits in the nerve-oriented and neurofibromatosis-related types of gigantism. Kelikian (1974) has recommended excision of the large tortuous segment of nerve, resection of redundancies, and end to end repair. Others have resected these nerves at very early ages, hoping to decrease the trophic influence on growth (McCarroll, 1950; Paletta and Rybka, 1972). Clearly, these are difficult problems with no clear-cut solutions.

In the grotesquely enlarged digit, shortening may be the most practical treatment. The simplest method involves ablation of the distal phalangeal segment and debulking of the remainder of the digit. Others have retained a portion of this segment, creating a dog-ear to be excised in a second stage (Barsky, 1967; Tsuge and Ikuta, 1973) (Fig. 128–91*A* and *B*). Barsky (1967) leaves the excess tissue on the palmar skin bridge, and Tsuge and Ikuta (1973) prefer to leave it on the dorsal surface. There is a potential for nail deformities. None of the illustrations in current textbooks adequately portrays this deformity as it actually exists, and case reports and large series do not show long-term postoperative results, which are never normal (Dell, 1985). For correction of lateral deviation, closing wedge osteotomies through the metaphyses of the involved phalanges are effective, especially

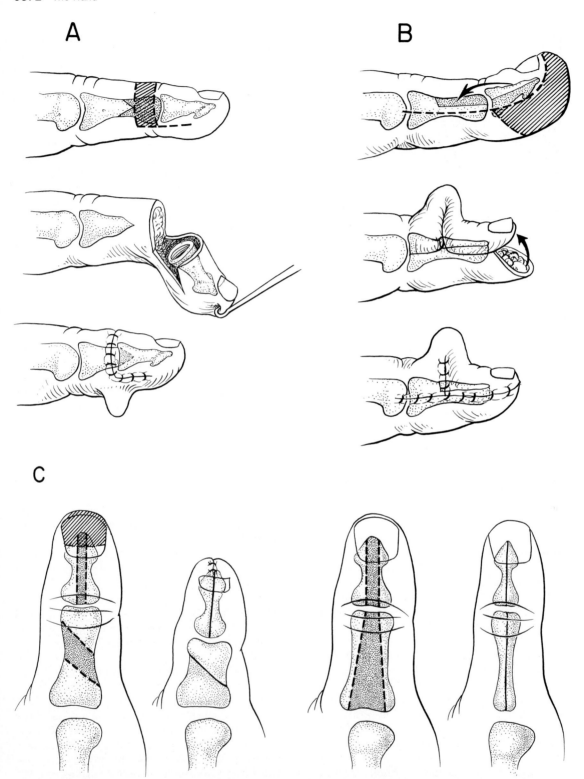

Figure 128–91. Macrodactyly. There are three conceptual approaches for correction of the enlarged digit or thumb. *A,* Resection of dorsal soft tissue, bone excision and arthrodesis, and creation of a palmar dog-ear (Barsky, 1967); *B,* distal and palmar soft tissue reduction, a split bone resection and recession, and creation of a dorsal dog-ear (Tsuge, 1973); and *C,* distal nail and soft tissue ablation, preservation of paronychial flaps, midline and oblique bone resection, and primary closure without skin redundancy. The first two methods require soft tissue resections as second stages (Milessi, 1974). These alternatives can be carefully individualized to the particular anatomic abnormality seen.

in the slowly progressing types of gigantism. Frequently, arthrodeses of the proximal and middle phalanges are done at the same time. Restoration of motion to stiff joints after multiple previous operations is impractical because of adherence of flexor and extensor tendons. Partial digital amputation or ray resection must always be considered (1) in severe enlargement for grotesque deformities, (2) after multiple failed previous operations, and (3) in the insensate digit (Wood, 1969; Boyes, 1977).

The enlarged thumb has evoked innovative alternative approaches. Millesi (1974) has advocated a central en bloc resection of the distal phalangeal segment combined with a oblique skeletal shortening of the proximal phalangeal segment (Fig. 128–91C). This principle can be applied further to central soft tissue and bone reduction in the grotesquely enlarged digit, where amputation with ray resection is the only other practical treatment. In all the radical resection procedures mentioned, skin and flap necrosis is the primary complication, coupled with loss of sensation. Some have even recommended removing all marginal skin and replacing the defatted tissue as a full-thickness skin graft so that it will survive as a graft rather than fail as a flap (Edgerton and Tuerk, 1974). This tissue is not normal.

In the neurofibromatosis and hyperostotic forms, surgical resection of the large osteochondral masses should be performed before significant joint restriction has occurred. The palmar plate usually must be removed, and interphalangeal joint motion is often reduced after these resections. Early gains in motion following resection are often lost with growth of the child. In adolescents and adults, arthrodesis is more practical. Metacarpophalangeal joint implant arthroplasty should be considered for preservation of motion at this level.

Patients with hemihypertrophy are difficult to treat. As long as the hand is functional and all joints are passively mobile, no surgery is recommended. If the patient is seen as an infant or during the first year of life, passive stretching exercises and static night splints should be started. Progressive ulnar drift and flexion of the digits may require centralization of the extensor mechanism and release of abnormal intrinsic muscles on the palmar side. Severe flexion contractures combined with ulnar drift and loss of function are

treated in stages. First, the splayed-out metacarpals are brought toward the midline of the hand with closing wedge osteomies; as a second stage, deforming forces are released by excision of abnormal intrinsic muscles, lengthening of extrinsic flexor tendons, and centralization of the extensors at the metacarpophalangeal joint level. Debulking of massive thenar and especially hypothenar muscle masses can be done as a third stage and is often considered for aesthetic reasons. For gigantism recognized during infancy, passive range of motion exercises and night splinting has been recommended. Occasionally, progressive, unrelating contractures of the metacarpophalangeal joint and wrist require early release and subsequent splinting.

CONGENITAL CONSTRICTION RING SYNDROME

Numerous terms have been used to describe this syndrome: annular bands, constriction rings or grooves, annular defects, intrauterine or fetal amputations, and Streeter's dysplasia. Despite many similarities to anomalies seen with undergrowth and syndactyly (failure of differentiation), a separate category has been designated for these special cases.

Clinical Presentation

The etiology of constriction rings has been the subject of great interest for centuries. The early work of Streeter (1930), whose namesake is commonly associated with this syndrome, and others implicates "defective germ plasm," whereas more recent work has documented the presence of amnionic tissue at the depths of these grooves and has implicated mechanical constriction of an otherwise normal fetal limb (Field and Krag, 1973; Kino, 1975; Rowsell, 1988). Present-day developmentalists invoke disruption and deformation sequences in the etiology of these deformities (Smith, 1982; Granick and associates, 1987) (see earlier section in this chapter). This evidence supports the concept that early rupture of the amnion produces fibrous bands that become entangled with fetal parts such as limbs. It does not adequately explain associated malformations such as cleft lip or palate and club feet. Normal anatomy proximal to the defect, the sporadic nature of the deformity, and the low incidence of associated anomalies add weight to the latter hypothesis (Wynne-Davies and Lamb, 1985).

Inheritance is sporadic, and the incidence varies from one in 5000 to one in 15,000 live births (Patterson, 1961; Dobyns, 1985) for greater involvement of the larger digits and toes. Associated defects primarily consist of missing toes, clubbed feet, and severe constriction rings around other parts of the body, pseudoarthrosis of the tibia and fibula, and, occasionally, an amputation. Facial clefts and other craniofacial abnormalities have been reported to occur in between 10 and 40 per cent of patients but their appearance may well be coincidental (Patterson, 1961; Fishl, 1971; Casaubon, 1983). Neurovascular structures may be compressed distal to the area of involvement, particularly in cases of acrosyndactyly. There may be progression of the distal swelling or neurologic symptoms as the scar tissue at the base of the band contracts or does not expand with growth. Peripheral vascular insufficiency is invariably present distal to constrictions and is rarely symptomatic.

Tight constriction rings or annular bands may be found around part or all of the extremities of newborn infants, just as they can affect other parts of the body. The depth of the groove may vary from a partial defect with a mild deficiency of subcutaneous tissue to a deep circumferential indentation that may interrupt veins, lymphatic channels, tendons, and even nerves (Farmer, 1948). Occasionally, a missing fingertip or finger or an auto-amputated part will be found within the amniotic sac (Field and Krag, 1973; Clavert and associates, 1978). With moderate and severe involvement, a side to side soft tissue fusion of hypoplastic digits is present, signifying an acrosyndactyly (see "Syndactyly"). The tiny or large dorsal to palmar epithelium-lined clefts always present represent web commissures, which are never located at their normal level. Adjacent phalanges do not have osseous fusion but are joined by a common band of scar tissue; this is thought to be the result of an ischemic insult, which most postulate to occur after creation of the cleft by the process of programmed cell death. In contrast to other conditions, in which there are acral absences, all tissue up to the abnormal constriction ring or acrosyndactyly is normal (Patterson, 1961).

Constriction ring syndrome may be confused with many other entities. For this reason Patterson (1961) has set strict diagnostic criteria. The following features, which may appear alone or in combination, must be present for this diagnosis: (1) a simple constriction ring, (2) constriction ring accompanied by a distal deformity with or without lymphedema, (3) constriction ring with soft tissue fusion of distal parts (acrosyndactyly), and (4) (congenital) intrauterine amputations. The most comprehensive discussion of amputations is contained in Torpin's (1968) book. Bilateral asymmetric involvement of upper limbs is common, and a given patient may have an incomplete band on one digit, a very deep band with lymphedema in another, and amputation or acrosyndactyly of yet others. Bilateral hand deformities are commonly accompanied by toe or major foot anomalies. The entire spectrum, ranging from a shallow groove to a deep groove, to a deeper groove with distal lymphedema, to a transverse amputation, may be seen in a single patient and may affect one or all of the fingers or toes (Fig. 128–92). Despite their diminutive length, most of these digits can be quite useful. Many of these deformities would be classified in the failure of formation—transverse absence category if no other stigmata of the constriction ring syndrome were present. Isolated unilateral transverse amputations with no other stigmata of the constriction ring syndrome belong in the failure of formation category (Ogino and Saitsu, 1987).

Severe distal lymphedema beyond the constriction band denotes a more urgent situation. Here, circulation and neurologic function may be impaired and should be carefully monitored by measuring temperature gradients, the adherence test for sensation (Harrison, 1974), and spontaneous movement. Increasing edema will require earlier surgical correction (Moses, Flatt, and Cooper, 1979). Usually, the edematous tissue is firm and indurated and grows proportionately with the rest of the body.

Treatment

Appropriate treatment varies with the severity of the deformity, number of functional digits, and presence or absence of the thumb. Excision of the annular groove and Z-plasty may be required for lymphedematous digits

CONSTRICTION RING VARIATIONS

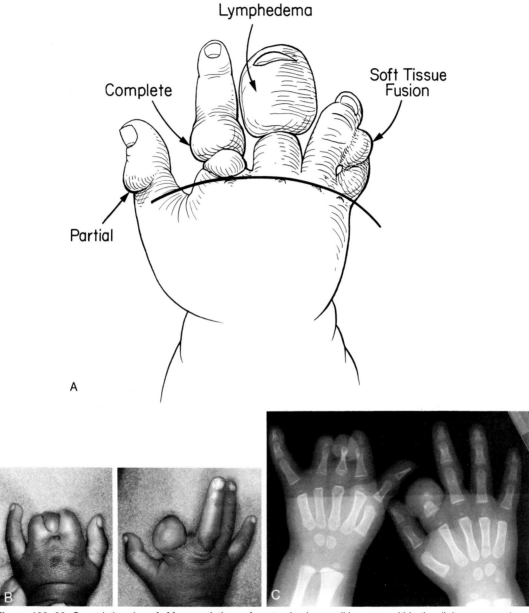

Figure 128–92. Constriction ring. *A,* Many variations of anatomic abnormalities seen within the digits may consist of a ring or a groove extending partially around the part (thumb), multiple complete and/or partial grooves in the same digit with interposed lymphedematous soft tissue (index), severe complete groove with distal edema and compromise of circulation (long), side-to-side coalescence of two digits with scar tissue (ring and fifth), and partial digital amputation (fifth). A dorsal palmar sinus is usually present in instances of distal fusion in acrosyndactyly. *B* and *C,* Clinical appearance and radiographs in a youngster show many of the preceding variations, which may occur alone or in combination in the same patient. Mirror image deformities of both hands do not occur in this syndrome.

in extremities with impending circulatory compromise. For correction of the simplest shallow bands, small Z-plasties are sufficient. In such cases, most authors recommend release of only 50 per cent of the circumference of the digit at a time (Farmer, 1948; Blackfield and Hause, 1951), whereas others do not hesitate to perform a one stage total release (Buck-Gramcko, 1981). Several principles are important in the surgical correction. The depth of the groove should be completely excised, local tissue defatted and advanced into the defect to correct the ultimate contour deficiency, and Z-plasties placed in the high mid-lateral line of the digit. Careful dissection is required at the base of all grooves to avoid injury to nerves, arteries, and tendons. Magnification is very useful for the preservation of nerves, digital arteries, and dorsal veins in these small hands (Figs. 128–93, 128–94).

The treatment of acrosyndactyly is discussed in the syndactyly section. Management of the individual digits depends upon the severity and pattern of involvement in the rest of the hand. Because the majority of cases are moderate to severe, almost all will need secondary reconstruction. The general principle is to start with early release of coalesced tips, in conjunction with or followed by commissure construction to allow unrestricted growth of individual digits. Soft tissue nubbins with or without nails can be debulked and often rotated into place to provide coverage or can be used as sources of full-thickness skin grafts (Flatt, 1977). Tiny, functionless nubbins at the end of amputation stumps are satisfactory sources of skin grafts only if they do not contain lymphedematous tissue. Digit length and mobility may be improved by local digital transposition procedures, which must be carefully executed

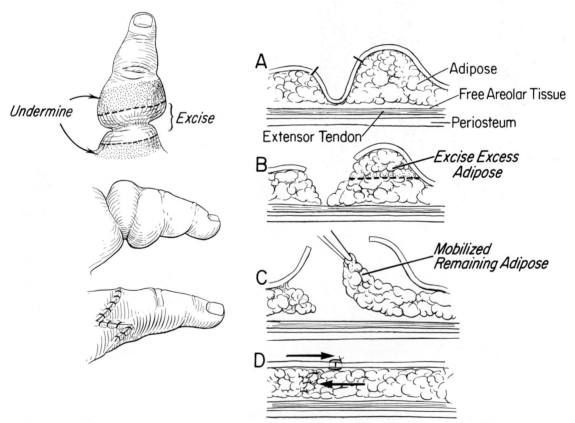

Figure 128–93. Constriction ring. Excision and restoration of contour involves more than a simple series of Z-plasties. *A* and *B,* A complete excision of skin within the entire depth of the groove is usually possible, as excess tissue is present. *C,* Dorsal and distal adipose tissue is debulked while a tongue is retained and mobilized into the defect created by the groove. *D,* Differential closures of the skin and underlying fat will help minimize a residual groove or ring. Z-plasties in the midlateral or midaxial lines of the digit conform better than multiple smaller Z-plasties around the entire circumference of a digit or thumb.

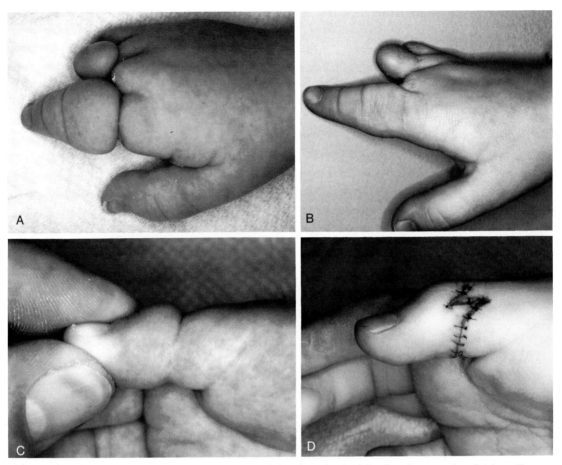

Figure 128–94. *A,* Appearance of multiple deep constriction rings that had developed progressive distal swelling over the first three months of life. *B,* Appearance several years after single staged band excision, soft tissue advancement, and Z-plasty. No dorsal veins were visualized under the microscope. *C* and *D,* Z-plasties are effectively placed in the midaxial or high midlateral line along the side of a digit or thumb. Most scars migrate in a palmar direction with time and growth in these children.

(Carroll, 1959; Peacock, 1962; Kaplan, 1966). Proper identification of neurovascular structures is mandatory during staged transpositions of partial rays from one part of the hand to another, in which circulatory compromise is the primary problem.

Ray resection of residual digital stumps may improve function. Most amputations (about 70 per cent) require no surgery, but some benefit from web deepening, distraction lengthening (Kessler, Baruch, and Hecht, 1978; Matev, 1979), and local transpositions (Dobyns, 1985). Local flaps and full-thickness skin grafts are frequently necessary for creation of a functional hand.

Complete or partial absence of the thumb is a challenging problem frequently seen in patients with constriction ring syndrome. The reconstruction chosen depends upon the pres-ence or absence of the carpometacarpal joint, the existing digital length, thenar intrinsic muscles, and the presence and length of other digits. When the proximal portion is present, options include lengthening with or without bone graft (Matev, 1979; Cowen and Loftus, 1978), toe to thumb transfer (Yoshimura, 1980), and local transposition using the "on-top-plasty" (Soiland, 1961; Dobyns, 1985). Toe transfer is an attractive option in these patients with partial thumb absence, because there is a higher probability that a more normal complement of muscles, tendons, and nerves will be found in the forearm, which is not the case in patients with transverse am-putations group, discussed earlier in this chapter (Gilbert, 1982). Although experience with distraction lengthening is limited and long-term follow-up greater than 10 years

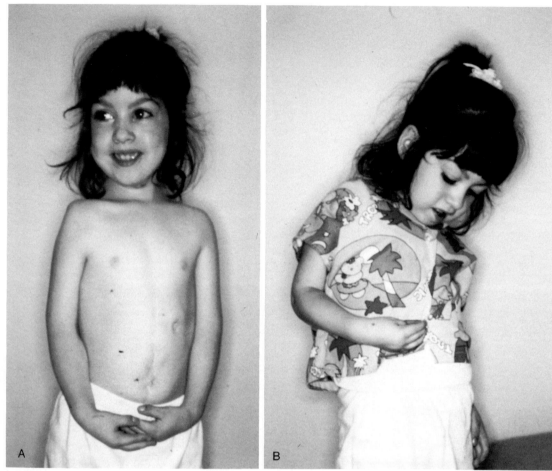

Figure 128–95. Arthrogryposis. *A,* The child with upper limb involvement demonstrates thin musculature of the shoulder with the humerus held in adduction and internal rotation. Elbows are extended and wrists held in semi-flexed pronated postures. *B* and *C,* Attempts to flex the elbows to perform simple tasks are difficult, but affected children continuously adapt by positioning their upper bodies and necks and assisting with their legs. *D,* Thumbs are often characterized by adduction into the palms with tight first web spaces. Long slender digits are usually held in slight ulnar deviation and have very little interphalangeal joint motion, as noted by the lack of flexion creases.

has not been achieved, this technique is more predictable at the metacarpal level than with hypoplastic phalanges often seen in this syndrome. Radiographs of the transverse amputations at the digital level seen within this syndrome often show a broad metaphysis and hypoplastic and often nonossified epiphyses, which funnel down to a pencil-thin diaphysis that ends without a condyle. These bones provide poor stock for distraction lengthening. Methods for thumb reconstruction are described more thoroughly in Chapters 123 to 127.

The major complications of procedures to enhance function in these hands are inadequate correction and circulatory compromise of flaps or transferred segments of bone or soft tissue. It is easy to injure digital nerves and flexor and extensor tendons during correction of deep grooves. Early, aggressive osteotomies to correct skeletal deformities will yield a plethora of nonunions, fortunately at the phalangeal level.

ARTHROGRYPOSIS

Clinical Presentation

Arthrogryposis multiplex congenita is a syndrome of unknown etiology that is always present at birth and manifests with persistent joint contractures (Lewin, 1925). It is not a disease per se, but presents as a syndrome with variable joint contractures, both multi-

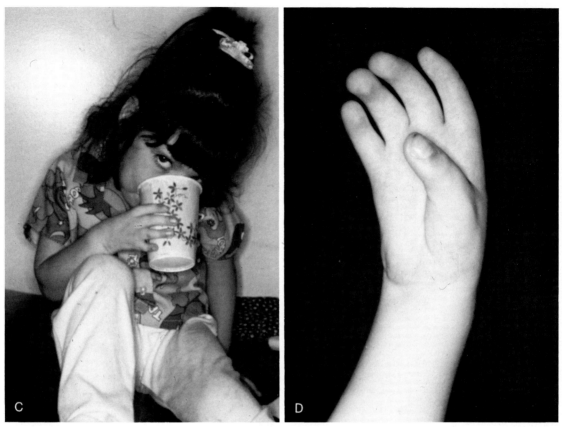

Figure 128–95 *Continued*

ple and protean, which are caused by abnormalities of muscle and nerves. The degree of disability varies from mild to total (Lloyd-Roberts and Leitin, 1970).

The cause is unknown, but striated muscles and the central nervous system seem to be sites of most interest to researchers. A decrease in numbers of muscle fibers and all degrees of degeneration and fatty infiltration are seen (Sheldon, 1932; Kite, 1955; Banker, 1957), and reduction in both the number and size of anterior horn cells has been noted within the spinal cord (Whitten, 1957; Drachman and Banker, 1961). Secondary joint contractures are the result of thickening and contracture of joint capsules and collateral ligaments. If primary joint pathology is present, arthrogryposis can be ruled out.

Classification into *neuropathic* and *myopathic* types can be determined on the basis of muscle biopsy, peripheral nerve biopsy, and electromyographic studies. The neuropathic form is more common, involves C5 to C7 segments, displays neuro-segmented involve-

ment patterns, and has no hereditary association. Myopathic forms are less common, demonstrate positive hereditary pedigrees, have profound muscle atrophy and progressive muscular dystrophy, tend to develop flexion contractures, and have associated chest wall and spinal deformities (Brown, Robson, and Sharrard, 1980). Intelligence is not affected in either type. An incidence of three in 10,000 live births has been reported (Laitinen, 1966). The differential diagnosis is often hard to determine at birth, and is confirmed by muscle and nerve biopsies, serum enzymes determinations, electromyography, and genetic consultation.

The clinical appearance is easy to diagnose. Arthrogryposis, in particular, is a diagnosis of exclusion based primarily on physical examination (Fig. 128–95). Shoulders have thin muscles and are held in adduction and internal rotation. Symmetric involvement of upper limbs, varying in degree from minimal to severe, is common. Elbows are usually extended, and the forearms may be held in a semi-flexed and pronated posture. Passive elbow flexion is moderate, and severe deformities lack active motion.

In severe cases, the wrist is held in palmar flexion and ulnar deviation while the thumb assumes a tightly flexed and adducted position within the palm. Active thumb extension is lacking. The digits are flexed and ulnarly deviated at the metacarpophalangeal joints and demonstrate very little, if any, interphalangeal joint motion. The upper limb skin is atrophied and waxy in appearance, flexion and extension creases are absent, and skin dimples may signify underlying joints (Tachdjian, 1972). There are usually extensive abnormalities of the lower limbs, primarily the feet, and of the spine (Kite, 1955; Hansen, 1961; Friedlander, Westin, and Wood, 1968). The distal limb parts—hands and feet—are involved to a much greater degree than the proximal.

Treatment

Once the diagnosis is made, parents should be told that splinting and stretching exercises are the hallmarks of treatment. Surgical priorities are usually given to the lower extremities during the first 18 months of life so that the child may eventually ambulate with or without crutches or braces. During this time, range of motion in the upper limb and hand can be maintained or improved. The general principles of treatment are to increase passive range of motion, to correct disabling deformities, and to encourage use of adaptive aids.

More proximal positioning of the shoulder and elbow must precede any hand surgery, which will be of little value if the shoulder is adducted and the elbow fully extended. Treatment of the shoulder is determined by its position and by the integrated function of the elbow, forearm, wrist, and hand in the child's daily activities. Muscle transfers to provide shoulder abduction have limited value and must be accompanied by aggressive joint release. Just as much progress is usually made with splints that mobilize the shoulder in extension and external rotation. Derotational osteotomies of the humerus are more predictable.

Surgery at the elbow level is infrequently done, because elastic harnesses are useful to maintain 75 degrees of elbow flexion so the child can get the hand to the mouth (Bayne, 1982). After age 4, the child can wear commercially available, dynamic, flexion assisted splints. When conservative measures fail in patients with moderate and severe extension contractures, a posterior release and step lengthening of the triceps allow more passive flexion. These procedures are best done early, at age 2 or 3 years. Biceps function can be substituted with anterior transfer of the triceps (Carroll and Hill, 1970) or the pectoralis major muscle (Clark, 1946; Lloyd-Roberts and Leitin, 1970). A third option is a proximal advancement of the flexor-pronator origin into the distal humerus, just above the elbow joint (Steindler, 1949). Operating on both elbows is never recommended, so that the child will have at least one limb extended for perineal care and pushing up from a sitting position. Functional predictability of these transfers is low because the muscle being transferred is not always normal and preoperative passive range of motion may be limited. Night splinting is always necessary to maintain correction. Elbow flexion contractures are unusual and rarely require surgery.

The wrist and hand present more areas for surgical rehabilitation than more proximal regions of the upper limb. The condition of the hand determines to a great degree the treatment of the shoulder and elbow (Tachdjian, 1972). Stiff fingers and wrists with no passive motion are a grave prognostic sign. In more supple hands, the tightly flexed and ulnarly deviated hand can be repositioned, with release of the volar capsular ligaments and transfer of the flexor carpi ulnaris to the extensor carpi radialis brevis to maintain wrist dorsiflexion (Meyn and Ruby, 1976). When hand function is limited, the wrist is often best left in flexion and ulnar deviation, a position in which hook and grasping as with a shovel or rake can be effective (Cooney and Schutt, 1986). With severe flexion contractures of the digits and thumb, proximal row carpectomy may be useful (Smith, 1973; Williams, 1978). Soft tissue release of the thumb-index web space with Z-plasties or grafts, and adductor lengthening, if needed, are the procedures of greatest benefit in these hands. If thumb alignment is poor, ostectomy is much more predictable than tendon transfer. If flexion and ulnar deviation of the digits obstruct functional grasp, soft tissue release and rebalancing of dynamic forces with crossed intrinsic transfers may be helpful. Once skeletal maturity has been reached, metacarpal head resection and implant arthroplasty can be done. Syndactyly release and metacarpophalangeal capsulotomy will improve finger position. All authors emphasize that patients with arthrogryposis rarely require operation, which may do great harm because one is not working with normal muscles, tendons, or joints. Although many question the advisability of any hand surgery in these patients, the specific goals of independent feeding, self care, and object handling can be improved with limb surgery in patients with supple hands, adequate passive motion, and satisfactory overall function.

REFERENCES

Introduction

Bardeen, D. R., and Lewis, W. H.: Development of the limbs, body wall, and back in man. Am. J. Anat., *1:*1, 1901–1902.

Boinet, E.: Polydactylie et atavism. Rev. Med. (Paris), *18:*316, 1898.

Caffey, J.: Pediatric X-ray Diagnosis: A Textbook for Students and Practitioners of Pediatrics, Surgery and Radiology. 7th Ed. Chicago, Year Book Medical Publishers, 1978.

Felizet, G.: Opération de la syndactylie congénitale (procédé autoplastique). Rev. d'Orthop., *10:*49, 1892.

Flatt, A. E.: The Care of Congenital Hand Anomalies. St. Louis, C. V. Mosby Company, 1977.

Lewis, W. H.: The development of the arm in man. Am. J. Anat., *1:*146, 1901–1902.

Lister, G.: The Hand: Diagnosis and Indications. New York, Churchill-Livingstone, 1984.

Paré, A.: The Works of That Famous Chirurgion Ambroise Parey. Translated out of Latin and compared with the French by Thomas Johnson. London, T. Cotes and R. Young, 1634.

Persaud, T. V. N.: Classification and epidemiology of developmental defects. *In* Basic Concepts in Teratology. New York, A. R. Liss, Inc., 1985.

Smith, R. J., and Lipke, R.: Treatment of congenital deformities of the hand and forearm. N. Engl. J. Med., *300:*344, 1979.

St. Hilaire, I. G.: Histoire Générale et Particulière des Anomalies de l'Organisation chez l'Homme et les Animaux. Paris, J. B. Ballière, 1832.

Stuart, H. C., Pyle, S. I., Cornol, J., Reed, R. B.: Onsets, completions and spans of ossification in the 29 bone growth centers of the hand and wrist. Pediatrics, *29:*237, 1962.

Temtamy, S. A., and McKusick, V.: The Genetics of Hand Malformations. New York, Alan R. Liss, 1982.

Velpeau, A. A. L. M.: New Elements of Operative Surgery. Vol. I trans. by P. S. Townsend. New York, Samuels and Woods, 1847 (cited by Kelikian, 1974).

Vrolik, W.: Teratology. *In* Todd, R. B. (Ed.): Cyclopaedia of Anatomy and Physiology. Vol. IV. London, Longman, Brown, Green, Longman, and Roberts, 1849 (cited by Kelikian, 1974).

Embryology

Adamson, K., Jr.: Fetal surgery. N. Engl. J. Med., *275:*204, 1966.

Bardeen, D. R., and Lewis, W. H.: Development of the limbs, body wall, and back in man. Am. J. Anat., *1:*1, 1901–1902.

Bogusch, G.: Muscle development during normal and disturbed skeletogenesis. *In* Merker, H. J., and Nau, H. (Eds.): Teratology of the Limbs. Berlin, Walter de Gruyter and Company, 1980.

Boinet, E.: Polydactylie et atavism. Rev. Med., *18:*316, 1898.

Caplan, A. I., and Koutroupas, S.: The control of muscle and cartilage development in the chick limb: The role of differential vascularization. J. Embryol. Exp. Morphol., *29:*571, 1973.

Chevallier, A., Kieny, M., and Mauger, A.: Limb-somite relationship: Origin of limb musculature. J. Embryol. Exp. Morphol., *41:*245, 1977.

Chevallier, A., Kieny, M., and Mauger, A.: Limb-somite relationship: Effect of removal of somatic mesoderm in the wing musculature. J. Embryol. Exp. Morphol., *43:*263, 1978.

Cihak, R.: Connections of the abductor pollicus longus and brevis in the ontogenesis of the human hand. Folia Morphol., *20:*102, 1972a.

Cihak, R.: Ontogenesis of the skeleton and intrinsic muscles of the human hand and foot. Ergeb. Anat. Entwicklungsgesch, *46:*1, 1972b.

Cihak, R.: Reduction of insertion of M. interosseous dorsalis accessorius in human ontogenesis. Folia Morphol., *21:*228, 1973.

Cihak, R.: Differentiation and rejoining of muscular layers in the embryonic hand. *In* Bergsma, D., and Wicklind, L. (Eds.): Morphogenesis and Malformation of the Limb. Vol. 13. New York, Alan R. Liss, 1977.

Coleman, S. S., and Anson, B. J.: Arterial patterns in the hand. Surg. Gynecol. Obstet., *113:*409, 1961.

Drachman, D. B., and Sokoloff, L.: The role of movement in embryonic joint development. Dev. Biol., *14:*401, 1966.

Edwards, E. A.: Organization of the small arteries of the hand and digits. Am. J. Surg., *99:*837, 1960.

Feinberg, R. M., and Saunders, J. W., Jr.: Effects of excising the apical ectodermal ridge in the development of the marginal vasculature in the wing bud of the chick embryo. J. Exp. Zool., *219:*345, 1982.

Fraser, F. C.: Causes of congenital malformations in human beings. J. Chronic Dis., *10:*97, 1959.

Goldberg, M. J., and Bartoshesky, L. E.: Congenital hand anomaly: Etiology and associated malformations. Hand Clin. *1:*405, 1985.

Graham, J. H., Stephens, T. D., Siebert, G. R., et al.: Determinants in the morphogenesis of muscle tendon insertions. J. Pediatr., *101:*825, 1982.

Gray, D. J., Gardner, E., and O'Rahilly, R.: The prenatal development of the skeleton and joints of the human hand. Am. J. Anat., *101:*169, 1957.

Haines, R. W.: The development of joints. J. Anat., *81:*33, 1947.

Harrison, R. G.: Experiments on the development of the fore limb of Amblystoma, a self-differentiating equipotential system. J. Exp. Zool., *25:*413, 1918.

Hodgen, G. D.: Antenatal diagnosis and treatment of fetal skeletal malformations. With emphasis on in utero surgery for neural tube defects and limb bud regeneration. J. A. M. A., *246:*1079, 1981.

Hollyday, M.: Development of motor innervation of chick limbs. *In* Fallon, J. F., and Caplan, A. I. (Eds.): Limb Development and Regeneration, Part A. New York, Alan R. Liss, 1983.

Hootnick, D. R., Levinsohn, E. M., Randall, P. A., et al.: Vascular dysgenesis associated with skeletal dysplasia of the lower limb. J. Bone Joint Surg., *62A:*1123, 1980.

Horder, T. J., and Martin, K. A. C.: Some determinants of often terminal localization and retinotopic polarity within fibre populations in the tectum of goldfish. J. Physiol., *333:*481, 1982.

Jacob, H. J., and Christ, B.: On the formation of muscular pattern in the chick limb. *In* Merker, H. J., and Nau, H. (Eds.): Teratology of the Limbs. Berlin, Walter de Gruyter and Company, 1980.

Kieny, M., and Chevallier, A.: Autonomy of tendon development in the embryonic chick wing. J. Embryol. Exp. Morphol., *49:*153, 1979.

Klein, K. L., Scott, W. J., and Wilson, J. G.: Aspirin induced teratogenesis: A unique pattern of cell death and subsequent polydactyly in the rat. J. Exp. Zool., *216:*107, 1981.

Krey, A. K., Dayton, D. H., and Goetnick, P. F.: NICHD Research Workshop: Normal and abnormal development of the limb. Teratology, *29:*315, 1984.

Lewis, W. H.: The development of the arm in man. Am. J. Anat., *1:*145, 1901–1902.

Michejda, M., Bacher, J., Kuwabara, T., et al.: In utero allogeneic bone transplantation in primates. Transplantation, *32:*96, 1981.

Michejda, M., and Hodgen, G. D.: In utero diagnosis and treatment of non-human primate fetal skeletal anomalies. J. A. M. A., *246:*1093, 1981.

Milaire, J.: Aspects of limb morphogenesis in mammals. *In* DeHaan, R. L., and Ursprung, H. (Eds.): Organogenesis. New York, Holt, Rinehart and Winston, 1965.

Moffett, B. C.: The morphogenesis of joints. *In* DeHaan, R. L., and Ursprung, H. (Eds.): Organogenesis. New York, Holt, Rinehart and Winston, 1965.

Mrazkova, O.: Ontogenesis of arterial trunks in the human forearm. Folia Morph., *21:*193, 1973.

Newman, S. A.: Lineage and pattern in the developing wing bud. *In* Ede, D. A., Hinchliffe, J. R., and Balls, M. (Eds.): Vertebrate Limb and Somite Morphogenesis. Cambridge, Cambridge University Press, 1977.

Newman, S. A., and Frisch, H. L.: Dynamics of skeletal pattern formation in developing chick limb. Science, *205:*662, 1979.

O'Rahilly, R., Gray, D. J., and Gardner, E.: Chondrification in the hand and feet of staged human embryos. Contrib. Embryol., *36:*183, 1957.

O'Rahilly, R., and Gardner, E.: The timing and sequence of events in the development of the limbs in the human embryo. Anat. Embryol., *148:*1, 1975.

Saunders, J. W., Jr., Gasseling, M. T., and Saunders, L. C.: Cellular death in morphogenesis of the avian wing. Develop. Biol., *5:*147, 1962.

Shellswell, G. B., and Wolpert, L.: The pattern in muscle and tendon development in the chick wing. *In* Ede, D. A., Hinchcliff, J. R., and Balls, M. (Eds.): Vertebrate Limb and Somite Morphogenesis. Cambridge, Cambridge University Press, 1977.

Smith, D. W.: Recognizable Patterns of Human Malformation. Genetic, Embryologic and Clinical Aspects. 3rd Ed. Philadelphia, W. B. Saunders Company, 1982.

Smith, R. J.: Preventive surgery for congenital deformities of the hand. Hand Clin., *1:*373, 1985.

Streeter, G. L.: Focal deficiencies in fetal tissues and their relation to intrauterine amputations. Carnegie Contrib. Embryol., *22:*1, 1930.

Streeter, G. L.: Developmental horizons in human embryos IV. A review of histogenesis of cartilage and bone. Contrib. Embryol., *33:*149, 1949.

Temtamy, S., and McKusick, V.: The Genetics of Hand Malformations. Birth Defects, *14:*25, 1978.

Thaller, L., and Eichele, G.: Identification and spatial distribution of retinoids in the developing chick limb bud. Nature, *327:*625, 1987.

Tickle, C.: Experimental embryology as applied to the upper limb: Review article. J. Hand Surg. *12B:*294, 1987.

Tridon, P., and Thiret, M.: Malformations associées de la tête et des extrémitées. Paris, Masson et cie, 1966.

Van Allen, M. I., Hoyme, H. E., and Jones, K. L.: Vascular pathogenesis of limb defects I: Radial artery anatomy in radial aplasia. J. Pediatr., *101:*832, 1982.

Vrolik, W.: Teratology. *In* Todd, R. B. (Ed.): Encyclopedia of Anatomy and Physiology. Vol. IV. London, Longman, Brown, Green, Longman, and Roberts, 1849 (cited by Kelikian, 1974).

Wolpert, L., Lewis, J., and Summerbell, D.: Morphogenesis of the vertebrate limb. Ciba Found. Symp., *29:*95, 1975.

Wolpert, L.: Mechanisms of limb development and malformation. Brit. Med. Bull., *32:*65, 1976.

Wolpert, L.: Positional information, pattern formation, and morphogenesis. *In* Connelly, T. G. (Ed.): Morphogenesis and Pattern Formation. New York, Raven Press, 1981.

Yasuda, M.: Pathogenesis of pre-axial polydactyly of the hand in human embryos. J. Embryol. Exp. Morphol., *33:*745, 1975.

Zaleskie, D. J., and Holmes, L. B.: Vascular patterns in the malformed hindlimb of DH/+ mice. *In* Fallon, J. F., and Caplan, A. I. (Eds.): Limb Development and Regeneration, Part A. New York, Alan R. Liss, 1983.

Zwilling, E.: Ectoderm mesoderm relationship in the development of the chick embryo limb bud. J. Exp. Zool., *128:*423, 1955.

Zwilling, E.: Limb morphogenesis. Adv. Morphol., *1:*301, 1960.

Zwilling, E.: Morphogenetic phases in development. Dev. Biol. Suppl., *2:*184, 1968.

Incidence

Birch-Jensen, A.: Congenital Deformities of the Upper Extremities. Copenhagen, Ejnar Munksgaard, 1949.

Bod, M., Dzeizel, A., and Lenz, W.: Incidence at birth of different types of limb reduction abnormalities in Hungary 1975–1977. Hum. Genet., *65:*27, 1983.

Centers for Disease Control: Congenital Malformation Surveillance Report. Atlanta, U.S. Public Health Service, U.S. Department of Health and Social Services, 1984.

Cheng, J. C. Y., Chow, S. K., and Leung, P. C.: Classification of 578 cases of congenital upper limb anomalies with the IFSSH system—a 10 years' experience. J. Hand Surg., *12A:*1055, 1987.

Conway, H., and Bowe, J.: Congenital deformities of the hands. Plast. Reconstr. Surg., *18:*286, 1956.

Erickson, J. D., Mulinare, J., McClain, P. W., et al.: Viet Nam veterans' risks for fathering babies with birth defects. J. A. M. A., *252:*903, 1984.

Flatt, A. E.: A test of a classification of congenital

anomalies of the upper extremity. Surg. Clin. North Am., *50*:509, 1970.

Flatt, A. E.: The Care of Congenital Hand Anomalies. St. Louis, C. V. Mosby Company, 1977.

Flatt, A. E.: Restoration of Function to Congenitally Deformed Hands. Final Report. National and Child Health Service Grant No. MC-R-190356. Copyright 1980, A. E. Flatt, M. D.

Garn, S. M., Frisancho, A. R., Pozanski, A. K., et al.: Analysis of triquetral-lunate fusion. Am. J. Phys. Anthropol., *34*:431, 1971.

Goldberg, M. J., and Bartoshesky, L. E.: Congenital hand anomaly: Etiology and associated malformations. Hand Clin., *1*:405, 1985.

Holmes, L. B.: Congenital malformations. *In* Cloherty, J. P., and Stack, A. R. (Eds.): Manual of Neonatal Care. Boston, Little, Brown and Company, 1980.

Hoyme, H. E., Jones, K. L., Van Allen, M. I., et al.: Vascular pathogenesis of transverse limb reduction defects. J. Pediatr., *101*:839, 1982.

Jurczock, F., and Shollmeyer, R.: Classification of limb anomalies in the newborn. Geburtsch. Frauenheick, *22*:400, 1962.

Kallen, B., Tamereh, M. Z., and Winberg, J.: Infants with congenital limb reductions registered in the Swedish registry of congenital malformations. Teratology, *29*:73, 1984.

Lamb, D. W., Wynne-Davies, R., and Soto, L.: An estimate of the population frequency of congenital malformations of the upper limb. J. Hand Surg., *7*:557, 1982.

Leung, P. C., Chan, K. M., and Cheng, J. C. Y.: Congenital anomalies of the upper limb among the Chinese population in Hong Kong. J. Hand Surg., *7*:563, 1982.

Marden, P. M., Smith, D. W., and McDonald, M. J.: Congenital anomalies in the newborn infant, including minor variations: A study of 4,412 babies by surface examination for anomalies and buccal smear for sex chromatin. J. Pediatr., *64*:357, 1964.

Ogino, T., Minami, K., Fukuda, K., and Kato, H.: Congenital anomalies of the upper limb among the Japanese in Sapporo. J. Hand Surg., *11B*:364, 1986.

Temtamy, S., and McKusick, V.: The Genetics of Hand Malformations. Birth Defects, *Vol. 14*, 1978.

Woolf, R. M., Broadbent, T. R., and Woolf, G. M.: Practical genetics of congenital hand abnormalities. *In* Littler, J. W., et al. (eds.): Symposium on Reconstructive Hand Surgery. St. Louis, C. V. Mosby Company, 1974.

Wynne-Davies, R.: Genetics and malformations of the hand. Hand, *3*:184, 1971.

Wynne-Davies, R., and Lamb, D. W.: Congenital upper limb anomalies: An etiologic grouping of clinical, genetic, and epidemiologic data from 387 patients with "absence" defects, constriction bands, polydactylies, and syndactylies. J. Hand Surg., *10A*:958, 1985.

Yamaguchi, S., Hozumi, Y., Kurosaka, T., et al.: Incidence of various congenital anomalies of the hand from 1961–1972. Proceedings of Sixteenth Annual Meeting, Japanese Society for Surgery of the Hand, Fukuoka, 1973.

Dysmorphology Approach

Holmes, L. B.: Congenital malformation. *In* Cloherty, J. P., and Stark, A. R. (Eds.): Manual of Neonatal Care. Boston, Little, Brown and Company, 1980.

Marden, P. M., Smith, D. W., and McDonald, M. J.: Congenital anomalies in the newborn infant, including minor variations. J. Pediatr., *64*:358, 1904.

McKusick, V. A.: On lumpers and splitters, or the morphology of genetic disease. Perspect. Biol. Med., *12*:298, 1969.

Poswillo, D.: Mechanisms and pathogenesis of malformation. Brit. Med. Bull., *32*:59, 1976.

Smith, D. W.: Recognizable Patterns of Human Malformation. Philadelphia, W. B. Saunders Company, 1982.

Temtamy, S. A., and McKusick, V. A.: The Genetics of Hand Malformations. Birth Defects, *14*:1, 1978.

Warkeny, J.: Congenital Malformations: Notes and Comments. Chicago, Year Book Medical Publishers, 1971.

Genetics and Etiology; Syndromes

Bouwes-Bavinck, J. N., and Weaver, D. D.: Subclavian artery supply disruption sequence: Hypothesis of a vascular etiology for Poland, Klippel-Feil, and Mobius anomalies. Am. J. Med. Genet., *23*:903, 1986.

Flatt, A. E.: The Care of Congenital Hand Anomalies. St. Louis, C. V. Mosby Company, 1977.

Frazier, T. M.: A note on race-specific congenital malformation rates. Am. J. Obstet. Gynecol., *80*:184, 1960.

Friedman, J. M.: Does Agent Orange cause birth defects? Teratology, *29*:193, 1984.

Garn, S. M., Silverman, F. N., and Rohmann, C. G.: A rational approach to the assessment of skeletal maturation. Ann. Radiol., *7*:297, 1964.

Goldberg, M. J., and Bartoshesky, L. E.: Congenital hand anomaly: Etiology and associated malformations. Hand Clin., *1*:405, 1985.

Goldberg, M. J., Bartoshesky, L. E., and O'Toole, D.: The pediatric amputee, an epidemiologic survey. Orthop. Rev., *10*:49, 1981.

Graham, J. M., Miller, M. E., Stephan, M. J., et al.: Limb reduction anomalies and early in utero limb compression. J. Pediatr., *96*:1052, 1980.

Greulich, W. S., and Pyle, S. I.: Radiographic Atlas of Skeletal Development of the Hand and Wrist. 2nd Ed. Stanford, CA, Stanford University Press, 1959.

Hall, J. G., Pauli, R. M., and Wilson, K. M.: Maternal and fetal sequelae of anti-coagulation during pregnancy. Am. J. Med., *68*:122, 1980.

Hanson, J. W., Myrianthopoulos, N. C., Sedgwick, M. A., et al.: Risks to offspring of women treated with hydantoin anticonvulsants. J. Pediatr., *89*:662, 1976.

Higginbottom, M. C., Jones, K. L., Hall, B. D., et al.: The amniotic rupture and variable spectra of consequent defects. J. Pediatr., *95*:544, 1979.

Holmes, L. B.: Teratogen update: Benedectin. Teratology, *27*:277, 1983.

Hoyme, H. E., Jones, H. K., Van Allen, M. F., et al.: Vascular pathogenesis of transverse limb reduction defects. J. Pediatr., *101*:839, 1982.

Lamb, D. W., Wynne-Davies, R., and Soto, L.: An estimate of the population frequency of congenital malformations of the upper limb. J. Hand Surg., *7*:557, 1982.

Mahony, B. S., and Filly, R. A.: High resolution sinographic assessment of the fetal extremities. J. Ultrasound Med., *3*:489, 1982.

McBride, W. G.: Thalidomide embryopathy. Teratology, *16*:79, 1977.

McKusick, V. A.: Mendelian Inheritance in Man, 6th Ed. Baltimore, Johns Hopkins University Press, 1983.

Pearn, J. H.: Teratogens and the male. An analysis with special reference to herbicide exposure. Med. J. Aust., *2*:16, 1983.

Poznanski, A. K.: The Hand in Radiologic Diagnosis with Gamuts and Pattern Profiles. 2nd Ed. Philadelphia, W. B. Saunders Company, 1984.

Schardein, J. L.: Congenital abnormalities and hormones during pregnancy. A clinical review. Teratology, 22:251, 1980.

Shepherd, T. H.: Detection of human teratogenic agents. J. Pediatr., 101:810, 1982.

Smith, D. W.: Recognizable Patterns of Human Malformation. Genetic, Embryologic and Clinical Aspects. Philadelphia, W. B. Saunders Company, 1982.

Soyka, L. E.: Influences of drug exposure of the father on perinatal outcome. Clin. Perinatol., 6:21, 1979.

Temtamy, S. A., and McKusick, V. A.: The Genetics of Hand Malformations. New York, Alan R. Liss, 1978.

Wilson, J. G., and Fraser, F. C. (Eds.): Handbook of Teratology. New York, Plenum Press, 1978.

Classification

Blauth, W., and Gekeler, J.: Zur morphologie und klassifikation der symbrachydaklylie. Hand Chir., 3:125, 1971.

Frantz, C. H., and O'Rahilly, R.: Congenital skeletal limb deficiencies. J. Bone Joint Surg., 43A:1202, 1961.

Hall, C. B., Brooks, M. B., and Dennis, J. F.: Congenital skeletal deficiencies of the extremities: Classification and fundamentals of treatment. J. A. M. A., 180:590, 1962.

Kanavel, A. B.: Congenital malformations of the hand. Arch. Surg., 25:1, 1932.

Kelikian, H.: Congenital Deformities of the Hand and Forearm. Philadelphia, W. B. Saunders Company, 1974.

Miura, T.: Syndactyly and split hand. Hand (Suppl.) 10:99, 1978.

Ogino, T.: Clinical and experimental study on the teratogenic mechanisms of cleft hand, polydactyly, and syndactyly. J. Jap. Orthop. Assn., 53:535, 1979.

Ogino, T., Minami, A., Fukuda, K., and Kato, H.: Congenital anomalies of the upper limb among the Japanese in Sapporo. J. Hand Surg., 11B:364, 1986.

O'Rahilly, R.: Morphological patterns in limb deficiencies and duplications. Am. J. Anat., 89:135, 1951.

St. Hillaire, I. G.: Histoire Générale et Particulière des Anomalies de l'Organisation chez l'Homme et les Animaux. Paris, J. B. Baillière, 1832.

Swanson, A. B.: A classification for congenital limb malformations. J. Hand Surg., 1:8, 1976.

Swanson, A. B., Barsky, A. J., and Entin, M. A.: Classification of limb malformations on the basis of embryology failure. Surg. Clin. North Am. 48:1169, 1968.

Timing of Surgery

Buck-Gramcko, D. B.: Congenital malformations of the hand: Indications, operative treatment and results. Scand. J. Plast. Reconstr. Surg., 9:190, 1975.

Buck-Gramcko, D. B.: Hand surgery in congenital malformations. In Jackson, I. (Ed.): Recent Advances in Plastic Surgery. Edinburgh, Churchill Livingstone, 1981.

Eaton, R. G.: Hand problems in children: A timetable for management. Pediatr. Clin. North Am., 14:643, 1967.

Flatt, A. E.: The Care of Congenital Hand Anomalies. St. Louis, C. V. Mosby Company, 1977.

McGraw, M.: The Neuromuscular Maturation of the Human Infant. New York, Hafner Publishing Company, 1943.

Zaricznyj, B.: Centralisation of the ulna for congenital radial hemimelia. J. Bone Joint Surg., 59A:694, 1977.

Transverse Absence: Upper Arm; Intercalated "Phocomelia"

Aitkin, G. I., and Frantz, C. H.: Management of the child amputee. In American Academy of Orthopedic Surgeons: Instructional Course Lectures. Ann Arbor, Michigan, J. W. Edwards, 1960.

Clippinger, F. W., Avery, R., and Titus, B. R.: A sensory feedback system for an upper-limb amputation prosthesis. Bull. Prosth. Res., 10:247, 1974.

Dick, H. M., and Tietjen, R.: Humeral lengthening for septic neonatal growth arrest: Case report. J. Bone Joint Surg., 60:1138, 1978.

Downie, C. R.: Limb deficiencies and prosthetic devices. Orthop. Clin. North Am., 7:465, 1976.

Fletcher, I.: Review and treatment of thalidomide children with limb deficiencies in Great Britain. Clin. Orthop., 148:18, 1980.

Frantz, C. H., and O'Rahilly, R.: Congenital skeletal limb deficiencies. J. Bone Joint Surg., 43A:1202, 1961.

Kadefors, R., and Taylor, C. J. M.: On the feasibility of myoelectric control of multi-functional orthoses. Scand. J. Rehab. Med., 5:134, 1973.

Kay, A. E., Day, H. S. B., Henkel, H. L., et al.: A proposed international terminology of the classification of congenital limb deficiences. Orthot. Prosth., 28:33, 1974.

Kelikian, H.: Congenital Deformities of the Hand and Forearm. Philadelphia, W. B. Saunders Company, 1974.

Kritter, A. F.: The bilateral upper extremity amputee. Orthop. Clin. North Am., 3:419, 1972.

Marquardt, E.: The Heidelberg pneumatic arm prosthesis. J. Bone Joint Surg., 47B:425, 1965.

Murray, J. F., Shore, B., and Trefler, P.: Prostheses for children with unilateral congenital absence of the hand. J. Bone Joint Surg., 54A:1658, 1972.

Pellicore, R. J., and Lambert, C. N.: Congenital limb deficiencies: Upper limb deficiencies. In Atlas of Limb Prosthetics: Surgical and Prosthetic Principles, American Academy of Orthopaedic Surgeons. St. Louis, C. V. Mosby Company, 1981.

Posner, M. A.: Upper limb prosthesis. In Bora, F. W., Jr. (Ed.): The Pediatric Upper Extremity. Philadelphia, W. B. Saunders Company, 1985.

Setoguchi, Y., Sumida, C., and Shaperman, J.: Child Amputee Prosthetic Project—Research. Los Angeles, University of California Rehabilitation Center, 1982.

Shaperman, J.: Learning patterns of young children with above elbow prostheses. Am. J. Occup. Ther., 33:299, 1979.

Sulamaa, M., and Ryoppy, S.: Early treatment of congenital bone defects of the extremities: Aftermath of thalidomide disaster. Lancet, Original Articles, 1964.

Swanson, A.: Phocomelia and congenital limb malformation: Reconstruction and prosthetic replacement. Am. J. Surg., 109:294, 1965.

Taussig, H. B.: A study of the German outbreak of phocomelia: The thalidomide syndrome. J. A. M. A., 180:1106, 1962.

Temtamy, S. A., and McKusick, V. A.: Absence deformities as a part of syndromes. Birth Defects, 14:73, 1978.

Temtamy, S. A., and McKusick, V. A.: The Genetics of Hand Malformations. New York, Alan R. Liss, 1978.

Tsai, T.-M., Ludwig, L., and Tonkin, M.: Free vascularized epiphyseal transfer. In Urbaniak, J. R. (Ed.): Microsurgery For Major Limb Reconstruction. St. Louis, C. V. Mosby Company, 1987.

Transverse Absence: Forearm

Aitkin, G. I.: Management of severe bilateral upper limb deficiencies. Clin. Orthop., *37:*53, 1964.

Aitkin, G. I.: The child amputee: an overview. Orthop. Clin. North Am., *3:*447, 1972.

Celikyol, F.: The upper limb deficient child: A brief review of treatment strategies, and modifications as the child grows. Phys. Disabil. Spec., *2:*6, 1979.

Chan, K. M., et al.: The Krukenberg procedure: A method of treatment for unilateral anomalies of the upper limb in Chinese children. J. Hand Surg., *9A:*548, 1984.

Childress, D. S., et al.: Myoelectric immediate postsurgical procedure: A concept for fitting the upper extremity amputee. Artif. Limbs *9:*2, 1965.

Epps, C., Burkhalter, W., and McCollough, N. C.: Modern amputation surgery and prosthetic techniques. American Academy of Orthopedic Surgeons Instructional Course Lecture. Presented in Atlanta, Georgia, 1980.

Gillespie, R.: Congenital limb deformities amputation surgery in children. *In* Kostvia, J. P., and Gillespie, R. (Eds.): Amputation Surgery and Rehabilitation: The Toronto Experience. New York, Churchill Livingstone, 1981.

Kritter, A. E.: The bilateral upper extremity amputee. Orthop. Clin. North Am., *3:*419, 1972.

Krukenberg, H.: Über plastiche Umwertung von Amputationsstumpfen. Stuttgart, Ferdinand Enke, 1917.

Laboriel, M. M., and Setoguchi, Y.: Research in juvenile prosthetics. *In* Atlas of Limb Prosthetics: Surgical and Prosthetic Principles. The American Academy of Orthopedic Surgeons. St. Louis, C. V. Mosby Company, 1981.

Lamb, D. W.: Prosthetics in the upper extremity. J. Hand Surg., *8:*774, 1983.

Lamb, D. W., and Law, H. T.: Upper-Limb Deficiences in Children: Prosthetic, Orthotic, and Surgical Management. Boston, Little, Brown and Co., 1987.

MacDonell, J. A.: Age of fitting upper extremity prostheses in children. J. Bone Joint Surg., *40A:*655, 1958.

Marquardt, E.: The Heidelberg pneumatic arm prosthesis. J. Bone Joint Surg., *47B:*425, 1965.

Marquardt, E.: The multiple limb-deficient child. *In* Atlas of Limb Prosthetics: Surgical and Prosthetic Principles. The American Academy of Orthopedic Surgeons. St. Louis, C. V. Mosby Company, 1981.

Murray, J. F., Shore, B., and Trefler, E.: Prostheses for children with unilateral congenital absence of the hand. J. Bone Joint Surg., *54A:*1658, 1972.

Nathan, P. A., and Trung, N. B.: The Krukenberg operation: A modified technique avoiding skin grafts. J. Hand Surg., *2:*127, 1977.

Pellicore, R. J., and Lamberg, C. N.: Congenital limb deficiencies: upper limb deficiencies. *In* Atlas of Limb Prosthetics: Surgical and Prosthetic Principles. The American Academy of Orthopedic Surgeons. St. Louis, C. V. Mosby Company, 1981.

Pellicore, R., Sciora, J., et al.: Incidence of bone overgrowth in the juvenile amputee population. Inter-Clin. Info. Bull. *13:*1, 1974.

Sauter, W. F.: Prostheses for the child amputee. Orthop. Clin. North Am., *3:*483, 1972.

Sorbye, R.: Myoelectric prosthetic fitting in young children. Clin. Orthop. *148:*34, 1980.

Sung, R. Y.: Experience with the Krukenberg plastic operation. Chin. Med. J., *7:*212, 1957.

Swanson, A. B.: The Krukenberg procedure in the juvenile amputee. J. Bone Joint Surg., *46A:*1540, 1964.

Swanson, A. B.: Phocomelia and congenital limb malformations: Reconstruction and prosthetic replacement. Am. J. Surg., *109:*294, 1965.

Temtamy, S. A.: Classification of hand malformations as isolated defects: An overview. J. Genet. Hum., *30:*281, 1982.

Transverse Absence: Carpal and Metacarpal; Phalangeal

Bos, G. D., Goldberg, V. M., Powell, A. E., et al.: The effect of histocompatibility matching on canine frozen bone allografts. J. Bone Joint Surg., *65A:*89, 1983.

Buck-Gramcko, D.: *In* Nigst, H., Buck-Gramcko, D., and Millesi, H. (Eds.). Hand Chirurgie. Stuttgart, Geo. Thieme, 1981.

Carroll, R. E.: Construction of functioning unit in congenital absence of the hand. J. Bone Joint Surg., *55A:*879, 1973.

Carroll, R. E., and Green, D. P.: Reconstruction of hypoplastic digits using toe phalanges. J. Bone Joint Surg., *57A:*727, 1975.

Codivilla, A.: On the means of lengthening in the lower limbs, the muscles and tissues which are shortened through deformity. Am. J. Orthop. Surg., *2:*353, 1905.

Cowen, N. J.: Surgical management of the hypoplastic hand. *In* Cowen, N. J. (Ed.): Practical Hand Surgery. Miami, Symposium Specialists Inc., 1980.

Cowen, N. J., and Loftus, J. M.: Distraction augmentation manoplasty. Technique for lengthening digits of entire hands. Orthop. Rev., *7:*45, 1978.

Dobyns, J. H.: *In* Green, D. P. (Ed.): Operative Hand Surgery. Vol. 1. New York, Churchill Livingstone, 1982.

Entin, M. A.: Reconstruction of congenital anomalies of the upper extremities. J. Bone Joint Surg., *41A:*681, 1959.

Entin, M. A.: Reconstruction of congenital aplasia of phalanges in the hand. Surg. Clinc North Am., *48:*1155, 1968.

Flatt, A. E.: The Care of Congenital Hand Anomalies. St. Louis, C. V. Mosby Company, 1977.

Freeman, B. S.: Results of epiphyseal transplants by flap and by free graft: A brief survey. Plast. Reconstr. Surg., *36:*227, 1965.

Gilbert, A.: Toe transfers for congenital hand defects. J. Hand Surg., *7:*118, 1982.

Gilbert, A.: Reconstruction of congenital hand defects with microvascular toe transfers. Hand Clin., *1:*351, 1985.

Goldberg, N. H., and Watson, H. K.: Composite toe (phalanx and epiphysis) transfers in the reconstruction of the aphalangic hand. J. Hand Surg., *7:*454, 1982.

Hentz, V. R., and Littler, J. W.: The surgical management of congenital hand anomalies. *In* Converse, J. M. (Ed.): Reconstructive Plastic Surgery. 2nd Ed. Vol. VI. Philadelphia, W. B. Saunders Company, 1977.

Kelikian, H.: Congenital Deformities of the Hand and Forearm. Philadelphia, W. B. Saunders Company, 1974.

Kessler, I., Baruch, A., and Hecht, O.: Experience with distraction lengthening of digital rays in congenital anomalies. J. Hand Surg., *2:*394, 1977.

Lamb, D. W.: Prosthetics in the upper extremity. J. Hand Surg., *8:*774, 1983.

Lamb, D. W., and Kuczynski, K.: The Practice of Hand Surgery. Edinburgh, Blackwell Scientific Publications, 1981.

Leung, P. C.: Problems in toe-to-hand transfer. Ann. Acad. Med. Singapore, *12*(Suppl.):377, 1982.

Leung, P. C.: Thumb reconstruction using second toe transfer. Hand Clin., *1:*2852, 1985.

Lipton, H. A., May, J. W., Jr., and Simon, S. R.: Preoperative and postoperative gait analyses of patients undergoing great toe-to-thumb transfer. J. Hand Surg., *12A:*66, 1987.

Lister, G.: The Hand: Diagnosis and Indications, 2nd Ed. New York: Churchill Livingstone, 1984.

Littler, J. W.: Introduction to surgery of the hand. Plast. Reconstr. Surg., *4:*1543, 1964.

Matev, I. B.: Thumb reconstruction after amputation at the metacarpophalangeal joint by bone lengthening. J. Bone Joint Surg., *52A:*957, 1970.

Matev, I. B.: Gradual elongation of the first metacarpal as a method of thumb reconstruction (1967). *In* Stack, J. B., and Bolton, H. (Eds.): The Second Hand Club. London, British Society for Surgery of the Hand, 1975.

Matev, I. B.: Thumb reconstruction in children through metacarpal lengthening. Plast. Reconstr. Surg., *64:*665, 1979.

Matev, I. B.: The distraction method in reconstructive surgery of the hand. *In* Tubiana, R. (Ed.): The Hand. Vol. II. Philadelphia, W. B. Saunders Company, 1985.

May, J. W., Smith, R. J., and Peimer, C. A.: Toe-to-hand free tissue transfer for thumb reconstruction with multiple digit aplasia. Plast. Reconstr. Surg., *67:*205, 1981.

Mulliken, J. B., and Curtis, R. M.: Thumb lengthening by metacarpal distraction. J. Trauma, *20:*250, 1980.

O'Brien, B. McC., Black, M. J. M., Morrison, W. A., and MacLeod, A. M.: Microvascular great toe transfer for congenital absence of the thumb. Hand, *10:*113, 1978.

Paneva-Holevich, E., and Yankov, E.: A distraction method for lengthening of the finger metacarpals: A preliminary report. J. Hand Surg., *5:*160, 1980.

Peltomen, J. I., Karaharju, E. O., and Alitalo, I.: Experimental epiphyseal distraction producing and correcting angular deformities. J. Bone Joint Surg., *66B:*598, 1984.

Pillet, J.: Esthetic hand prostheses. J. Hand Surg., *8:*778, 1973.

Rank, B. K.: Longterm results in epiphyseal transplants in congenital deformities of the hand. Plast. Reconstr. Surg., *61:*321, 1978.

Reid, D. A. C.: The Gillies thumb lengthening operation. Hand, *12:*123, 1980.

Smith, R. J., and Dworecka, F.: Treatment of the one digit hand. J. Bone Joint Surg., *55A:*113, 1973.

Smith, R. J., and Gumley, G.: Metacarpal distraction lengthening. Clin. Hand Surg., *1:*417, 1985.

Ulitskyi, G. I., and Malygin, G. D.: Roentgenological dynamics of reparative regeneration in lengthening of metacarpals by the distraction method. Acta Chir. Plast., *15:*82, 1973.

Upton, J., Boyajian, M., Mulliken, J. B., and Glowacki, J.: The use of demineralized xenogenic bone implants to correct phalangeal defects: A case report. J. Hand Surg., *9A:*388, 1984.

Longitudinal Absence: Preaxial (Radial)

Albee, F. H.: Formation of radius congenitally absent: Condition seven years after implantation of bone graft. Ann. Surg., *87:*105, 1928.

Bayne, L. G.: Radial club hand. *In* Green, D. P. (Ed.): Operative Hand Surgery. New York, Churchill Livingstone, 1982.

Bayne, L. B., and Klug, W. S.: Long-term review of the surgical treatment of radial deficiencies. J. Hand Surg., *12A:*169, 1987.

Blauth, W., and Schmidt, H.: The implication of arteriographic diagnosis in malformation of the radial marginal ray. Z. Orthop., *106:*102, 1969.

Bora, F. W., Jr., Nicholson, J. T., and Cheema, H. M.: Radial meromelia: The deformity and its treatment. J. Bone Joint Surg., *51A:*966, 1970.

Bora, F. W., Jr., Osterman, A. L., Kaneda, R. R., and Esterhai, J.: The radial club hand deformity. J. Bone Joint Surg., *63A:*741, 1981.

Buck-Gramcko, D.: Hand surgery in congenital malformations. *In* Jackson, I. (Ed.): Recent Advances in Plastic Surgery (2). London, Churchill Livingstone, 1981.

Buck-Gramcko, D.: Radialization as a new treatment for radial club hand. J. Hand Surg., *10A:*964, 1985.

Bunnell, S.: Restoring flexion to the paralytic elbow. J. Bone Joint Surg., *33A:*566, 1951.

Carroll, R. E., and Louis, D. S.: Anomalies associated with radial dysplasia. J. Pediatr., *84:*409, 1974.

Davidson, A. J., and Horwitz, M. T.: Congenital club hand deformity associated with absence of radius; its surgical correction, case report. J. Bone Joint Surg., *21:*462, 1939.

Dell, P. C., and Sheppard, J. E.: Thrombocytopenia, absent radius syndrome. Report of two siblings and a review of the hematologic and genetic features. Clin. Orthop., *162:*129, 1982.

DeLorme, T. L.: Treatment of congenital absence of the radius by transepiphyseal fixation. J. Bone Joint Surg., *51A:*117, 1969.

Dick, H. M., Petzoldt, R. L., Bowers, W. R., et al.: Lengthening of the ulna in radial agenesis: A preliminary report. J. Hand Surg., *2:*175, 1977.

Duraiswami, P. K.: Experimental causation of congenital skeletal defects and its significance in orthopedic surgery. J. Bone Joint Surg., *34B:*646, 1952.

Fanconi, G.: Familial constitutional panmyelocytopathy. Fanconi's anemia (F. A.). I. Clinical aspects. Semin. Hematol., *4:*233, 1967

Flatt, A. E.: The Care of Congenital Hand Anomalies. St. Louis, C.V. Mosby Company, 1977.

Forbes, G: A case of congenital club hand with a review of the etiology of the condition. Anat. Rec., *71:*181, 1938.

Gmyrek, D., and Sullum-Rapopoa, I.: Zur Fanconi anamie. Analyse von 129 Beschrieben Fallen. Z. Kinderheilkd., *91:*297, 1964.

Goldberg, M. J., and Bartoshesky, L. E.: Congenital hand anomaly: Etiology and associated malformations. Hand Clin. *1:*405, 1985.

Goldberg, M. J., and Meyn, M.: The radial club hand. Orthop. Clin. North Am. 7:341, 1976.

Goldenberg, R. R.: Congenital bilateral complete absence of the radius in identical twins. J. Bone Joint Surg., *30A:*1001, 1948.

Hall, J. G., Levin, J., Kuhn, J. P., Ottenheimer, E. J., Van Berkum, K. A. P., and McKusick, V. A.: Thrombocytopenia with absent radius (TAR). Medicine, *48:*411, 1969.

Hays, R. M., Bartoshesky, L. E., and Feingold M.: New features of thrombocytopenia and absent radius syndrome. Birth Defects, *18:*115, 1982.

Heikel, H. V. A.: Aplasia and hypoplasia of the radius. Acta Orthop. Scand. (Suppl.) *39:*1, 1959.

Holt, M., and Oram, S.: Familial heart disease with skeletal malformations. Br. Heart J., *22:*236, 1960.

Huber, E.: Hilssoperation bei medianuslahung. Dtsch. Z. Chir., *162:*271, 1921.

Kato, K.: Congenital absence of the radius, with review of the literature and report of three cases. J. Bone Joint Surg., *6:*589, 1924.

Kelikian, H., and Doumanian, A.: Congenital anomalies of the hand. Part I. J. Bone Joint Surg., *39A:*1002, 1957.

Lamb, D. W.: Radial club hand: A continuing study of sixty-eight patients with one hundred and seventeen club hands. J. Bone Joint Surg., *59A:*1, 1977.

Lidge, R. T.: Congenital radial deficient club hand. J. Bone Joint Surg., *51A:*1041, 1969.

Lin, A. E., and Perloff J. K.: Upper limb malformations associated with congenital heart disease. Am. J. Cardiol., *55:*1576, 1985.

Manske, P., and McCarroll, H. R., Jr.: Abductor digiti minimi opponensplasty in congenital radial dysplasia. J. Hand Surg., *3:*552, 1978.

Menelaus, M. B.: Radial club hand with absence of the biceps muscle treated by centralization of the ulna and triceps transfer: Report of two cases. J. Bone Joint Surg., *58B:*488, 1976.

O'Rahilly, R.: Morphologic patterns in limb deficiencies and duplications. Am. J. Anat., *89:*135, 1951.

Quan, L., and Smith, D. W.: The VATER association: Vertebral defects, anal atresia, T-E fistula with esophageal atresia, radial and renal dysplasia: A spectrum of associated defects. J. Pediatr., *82:*104, 1973.

Riordan, D. C.: Congenital absence of the radius. J. Bone Joint Surg., *37A:*1129, 1955.

Riordan, D. C.: Congenital absence of the radius: A fifteen year follow-up. J. Bone Joint Surg., *45A:*1783, 1963.

Rosa, G., and Peluso, F.: Surgical treatment of congenital radial club hand. Ital. J. Orthop. Traumatol., *3:*341, 1977.

Sayer, R. H.: A contribution to the study of the club hand. Trans. Am. Orthop. Assoc., *6:*208, 1893.

Schaeffer, J. P., and Nachamopsky, L. H.: Some observations on the anatomy of the upper extremities of an infant with complete bilateral absence of the radius. Anat. Rec., *8:*1, 1914.

Skerik, S. K., and Flatt A. E.: The anatomy of congenital radial dysplasia. Clin. Orthop., *66:*125, 1969.

Smith, D. W.: Recognizable Patterns of Human Malformations: Genetic, Embryologic and Clinical Aspects. 3rd Ed. Philadelphia, W. B. Saunders Company, 1982.

Starr, D. E.: Congenital absence of the radius: A method of surgical correction. J. Bone Joint Surg., *27:*572, 1945.

Stoffel, A., and Stempel, E.: Anatomische studien uber die klumphand. Z. Orthop. Chir., *23:*1, 1909.

Tsai, T. M., Ludwig, L., and Tonkin, M.: Free vascularized epiphyseal transfer. *In* Urbaniak, J. R. (Ed.): Microsurgery for Major Limb Reconstruction. St. Louis, C.V. Mosby Company, 1987.

Watson, H. K., Beebe, R. D., and Cruz, N. I.: A centralization procedure for radial club hand. J. Hand Surg., *9A:*541, 1984.

Weiland, A. J., Kleinert, H. E., Kutz, J. E., et al.: Application of free vascularized bone grafts in reconstructive surgery. J. Hand Surg., *3:*289, 1978.

Longitudinal Absence: Central

Ahstrom, J. P.: Surgical treatment of the cleft hand. Orthop. Trans., *1:*92, 1977.

Barsky, A. J.: Cleft hand: Classification, incidence and treatment. Review of the literature and report of nineteen cases. J. Bone Joint Surg., *46A:*1707, 1964.

Birch-Jensen, A.: Congenital Deformities of the Upper Extremities. Copenhagen, Ejnar Munksgaard, 1949.

Buck-Gramcko, D.: Cleft hands: Classification and treatment. Hand Clin., *1:*467, 1985.

Buck-Gramcko, D.: Congenital malformations. *In* Nigst, H., Buck-Gramcko, D., Millesi, H., and Lister, G. O. (Eds.): Hand Surgery. Vol. 1. Stuttgart, Geo. Thieme, 1988.

David, T. J.: The differential diagnosis of the cleft hand and cleft foot malformations. Hand, *6:*58, 1974.

Dobyns, J. H.: Segmental digital transposition in congenital hand deformities. Hand Clin., *1:*475, 1985.

Dowd, Ch. M.: Cleft hand: A report of a case successfully treated by the use of periosteal flaps. Ann. Surg., *24:*211, 1986.

Flatt, A. E.: The Care of Congenital Hand Anomalies. St. Louis, C.V. Mosby Company, 1977.

Jaworska, M., and Popiolek, J.: Genetic counseling in lobster-claw anomaly: Discussion of variability of genetic influence in different families. Clin. Pediatr., *7:*396, 1968.

Kelikian, H., and Doumanian, A.: Congenital anomalies of the hand. J. Bone Joint Surg., *39A:*1002, 1957.

Lister, G.: The Hand: Diagnosis and Indications. 2nd Ed. London, Churchill Livingstone, 1985.

Lister, G., and Scheker, L.: The role of microsurgery in the reconstruction of congenital deformities of the hand. Hand, *1:*431, 1985.

Maisels, D. O.: Theory of pathogenesis of lobster claw deformities. Hand, *2:*79, 1970.

Manske, P. R.: Cleft hand and central polydactyly in identical twins: A case report. J. Hand Surg., *8:*906, 1983.

May, J. W., Smith, R. J., and Peimer, C. A.: Toe-to-hand free tissue transfer for thumb reconstruction with multiple digit aplasia. Plast. Reconstr. Surg., *67:*205, 1981.

Miura, T., and Komada, T.: Simple method for reconstruction of the cleft hand with an adducted thumb. Plast. Reconstr. Surg., *64:*65, 1979.

Miura, T., and Suzuki, M.: Clinical differences between typical and atypical cleft hand. J. Hand Surg., *9B:*311, 1984.

Muller, W.: Die angeborenen Fehlbildungen der menschlichen Hand. Leipzig, Thieme, 1937.

Nutt, J. N., and Flatt, A. E.: Congenital central hand deficit. J. Hand Surg., *6:*48, 1981.

Ogino, T.: Clinical and experimental study on the teratogenic mechanisms of cleft hand, polydactyly, and syndactyly. J. Jap. Orthop. Assn., *53:*535, 1979.

Reid, D. A. C.: Reconstruction of the thumb. J. Bone Joint Surg. *42B:*444, 1960.

Reid, D. A. C.: The Gilles thumb lengthening operation. Hand, *12:*123, 1980.

Rudiger, R. A., Haase, W., and Passarge, E.: Association of ectrodactyly, ectodermal dysplasia, and cleft lip-palate. Am. J. Dis. Child., *120:*160, 1970.

Sandzen, S. C., Jr.: Classification and functional management of congenital central defect of the hand. Hand Clin., *1:*483, 1985.

Snow, J. W., and Littler, J. W.: Surgical treatment of the cleft hand. *In* Transactions of the International Society for Plastic and Reconstructive Surgery, 4th Congress, Rome, 1967. New York, Excerpta Medica Foundation, 1969.

Tada, K., Yonenobu, K., and Swanson, A. B.: Congenital central ray deficiency in the hand—a survey of 59 cases and subclassification. J. Hand Surg., *6:*434, 1981.

Ueba, Y.: Plastic surgery for the cleft hand. J. Hand Surg., *6:*557, 1981.

Upton, J.: Current trends in congenital hand surgery. *In* Advances in Plastic Surgery. New York, Year Book Medical Publishers, 1989.

Watari, S., and Tsuge, K.: A classification of cleft hands based on clinical findings. Plast. Reconstr. Surg., *64:*381, 1979.

Watari, S., Hagiyama, Y., and Tsuge, K.: Recent knowledge on the cleft hand. Hiroshima J. Med. Sci., *33:*81, 1984.

Wood, V. E.: The cleft hand (central deficiencies). *In* Green, D. P. (Ed.): Operative Hand Surgery. New York, Churchill Livingstone, 1982.

Longitudinal Absence: Ulnar

Bayne, L. G.: Ulnar club hand (ulnar deficiencies). *In* Green, D. P. (Ed.): Operative Hand Surgery. New York, Chruchill Livingstone, 1982.

Birch-Jensen, A.: Congenital Deformities of the Upper Extremities. Copenhagen, Ejnar Munksgaard, 1949.

Blair, W. F., Shurr, D. B., and Buckwalter, J. A.: Functional status of ulnar deficiency. J. Pediatr. Orthop., *3:*37, 1983.

Broudy, A. S., and Smith, R. J.: Deformities of the hand and wrist with ulnar deficiency. J. Hand Surg., *4:*304, 1979.

Burck, U., Schaefer, E., and Held, K. R.: Mesomelic dysplasia with short ulna, long fibula, brachymetacarpy, and micrognathia. Clinical and radiological differential diagnostic features. Pediatr. Radiol., *9:*161, 1980.

Carroll, R. E., and Bowel, W. H.: Congenital deficiency of the ulna. J. Hand Surg., *2:*169, 1977.

Dick, H. M., Petzoldt, R. C., and Bowers, W. R.: Lengthening of the ulna in radial agenesis: A preliminary report. J. Hand Surg., *2:*175, 1977.

Flatt, A. E.: Ulnar club hand. *In* Flatt, A. E.: The Care of Congenital Hand Anomalies. St. Louis, C.V. Mosby Company, 1977.

Harrison, R. G., Pearson, M. A., and Roaf, R.: Ulnar dimelia. J. Bone Joint Surg., *42B:*549, 1960.

Johnson, J., and Omer, G. E.: Congenital ulnar deficiency: Natural history and therapeutic implications. Hand Clin., *1:*499, 1985.

Kummel, W.: Die Missbildungen der Extremitaten durch Delekt, Verwachsung und Ueberzahl. Hefte 3. Kassel, Bibliotheca Medica, 1895.

Laurin, C. A., and Farmer, A. W.: Congenital absence of ulna. Can. J. Surg., *2:*204, 1959.

Lloyd-Roberts, G. C.: Treatment of defects of the ulna by establishing a cross-union with the radius. J. Bone Joint Surg., *55B:*327, 1973.

Marcus, N. A., and Omer, G. E., Jr.: Carpal deviation in congenital ulnar deficiency. J. Bone Joint Surg., *66A:*1003, 1984.

Miller, J. K., Wenner, S. M., and Kruger, L. M.: Ulnar deficiency. J. Hand Surg., *11A:*822, 1986.

Ogden, J. A., Watson, H. K., and Bohne, W.: Ulnar dysmelia. J. Bone Joint Surg., *58A:*467, 1976.

Ogden, J. A., Beall, J. K., Conlogue, G. J., and Light, T. R.: Radiology of postnatal skeletal development. IV. Distal radius and ulna. Skeletal Radiol., *6:*255, 1981.

Riordan, D. C., Mills, E. H., and Aldredge, R. H.: Congenital absence of the ulna: Proceedings of the American Society for Surgery of the Hand. J. Bone Joint Surg., *43A:*614, 1961.

Southwood, A. R.: Partial absence of the ulna and associated structures. J. Anat., *61:*346, 1926–1927.

Spinner, M., Freundlich, B. D., and Abeles, E. D.: Management of moderate longitudinal arrest of development of the ulna. Clin. Orthop., *69:*199, 1970.

Straub, L. R.: Congenital absence of the ulna. Am. J. Surg., *109:*300, 1965.

Swanson, A. B., Tada, K., and Yonenobu, K.: Ulnar ray deficiency: Its various manifestations. J. Hand Surg., *9A:*658, 1984.

Tachdjian, M. O.: Defects of the neck and upper limb. *In* Tachdjian, M. O.: Pediatric Orthopedics. Philadelphia, W. B. Saunders Company, 1972.

Temtamy, S., and McKusick, V.: Ulnar defects. Birth Defects, *14:*48, 1978.

Vitale, C. C.: Reconstructive surgery for defects in the shaft of the ulna in children. J. Bone Joint Surg., *34A:*804, 1952.

Watson, H. K., and Bohne, W. H.: The role of the fibrous hand in ulnar deficient extremities. Proceedings of the American Society for Surgery of the Hand. J. Bone Joint Surg., *53A:*816, 1971.

Syndactyly; Syndactyly-Related Syndromes

Agnew, D. H.: The Principles and Practice of Surgery. Being a Treatise on Surgical Diseases and Injuries. Vol. 3. Philadelphia, J. B. Lippincott Company, 1883.

Barot, L. R., and Caplan, H. S.: Early surgical intervention in Apert's syndactyly. Plast. Reconstr. Surg., *77:*282, 1986.

Bauer, T. B., Tondra, J. M., and Trusler, H. M.: Technical modification in repair of syndactylism. Plast. Reconstr. Surg., *17:*385, 1956.

Beals, R., and Crawford, S.: Congenital absence of the pectoral muscles. A review of twenty-five patients. Clin. Orthop. Rel. Res., *119:*166, 1976.

Belfer, M. D., Harrison, A. M., and Murray, J. E.: Body image and the process of reconstructive surgery. Am. J. Dis. Child., *133:*532, 1979.

Bidwell, L. A.: Minor Surgery. 2nd Ed. New York, William Wood and Company, 1913.

Blackfield, H. M., and Hause, D. P.: Syndactylism. Plast. Reconstr. Surg., *16:*37, 1955.

Blank, C. E.: Apert's syndrome (a type of acrocephalosyndactyly)—observations on a British series of thirty-nine cases. Ann. Hum. Genet., *24:*151, 1960.

Blauth, W.: Das Syndaktylie-Rezidiv. Handchirurgie, *2:*95, 1970.

Blauth, W.: Syndactylien der hand. Dtsch. Argtebl., *69:*2013, 1972.

Blauth, W., and Schneider-Sickert, F.: Congenital Deformities of the Hand: An Atlas of Their Surgical Treatment. Translated by U. H. Weil. Berlin, Springer-Verlag, 1981.

Bouvet, J., Levesque, D., Bernetieres, F., and Gros, J.: Vascular origin of Poland syndrome: A comparative rheographic study of the vascularization of the arms in eight patients. Eur. J. Pediatr., *128:*17, 1978.

Bouvet, J. P., Maroteaux, P., and Briard-Guillemot, M. L.: Le syndrome de Poland. Etudes cliniques et génétiques—Considerations physiopathologiques. Nouv. Presse Med., *5:*185, 1976.

Brown, P. M.: Syndactyly—a review and long term results. Hand, *9:*16, 1977.

Buck-Gramcko, D.: Indikation und Zeitpunkt der operativen Behandlung angeborener Handfehibildungen. Z. Kinderchir., *10:*220, 1971.

Buck-Gramcko, D.: Correspondence Newsletter 1986–47. American Society for Surgery of the Hand, 1986.

Bunnell, S.: Surgery of the Hand. 2nd Ed. Philadelphia, J. B. Lippincott Company, 1948.

Bunnell, S.: Surgery of the Hand. 3rd Ed. Philadelphia, J. B. Lippincott Company, 1956.

Clarkson, P.: Poland's syndactyly. Guy's Hosp. Rep., *111:*335, 1962.

Cogswell, H. D., and Trusler, H. M.: A modified Agnew's operation for syndactylism. Surg. Gynecol. Obstet., *64:*792, 1937.

Cronin, T. D.: Syndactylism. Experiences in its correction. Tri State Med. J., *15:*2869, 1943.

Cronin, T. D.: Syndactylism: Results of zig-zag incision to prevent postoperative contracture. Plast. Reconstr. Surg., *18:*460, 1956.

Davis, J. S., and German, W. J.: Syndactylism. Coherence of the fingers and toes. Arch. Surg., *21:*32, 1930.

Didot, A.: Note sur la séparation des doigts palmes, et sur un nouveau procédé anaplastiques destiné à prévenir la réproduction de la difformité. Bull. Acad. Roy. Méd. Belgique, *9:*351, 1849.

Dieffenbach, F. J.: Chirurgische Erfahrungen besonders ueber die Wiederherstellung zerstoerter Teile des menschlichen Koerpers nach neuen methoden. Berlin, T. C. F. Enslin, 1834.

Dobyns, J. H.: Syndactyly. *In* Green, D. P. (Ed.): Operative Hand Surgery. Vol. 1. New York, Churchill Livingstone, 1982.

Ebskov, B., and Zachariae, L.: Surgical methods in syndactylism. Evaluation of 208 Operations. Acta Chir. Scand., *131:*258, 1966.

Faniel, H.: Syndactylie: Modification du procédé de Didot. Scalpel, *64:*254, 1911.

Felizet, G.: Opération de la syndactylie congénitale (procédé autoplastique). Rev. d'Orthop., *10:*49, 1892.

Flatt, A. E.: Treatment of syndactylism. Plast. Reconstr. Surg., *29:*336, 1962.

Flatt, A. E.: Practical factors in the treatment of syndactyly. *In* Littler, J. W., Cramer, L. M., and Smith, J. W. (Eds.): Symposium on Reconstructive Hand Surgery. St. Louis, C.V. Mosby Company, 1974.

Flatt, A. E.: The Care of Congenital Hand Anomalies. St. Louis, C.V. Mosby Company, 1977.

Forgues, L. D.: Syndactylie membraneuse congénitale du médius et de l'annulaire de deux mains: Opération. Arch. Med. Pharm. Mil., *27:*128, 1896.

Furnas, D. W., and Fischer, G. W.: The Z-plasty: Biomechanics and mathematics. Br. J. Plast. Surg., *24:*144, 1971.

Gesell, A., Halverson, H. M., Thompson, H., Ilg, F. L., Castner, B. M., et al.: The First Five Years of Life: A Guide to the Study of the Preschool Child. New York, Harper & Row, 1940.

Goldberg, M. J., and Bartoshesky, L. E.: Congenital hand anomaly: Etiology and associated malformations. Hand. Clin., *1:*405, 1985.

Goldberg, M. J., and Mazzei, R. J.: Poland syndrome: A concept of the pathogenesis based on limb bud embryology. Birth Defects, *8:*103, 1977.

Granick, M. S., Ramasastry, S., Vries, J., and Cohen, M. M.: Severe amniotic band syndrome occurring with unrelated syndactyly. Plast. Reconstr. Surg., *80:*829, 1987.

Heinrich, R., and Vavuras, E.: Zum Problem der Syndaktylie der Kinderhand. Z. Kinderchir., *6:*216, 1968.

Hentz, V. R.: Correspondence Newsletter 65. American Society for Surgery of the Hand, 1985.

Hentz, V. R., and Littler, J. W.: The surgical management of congenital hand anomalies. *In* Converse, J. M. (Ed.): Plastic and Reconstructive Surgery. Vol. 6. Philadelphia, W. B. Saunders Company, 1977.

Hirshowitz, B., Karev, A., and Rousso, M.: Combined double Z-plasty and Y-V advancement for thumb web contracture. Hand, *7:*291, 1975.

Hoover, G. H., Flatt, A. E., and Weiss, M. W.: The hand and Apert's syndrome. J. Bone Joint Surg., *52A:*878, 1970.

Ireland, D. C. R., Takayama, N., and Flatt, A. E.: Poland's syndrome: A review of forty-three cases. J. Bone Joint Surg., *58A:*52, 1976.

Iselin, M.: Chirurgie der Hand: Atlas der operationstechnik. Stuttgart, Geo. Thieme Verlag, 1959.

Johannsen, S. H.: Nagelwallbidung dirch thenarlappen bei kompletter syndactylie. Handchir., *14:*199, 1982.

Kanavel, A. B.: Congenital malformations of the hand. Arch. Surg., *28:*1, 1932.

Kelikian, H.: Congenital Deformities of the Hand and Forearm. Philadelphia, W. B. Saunders Company, 1974.

Kettlekamp, D. B., and Flatt, A. E.: An evaluation of syndactylia repair. Surg. Gynecol. Obstet., *113:*471, 1961.

Kummer, E.: Syndactylie congénitale: Anaplastie d'après la méthode italienne. Rev. d'Orthop., *2:*129, 1891.

Lennander, K. G.: Fall af kongenital syndaktyli, opereadt med, hjelp af Thiersch's hudtransplantationmetod. Upsala Lakaref. Forhandlingar, *26:*151, 1891.

Littler, J. W.: Principles of reconstructive surgery of the hand. *In* Converse, J. M. (Ed.): Plastic and Reconstructive Surgery. Vol. 6. Philadelphia, W. B. Saunders Co., 1977.

Littler, J. W.: Personal communication, 1978.

Lösch, G. M., and Duncker, H. R.: Acrosyndactylism. *In* Transactions of the International Society of Plastic and Reconstructive Surgery, 5th Congress, Australia. Butterworths Pty. Ltd., 1971.

Lösch, G. M., and Duncker, H. R.: Anatomy and surgical treatment of syndactyly. Plast. Reconstr. Surg., *50:*167, 1972.

MacCollum, D. W.: Webbed fingers. Surg. Gynecol. Obstet., *71:*782, 1940.

Mah, J., Kasser, J., Upton, J., and Griffin, P.: Foot, shoulder and elbow in Apert's syndrome. J. Bone Joint Surg (in press).

Maisels, D. O.: Acrosyndactyly. Br. J. Plast. Surg., *15:*166, 1962.

Mansfield, O. T.: Syndactyly. Br. J. Plast. Surg., *13:*249, 1961.

McGraw, M.: The Neuromuscular Maturation of the Human Infant. New York, Hafner Publishing Company, 1943.

Millesi, H.: Kritische Betrachtungen zur Syndaktylie Operation. Chir. Plast. Reconstr., *7:*99, 1970.

Nelaton, A.: Eléments de Pathologie Chirurgicale. Vol. 16. Paris, G. Baillière et Cie, 1884.

Norton, A. T.: A new and reliable operation for the cure of webbed fingers. Br. Med. J., *2:*931, 1881.

Nylen, B.: Repair of congenital finger syndactyly. Acta Chir. Scand., *113:*310, 1957.

Ohmori, K., and Takada, H.: Correction of Poland's pectoralis major muscle anomaly with latissimus dorsi musculocutaneous flaps. Plast. Reconstr. Surg., *65:*400, 1980.

Oldfield, M. C.: The "horse-shoe" web flap in the treatment of syndactyly. Br. J. Plast. Surg., *1:*69, 1948.

Patterson, T. J. S.: Congenital ring constrictions. Br. J. Plast. Surg., *14:*1, 1961.

Pieri, G.: Plastica cutanea per le retrazioni cicatriziali delle ditta. Chir. Organi Mov., 4:303, 1920.

Pieri, G.: Processo operatorio per la cura sindattilia grave. Chir. Ital., 3–4:258, 1949.

Poland, A.: Deficiency of the pectoral muscles. Guy's Hosp. Rep., 6:191, 1841.

Posch, J. L., Dela Cruz-Saddul, F. A., Posch, J. L., Jr., et al.: Congenital syndactylism of fingers in 262 cases. Orthop. Rev., 10:23, 1981.

Poznanski, A. K.: The Hand in Radiologic Diagnosis. 2nd Ed. Philadelphia, W. B. Saunders Company, 1984.

Radulesco, A. D.: Un nouveau procédé opératoire digitocommissural comme traitement de la syndactylie congénitale. Rev. d'Orthop., 10:499, 1923.

Raus, E. E.: Repair of simple syndactylism in the healthy neo-newborn. Orthop. Rev., 13:33, 1984.

Ravitch, M. M.: Poland's syndrome—a study of an eponym. Plast. Reconstr. Surg., 59:508, 1977.

Rowsell, A. R., and Godfrey, A. M.: A fortuitous donor site for full thickness skin grafts in the correction of syndactyly. Br. J. Plast. Surg., 37:31, 1984.

Rudtorffer, F. X.: Abhandling uber die Einjackste und Sicherste Operations—Method eingesperrter Leisten und Schenkelbrucke. Vienna, J. U. Degan, 1808.

Rypalkova, B.: Dnesmi stav operaci syndaktylie. Cas. Lek. Ces., 90:1081, 1951.

Shaw, D. T., Li, C. S., Rickey, D. C., et al.: Interdigital butterfly flap in the hand (the double-opposing Z-plasty). J. Bone Joint Surg., 55A:1677, 1973.

Skoog, T.: Syndactyly: A clinical report on repair. Acta Chir. Scand., 130:537, 1965.

Stone, J. S.: American Practice of Surgery. Vol. 4. New York, William Wood and Company, 1908.

Suguira, Y.: Poland's syndrome: Clinico-roentgenographic study of 45 cases. Cong. Anom., 16:17, 1976.

Swanson, A. B.: A classification for congenital limb malformations. J. Hand Surg., 1:8, 1976.

Temtamy, S. A., and McKusick, V. A.: Syndactyly as an isolated malformation. Birth Defects, 14:301, 1978.

Torpin, R., and Faulkner, A.: Intrauterine amputation with the missing member found in the fetal membranes. J.A.M.A., 198:185, 1966.

Tubby, A. H.: An operation for webbed fingers. Br. Med. J., 2:1464, 1912.

Upton, J.: Early surgical intervention in Apert's syndactyly: A discussion. Plast. Reconstr. Surg., 77:286, 1986.

Velasco, J. G., Broadbent, T. R., and Woolf, R. M.: Syndactylism. Br. J. Plast. Surg., 20:364, 1967.

Velpeau, A. L. M.: New Elements of Operative Surgery. Vol. 2. Translated by P. S. Townsend. New York, Samuels and Wood, 1847.

Villeschaise, H. M., and Jean, G.: Quelques points de technique concernant la chirurgie de la syndactylie. Rev. d'Orthop., 14:241, 1927.

Walsh, R. J.: Acrosyndactyly. A study of 27 patients. Clin. Orthop. Rel. Res., 71:99, 1970.

Woolf, C. M., and Woolf, R. M.: A genetic study of syndactyly in Utah. Soc. Biol., 20:335, 1973.

Woolf, R. M., and Broadbent, T. R.: The four-flap Z-plasty. Plast. Reconstr. Surg., 49:48, 1972.

Zachariae, L.: Syndactylia. J. Bone Joint Surg., 37B:356, 1955.

Zeller, S.: Abhandung uber die ersten erscheinunger venerischer lokalkrankheits—Formen und deren Behandlung, Sammt einer Kurzen Arzeigo zweir neuen Operation-Methoden, namlich: die angeborenen verwachsenen Finger und die kastrizion. Wien, J. G. Binz, 1810.

Symphalangism

Bell, J.: On hereditary digital anomalies. On brachydactyly and symphalangism. In Penrose, L. S. (Ed.): The Treasury of Human Inheritance. Vol. 5, Part 1. London, Cambridge University Press, 1951.

Cushing, H.: Hereditary ankylosis of the proximal interphalangeal joints (symphalangism). Genetics, 1:90, 1916.

Dobyns, J. H., et al.: Congenital hand deformities. In Green, D. (Ed.): Operative Hand Surgery. London, Churchill Livingstone, 1982.

Drinkwater, H.: Phalangeal anarthrosis (synostosis, ankylosis) transmitted through fourteen generations. Proc. Roy. Soc. Med., 10:60, 1917.

Elkington, S. G., and Huntsman, R. G.: The Talbot fingers: A study in symphalangism. Br. Med. J., 1:407, 1967.

Flatt, A. E.: The Care of Congenital Hand Anomalies. St. Louis, C.V. Mosby Company, 1977.

Flatt, A. E., and Wood, V. E.: Rigid digits or symphalangism. Hand, 7:197, 1975.

Goldberg, M. J., and Bartoshesky, L. E.: Congenital hand anomaly: Etiology and associated malformations. Hand Clin., 1:405, 1985.

Lister, G.: The Hand: Diagnosis and Indications. 2nd Ed. New York, Churchill Livingstone, 1984.

Palmieri, T. J.: The use of silicone rubber implants arthroplasties in treatment of true symphalangism. J. Hand Surg., 5:242, 1980.

Strasburger, A. K., Hawkins, M. R., Eldridge, R., et al.: Symphalangism: Genetic and clinical aspects. Bull. Johns Hopkins Hosp., 117:108, 1965.

Temtamy, S. A., and McKusick, V. A.: Symphalangism as an essentially isolated malformation. Birth Defects, 14:495, 1978.

Upton, J., Sohn, S., and Glowacki, J.: Neocartilage derived from transplanted perichondrium: What is it? Plast. Reconstr. Surg., 68:166, 1981.

Radioulnar Synostosis

Blaine, E. S.: Congenital radio-ulnar synostosis, with report of a case. Am. J. Surg., 7:429, 1930.

Brady, L. P., and Jewett, E. L.: A new treatment of radio-ulnar synostosis. South. Med. J., 53:507, 1960.

Clearly, J. E., and Omer, G. E.: Congenital proximal radioulnar synostosis. Natural history and functional assessment. J. Bone Joint Surg., 67A:539, 1985.

Dawson, H. G.: A congenital deformity of the forearm and its operative treatment. Br. Med. J., 2:833, 1912.

Fahlstrom, S.: Radio-ulnar synostosis. J. Bone Joint Surg., 14:395, 1932.

Feidt, W. S.: Congenital radio-ulnar synostosis. Surg. Gynecol. Obstet., 24:696, 1917.

Green, W. T., and Mital, M. A.: Congenital radio-ulnar synostosis: Surgical treatment. J. Bone Joint Surg., 61A:738, 1979.

Hansen, O. H., and Anderson, N. O.: Congenital radioulnar synostosis: Report of 37 cases. Acta Orthop. Scand., 41:225, 1970.

Kelikian, H., and Doumanian, A.: Swivel for proximal radio-ulnar synostosis. J. Bone Joint Surg., 39A:945, 1957.

Lewis, W. H.: The development of the arm in man. Am. J. Anat., 1:169, 1901.

Lunn, J. R.: Congenital synostosis of radio-ulnar articulations. Br. Med. J., 1:499, 1906.

Mardam-Bey, T., and Ger, E.: Congenital radial head dislocation. J. Hand Surg., 4:316, 1979.

McCredie, J.: Congenital fusion of bones: Radiology, embryology, and pathogenesis. Clin. Radiol., 26:47, 1975.

Mital, M. A.: Congenital radioulnar synostosis and congenital dislocation of the radial head. Orthop. Clin. North Am., 7:375, 1976.

Robinson, G. C., Miller, J. R., Dill, F. J., et al.: Kleinfelter's syndrome with the XXYY sex chromosome complex. J. Pediatr., 65:226, 1964.

Sever, J. W.: Congenital radio-ulnar synostosis. Surg. Gynecol. Obstet., 24:203, 1969.

Simmons, B. P., Southmayd, W. W., and Riseborough, E. J.: Congenital radioulnar synostosis. J. Hand Surg., 8:829, 1983.

Wilkie, D. P. D.: Congenital radio-ulnar synostosis. Br. J. Surg., 1:366, 1914.

Wynne-Davies, R.: Heritable Disorders in Orthopedic Practice. Oxford, Blackwell Scientific, 1973.

Vascular Malformations

Boyd, J. B., Mulliken, J. B., Kaban, L. B., Upton, J., and Murray, J. E.: Skeletal changes associated with vascular malformations. Plast. Reconstr. Surg., 74:789, 1984.

Branham, H. H.: Aneurismal varix of the femoral artery and vein following a gunshot wound. Int. J. Surg., 3:250, 1890.

Burrows, P. E., Mulliken, J. B., Fellows, K. E., and Strand, R. D.: Childhood hemangiomas and vascular malformations—angiographic differentiation. Am. J. Roentgenol., 141:483, 1983.

Callander, C. L.: Study of arteriovenous fistula with an analysis of four hundred and forty seven cases. Johns Hopkins Hosp. Rep., 19:259, 1920.

Charles, R. H.: A System of Treatment. Vol. 3. London, Churchill Livingstone, 1912.

Clodius, L.: Excision and grafting of extensive facial hemangiomas. Br. J. Plast. Surg., 30:185, 1977.

Coursley, G., Ivins, J. C., and Barker, N. W.: Congenital arteriovenous fistulas in extremities: Analysis of 69 cases. Angiology, 7:201, 1956.

Cross, F. S., Glover, D. M., Simeone, F. A., and Oldenburg, F. A.: Congenital arteriovenous aneurysms. Ann. Surg., 148:649, 1958.

Curtis, R. M.: Congenital arteriovenous fistulae of the hand. J. Bone Joint Surg., 35A:917, 1953.

deTakats, G.: Vascular anomalies of the extremities. Report of five cases. Surg. Gynecol. Obstet., 55:227, 1932.

Finn, M. C., Glowacki, J., and Mulliken, J. B.: Congenital vascular lesions: Clinical application of a new classification. J. Pediatr. Surg., 18:894, 1983.

Fonkalsrud, E. W., and Coulson, W. F.: Management of congenital lymphedema in infants and children. Ann. Surg., 177:280, 1973.

Gelberman, R. H., and Goldner, J. L.: Congenital arteriovenous fistulas of the hand. J. Hand Surg., 3:451, 1978.

Glowacki, J., and Mulliken, J. B.: Mast cells in hemangiomas and vascular malformations. Pediatrics, 70:48, 1982.

Gomes, M. R., and Bernatz, P. E.: Arteriovenous fistulas: A review and ten year experience at the Mayo Clinic. Mayo Clin. Proc., 45:81, 1970.

Griffin, J. M., Vasconez, L. O., and Schatten, W. E.: Congenital arteriovenous malformations of the upper extremity. Plast. Reconstr. Surg., 62:49, 1978.

Hall, R. R., Beach, A. D., Baker, E., and Morrison, P.: Incision of tissue by carbon dioxide laser. Nature, 232:131, 1971.

Jarzab, G.: Clinical experience in the cryo-surgery of hemangioma. J. Maxillofac. Surg., 3:146, 1975.

Kasabach, H. H., and Merritt, K. K.: Capillary hemangiomata with extensive purpura: Report of a case. Am. J. Dis. Child., 59:1063, 1940.

Klippel, M., and Trenaunay, P.: Mémoires originaux du noevus variqueux ostéohypertrophique. Arch. Gen. Med., 3:641, 1900.

Lister, W. A.: Natural history of strawberry nevi. Lancet, 1:1429, 1938.

Malan, E., and Puglionisi, A.: Congenital angiodysplasias of the extremities (Note I: Generalities and classification; venous dysplasias). J. Cardiovasc. Surg., 5:87, 1964.

Malan, E., and Puglionisi, A.: Congenital angiodysplasias of the extremities (Note II: Arterial, arterial and venous, and haemolymphatic dysplasias). J. Cardiovasc. Surg., 6:255, 1965.

McNeil, T. W., Chan, G. E., Capek, V., and Ray, R. D.: The value of angiography in the surgical management of deep hemangiomas. Clin. Orthop., 101:176, 1974.

Miller, S. H., Smith, R. L., and Shochat, S. J.: Compression treatment of hemangiomas. Plast. Reconstr. Surg., 58:573, 1976.

Miller, T. A.: Surgical management of lymphedema of the extremity. Plast. Reconstr. Surg., 56:633, 1975.

Moore, J. R., and Weiland, A. J.: Embolotherapy in the treatment of congenital arteriovenous malformations of the hand: A case report. J. Hand Surg., 10A:135, 1985.

Mulliken, J. B., and Glowacki, J.: Hemangiomas and vascular malformations in infants and children: A classification based on endothelial characteristics. Plast. Reconstr. Surg., 69:412, 1982.

Newmeyer, W. L.: Vascular disorders. In Green, D. P. (Ed.): Operative Hand Surgery. New York, Churchill Livingstone, 1982.

Nicoladoni, C.: Phlebarteriectasie der rechten oberen extremitat. Arch. Klin. Chir., 18:252, 1875.

Noe, J. M., Barsky, S. H., Geere, D. E., and Rosen, S.: Portwine stains and the response to argon laser therapy: Successful treatment and the predictive role of color, age and biopsy. Plast. Reconstr. Surg., 65:130, 1980.

Owens, N., and Stephenson, K. L.: Hemangiomas: An evaluation of treatment by injection and surgery. Plast. Reconstr. Surg., 3:109, 1948.

Rodriguez-Erdman, F., Burron, L., Murray, J. E., and Moloney, W. L.: Kasabach-Merritt syndrome: Coagulo-analytical observations. Am. J. Med. Sci., 261:9, 1971.

Szilagyi, D. E., Elliott, J. P., DeRusso, F. J., and Smith, R. F.: Peripheral congenital arteriovenous fistulas. Surgery, 57:61, 1965.

Szilagyi, D. E., Smith, R. F., Elliott, J. P., and Hageman, J. H.: Congenital arteriovenous anomalies of the limbs. Arch. Surg., 111:423, 1976.

Upton, J.: Vascular anomalies of the upper extremity. In Mulliken, J. B., and Young, A. E. (Eds.): Vascular Birthmarks: Hemangiomas and Malformations. Philadelphia, W. B. Saunders Company, 1988.

Upton, J., Mulliken, J. B., and Murray, J. E.: Classification and rationale for management of vascular anomalies in the upper extremity. J. Hand Surg., 10A:970, 1985.

Wakim, K. G., and Janes, J. M.: Influence of arteriovenous fistula on the distal circulation in the involved extremity. Arch. Phys. Med. Rehabil., 39:431, 1958.

Watson, W. L., and McCarthy, W. D.: Blood and lymph vessel tumors. A report of 1056 cases. Surg. Gynecol. Obstet., 71:569, 1940.

Weber, F. P.: Hemangiectatic hypertrophy of limbs—congenital phlebarteriectasis and so called congenital varicose veins. Br. J. Child. Dis., 15:13, 1918.

Zarem, H. A., and Edgerton, M. T.: Induced resolution of cavernous hemangiomas following prednisolone therapy. Plast. Reconstr. Surg., 39:76, 1967.

Flexion Deformities; Flexion Deformity of Digits Secondary to Extensor Hypoplasia

Crawford, H. H., Horton, C. E., and Adamson, J. E.: Congenital aplasia or hypoplasia of the thumb and finger extensor tendons. Report of six cases. J. Bone Joint Surg., 48A:82, 1966.

Crenshaw, A. H.: Campbell's Operative Orthopedics. 5th Ed. St. Louis, C. V. Mosby Company, 1971.

Flatt, A. E.: The Care of Congenital Hand Anomalies. St. Louis, C. V. Mosby Company, 1977.

Gold, A. M., and Perlman, R. D.: Congenital clasped thumb deformity. Case report. Bull. Hosp. Joint. Dis., 29:255, 1968.

Granberry, W. M.: Correspondence Newsletter #1975–36. American Society for Surgery of the Hand, 1975.

Inokuchi: Congenital aplasia of the extensor digitorum communis. Clin. Orthop. Surg. (Tokyo), 8:877, 1973.

Kelikian, H.: Congenital Deformities of the Hand and Forearm. Philadelphia, W. B. Saunders Company, 1974.

Loomis, L. K.: Congenital "clasped thumb." J. La. State Med. Soc., 110:23, 1958.

McCarroll, H. R.: Congenital flexion deformities of the thumb. Hand Clin., 1:567, 1985.

McMurtry, R. Y., and Jochims, J. L.: Congenital deficiency of the extrinsic extensor mechanism of the hand. Clin. Orthop., 125:36, 1977.

Neviaser, R. J.: Congenital hypoplasia of the thumb with absence of the extrinsic extensors, abductor pollicis longus and thenar muscles. J. Hand Surg., 4:301, 1979.

Rinsky, L. A., and Bleck, E. E.: Freeman-Sheldon ("whistling face") syndrome. J. Bone Joint Surg., 58A:148, 1976.

Sallis, J. G.: Dominantly inherited digito-talar dysmorphism. J. Bone Joint Surg., 54B:509, 1972.

Snow, J. W.: A method for reconstruction of the central slip of the extensor tendon of a finger. Plast. Reconstr. Surg., 57:455, 1976.

Tajima, T.: Classification of thumb hypoplasia. Clin. Hand Surg., 1:577, 1985.

Tsuge, K.: Congenital aplasia or hypoplasia of the finger extensors. Hand, 7:15, 1975.

Tsuge, K., Kawanishi, T., Baba, I., and Koyama, K.: Congenital aplasia of the finger extensors. Orthop. Surg. (Tokyo), 20:1353, 1969.

Tsuyuguchi, Y., Masada, K., Kawabata, H., Kawai, H., and Ono, K.: Congenital clasped thumb: A review of forty-three cases. J. Hand Surg., 10A:613, 1985.

Weckesser, E. C.: Congenital flexion-adduction deformity of the thumb (congenital "clasped thumb"). J. Bone Joint Surg., 37A:977, 1955.

Weckesser, E. C., Reed, J. R., and Heiple, K. G.: Congenital clasped thumb (congenital flexion-adduction deformity of the thumb). J. Bone Joint Surg., 50A:1417, 1968.

White, J. W., and Jensen, W. E.: The infant's persistent thumb clutched hand. J. Bone Joint Surg., 34A:680, 1952.

Wood, V. E.: Thumb clutched hand: In Green, D. P. (Ed.): Operative Hand Surgery. New York, Churchill-Livingstone, 1982.

Zadek, I.: Congenital absence of the extensor pollicis longus of both thumbs, operation and cure. J. Bone Joint Surg., 16:432, 1934.

Camptodactyly

Anderson, W.: Lectures on contractions of the fingers and toes; their varieties, pathology and treatment. Lancet 2:1, 1891.

Baraitser, M., Burn, J., and Fixsen, J.: A recessively inherited windmill-vane camptodactyly/ichthyosis syndrome. J. Med. Genet., 20:125, 1983.

Barinka, L.: Kampylodaktylie (predbezne sdeleni). Acta Chir. Orthop. Traumatol. Cech., 28:279, 1961.

Barletta, L. P. A.: Campilodactilia. Prensa Med., 46:758, 1959.

Berger, A., and Millisi, H.: Spatergebnisse der operativen Behandlung der Kamptodaktylie. Handchirurgie, 7:75, 1975.

Buck-Gramcko, D.: Congenital and developmental conditions. In Lamb, D. S. (Ed.): The Interphalangeal Joints. London, Churchill Livingstone, 1986.

Courtemanche, A. D.: Camptodactyly: Etiology and management. Plast. Reconstr. Surg., 44:451, 1969.

Currarino, G., and Waldman, I.: Camptodactyly. Am. J. Roentgenol., 92:1312, 1964.

DeHaas, W. H. D.: Camptodactylie. Ned. Tijdschr. Geneeskd., 101:2121, 1957.

Eaton, R. G.: Hand problems in children; a timetable for management. Pediatr. Clin. North Am., 14:643, 1967.

Engber, W. M., and Flatt, A. E.: Camptodactyly: An analysis of sixty-six patients and twenty-four operations. J. Hand Surg., 2:216, 1977.

Eyler, D. L., and Markee, J. E.: The anatomy and function of the intrinsic musculature of the fingers. J. Bone Joint Surg., 36A:1, 1954.

Faher, M.: Considérations sur les insertions d'origine des muscles lumbricaux: Les systèmes digastriques de la main. Ann. Chir., 29:979, 1975.

Flatt, A. E.: The Care of Congenital Hand Anomalies. St. Louis, C. V. Mosby Company, 1977.

Furnas, D. W.: Muscle-tendon variations in the flexor compartment of the wrist. Plast. Reconstr. Surg., 36:320, 1965.

Gollop, T., et al.: New manifestations observed in the Tel Hashomer camptodactyly syndrome. Prog. Clin. Biol. Res., 104:269, 1982.

Hori, M., Nakamura, R., Inoue, G., et al.: Nonoperative treatment of camptodactyly. J. Hand Surg., 12A:1061, 1987.

Hueston, J. T.: Dupuytren's Contracture. Edinburgh, Churchill Livingstone, 1963.

Humphrey, G. M.: Observations in Myology. Cambridge/London, MacMillan, 1872.

Jones, K. G., Marmor, L., and Lankford, L. L.: An overview on new procedures in surgery of the hand. Clin. Orthop., 99:154, 1974.

Landsmeer, J. M. F.: Atlas of Anatomy of the Hand. New York, Churchill-Livingstone, 1976.

Lankford, L. L.: Correspondence Club Letter, #1975–I. Dallas, May, 1975.

Lister, B.: The Hand: Diagnosis and Indications. 2nd Ed. New York, Churchill-Livingstone, 1984.

Littman, A., Yates, J. W., and Treger, A.: Camptodactyly, a kindred study. J.A.M.A., *206:*565, 1968.

Maeda, M., and Matsui, T.: Camptodactyly caused by an abnormal lumbrical muscle. J. Hand Surg., *10B:*95, 1985.

McCash, C., and Backhouse, K.: Demonstration of a Representative Series of Congenital Hand Deformities in Children. Presented at the British Club for Surgery of the Hand, London, 1966.

McFarlane, R. M., Curry, G. I., and Evans, H. B.: Anomalies of the intrinsic muscles in camptodactyly. J. Hand Surg., *9:*531, 1983.

McGraw, M.: The Neuromuscular Maturation of the Human Infant. New York, Hafner Publishing Company, 1943.

Mehta, H. J., and Gardner, W. V.: A study of lumbrical muscles in the human hand. Am. J. Anat., *109:*227, 1961.

Millesi, H.: Camptodactyly. *In* Littler, J. W., Cramer, L. M., and Smith, J. W. (Eds.): Symposium on Reconstructive Hand Surgery. St. Louis, C. V. Mosby Company, 1974.

Miura, T.: Non-traumatic flexion deformity of the proximal interphalangeal joint—its pathogenesis and treatment. Hand, *15:*25, 1983.

Montant, R., and Baumann, A.: Recherches anatomiques sur le système tendineux extensor des doigts de la main. Ann. Anat. Pathol., *14:*311, 1937.

Murphy, D. P.: Familial finger contracture and associated familial knee-joint subluxation. J.A.M.A., *86:*395, 1926.

O'Brien, J. P., and Hodgson, A. R.: Congenital abnormality of the flexor digitorum profundus, a cause of flexion deformity of the long and ring fingers. Clin. Orthop., *104:*206, 1974.

Ochi, T., Iwasi, R., Okabe, N., Fink, C. W., and Ono, K.: The pathology of the involved tendons in patients with familial arthropathy and congenital camptodactyly. Arthritis Rheum., *26:*896, 1983.

Oldfield, M. C.: Camptodactyly: Flexor contracture of the fingers in young girls. Br. J. Plast. Surg., *8:*312, 1956.

Poznanski, A. K.: The Hand in Radiologic Diagnosis. Vol. 4. Philadelphia, W. B. Saunders Company, 1974.

Rabischong, P.: L'innervation proprioceptive des muscles lombriceaux de la main chez l'homme. Rev. Chir. Orthop., *48:*234, 1962.

Smith, R. J., and Kaplan, E. B.: Camptodactyly and similar atraumatic flexion deformities of the proximal interphalangeal joints of the fingers. J. Bone Joint Surg., *50A:*1187, 1968.

Stack, H. G.: A study of muscle function in the fingers. Ann. Roy. Coll. Surg. Engl., *33:*307, 1963.

Stark, H. H.: Discussion of camptodactyly. J. Bone Joint Surg., *50A:*1203, 1968.

Steindler, A.: Congenital malformations and deformities of the hand. Orthop. Surg., *2:*639, 1920.

Stoddard, S. E.: Nomenclature of hereditary crooked fingers. J. Hered., *30:*511, 1939.

Tamplin, R. W.: Lecture on the Nature and Treatment of Deficiencies. London, Longman, Brown, Green, Longman and Roberts, 1846.

Todd, A. H.: Case of hereditary contracture of the little fingers. Lancet, *2:*1088, 1929.

Watson, K. H., Light, T. D., and Johnson, T. R.: Checkrein resection for flexion contracture of the middle joint. J. Hand Surg., *4:*67, 1979.

Welch, J. P., and Temtamy, S. A.: Hereditary contractures of the fingers (camptodactyly). J. Med. Genet., *3:*104, 1966.

Wilhelm, A., and Kleinschmidt, W.: Neue atiologische und therapeutische gesichtspunkte bei der kamptodacktylie und tendovaginitis stenosans. Chir. Plast. Reconstr., *5:*62, 1968.

Clinodactyly; Delta Phalanx

Ashley, L. M.: The inheritance of streblomicrodactyly. J. Hered., *38:*93, 1947.

Barsky, A. J.: Congenital Anomalies of the Hand and Their Surgical Treatment. Springfield, IL, Charles C. Thomas, 1958.

Burgess, R. C.: Use of an H-graft in the treatment of a delta phalanx. J. Hand Surg., *13A:*297, 1988.

Burke, F., and Flatt, A. E.: Clinodactyly. A review of a series of cases. Hand, *11:*269, 1979.

Carstam, N., and Theander, G.: Surgical treatment of clinodactyly caused by longitudinally bracketed diaphysis. Scand. J. Plast. Reconstr. Surg., *9:*199, 1975.

Flatt, A. E.: The Care of Congenital Hand Anomalies. St. Louis, C. V. Mosby Company, 1977.

Fort, J. A.: Des Difformites Congénitales et Acquises des Doigts et des Moyens d'y Remédier. Thèse. Paris, A. Delahaye, 1869.

Hersch, A. H., DeMarinis, F., and Stecher, R. M.: On the inheritance and development of clinodactyly. Am. J. Human Genet., *5:*257, 1953.

Hoover, G. H., Flatt, A. E., and Weiss, M. W.: The hand and Apert's syndrome. J. Bone Joint Surg., *52A:*878, 1970.

Jaeger, M., and Refior, H. J.: Congenital triangular deformity of the tubular bones of hand and foot. Clin. Orthop., *81:*139, 1971.

Jones, G. B.: Delta phalanx. J. Bone Joint Surg., *46B:*226, 1964.

Kelikian, H.: Congenital Deformities of the Hand and Forearm. Philadelphia, W. B. Saunders Company, 1974.

Light, T., and Ogden, J.: The longitudinal epiphyseal bracket: Implications for surgical correction. J. Paediatr. Orthop., *1:*299, 1981.

Ogden, J. A., Light, T. R., and Conlogue, G. J.: Correlative roentgenography and morphology of the longitudinal epiphyseal bracket. Skeletal Radiol., *6:*109, 1981.

Pol, R.: Brachydacktylie- klinodacktylie- hyperphalangie und ihre Grundlagen. Form und Eustelung der meist unter dem Bild der Brachydocktylie auftrenden Varietaten, Anomalien und Misbildungen der hand und des fuses. Arch. Path. Anat. U. Klin. Med., *229:*388, 1921.

Poznanski, A. K., Pratt, G. B., Manson, G., and Weiss, L.: Clinodactyly, camptodactyly, Kirner's deformity and other crooked fingers. Radiology, *93:*573, 1969.

Poznanski, A. K., Garn, S. M., and Holt, J. F.: The thumb in the congenital malformation syndromes. Radiology, *100:*115, 1971.

Rubinstein, J. H.: The broad thumbs syndrome—progress report 1968. Birth Defects, *5:*25, 1969.

Schatzki, P.: Uber verdeckte syndaktyle Polydaktylie und uber "Triangelbildung" in dermenschlichen Mittlehand. Arch. Orthop. Unfall-Chir., *34:*637, 1934.

Sella, E. J.: Delta phalanx. Conn. Med., *36:*437, 1972.

Skvarilova, B., and Smahel, Z.: Clinodactyly: Frequency and morphological implications. Acta Chir. Plast. (Prague), *26:*72, 1984.

Smith, R. J.: Osteotomy for "delta phalanx" deformity. Clin. Orthop. Rel. Res., *123:*91, 1977.

Theander, G., and Carstam, N.: Longitudinally bracketed diaphysis. Ann. Radiol., *17:*355, 1974.

Theander, G., Carstam, N., and Rausing, A.: Longitudinally bracketed diaphysis in young children: Radiologic-histopathologic correlation. Acta Radiol. Diag., *23*:293, 1982.

Vickers, D. W.: Premature incomplete fusion of the growth plate: Causes and treatment by resection (physolysis) in fifteen cases. Aust. N.Z. J. Surg., *50*:393, 1980.

Vickers, D.: Clinodactyly of the little finger: A simple operative technique for reversal of the growth abnormality. J. Hand Surg., *12B*:335, 1987.

Watson, H. K., and Boyes, J. H.: Congenital angular deformity of the digits. Delta phalanx. J. Bone Joint Surg., *49A*:333, 1967.

Wood, V. E.: Treatment of the triphalangeal thumb. Clin. Orthop. Rel. Res., *120*:188, 1976.

Wood, V. E.: Clinodactyly. In Green, D. P. (Ed.): Operative Hand Surgery. New York, Churchill Livingstone, 1982.

Wood, V. E., and Rubinstein, J. H.: Surgical treatment of the thumb in the Rubinstein-Taybi syndrome. J. Hand Surg., *12B*:166, 1987.

Wynne-Davies, R., and Lamb, D. W.: Congenital upper limb anomalies: An etiologic grouping of clinical, genetic, and epidemiologic data from 387 patients with "absence defects, constriction bands, polydactylies, and syndactylies." J. Hand Surg., *10A*:958, 1985.

Duplication: Central; Postaxial

Barsky, A. J.: Congenital Anomalies of the Hand and Their Surgical Treatment. Springfield, IL, Charles C Thomas Company, 1958.

Bilhaut, M.: Guérison d'un pouce bifide par un nouveau procédé opératoire. Congrès Français de Chirurgie, *4*:576, 1890.

Burman, M.: Note on duplication of the index finger. J. Bone Joint Surg., *54A*:884, 1972.

Carstam, N., and Theander, G.: Surgical treatment of clinodactyly caused by longitudinally bracketed diaphysis (delta phalanx). Scand. J. Plast. Reconstr. Surg., *9*:199, 1975.

Centers for Disease Control: Congenital Malformation Surveillance Report. Atlanta, U.S. Public Health Service, U.S. Department of Health and Social Service, 1984.

Dobyns, J. H.: Duplicate thumbs (pre-axial polydactyly). In Green, D. P. (Ed.): Operative Hand Surgery. New York, Churchill Livingstone, 1982.

Egawa, T.: Surgical treatment of the polydactyly of the thumb. Plast. Reconstr. Surg. (Japan), *9*:97, 1966.

Flatt, A. E.: Problems in polydactyly. In Cramer, I. M., and Chase, R. A. (Eds.): Symposium on the Hand. Vol. 3. St. Louis, C. V. Mosby Company, 1971.

Flatt, A. E.: The Care of Congenital Hand Anomalies. St. Louis, C. V. Mosby Company, 1977.

Frazier, T. M.: A note on race-specific congenital malformation rates. Am. J. Obstet. Gynecol., *80*:184, 1960.

Goldberg, M. J., and Bartoshesky, L. E.: Congenital hand anomaly: Etiology and associated malformations. Hand Clin., *1*:405, 1985.

Goodman, R. M.: A family with polysyndactyly and other anomalies. J. Hered., *56*:37, 1965.

Goodwin, A. W., and Darian-Smith, I. (Eds.): Hand function and the neocortex. Exp. Brain Res. Suppl. 10, 1985.

Handforth, J. R.: Polydactylism of the hand in southern Chinese. Anat. Rec., *106*:119, 1950.

Hanson, J. W., Myrianthopoulos, N. C., and Sedgwick, M. A., et al: Risks of offspring to women treated with hydantoin anticonvulsants. J. Paediatr., *89*:662, 1976.

Hefner, R. A.: Hereditary polydactyly associated with extra phalanges in the thumbs. J. Hered., *31*:25, 1940.

The Holy Bible, King James Version. II Samuel 21:20.

James, J. I. P., and Lamb, D. W.: Congenital abnormalities of the limbs. Practitioner, *191*:159, 1962.

Kanavel, A. B.: Congenital malformations of the hands. Arch. Surg., *25*:282, 1932.

Kelikian, H.: Congenital Deformities of the Hand and Forearm. Philadelphia, W. B. Saunders Company, 1974.

Kelikian, H., and Doumanian, A.: Congenital anomalies of the hand. J. Bone Joint Surg., *39A*:1002, 1957.

Leung, P. C., Chan, K. M., and Cheng, J. C. Y.: Congenital anomalies of the upper limb among the Chinese population in Hong Kong. J. Hand Surg., *7*:563, 1982.

Marks, T. W., and Bayne, L. G.: Polydactyly of the thumb: Abnormal anatomy and treatment. J. Hand Surg., *3*:107, 1978.

McClintic, B. S.: Five generations of polydactylism. J. Hered., *26*:141, 1935.

Mellin, G. W.: The frequency of birth defects. In Fishbein, M. (Ed.): Birth Defects. Philadelphia, J. B. Lippincott Company, 1963.

Milessi, H.: Fingerverformung nach Operationen wegen Polydaktylie. Klin. Med. (Wein), *22*:266, 1967.

Miura, T.: An appropriate treatment for postoperative Z-formed deformity of the duplicated thumb. J. Hand Surg., *2*:380, 1977.

Miura, T.: Duplicated thumb. Plast. Reconstr. Surg., *69*:470, 1982.

Nathan, P. A., and Keniston, R. C.: Crossed polydactyly. J. Bone Joint Surg., *57A*:847, 1975.

Nicolai, J. A., and Schoch, S. L.: Polydactyl in the Bible. J. Hand Surg., *11A*:293, 1986.

Odiorne, J. M.: Polydactylism in related New England families. J. Hered., *34*:45, 1943.

Ruby, L., and Goldberg, M. J.: Syndactyly and polydactyly. Orthop. Clin. North Am., *7*:361, 1976.

Stelling, F.: The upper extremity. In Ferguson, A. B. (Ed.): Orthopedic Surgery in Infancy and Childhood. Vol. 2. Baltimore, The Williams & Wilkins Company, 1963.

Strickland, A.: Lives of the Queens of England. Vol. II. London, H. Colburn, 1840–1848.

Sverdrup, A.: Postaxial polydactylism in six generations of a Norwegian family. J. Genet., *12*:217, 1922.

Swanson, A. B., and Brown, K. S.: Hereditary triphalangeal thumb. J. Hered., *53*:259, 1962.

Tada, K., Kurisaki, E., Yonenobu, K., Tsuyuguchi, Y., and Kawai, H.: Central polydactyly—a review of 12 cases and their surgical treatment. J. Hand Surg., *7*:460, 1982.

Temtamy, S., and McKusick, V. A.: Synopsis of hand malformations with particular emphasis upon genetic factors. Birth Defects, *3*:125, 1969.

Temtamy, S. A., and McKusick, V. A.: Polydactyly. Birth Defects, *14*:364, 1978.

Turek, S. L.: Orthopedic Principles and their Application. Philadelphia, J. B. Lippincott Company, 1967.

Upton, J.: Duplicated thumb: Discussion. Plast. Reconstr. Surg., *69*:480, 1982.

Walker, J. T.: A pedigree of extra digit V polydactyly in a Batutsi family. Ann. Hum. Genet., *25*:65, 1961.

Wassel, H. D.: The results of surgery for polydactyly of the thumb: A review. Clin. Orthop., *64*:175, 1969.

Wood, V. E.: Duplication of the index finger. J. Bone Joint Surg., 52A:569, 1970.

Wood, V. E.: Treatment of central polydactyly. Clin. Orthop., 74:196, 1971.

Wood, V. E.: Polydactyly and the triphalangeal thumb. J. Hand Surg., 3:436, 1978.

Woolf, C. M., and Myrianthopoulos, N. C.: Polydactyly in American Negroes and whites. Am. J. Hum. Genet., 25:397, 1973.

Mirror Hand (Ulnar Dimelia)

Barton, N. J., Buck-Gramcko, D. B., and Evans, D. M.: Soft tissue anatomy of mirror hand. J. Hand Surg., 11B:307, 1986.

Beasley, R. W.: Reconstructive surgery in upper extremity anomalies. In Swinyard, C. E. (Ed.): Limb Development and Deformity. Problems of Evaluation and Rehabilitation. Springfield, IL, published for the Association for Aid of Crippled Children by Charles C Thomas Company, 1969.

Boyes, J. (Ed.): Bunnell's Surgery of the Hand. 5th Ed. Philadelphia, J. B. Lippincott Company, 1970.

Burman, M.: An historical perspective of double hands and double feet. Bull. Hosp. Joint Dis., 29:241, 1968.

Davis, R. G., and Farmer, A. W.: Mirror hand anomaly; a case presentation. Plast. Reconstr. Surg., 21:80, 1958.

Dwight, T.: Fusion of Hands. Mem. Boston Soc. Nat. Hist., 4:473, 1892.

Entin, M. A.: Reconstruction of congenital anomalies of the upper extremities. J. Bone Joint Surg., 41A:681, 1959.

Giraldes, J.: Fusion de deux mains. Bill Soc. Chir., 2:505, 1866; cited in Kelikian, H.: Congenital Deformities of the Hand and Forearm. Philadelphia, W. B. Saunders Company, 1974.

Gorriz, G.: Ulnar dimelia—a limb without anteroposterior differentiation. J. Hand Surg., 7:466, 1982.

Harrison, R. G., Pearson, M. A., and Roaf, R.: Ulnar dimelia. J. Bone Joint Surg., 42B:549, 1960.

Jackson, B.: Malformation in an adult subject consisting of fusion of two upper extremities. Am. J. Med. Science 25:91, 1853; cited in Kelikian, H.: Congenital Deformities of the Hand and Forearm. London, W. B. Saunders Company, 1974.

Kanavel, A. B.: Congenital malformations of the hands. Arch. Surg., 25:282, 1932.

Kelikian, H.: Congenital Deformities of the Hand and Forearm. Philadelphia, W. B. Saunders Company, 1974.

Kelley, J. W.: Mirror hand. Plast. Reconstr. Surg., 30:374, 1962.

Mau, C.: Ein Weiterer Fall von Doppelbilding der ulna de fehlenden radius. Z. Orthop. Chir., 42:355, 1922; cited in Kelikian, H.: Congenital Deformities of the Hand and Forearm. Philadelphia, W. B. Saunders Company, 1974.

Mukerji, M.: Congenital anomaly of the hand: "Mirror hand." Br. J. Plast. Surg., 9:222, 1956–1957.

Pintilie, D., Hatmanu, D., Olaru, I., and Panoza, G. H.: Double ulna with symmetrical polydactyly. J. Bone Joint Surg., 46B:89, 1964.

Sandrow, R., Sullivan, R., and Steel, H.: Hereditary ulna and fibular dimelia with peculiar facies. J. Bone Joint Surg., 52A:367, 1970.

Santero, N.: Dichiria con duplicata dell ulna e assenza del radio. Arch. Ital. Chir., 43:173, 1936; cited in

Kelikian, H.: Congenital Deformities of the Hand and Forearm. Philadelphia, W. B. Saunders Company, 1974.

Saunders, J. W.: The proximo-distal sequence of origin of the parts of the chick wing and the role of ectoderm. J. Exp. Zool., 108:363, 1948.

Saunders, J. W., and Gasseling, M. T.: Ectodermal-mesenchymal interactions in the origin of limb symmetry. In Fleischmajer, R., and Billingham, R. E. (Eds.): Epithelial-Mesenchymal Interactions. Baltimore, Williams & Wilkins, 1968.

Summerbell, P.: The zone of polarizing activity: Evidence for a role in normal chick limb morphogenesis. J. Embryol. Exp. Morph., 50:217, 1979.

Tickle, C., and Wolpert, L.: Limb development. In Davis, J. A. (Ed.): Scientific Foundations of Paediatrics. 2nd Ed. London, Heinemann, 1981.

Tsuyuguchi, Y., Tada, K., and Yonenobu, K.: Mirror hand anomaly; reconstruction of the thumb, wrist, forearm and elbow. Plast. Reconstr. Surg., 70:384, 1982.

Wolpert, L.: Position and pattern formation. Dev. Biol., 6:183, 1971.

Wolpert, L.: Pattern formation in biological development. Sci. Am., 239:124, 1978.

Wolpert, L., and Hornbruch, A.: Positional signalling along the anteroposterior axis of the chick wing: The effects of multiple polarizing region grafts. J. Embryol. Exp. Morphol., 63:145, 1981.

Overgrowth (Gigantism)

Allende, B. T.: Macrodactyly with enlarged median nerve associated with carpal tunnel syndrome. Plast. Reconstr. Surg., 39:578, 1967.

Appenzeller, O., and Kornfeld, M.: Macrodactyly and localized hypertrophic neuropathy. Neurology, 24:767, 1974.

Barsky, A. J.: Macrodactyly. J. Bone Joint Surg., 49A:1255, 1967.

Ben-Bassat, M., Casper, J., Kaplan, I., and Laron, Z.: Congenital macrodactyly. A case report with a three year follow-up. J. Bone Joint Surg., 48B:359, 1966.

Bjorklund, S. I.: Hemihypertrophy and Wilms' tumor. Acta Paediatr., 44:287, 1955.

Boyes, J. G.: Macrodactylism—a review and proposed management. Hand, 9:172, 1977.

Brihayek, J., Milaire, J., Dustin, P., and Retif, J.: Local gigantism of the hand associated with a plexiform neurofibroma of the ulnar nerve. Report of a case. J. Neurosurg. Sci., 18:271, 1974.

Brooks, B., and Lehman, E. P.: The bone changes in Recklinghausen's neurofibromatosis. Surg. Gynecol. Obstet., 38:587, 1964.

Clifford, R. H.: The treatment of macrodactylism; a case report. Plast. Reconstr. Surg., 23:245, 1959.

DeLaurenzi, V.: Macrodattilia de medio. Gior. Med. Mil., 112:401, 1962.

Dell, P. C.: Macrodactyly. Hand Clin., 1:511, 1985.

Edgerton, M. T., and Tuerk, D. B.: Macrodactyly (digital gigantism): Its nature and treatment. In Littler, J. W., Cramer, L. M., and Smith, J. W. (Eds.): Symposium on Reconstructive Hand Surgery, Vol. 9. St. Louis, C. V. Mosby Company, 1974.

El-Shami, I. N.: Congenital partial gigantism. Case report and review of literature. Surgery, 65:683, 1969.

Flatt, A. E.: The Care of Congenital Hand Anomalies. St. Louis, C. V. Mosby Company, 1977.

Fraumeni, J. F., Jr., and Miller, R. W.: Adrenocortical neoplasms and hemihypertrophy, brain tumors, and other disorders. J. Paediatr., 70:129, 1967.

Frykman, G. K., and Wood, V. E.: Peripheral nerve hamartomas with macrodactyly in the hand: Report of three cases and review of the literature. J. Hand Surg., 3:307, 1978.

Frykman, G. K., and Wood, V. E.: Macrodactyly. In Green, D. P. (Ed.): Operative Hand Surgery. New York, Churchill Livingstone, 1982.

Greulich, W. S., and Pyle, S. I.: Development of the Hand and Wrist. Radiologic Atlas of the Skeleton. Stanford, CA, Stanford University Press, 1966.

Heiple, K. B., and Elmer, R. M.: Chondromatous hamartomas arising from the volar digital plates. J. Bone Joint Surg., 54A:393, 1972.

Hensinger, R. N., and Rhyne, D. A.: Multiple enchondromatous hamartomas. Report of a case. J. Bone Joint Surg., 56A:1068, 1974.

Holt, J. F., and Wright, E. M.: The radiologic features of neurofibromatosis. Radiology, 51:647, 1948.

Hueston, J. T., and Millray, B.: Macrodactyly associated with hamartoma of major peripheral nerves. Aust. N.Z. J. Surg., 37:394, 1968.

Inglis, K.: Local gigantism (a manifestation of neurofibromatosis): Its relation to general gigantism and to acromegaly. Am. J. Pathol., 26:1059, 1950.

Johnson, R. J., and Bonfiglio, M.: Lipofibromatous hamartoma of the median nerve. J. Bone Joint Surg., 51A:984, 1969.

Jones, K. G.: Megadactylism: Case report of a child treated by epiphyseal resection. J. Bone Joint Surg., 45A:1704, 1963.

Kelikian, H.: Congenital Deformities of the Hand and Forearm. Philadelphia, W. B. Saunders Company, 1974.

Khanna, N., Gupta, S., Khanna, S., and Tripathi, F.: Macrodactyly. Hand, 7:212, 1975.

McCarroll, H. R.: Clinical manifestations of congenital neurofibromatosis. J. Bone Joint Surg., 32A:601, 1950.

Millesi, H.: Macrodactyly: A case study. In Littler, J. W., Cramer, L. M., and Smith, J. W. (Eds.): Symposium of Reconstructive Hand Surgery. Vol. 9. St. Louis, C. V. Mosby Company, 1974.

Minkowitz, S., and Minkowitz, F.: A morphological study of neurodactylism: A case report. J. Pathol. Bacteriol., 90:323, 1965.

Moore, B. H.: Peripheral nerve changes associated with congenital deformities. J. Bone Joint Surg., 26A:282, 1944.

Paletta, F. X., and Rybka, F. J.: Treatment of hamartomas of the median nerve. Ann. Surg., 176:217, 1972.

Pho, R. W. H., Patterson, M., and Lee, Y. S.: Reconstruction and pathology in macrodactyly. J. Hand Surg., 13A:78, 1988.

Pulvertaft, R. G.: Unusual tumors of the median nerve. Report of two cases. J. Bone Joint Surg., 46B:731, 1964.

Ranawat, C. S., Arora, M. M., and Singh, R. G.: Neurodystrophia lipomatosa with carpal tunnel syndrome. J. Bone Joint Surg., 50A:1242, 1968.

Rosenberg, L., Yanai, A., and Mahler, D.: A nail island flap for treatment of macrodactyly. Hand, 15:167, 1983.

Rousso, M., Katz, S., and Khodadadi, D.: Treatment of a case of macrodactyly of the thumb. Hand, 8:131, 1976.

Rudolph, R., and Jaffee, S.: Painless fibrofatty hamartoma of the median nerve. Br. J. Plast. Surg., 28:301, 1975.

Streeter, G. L.: Focal deficiencies in fetal tissues and their relation to intrauterine amputations. Contrib. Embryol., 22:1, 1930.

Temtamy, S. A., and Rogers, J. G.: Macrodactyly, hemihypertrophy and connective tissue nevi: Report of a new syndrome and review of the literature. J. Pediatr., 89:924, 1976.

Thorne, F. L., Posch, J. L. and Mladick, R. A.: Megalodactyly. Plast. Reconstr. Surg., 41:232, 1968.

Tsuge, K.: Treatment of macrodactyly. Plast. Reconstr. Surg., 39:590, 1967.

Tsuge, K.: Treatment of macrodactyly. J. Hand Surg., 10A:968, 1985.

Tsuge, K., and Ikuta, Y.: Macrodactyly and fibrofatty proliferation of the median nerve. Hiroshima J. Med. Sci., 22:83, 1973.

Tuli, S. M., Khanna, N. N., and Sinha, G. P.: Congenital macrodactyly. Br. J. Plast. Surg., 22:237, 1969.

Wood, V. E.: Macrodactyly. J. Iowa Med. Soc., 59:922, 1969.

Yaghmai, I., McKowne, F., and Alizadeh, A.: Macrodactylia fibrolipomatosis. South. Med. J., 69:1565, 1976.

Yeoman, P. M.: Fatty infiltration of the median nerve. J. Bone Joint Surg., 46B:737, 1964.

Congenital Constriction Ring Syndrome

Baker, C. J., and Rudolph, A. J.: Congenital ring constrictions and intrauterine amputations. Am. J. Dis. Child., 121:393, 1971.

Blackfield, H. M., and Hause, D. P.: Congenital constricting bands of the extremities. Plast. Reconstr. Surg., 8:101, 1951.

Browne, D.: The pathology of congenital ring constrictions. Arch. Dis. Child., 32:517, 1957.

Buck-Gramcko, D.: Hand surgery in congenital malformations. In Jackson, I. (Ed.): Recent Advances in Plastic Surgery. London, Churchill Livingstone, 1981.

Carroll, R. E.: Transposition of the index finger to replace the middle finger. Clin. Orthop., 15:27, 1959.

Casaubon, J. N.: Congenital band about the pelvis. Plast. Reconstr. Surg., 71:120, 1983.

Chemke, J., Graff, G., Hurwitz, N., and Liban, E.: The amniotic band syndrome. Obstet. Gynecol., 41:332, 1973.

Clavert, J. M., Berlizon, A., Clavert, A., and Buck, P.: Étude expérimentale: Les amputations de membre obtenues par injection intra-annexielle de glucose chez le foetus de lapin. Ann. Chir. Infant., 18:405, 1977.

Clavert, J. M., Clavert, A., Berlizon, A., and Buck, P.: Abnormalities resulting from intra-adnexal injection of glucose in rabbit embryo—an experimental model of "Amniotic Disease." Prog. Pediatr. Surg., 12:143, 1978.

Clavert, J. M., Clavert, A., Issa, W. N., and Buck, P.: Experimental approach to the pathogenesis of the anomalies of amniotic disease. J. Pediatr. Surg., 15:63, 1980.

Cowen, N., and Loftus, J. M.: Distraction augmentation manoplasty. Technique for lengthening digits or entire hands. Orthop. Rev., 6:45, 1978.

DeMyer, W., and Baird, I.: Mortality and skeletal malformations from amniocentesis and oligohydramnios in rats: Cleft palate, clubfoot, microstomia, and adactyly. Teratology, 2:33, 1969.

Dobyns, J. H.: Segmental digital transpositions in congenital hand deformities. Hand Clin., *1:*475, 1985.

Farmer, A. W.: Congenital elephantiasis associated with constriction by anomalous bands. J. Bone Joint Surg., *30B:*606, 1948.

Field, J. H., and Krag, D. O.: Congenital constricting band and congenital amputation of the fingers: Placental studies. J. Bone Joint Surg., *55A:*1035, 1973.

Fischl, R. A.: Ring constriction syndrome. *In* Transactions of the International Society of Plastic and Reconstructive Surgeons, 5th Congress. Melbourne, Australia, Butterworths Pty. Ltd., 1971.

Flatt, A. E.: The Care of Congenital Hand Anomalies. St. Louis, C. V. Mosby Company, 1977.

Gellis, S. S.: Constrictive bands in the human. Birth Defects, *13:*259, 1977.

Gilbert, A.: Toe transfers for congenital hand defects. J. Hand Surg., *7:*118, 1982.

Granick, M. S., Ramasastry, S., Vries, J., and Cohen, M. M.: Severe amniotic band syndrome occurring with unrelated syndactyly. J. Plast. Reconstr. Surg., *80:*829, 1987.

Harrison, S. H.: The tactile adhesion test estimating loss of sensation after nerve injury. Hand, *6:*148, 1974.

Higgenbottom, M. C., Jones, K. L., Hall, B. D., and Smith, D. W.: The amniotic band disruption complex: Timing of amniotic rupture and variable spectra of consequent defects. J. Pediatr., *95:*544, 1979.

Isacsohn, M., Aboulafia, Y., Horowitz, B., and Ben-Hur, N.: Congenital annular constrictions due to amniotic bands. Acta Obstet. Gynecol. Scand., *55:*179, 1976.

Jones, K. L., Jones, M., and Fisher, J. C.: A developmental approach to the classification of birth defects. Ann. Plast. Surg., *14:*135, 1985.

Jones, M. C.: The spectrum of structural defects produced as a result of amnion rupture. Semin. Perinatol., *7:*281, 1983.

Kaplan, E. B.: Replacement of an amputated middle metacarpal and finger by transposition of the index finger. Bull. Hosp. Joint Dis., *27:*103, 1966.

Kelikian, H.: Congenital Deformities of the Hand and Forearm. Philadelphia, W. B. Saunders Company, 1972.

Kessler, I., Baruch, A., and Hecht, O.: Experience with distraction lengthening of digital rays in congenital anomalies. J. Hand Surg., *2:*394, 1978.

Kino, Y.: Clinical and experimental studies of the congenital constriction band syndrome with an emphasis on its etiology. J. Bone Joint Surg., *57A:*636, 1975.

Matev, I.: Thumb reconstruction in children through metacarpal lengthening. Plast. Reconstr. Surg., *64:*665, 1979.

Miura, T.: Congenital constriction band syndrome. J. Hand Surg., *9A:*82, 1984.

Moessinger, A. C., Blanc, W. A., et al.: Amniotic band syndrome associated with amniocentesis. Am. J. Obstet. Gynecol., *141:*588, 1981.

Moses, J. M., Flatt, A. E., and Cooper, R. R.: Annular constricting bands. J. Bone Joint Surg., *61A:*562, 1979.

Ogino, T., and Saitou, Y.: Congenital constriction band syndrome and transverse deficiency. J. Hand Surg., *12B:*343, 1987.

Patterson, T. J. S.: Congenital constrictions. Br. J. Plast. Surg., *14:*1, 1961.

Peacock, E. E., Jr.: Metacarpal transfer following amputation of a central digit. Plast. Reconstr. Surg., *29:*345, 1962.

Poswillo, D.: Observations of fetal posture and causal

mechanisms of congenital deformity of palate, mandible, and limbs. J. Dent. Res. *45:*584, 1966.

Rehder, H.: Fetal limb deformities due to amniotic constrictions: A possible consequence of preceding amniocentesis. Pathol. Res. Pract., *162:*316, 1978.

Rowsell, A. R.: The amniotic band disruption complex. The pathogenesis of congenital limb ring-constrictions; experimental study in the foetal rat. Br. J. Plast. Surg., *41:*45, 1988.

Soiland, H.: Lengthening a finger with the "on the top" method. Acta Chir. Scand., *122:*184, 1961.

Stevenson, T. W.: Release of circular constricting scar by Z flaps. Plast. Reconstr. Surg., *1:*39, 1946.

Streeter, G. L.: Focal deficiencies in fetal tissues and their relation to intrauterine amputation. Contrib. Embryol., *22:*1, 1930.

Temtamy, S. A., and McKusick, V. A.: Digital and other malformations associated with congenital ring constrictions. Birth Defects, *14:*547, 1978.

Torpin, R.: Amniochorionic mesoblastic fibrous strings and amnionic bands. Am. J. Obstet. Gynecol., *91:*65, 1965.

Torpin, R.: Fetal Malformations Caused by Amnion Rupture During Gestation. Springfield, IL, Charles C Thomas, 1968.

Upton, J., and Tan, C.: Correction of constriction rings. J. Hand Surg., 1989 (in press).

Weeks, P. M.: Radial, median and ulnar nerve dysfunction associated with a congenital constricting band of the arm. Plast. Reconstr. Surg., *69:*333, 1982.

Wynne-Davies, R., and Lamb, D. W.: Congenital upper limb anomalies: An etiologic grouping of clinical, genetic, and epidemiologic data from 387 patients with "absence defects, constriction bands, polydactylies, and syndactylies." J. Hand Surg., *10A:*958, 1985.

Yoshimura, M.: Toe-to-hand transfer. Plast. Reconstr. Surg., *66:*74, 1980.

Arthrogryposis

Banker, B. Q., Victor, M., and Adams, R. D.: Arthrogryposis multiplex due to a congenital muscular dystrophy. Brain, *80:*319, 1957.

Bayne, L. G.: Arthrogryposis. *In* Green, D. P., (Ed.): Operative Surgery of the Hand. New York, Churchill Livingstone, 1982.

Brown, L. M., Robson, M. J., and Sharrard, W. J. W.: The pathology of arthrogryposis multiplex congenita neurologica. J. Bone Joint Surg., *62B:*291, 1980.

Carroll, R. E., and Hill, N. A.: Triceps transfer to restore elbow flexion. J. Bone Joint Surg., *52A:*239, 1970.

Clark, J. M. P.: Reconstruction of biceps brachii by pectoralis muscle transplantation. Br. J. Surg., *34:*180, 1946.

Cooney, W. P., and Schutt, A. H.: Arthrogryposis multiplex congenita. *In* Bora, F. W. (Ed.): The Pediatric Upper Extremity: Diagnosis and Management. Philadelphia, W. B. Saunders Company, 1966.

Doyle, J. R., James, P. M., Larsen, L. J., and Ashley, P. K.: Restoration of elbow flexion in arthrogryposis multiplex congenita. J. Hand Surg., *5:*149, 1980.

Drachman, D. B., and Banker, B. Q.: Arthrogryposis multiplex congenita. A case due to disease of the anterior horn cells. Arch. Neurol., *5:*77, 1961.

Friedlander, H. L., Westin, G. W., and Wood, W. L.: Arthrogryposis multiplex congenita. J. Bone Joint Surg., *50A:*89, 1968.

Hansen, O. M.: Surgical anatomy and treatment of patients with arthrogryposis. J. Bone Joint Surg., *43B:*855, 1961.

Hillman, J. W., and Johnson, J. T. H.: Arthrogryposis multiplex congenita in twins. J. Bone Joint Surg., *34A:*211, 1952.

Holtman, B., Wray, R. C., Lowrey, R., and Weeks, P.: Restoration of elbow flexion. Hand, *7:*256, 1975.

Kite, J. H.: Arthrogryposis multiplex congenita: Review of 54 cases. South. Med. J., *48:*1141, 1955.

Laitinen, O., and Hirvensalo, M.: Arthrogryposis multiplex congenita. Ann. Paediatr. Fenn., *12:*133, 1966.

Lewin, P.: Arthrogryposis multiplex congenita. J. Bone Joint Surg., *7:*630, 1925.

Lloyd-Roberts, G. C., and Leitin, A. W. F.: Arthrogryposis multiplex congenita. J. Bone Joint Surg., *52B:*494, 1970.

Meyn, M., and Ruby, L.: Arthrogryposis of the upper extremity. Orthop. Clin. North Am., 7:501, 1976.

Sheldon, W.: Anoplasia congenita. Arch. Dis. Child., *7:*117, 1932.

Smith, R. J.: Hand deformities with arthrogryposis multiplex congenita. J. Bone Joint Surg., *55A:*883, 1973.

Steindler, A.: Arthrogryposis. J. Int. Coll. Surg., *12:*21, 1949.

Tachdjian, M. O.: Pediatric Orthopedics. Philadelphia, W. B. Saunders Company, 1972.

Weeks, P. M.: Surgical correction of the upper extremity deformities in arthrogryposis. Plast. Reconstr. Surg., *36:*459, 1965.

Whitten, J. H.: Congenital abnormalities in calves: Arthrogryposis and hydroencephaly. J. Pathol., *73:*375, 1957.

Williams, P.: The management of arthrogryposis. Orthop. Clin., *9:*67, 1978.

Roger E. Salisbury

Acute Care of the Burned Hand

HISTORY

A historical review of the management of burns of the upper extremity invariably deals with the wound itself. In the preantibiotic era the emphasis was on covering the burn wound so that the upper extremity was protected from bacteria, mostly gram-positive streptococci and staphylococci thought to be transmitted by contact with other patients or hospital personnel. In World War I and shortly thereafter, paraffin wax was popularized for closed treatment of burns. Sherman (1918) wrote that over 3000 cases were treated by this technique, which was perfected by Barthe de Sandfordt and was first tested and popularized in French hospitals during World War I. Essentially the burns were dried and then sealed in paraffin wax, which excluded the air and maintained a constant temperature. It was felt that the wax, which was applied by an atomizer, best protected the regenerating epithelium and allowed healing to occur. Sherman, however, notes that "the odor at times in the severe

burns is rather nauseating" and it is obvious that it was not appreciated that the paraffin that kept organisms out also locked organisms in. As World War II approached, the issues of mobilization versus nonmobilization, early excision and grafting of the burn wound as opposed to delayed treatment with surgery, became matters of concern. Blair and Byars (1938) in America urged early active surgical repair of deep burns of any considerable size as early as was practical in order to achieve good skin coverage. Allen (1939), however, emphasized that the burned upper extremity should be cleaned and then dressed in a petroleum gauze, bulky sterile dressing and left in the same dressing for 14 days. He contended that daily dressing changes were not necessary and only caused repetitive trauma that injured healing tissue and risked infection. At the end of 14 days the dressings were changed and second degree burns were noted to be healed. Third degree burns were treated with a dilute solution of sodium hypochlorite dressings that were changed daily, and any wounds that were still open were skin grafted. Brown (1938, 1939), however, advocated that superficial burns be left open to allow for early joint movement. He emphasized that one should simply debride and keep the wounds clean, but not seal the area with any wound dressing or plaster for fear of producing stiff fingers. Brown definitely advocated early range of motion and active therapy to prevent secondary deformities of the hand. For deep burns, however, he suggested closed treatment with dressing changes once a day and grafting within three weeks. He allowed motion of the fingers only when the dressings were being changed. Brown emphasized that free grafts were more suitable than pedicle flaps, most closely simulating the patient's own unburned hand. Interestingly, he advocated full-thickness grafts and emphasized that they should be used in dorsal hand injuries, but admitted that there was absolutely no advantage in final function over that achieved by thick split-thickness skin grafts. For full-thickness injuries Brown did not advocate immediate excision and grafting, but the dressing changes as previously indicated, with grafting as soon as the wound was ready, invariably within three weeks. He stated: "When the full thickness of the skin has been lost even on small areas, in such a kinetic region as the hand the indication for treatment is to restore this loss as completely and as soon as possible."

Other investigators continued research to find a better wound dressing. They attempted to convert the burn wound into a closed coagulum or eschar that would allow for internal healing but would prevent entry of bacteria. This type of thinking persisted throughout World War II. Cohen (1940b) reviewed the advantages and disadvantages of tannic acid as a wound cover. He indicated that this coagulation treatment seemed to lessen toxemia, acted as an analgesic, cut fluid loss, and limited secondary infection and hypertrophic scar formation. The objections to it seemed to be the instability of the solutions, the stiffness of the coagulum, its unyielding nature (which could cause ischemia and gangrene in the hand and fingers if the wound was deep enough), and the necrosis and infection that could occur under the coagulum. Cohen cited other coagulant research that was being done with sodium carbonate, gentian violet, and silver nitrate. In using ferric chloride and comparing it with tannic acid, he found that the solution was more stable, that the coagulum was more consistent and more flexible, and that it would move over joints without cracking. Bettman (1937) used a solution of tannic acid and silver nitrate for treating burns. He emphasized that it gave the epithelial islands a chance to heal, and the wounds were always clean and dry. He too stressed that tannic acid by itself led to an unyielding coagulum that could be disastrous for the upper extremity burn. He specifically cited a case of a patient losing his upper extremity with the hand sloughing off at the wrist due to "leathery encasement." Silver nitrate added to the tannic acid prevented the eschar from being too tight. Bettman noted that no silver absorption was seen and that the 5 per cent tannic acid solution with 10 per cent silver nitrate solution seemed to speed up healing and shorten hospitalization.

Experiments were also made with compounds of aniline dyes. For instance, it was found that gentian violet would make a coagulum but was not an antiseptic, and contamination by gram-negative organisms occurred under the coagulum. From a combination of gentian violet and brilliant green, it was noted that an antiseptic resulted that would not injure cells. This combination did not seem to let bacteria in and yet formed a very tough eschar. In those instances in which the eschar developed an infection underneath, the eschar was excised, the wound was drained, and dye was reapplied. It is noteworthy that in all of these suggested treatments of the burn wound, no prospective studies were done comparing modalities of treatment, nor were patients grouped according to age, associated diseases, inhalation injury, or extent of total body burn. It is therefore somewhat difficult to analyze the results of the data.

A very important philosophical report about treating the burn wound was published by Hooker and Lam (1941), showing the absorption of sulfanilamide from the burned surfaces. It had been accepted by clinicians (since research by Underhill) that many substances did not pass through the burn wound. Specifically, absorption was inhibited into unburned areas through the eschar. Many thought, erroneously, that nothing would pass through the burn wound. Hooker and Lam (1941) suggested that for large infected wounds it might be possible to treat them appropriately if a drug were used that would easily penetrate the eschar. The importance of this line of reasoning is immense, since it is very different from the philosophy of painting the burn wound and creating a coagulum to prevent bacteria from crossing the wound. It would seem to recognize that bacteria could be trapped under the coagulum and present a danger to the patient. Thus, these authors sprinkled dry, powdered sulfanilamide on the burn wounds and measured blood levels, finding a marked elevation in the blood level of sulfanilamide. The report expressed the hope that the treatment could be used prophylactically to prevent infection as well as for patients who already had infection.

With the advent of World War II, a wealth of reports appeared in the literature for surgeons (especially British physicians) intimately involved with treating large numbers of casualties. Cohen (1940b) once again supported a case for tannic acid, pointing out that it was excellent for large groups of casualties in that the wounds could be easily sprayed, care was simple and minimal, and wounds would heal. He noted that the saline baths suggested by some would be very impractical for large numbers of casualties such as seen at Dunkirk and other major battles. The passion expressed by the authors in some of these papers is fascinating, seldom seen in today's rather sterile scientific presentations, and makes the study of the history of medicine very worthwhile. For instance, one should read Cohen's commentary and defense of the treatment of burns by tannic acid. Apparently the use of tannic acid was ordered to be discontinued in favor of saline baths, and Cohen took appropriate exception that "not a paper or a note has been published in any general medical journal either proving or even discussing" its validity. In discussing his treatment of 100 war wounds and burns, Ross (1941) wrote of his patients: "excited, with nerves still keyed to the highest pitch, with heads still spinning from the swift rush earthwards and with wounds bleeding freely from the battle, they formed a striking contrast to the Dunkirk soldiers with their grimy and inflamed wound holes often several days old."

Others continued investigation of tanning agents for use in large numbers of casualties. For instance, Wakely (1941) wrote about spraying on an aqueous solution of triple dye consisting of 2 per cent gentian violet, 1 per cent briliant green, and 0.1 per cent neutral acriflavine. His research found that the solution produced a more supple tan than tannic acid, no dressings were required, and second degree burns healed in ten days. With third degree burns the tannic coagulum fell off, leaving granulation tissues that could be skin grafted. Wakely also indicated that gentian violet jelly made an excellent emergency treatment and was carried in advance units, tanks, and field packs. Soldiers at sea might have to wait days before they could get to the hospital, but with application of gentian violet jelly the pain decreased, their wounds were covered and protected, and they could still keep working. For third degree burns

Wakely, too, advocated saline baths in the hospital and early excision and grafting. The envelope method of Bunyan (1941) received close scrutiny because of its painless application. Essentially, he irrigated the burned hand with a 10 per cent solution of hypochlorite at 100°F in a closed bag. This irrigation was believed to remove bacteria and dead tissue. The specially coated silk envelope put over the hand allowed irrigation with the hypochlorite that was painless and helped promote epithelization.

In view of the number of papers written on burns at that time, it is interesting that no attempts were made to group them clearly by total size body burn and depth, or to consider the problems of associated illnesses. Many of the reports failed to cover microbiology and some even boasted about this. Greeley (1940), discussing the plastic repair of cutaneous injuries of the hand, noted that "we do not ordinarily make bacterial counts, relying instead upon our experience and judgement to tell when the bed does or does not present an adequate healthy appearance."

The controversy over splinting versus early motion continued. Roulston (1941) used a closed plaster treatment of the extremities and even suggested that this treatment was the best for the worst burns, those with the most profuse drainage, indicating that they healed without problems in 10 to 14 days. All his patients healed within three weeks, which would indicate that the injuries were second degree and that no full-thickness burns were treated. Mason (1941) suggested keeping the burned hand splinted in the position of function and covering it with a dressing, but pointed out that there was nothing to be gained by continuing this treatment in patients with full-thickness injuries because contractures and loss of function would still occur. Those treating large numbers of casualties, such as Ross and Hulbert (1941), opted for dressings and immobilization, because preventing infection at that time seemed to be much more important than the fear of a stiff hand. The idea of preventing bacteria from getting through to the burn wound was paramount, and cultures that were taken almost uniformly grew *Streptococcus* (which in patients who died was also found in the blood and sputum). Ross and Hulbert therefore left dressings on for seven to ten days, and almost all of their 205 patients had full range of motion and healed in less than 30 days. Most important, 65 per cent of all upper extremity burns remained sterile on culture. In the case of third degree burns, these authors readily indicated that they should be excised and grafted as soon as possible to avoid edema, granulation tissue, and subsequent fibrosis. In patients with obvious full-thickness injuries, they applied penicillin cream dressings to rid the wound of the gram-positive bacteria. Cannon and Zuidema (1959) tried to explain to the neophyte when a burn would be ready for grafting and emphasized that experienced and less experienced clinicians could tell, if the following conditions existed: (1) decreased exudate, (2) granulation tissues that were bright red, and (3) visible marginal spread of epithelium. These authors also emphasized that skin grafts were overwhelmingly preferable to flaps for covering the burned hand. By the end of World War II and the postwar period, people such as Cope and associates (1947) recognized that coagulum treatment with tannic acid was injurious to the wound, especially in the case of second degree burns, and suggested protecting only the partial-thickness injuries with a simple dressing and splint. With this "undertreatment" these wounds would heal expeditiously. For full-thickness injuries, Cope urged excision and grafting as soon as possible. Braithwaite (1949) summarized the two prevalent schools of thought of the day as expressed by Trueta (1946) versus McIndoe (1944). Trueta made a plea for continued immobilization until healing occurred, whereas McIndoe emphasized that exercise was needed to maintain mobility, and healing would still occur. Exercise was not injurious to the healing wound. Braithwaite (1949) also suggested early excision of the eschar, granulations, and dermal remnants, followed by grafting. He felt that early surgery prevented deformities. He criticized Trueta for prolonged splinting, which caused the small muscles to lose their power and the hand to gradually become immobile. Truetta claimed that all his patients who were immobilized for three weeks obtained full range of motion and that almost all healed in four weeks; this was difficult for Braithwaite to believe. Braithwaite (1949) also emphasized that if the proximal interphalangeal joints were involved they should be splinted to avoid further tendon injury, while the metacarpophalangeal joints should be kept free and exercised.

PATHOLOGY

Thermal injury results in capillary damage, which causes an outpouring of protein-rich fluid and initiates an inflammatory response leading to increased fibrous protein synthesis. Edema may result from multiple causes including the initial injury, the inflammatory response, inadequate motion following injury, dependency, and lack of mobilization because of pain. All these factors cause prolonged edema and fibrosis of normal, initially uninjured structures. Internal scarring may result in shortening of the joint capsules, and adherence of gliding surfaces such as tendon sheaths to fascia and tendons to tendons. If wound contamination progresses to frank infection, the inflammatory response is prolonged and much greater scarring occurs. Infection may also result in conversion of partial- to full-thickness injury, which gives rise to still more scarring.

Aside from the initial injury itself, there are other contributing factors to postburn deformity, including persistent edema, wound infection, poor positioning, prolonged immobilization, and delayed or inadequate skin coverage. Each of these is discussed in detail later in this chapter. It is noteworthy that what may begin as purely a skin problem, if inappropriately treated, can affect all tissues of the hand including the extensor or flexor apparatus, intrinsic muscles, skeleton, and joints. A second degree burn that is immobilized for too long or with the hand in an inappropriate position can develop stiffness of the small joints that results in a far greater problem than the burn wound itself, which can heal within three weeks. The posthealing therapy for the second degree burn of the hand may be minimal compared with the efforts needed to mobilize joints that have become contracted from disuse and poor positioning. Likewise, edema that is uncontrolled in a circumferentially burned hand may result in necrosis of the intrinsic musculature with significant stiffness and marked loss of fine mobility that lasts long after the skin wound itself is healed.

In the freshly burned hand the most common position of comfort that the patient assumes is one that allows for adduction of the thumb, flexion of the proximal interphalangeal joints, hyperextension of the metacarpophalangeal joints, and flexion of the wrist (Fig. 129–1). If this habitus is not quickly

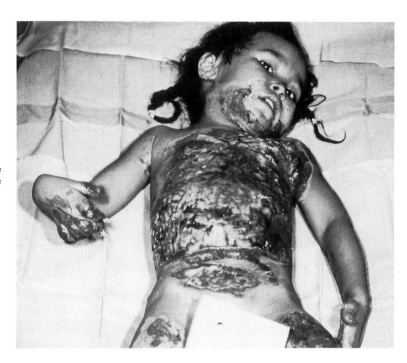

Figure 129–1. The position of comfort is usually the position of deformity.

corrected, irrevocable fibrosis occurs long before full healing of the hand has been accomplished. For example, by hyperextending the metacarpophalangeal joints, laxity occurs in the collateral ligaments, leading to shortening and fibrosis. The transverse metacarpal ligaments shorten and there is loss of the transverse metacarpal arch. Once fibrosis occurs, the long flexors are not able to flex the metacarpophalangeal joints. As long as these joints are held in hyperextension, the sagittal fibers of the extensor hood may become fixed and the central slip activity at the proximal interphalangeal joints is negligible. The flexor tendons act unopposed, since there is no extensor activity at this joint, and the proximal interphalangeal joints become fixed in flexion. If the burn is deep enough, direct injury may occur over the thin dorsal skin of the proximal interphalangeal joints and the extensor mechanism may become exposed and destroyed. With continued flexion a hole occurs in the extensor mechanism and the lateral bands slip below the axis of the joint, converting the finger extensor into a flexor. The distal interphalangeal joint may hyperextend as a result, and if this condition is allowed to persist changes to both joints result. Sometimes a wound that is neglected develops infection, causing full-thickness destruction of the skin and the underlying ex-

tensor mechanism, and the same type of deformity may result.

Prolonged extensive edema in the burned hand can lead to long-term changes in nerve function. Fissette, Onkelinx, and Fandi (1981), in a review of 22 patients with wrist burns, found a high incidence of conditions compatible with the carpal and Guyon tunnel syndrome. Electromyographic studies revealed that more than 50 per cent of the patients had motor and sensory involvement of the median nerve, and more than 60 per cent had involvement of the ulnar nerve. Significantly, none of these patients sustained direct injury to the nerves at the time of the burn: these changes were due to edema and resultant scar formation.

PHYSICAL EXAMINATION

The physical examination of burns of the hand should deal primarily with an estimate of the depth and extent of burn and the presence or absence of vascular integrity. If there is any history of associated trauma, x-rays should be taken. Because the skin on the back of the hand is so thin, it is difficult to ascertain the depth of burn merely by the color. For instance, a white eschar on the buttock or back may be partial thickness,

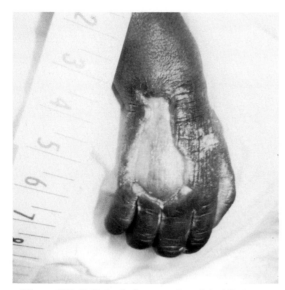

Figure 129–2. Burns in the neonate or infant that appear to be second degree are often full thickness.

deep second degree, but on the dorsum of the hand where the skin is thinner, it is invariably full thickness. A cherry-red color may indicate deep second degree on the back, but assuredly is a full-thickness burn on the dorsum of a child's hand (Fig. 129–2). Knowing the etiology of the injury helps the physician diagnose the depth of the burn. Short exposure scald burns are usually partial thickness, whereas flame burns are most frequently third degree. High voltage electrical injury (see Chap. 130) may well involve the deeper subfascial structures of the hand and upper extremity. Table 129–1 is meant as a helpful guide, but cannot be interpreted too

strictly. The presence or absence of sensation is almost impossible to ascertain in a child who is in pain from a large total body burn, and adults can be hardly more cooperative. Although investigations are presently being conducted to develop a test for diagnosing depth of injury, there is no uniformly accepted technique at this time.

It is crucial to diagnose vascular compromise in the circumferentially or severely burned upper extremity. First, it is uncommon to have arterial and venous interruptions unless the burn is circumferential. Second, the absence of pulses does not necessarily mean vascular compression secondary to the burn. One should first check the degree of resuscitation of the patient to be sure that there is adequate urine output, reflecting good internal organ perfusion. If, in a patient who is adequately resuscitated, there are circumferential burns and no pulse, there is a high index of suspicion of vascular compromise. The traditional signs of pain, pallor, pulselessness, and paralysis may not be apparent in burned patients. These patients are always in pain, and it may be difficult to differentiate pain due to vascular ischemia from that due to the cutaneous burn itself. Obviously, skin color is no help and it may be almost impossible to ask a patient who is in generalized pain to move his fingers through a range of motion to determine whether or not there is paresis or paralysis. The positive stretch test (demonstrating an increase in pain when the intrinsic muscles are stretched) can be suggestive, but again it is hard to get many patients to cooperate for

Table 129–1. Burn Depth Categories

Degree	Cause	Color	Pain Level	Surface Appearance
First	Flash flame, ultraviolet (sunburn)	Erythematous	Painful	Dry, no blisters; no or minimal edema
Second	Contact with hot liquids or solids, flash flame to clothing, direct flame, chemical, ultraviolet	Mottled white to pink, cherry red	Very painful	Moist blebs, blisters
Third (full-thickness)	Contact with hot liquids or solids, flame, chemical, electrical	Mixed white, waxy, pearly; dark, khaki, mahogany; charred	Little or no pain; hair pulls out easily	Dry with leathery eschar until debridement; charred vessels visible under eschar
Fourth (involves underlying structures)	Prolonged contact with flame, electrical injury	Same as third degree	Same as third degree	Same as third degree, possibly with exposed bone, muscle, or tendon

this test. Electromyography is impractical and compartmental pressure readings may be equivocal and unreliable, depending on who is doing the study. Therefore, in a patient who is adequately resuscitated, the Doppler flowmeter is used to check the presence of a radial and palmar arch pulse. If there is no palmar arch pulse, vascular compromise secondary to edema exists and escharotomy is indicated (see under Inpatient Treatment).

OUTPATIENT TREATMENT

Once the upper extremity burn has been assessed, the decision has to be made whether to treat it on an inpatient or outpatient basis. Obviously, if the patient has large burns other than those of the upper extremity, he will be admitted to the hospital for resuscitation and treatment. A patient with burns of both hands that are incapacitating, even though the total body burn size is small, might do best in the hospital environment if there is no one at home to be of assistance, since the patient is essentially helpless. For a patient with second degree and perhaps a small area of third degree burns involving one or both extremities that do not render him helpless, outpatient treatment is reasonable. Likewise, a patient who has burns of only one extremity that are second degree is a candidate for outpatient treatment. The very aged, the very young, and those without help at home or the intellectual ability to care for themselves might be candidates for admission even though their burns are not extensive. Several days of appropriate care heal some of these wounds, whereas several days of neglect may result in conversion of second to third degree burn and a larger problem. For immediate treatment of those burns to be treated in the outpatient clinic, it is sufficient merely to clean the wounds with a mild soap and to debride ruptured bulli and blebs. Small blisters are not ruptured, but large ones that retard movement of the fingers are. The choice of wound coverage is an interesting and somewhat controversial one. Topical chemotherapeutic agents are often suggested for outpatient use not because of medical necessity, but in deference to commercial and economic pressures. These agents, such as mafenide (Sulfamyalon) and silver sulfadiazine (Silvadene), were developed for inpatient burns and never intended

to be used for small outpatient-type injuries. Their outpatient use is a classic case of "overkill" and merely gives rise to resistant organisms. It is more reasonable to dress the burns with one of the readily available impregnated gauzes and a large bulky dressing and splint. The wound dressing should be changed by the physician every 72 hours. On this regimen, second degree burns are healed within 14 days, and it is rare for infection to occur. For portions of the wound that are deep, second degree healing may be somewhat slower. Third degree injuries gradually separate their eschar and the necessity for grafting can be evaluated.

Appropriate hand splinting is usually recommended, with the wrist in 30 degrees of extension, the metacarpophalangeal joints in 70 degrees of flexion, and the proximal interphalangeal joints in extension. If the thumb is involved, it should be placed in abduction and oral penicillin given to avoid a streptococcal infection. As far as possible the hand should be elevated in a sling and upon pillows at night to prevent swelling.

INPATIENT TREATMENT

During the first 24 hours after the burn, the injured extremity is elevated and pulses checked hourly. If vascular compromise is diagnosed, escharotomy for the injured extremity must include the burned arm, the wrist, and each involved finger as well as decompression of all intrinsic muscles. The extremity is held in the position of supplication to avoid confusion over the course of the incision. The incision is made in the midlateral plane (Fig. 129–3A) extending from the most proximal portion of the circumferential injury distally down to the wrist across the midlateral plane of the hand, and onto the hypothenar or thenar eminence. The incision should first be made laterally and extended deep enough to enter the normal soft tissue. The escharotomy can be performed with the electrocautery at the patient's bed; the operating room is not needed. Hemostasis is easily achieved with electrocautery and topical thrombin-soaked sponges. Once the limb is decompressed and increased blood flow enters the extremity, the bleeding from the escharotomy site can be prodigious; hemostasis therefore must be achieved at once. Once the escharotomy is made laterally, the extremity

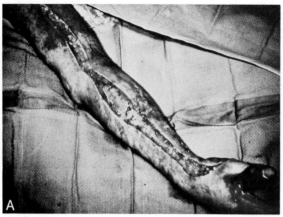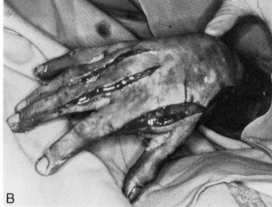

Figure 129–3. *A, B,* The escharotomy incision must extend the full length of the constricting burn and also decompress the fingers and intrinsic muscles.

is again checked with a Doppler for pulses. If no pulses are noted, the medial incision is made. If the escharotomy must extend proximal to the elbow, great care should be taken to make the incision anterior to the medial condyle, to avoid injury to the ulnar nerve. The incisions are carried across the thenar or hypothenar eminence and along the mid-lateral plane of each finger (Fig. 129–3B). It usually is not necessary to make an escharotomy incision on both sides of each finger unless the burns are very deep. Care is taken to extend the incision in each finger through the offending eschar and into viable soft tissue. The incision should not be deep enough to expose the neurovascular bundle, otherwise desiccation of the digital nerves will occur. Dorsal incisions are then made between each metacarpal down to the investing fascia of the intrinsic muscles. The investing fascia must be cut longitudinally to allow for decompression of the intrinsic musculature. It is imperative to note that the small intrinsic muscles become compromised very easily when edematous. Dorsal decompression should be enough to allow for adequate blood flow. Significantly, there are no deep venae comitantes accompanying the digital arteries, and therefore venous return depends on very small deep veins and on the superficial dorsal digital vessels, which are often burned. Thus, it is easy to see that the fingers are much at risk from venous compromise in a deep burn. In a prospective study, comparing digital escharotomy with none, there was a 3 to 1 increase in phalangeal loss in the group that did not have the digital escharotomy. Although it has been suggested that the ulnar

and median nerves should routinely be decompressed in their canals, this is impractical for all patients who need an escharotomy. Patients with high voltage electrical injuries and subfascial edema are usually those who benefit from this type of extensive decompression. Patients with nonelectrical injuries are usually decompressed adequately by the escharotomy described above.

During the first 48 hours following thermal injury, it is most common for the patient to be stabilized with intravenous resuscitation before any definitive surgical care is considered for the hand. During this time the upper extremity is best treated with continuous elevation and a towel sling from an intravenous pole, or elevation on several pillows, so that the hand is on a gentle incline above the level of the heart. The injured extremity is buttered with a topical chemotherapeutic agent and no dressings are applied, so that exercises can be performed such as extending and flexing the fingers. This milking action helps to diminish edema. If, however, the patient is uncooperative, a splint should be applied holding the hand in a functional position while the extremity is elevated. Achauer and associates (1974) fix the proximal interphalangeal joints in a neutral position at 24 hours with K-wires to ensure that a functional position is maintained, and exercise the metacarpophalangeal joints until grafting is performed.

Inpatient care of the burned upper extremity after 24 hours is a matter of great debate. The literature is replete with articles demonstrating superior results for early excision and grafting, tangential excision and grafting, enzymatic debridement and grafting, or simply the use of topical chemotherapeutic agents and grafting when necessary. These reports are very confusing to the neophyte or the person who sees the occasional upper extremity burn. Furthermore, there is an incredible overpreponderance of studies in the literature on the burned hand dealing with the one issue of whether or not dorsal burns should be excised, while almost no attention is paid to management problems of the severely burned palm or injuries involving the forearm, upper arm, and axilla.

The choices of treatment for dorsal burns include (1) topical enzymes, (2) topical chemotherapeutic agents and skin grafting if necessary; and (3) early excision and grafting. The most appealing simplistic solution to the problem of deep second or third degree burns of the hand is the use of a proteolytic enzyme to dissolve the dead tissue, spare the live tissue, and allow for more rapid healing. In

fact, several investigators have used sutilains (Travase) on the hands and found that in select instances it was very useful in rapidly removing the eschar and helping to achieve a healed wound. For instance, Gant (1980) pointed out that there was a zone of stasis between the deep viable tissue and the more superficial burn that could either go on to further tissue death, or be salvaged by rapid treatment of the burn wound before heavy contamination or infection occurred. He noted that there were multiple factors causing progression of necrosis of a dermal burn over 72 hours, including tissue edema, tension, severe external pressure, restrictive splints, shock, poor tissue oxygenation, and infection of the burn wound. By rapid removal of the eschar and grafting, Gant believed that many of these complicating factors that caused increased tissue death could be obviated. In 34 hands, he treated the second degree burns (Fig. 129–4A) with Travase for 24 hours, and

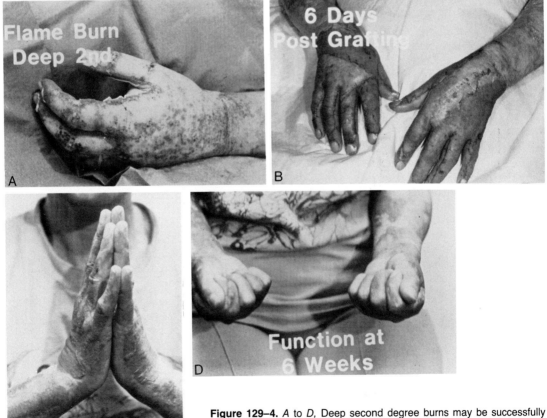

Figure 129–4. *A* to *D*, Deep second degree burns may be successfully treated with enzymes and grafting, with resultant rapid healing and return of function. (Courtesy of Dr. Thomas Gant.)

then scraped it off in the operating room and applied split-thickness skin grafts. He obtained 100 per cent graft take (Fig. 129–4B, C, D) and full range of motion one week after surgery in 31 out of 34 hands, with no hypertrophic scar formation. Cases were carefully selected and Gant discovered that the best result was predictable in deep second degree burns. With full-thickness burns, some mechanical excision of eschar in the operating room might be necessary, and for deeper burns (fourth degree) this treatment was not applicable. The advantages of Travase included: (1) it could be started immediately regardless of the status of the patient; (2) it required no special skills such as for surgery; (3) it was a fast and safe method, allowing skin grafting in 24 hours; (4) it helped promote early motion; and (5) it resulted in a satisfactory appearance. Others have used enzymatic debridement but have excluded very superficial burns and also third degree burns.

Travase obviously is not applicable for very superficial hand burns that heal anyway or for very deep injury that requires formal excision and grafting. One can understand this technique being very useful in a patient with a small total body burn, the hand burn being second degree. The technique may be very efficacious in the patient with a very large total body burn, including the hands, who is going to need a formal excision as a life-saving procedure. It may be appropriate during the first 24 hours, when the patient is being stabilized and resuscitated, to treat the hands with Travase and thus have the eschar removed in a matter of minutes when he is taken to the operating room for formal excision of the other burns. One would never spend two hours excising hands in a patient with a lethal body burn, but if Travase can accomplish the same procedure one may be inclined to graft the hands while the other burns are being excised.

The issue of whether to use topical chemotherapeutic agents and grafting when necessary, as opposed to early excision and grafting, has been fraught with confusing reports in the literature. Quite simply, there has been more passion than scientific fact. People have reported on a series of patients who have done well with one form of treatment, and used that information to criticize other forms of treatment without actually investigating them. Second, other studies have failed to

compare patients with comparable depth of burn, age, or systemic diseases. Some studies have described encouraging results without following the patients for a year or more, the necessary time interval to ascertain whether complications will develop. The published clinical series, however, are extremely worthwhile in emphasizing certain problems that the physician who only cares for an occasional hand burn might not otherwise appreciate. For example, Hunt and Sato (1982) performed early excision of full-thickness hand and digit burns in 50 patients and followed them for two to six years after surgery. They found that their patients fell neatly into two groups. Those who had no injury to the underlying extensor tendons or bone required only reconstructive surgery 12 per cent of the time in one year following injury, whereas of those who had underlying injury to extensors and bone, 75 per cent required further reconstructive surgery within the first year. Burke and associates (1976) wrote several papers comparing excised with nonexcised hands. The nonexcised group was treated with silver nitrate dressings and grafted when necessary. Burke and associates found a marked increase in complications in the silver nitrate–treated group. Seventy four out of 76 patients needed some type of secondary reconstruction, with complications occurring such as boutonnière deformity, hypertrophic scar, extension contractures, proximal and distal interphalangeal joint contractures, and contractures of the web spaces and the thumb. The study was not randomized in time, however, and one wonders if the treating physicians did not improve their care as time progressed, with a consequent difference in the quality of results. Levine and associates (1979) at the Army Institute of Surgical Research performed tangential excision and immediate autografting on deep second degree burns of the hand, using the style popularized by Janzekovic (1970). Interestingly, they found that the results were markedly better in patients who had total body burns of less than 40 per cent of body surface; they strongly urged against carrying out this procedure in patients with larger total body burns who were ill and could not comply with the postoperative therapy program.

Peacock, Madden, and Trier (1970), in their series of burned hands, noted that it was the proximal interphalangeal joint motion that was most difficult to maintain in someone who had sustained a severe thermal injury. They noted that immobilization can result in stiffness, and that immobilization plus edema from the injury itself can result in even worse edema. They appropriately emphasized that only the deep second degree burns cause controversy among treating physicians, but that everyone seems to excise third degree burns. The prolonged immobilization, the lengthy time for wound contraction to occur, the extensive synthesis of scar, and the poor results from a nonhealed wound cause progressive loss of hand function. For a combination of deep second and third degree dorsal burn, Peacock, Madden, and Trier excised everything, sacrificing some small bits of normal tissue in order to obtain more rapid healing of the wound. They made the very cogent point that it did not matter, in treating a burned thigh, if a wound treated by topical chemotherapy, took four weeks to heal. The hand, however, is very different, and gliding structures are in jeopardy during a prolonged period of nonhealing.

Edstrom and associates (1979), in a prospective study, took a series of 98 deep partial-thickness burned hands and divided them by random selection into those operated on immediately and those treated with topical chemotherapy and grafting when necessary. The results were most significant in that this was the first true prospective study for the management of deep second degree burns of the dorsum of the hand. These authors found that early function was excellent in both groups. The group that had surgery experienced an initial delay in their clinical progress, but caught up with the nonsurgery group by five weeks. Long-term results were the same in both groups, but there were different complications that were characteristic of each group. Some of the excised group developed web space contractures, linear scars, and pin tract infections. Some in the nonexcision group developed severe scar hypertrophy and unstable scars.

Salisbury and Wright (1982) divided a group of patients with deep burns on the dorsum of the hand into three groups. By random selection one group had early excision and grafting, and a second group was allowed to heal with topical chemotherapy and grafting if necessary. Those patients who required grafting were placed into a third group. Following the patients for a year, Salisbury and Wright noted that at discharge the group that healed spontaneously seemed to have the best range of motion, but that at 12 months there was no statistical difference among the operated groups and the group that healed with topical chemotherapy. At the end of 12 months, in studying the strength of key pinch and mass grip, there was no difference among groups. A very aggressive, closely supervised, splinting and therapy program that was carried on even beyond the hospitalization period may be the explanation for the lack of difference in results among groups. In this study, early excision and grafting did not shorten hospitalization time because the patients had other significant total body burns. The greatest gain in return of range of motion and power was in the six month period after discharge, with a gradual leveling off after this time. There was no increased instance of complications in any one group.

Magliacani, Bormioli, and Ceratti (1979) found in 467 patients over a ten year period that, of those whose burns of the hand took longer than 21 days to heal following injury, 100 per cent needed reconstructive surgery due to an anatomic deformity and/or the scar complications. The best results occurred when patients were operated on between five and ten days after the injury, only 26 per cent of these requiring further surgery.

It is obvious from reviewing the literature that no cookbook formula can be made for managing all burns of the hand in different populations of different ages. An inordinate amount of attention is given to burns of the dorsum of the hand, but almost nothing in the literature on the management of the difficult complications of the acutely burned hand or even burns of the palm, wrist, forearm, and upper arm. Burns of the hand in children should require special attention because of their very unique problems, yet very little has been written about these. The thinness of the skin on the upper extremity in children predisposes them to sustaining a deeper injury than adults exposed to a similar insult. A child's difficulty in understanding the severity of the problem and complying with treatment makes splinting, hand therapy, and especially outpatient therapy programs extremely difficult and usually ineffective. The smallness of the affected parts and the decreased strength leads to less ability to fight scar contractures. The mere act of elevating an arm to retard edema can be a nursing nightmare in a child who does not want to cooperate. Unlike adults, however, children are very rarely prone to developing contractures from splinting. Therefore, in uncooperative children, day and night splints in the position of function are very worthwhile to prevent secondary or iatrogenic contractures.

Likewise, elderly patients pose special problems in that they may not have the strength to comply with a program that requires their participation in performing exercises and applying and removing splints. In these patients, however, several hours of surgery and skin grafting may be impossible because of unassociated problems such as cardiovascular or renal disease. A full medical work-up to elucidate any systemic diseases must be carried out before excision and grafting of burns is performed in the elderly.

As Boswick (1974) indicated, there are certain well-defined factors that have been found to influence the prognosis for and also the method of treatment of the acutely burned hand. A review of these often clarifies the correct course of treatment.

Depth of Injury. It should be obvious that patients with a superficial or intermediate-thickness second degree burn heal quite well in less than two weeks as long as the wounds are not mismanaged, are kept clean, and do not become infected. Therefore, treatment with a topical chemotherapeutic agent, exercise, and splinting when necessary uniformly gives a good result. Likewise, in an outpatient burn, covering the wound with an impregnated gauze and a compression dressing and splint yield a good result. For an injury that is deeper than third degree, it is obvious that a poor result will be obtained regardless of the initial type of treatment. Any burn that destroys the tendons and bone is of such a magnitude as to guarantee chronic morbidity. Deep second degree burns can be treated by topical chemotherapeutic agents, exercise, and judicious splinting when a full team is available and the treating physician has an excellent support program. If the viable dermal elements are protected and the patient is given the attention that this type of injury needs, surgery can be avoided and a good result obtained. In the absence of a total team effort, such a patient does better with early excision and grafting provided that an experienced hand surgeon is available and feels comfortable in performing this procedure.

Extent of Hand Burn. A small patch of mixed second and third degree burn on the back of the hand may do very well with dressings and no immediate surgical attention or hospitalization. The patient may be treated in the clinic with dressing changes and use his fingers as tolerated, the decision to operate being made at the end of two and one-half weeks (when second degree burn has healed). This situation is far different from that of the individual who has burned the dorsal and volar surface of his hand completely in a mixed second and third degree pattern. This patient needs hospitalization and a decision about surgical intervention.

Extent of Total Body Thermal Injury. Early excision and grafting shorten hospitalization time only in patients who do not have a large total body burn. There is no evidence that excision and grafting shortens hospitalization time in patients with large burns. Furthermore, there is evidence that patients with large total body burns who are excised and grafted do not share the same functional gains as those with small total body burns, which should be an indication for caution in the individual who is considering a course of surgery. For the patient with a large, life-threatening injury, excision of the hands has a low priority because it is time consuming and uses valuable skin needed for total body coverage.

Location of Injury on Hands. Although more is written about dorsal burns of the hand, a deep second or third degree injury of the volar surface may be even more debilitating and difficult to treat surgically, with poorer long-term results. Thus, one is inclined to treat volar injuries nonsurgically unless it is obvious that healing will not occur.

Associated Injuries. Patients who have experienced significant trauma to other organs are not candidates for early excision and grafting of the associated burn wounds. Systemic considerations always take precedence over regional problems, and these patients are best treated with topical chemotherapeutic agents, splinting, and exercise.

Age of Patient. For any upper extremity problem, function is always the criteria by which results are judged. If the patient is an elderly citizen of a nursing home, it should be obvious that his functional needs are very different from the young blue collar worker who must use a jackhammer. Since the goals of success for the elderly may be simply the ability to eat and perform activities of daily living, a more conservative course of nonexcision may be in order if it saves the patient from several hours of general anesthesia that might be harmful for preexisting cardiac or renal problems. The very young patient with a diagnosed deep second degree or third degree burn, however, is an excellent candidate for early excision and grafting because it has been proved that the chances of cooperation are minimal, and it is highly desirable to achieve a healed wound within seven days. The young patient quickly resumes his preburn life style and usually creates his own hand therapy.

Cooperation of Patient. Regardless of the age of the patient or the type of treatment, lack of cooperation may doom the ultimate result. Patients with significant hand burns require an active hand therapy program after discharge from the hospital, and serial splinting as needed. If the patient will not help himself, the results will be very modest.

Thus, the choice of therapy is multifactorial and one cannot put down a strict rule that applies to every patient. If one decides on early surgical excision, the only issues become when and how. A review of the literature reveals very different opinions on when this procedure should be performed, but in general it seems reasonable to carry it out as soon as the patient is completely stabilized (48 to 72 hours post burn). The technique for excision can be tangential or down to the fascia. For a patient with a deep second degree burn it might indeed be reasonable to start with tangential excision of the burn wound and save any viable dermis and fat possible. To this end, a tourniquet is usually placed on the extremity but not elevated. Once the hand and upper extremity have been sterilely prepared and draped, a Braithwaite or Goullian knife is used to serially excise the burned tissue (Fig. 129–5) in the method popularized by Janzekovic (1970). A sequential excision of the eschar is performed down to punctate bleeding in the dermis. Parts of the wound may be full thickness, in which case the excision is carried down to the fat. Once the excision is completed, hemostasis is achieved with electrocautery or application of topical thrombin solution.

The surgeon is then confronted with several choices. For patients with a deep partial-thickness injury, should he cover the wounds with a biologic dressing and allow spontaneous healing to occur, or graft the wound? Second, should the grafting be done immediately or delayed 24 hours if there is a hemostasis problem? The answer to the first question is that the grafting should always be done. Wounds that heal from deep dermal elements from the back of the hand tend to develop bad hypertrophic scars (Fig. 129–6) and healing is also prolonged. If one is investing the time to operate on the patient, it is reasonable to try to achieve a healed wound as swiftly as possible. To that end, intermediate-thickness split skin grafts are applied to the dorsum of the hand. These grafts are sutured or Steri-stripped into place, the hand is placed on a sterile splint, the wounds are left open, and grafts are rolled regularly to express serum until the skin grafts have taken. If bleeding has been a problem, it is reasonable to mesh the grafts 1½:1 and merely open the mesh wide enough to create the pie crust effect and allow serum and blood

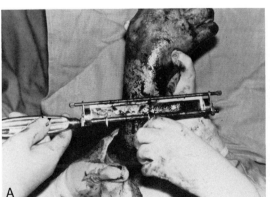
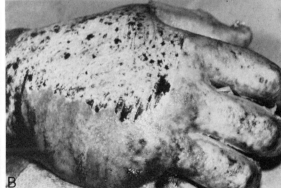

Figure 129–5. *A, B,* Tangential excision must be continued until punctate bleeding occurs. Nonviable tissue must be removed to ensure graft take.

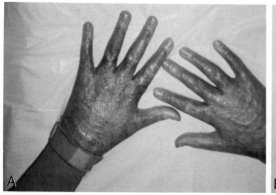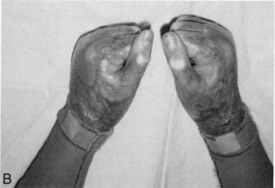

Figure 129–6. *A, B,* Spontaneous healing of deep second degree burns often results in hypertrophic scars. Although function may be good initially, range of motion may deteriorate as scarring worsens.

to escape through the interstices. These grafts should always be applied in the transverse direction so that longitudinal scars do not result over the dorsum of the fingers. No difference in function is noted between meshed and sheet skin as long as it is 1½:1. The cosmetic result obviously is better with sheet skin grafts. The decision whether or not to apply the grafts immediately depends on the hemostasis. The author has never encountered a situation in which hemostasis could not be achieved, provided that the surgeon was patient. Continuous elevation of the upper extremity for five minutes with topical thrombin-soaked sponges should give excellent control of bleeding. If the patient has also had the wrist and forearm excised, it might be worthwhile to place the extremity in biologic dressings such as porcine xenograft or Biobrane, and return to the operating room 24 hours later for definitive grafting. If the patient has been covered by meshed autograft, these wounds should not be left open; the hand should be covered with bulky dressings, and a volar splint, and the dressings should be wet down with silver nitrate, sulfa solution, or even saline to maintain graft viability.

For patients with obvious full-thickness burns, excision at the fascia level is indicated. The limb should be elevated and the pneumatic tourniquet raised to 250 mm. No attempt should be made to exsanguinate the extremity with the Esmarch bandage, or the milking of bacteria through lymphatics could occur, resulting in bacteremia. Excision should be carried down to the fascia (Fig. 129–7), taking great care to retain the dorsal venous network and the paratenon. Obliteration or injury of the dorsal venous network

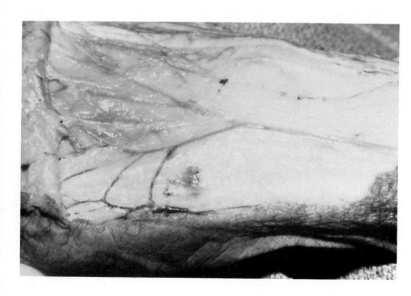

Figure 129–7. Excision must preserve the dorsal venous network and paratenon.

can result in a chronically edematous hand, and stripping the paratenon off the extensor tendons may cause difficulty with graft take and adhesions that make postoperative mobilization difficult. The excision should be carried out along the midlateral plane of the fingers and not more volarly, otherwise longitudinal contractures can occur on the volar surface of the fingers. Incision and excision in the web spaces should be done with darts or V's in order to avoid hooding postoperatively. It is useful to pin the metacarpophalangeal joints in 90 degrees of flexion and allow the interphalangeal joints to rest in very mild flexion. The goal is to provide the greatest amount of good skin on the dorsum of the hand following excision. If the wrist is placed in extension (intentionally or as a result of a bad dressing) and the finger joints in neutral, too little skin is grafted. This is a significant postoperative complication because the patient gets a very tight feeling when attempting to flex the wrist or make a fist. In fact, full flexion may be impossible. The grafts can be stapled or sewn on the recipient bed, but care should be taken not to place the seam of a graft over the joints. If the graft did not heal, the joints would be exposed, leading to significant morbidity. All seams should be transverse, not longitudinal, in order to discourage scar contracture formation. Postoperatively the hands should be maintained with the wrist in flexion, the metacarpophalangeal joints in 90 degrees of flexion, and the fingers in 10 degrees of flexion. If the burn is extended volarly onto the hypothenar or thenar eminence, these areas should be tangentially excised and grafted at the same time. Postoperatively the pins are left in the joints for one week, then removed and therapy begun. There is no necessity to start moving a hand three or five days postoperatively as some authors indicate. Irrevocable stiffness does not occur during a one week immobilization of the hand, and the first priority is to achieve total healing of the skin grafts.

Postoperatively a well-organized program of hand therapy should be instituted. It cannot be emphasized enough that surgery is only 50 per cent of the course of treatment and that no surgeon should suggest this operation unless there is good back-up support for the patient and himself. Patients should receive hand therapy twice a day during the first postoperative month, and splints should be applied according to individual needs. In many hospitals there is no person skilled in therapy for the burned hand. Therapists who are used to treating stroke and cerebral palsy patients may have small knowledge of the limits and the goals of the burned patient. A skin care program must be outlined that will soften grafts and provide lubrication so that cracking and ulceration does not occur. Splints are worn at night to maintain the gains achieved during the day. Day and night splinting with several sets of splints may be necessary to achieve optimal range of motion. The patient with a dorsal and a volar burn may need two separate sets of splints to achieve full range of motion: one to provide maximal extension of the wrist and fingers, and one to employ maximal flexion. All hands should be taken through range of motion exercises. Each joint is exercised individually, care being taken to protect the extensor mechanism. Active fist making can be allowed, for instance, but not passive fist making. Joints are exercised through their available range of motion but never forced into extension or flexion. Most important, measurements should be taken of each finger joint serially over time in the postoperative period to determine if gains are truly being made. Returning strength is determined by testing side and power pinch. If patients are lost to follow-up or an active program is not outlined and adhered to, they will never regain strength and may lose the opportunity for employment.

For individuals who do not require or are not candidates for early excision, the application of topical chemotherapy such as Silvadene should be made twice daily. A light dressing will keep the Silvadene from being rubbed off and yet allow for active range of motion of the fingers. With this regimen the eschar softens and gradually separates in the first 21 days after surgery. Application of biologic dressings and eventually skin grafting can be performed when clean, flat granulation tissue can be prepared.

The criteria for excising deep second or third degree burns of the upper arm or forearm are the same as those for the hand. If very deep second degree burns are allowed to heal spontaneously over four weeks, the result may be unstable skin or severe hypertrophy that is extremely disabling for the working person and esthetically inferior to skin grafting. Tangential excision of these burns is preferable to excision at the level of the fascia because of the severe resultant disfigurement from the latter. Bleeding can be a significant problem, however, if the entire upper extremity is tangentially excised, and several precautions must be taken. If the entire forearm and upper arm are to be excised, at least 500 ml of blood will be lost. A Foley catheter should be in place to monitor urine output during the procedure. Blood replacement should be begun when the patient is anesthetized and as the operation is started. Following excision, the entire wound is sprayed with topical thrombin and warm packs are applied. Elevation of the extremity for five minutes followed by electrocautery will control the bleeding. If there is still unsatisfactory hemostasis, pressure dressings may be applied and grafting done 24 hours later.

Circumferential grafting of the arm is a technically demanding procedure. The most common cause of graft loss is shearing of the splint against the graft in the postoperative period. Several alternative treatments increase the chances of success. Once the bulky dressing is applied, the splint may be placed on the extremity and attached to an overhead traction apparatus or intravenous pole. This maneuver decreases movement (rubbing of the splint against the dressing). If no splint is desirable, insertion of a radial pin and yoke

give superb immobilization. Occasionally, pins are placed also through the olecranon (Fig. 129–8). Pin tract infection has not been a complication, and the pin is removed in seven days when the graft has healed. All grafts must be applied transversely to discourage formation of scar contractures across the elbow or axilla. Use of overhead traction has been extremely helpful in straightening incipient elbow or axillary contractures. The patient with a burned axilla characteristically holds the extemity in adduction, and by two and one-half weeks after the burn, shortening of normal tissue has begun. Attempts to splint the patient (with ungrafted wounds) in abduction are usually unsuccessful because of pain. Once grafting has been done, wound pain diminishes and the patient must be overcorrected in an airplane splint or overhead traction.

In life-threatening burns, the secret of successful excision involves speed, limiting blood loss, and certainty of graft take. Thus, the upper extremities are often excised at the fascial level, using tourniquets to limit blood loss. The dissection can be hazardous unless the surgeon is respectful of anatomy. It is easy to injure the ulnar nerve behind the medial condyle or the median nerve at the cubital fossa or wrist. Dissection with electrocautery may be done if the power is kept low and the fascia is not violated.

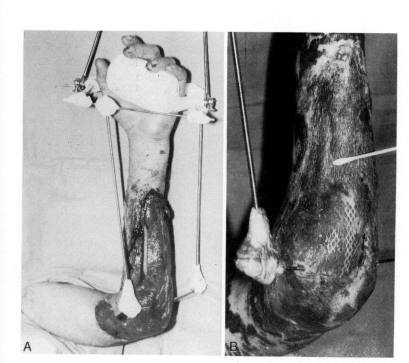

A   B

Figure 129–8. *A, B,* For a circumferential forearm burn with exposed ulnar nerve, pin traction through the olecranon and wrist provides excellent immobilization to achieve a healed wound.

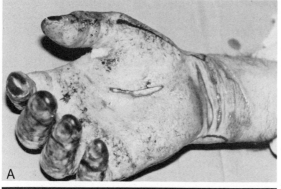
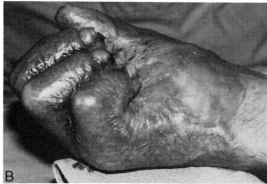
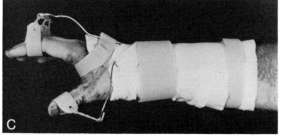

Figure 129–9. *A* to *C,* Deep burns of the palm heal with severe flexion contractures if exercise and splinting are neglected.

COMPLICATIONS

The management of early complications in the burned hand is a separate and very complex subject. These problems include (1) exposed joint capsule or tendons; (2) burned cortex; (3) combined palmar and extensor burn; (4) scar complications—wrist flexion, thumb adduction contracture, proximal interphalangeal flexion and metacarpophalangeal hyperextension, and retraction of interdigital webs; (5) boutonnière deformity; and (6) hypertrophic scars.

The exposed joint capsule may be treated by the application of bacitracin ointment to maintain the moistness of the vital structures, or by coverage with a biologic dressing such as porcine xenograft. The surrounding wound should be cared for in the routine fashion, and usually after a period of several weeks contraction of the local tissue takes place, covering the exposed joint. Mere application of topical chemotherapeutic agents may well result in desiccation of the joint, which would require debridement at a later date.

Burned cortex should be treated by debridement down to viable marrow. A series of dressing changes of wet saline result in granulations that can be skin grafted. If the debridement of the cortex reveals nonviable marrow, this can be a source of infection, and further debridement is done until viable bone

is reached. Exposed flexor or extensor tendons become desiccated if treated with Silvadene or Sulfamyalon; these should be kept wet with saline until covered by surrounding granulation tissue, and then skin grafted.

Deep palmar burns can be treated with topical chemotherapeutic agents until healing has occurred or skin grafting is necessary.

It is common for severe contractures of the palm to develop (Fig. 129–9*A,B*) and therefore it has to be splinted with the wrist in hyperextension (Fig. 129–9*C*), the thumb fully abducted, and all fingers hyperextended for at least a portion of the day. Excision of a palmar burn is rarely done as there is no natural plane for the excision and the bleeding is profuse. If contracture occurs, the wounds can always be opened and skin grafting performed. Scar complications can be avoided by a very vigorous exercise and splinting program. Interdigital web contractures can be prevented by inserts that fit between the fingers, applied under a Jobst glove. For any patient who has had a deep second degree burn or a grafted hand, a Jobst glove should be fitted immediately and applied as soon as healing occurs. This protocol has been found to markedly decrease the incidence of hypertrophic scar and scar complications. Hyperextension can be prevented by early splinting, with the metacarpophalangeal joints in 90 degrees of flexion. Even if the patient does not comply with this program, the application of fingerhook traction will be successful at holding the fingers in their proper position. Patients left to their own devices assume a position of maximal comfort, which is also the position of maximal deformity with the wrist in flexion, the metacarpophalangeal joints in extension, the proximal interphalangeal joints in flexion, and the thumb in adduction. Thus, for a patient with a dorsal burn, the wrist should be splinted in neutral or extension with the metacarpophalangeal joints in 90 degrees of flexion, the interphalangeal joints in neutral, and the thumb widely abducted. If the patient has a volar burn, a separate splint has to be designed to be worn at least part of the day or night; this will allow for full hyperextension of the wrist and fingers as well as abduction of the thumb. These scar deformities are far easier to prevent than they are to correct. Once shortening has occurred of deeply burned skin or wounds that have been skin grafted, it is almost impossible to stretch out the contractures, unlike the situation with normal skin that has merely shortened. Therefore, the key to avoiding these problems is early splinting and exercise, and daily attention to any incipient deformity formation. Occasionally, patients with severe burns of the upper extremity and large total body burns are unable to cooperate. Those on a ventilator are so sick that they cannot participate in their own care. Sometimes these patients' hands, in spite of excellent splinting, begin to contract and form secondary deformities. In this small group of patients, if one does not attack the problem immediately, the hand is destroyed by the time they are healed from their large total body burn and have survived. Therefore, it is best to perform internal splinting during a trip to the operating room for some other reason. These patients do well with early internal fixation with Steinman pins, the metacarpophalangeal joints being in 90 degrees and the interphalangeal joints in a neutral position. Internal splinting counteracts the tendency for contracture formation. Pin tract infection has not been a problem. The experience of Achauer and associates (1974) with children has been the same as the author's in that there has been no disturbance in growth to the fingers. When the patient is more responsive and can cooperate, the pins can be removed and range of motion begun. It is unwise to leave these pins in position longer than three weeks in adults, because fixed contractures may occur.

Extensor tendon destruction can be prevented in a severe burn on the dorsal aspect of the fingers by maintaining the interphalangeal joints in neutral. If destruction of the tendon has occurred and the patient has developed a boutonnière deformity, it is wise immediately to pin the interphalangeal joint in a hyperextended position. Once healing has occurred with this regimen, the patient may not need further surgery. If a boutonnière deformity develops, application of external splints is usually unsuccessful because the dorsal pressure needed to keep the proximal interphalangeal joint in neutral or extension is so great that the overlying skin is destroyed and infection occurs.

The development of hypertrophic scars is an extremely severe problem that, once present, is almost impossible to correct without extensive surgery. Its prevention should be paramount. It is the author's practice to order a Jobst glove for any patient who has had skin grafting of the hand or whose wounds have taken longer than 14 days to heal. It has been found that wounds that take a prolonged time to heal are most prone to developing hypertrophic scars. Patients with wounds that have been skin grafted (especially blacks and other dark-skinned people) are also liable to develop hypertrophic scars, and the glove is therefore applied as a prophylactic measure. Oiling of the skin with any of the commercially available preparations is extremely important in order to avoid ulcerations or tissue breakdown with new deposition of scar. The formation of heavy scar along suture lines where skin grafts have been applied can be treated judiciously by small injections of triamcinolone acetonide (Kenalog).

In summary, the history of management of the burned hand represents a fascinating survey of the basic concepts of wound healing in plastic surgery. The challenges have peaked the interest of some of our finest scientists and surgeons. Results have steadily improved. The clinician must be aware that multiple techniques are now available to give superior results. Choice of the correct modality of treatment for each patient remains the greatest challenge.

REFERENCES

Achauer, B., Bartlett, R., Furnas, D., Allyn, P., and Wingerson, E.: Internal fixation in the management of the burned hand. Arch. Surg., *108*:814, 1974.

Aldrich, R. H.: Treatment of burns with a compound of aniline dyes. N. Engl. J. Med., *217*:911, 1937.

Allen, H. S.: Treatment of superficial injuries and burns of the hand. J.A.M.A., *116*:1370, 1939.

Apfel, L. M., Synolegard, T., Wachtel, T., and Frank, H.: Functional hand assessment after enyzmatic debridement and early autografting. J. Burn Care Rehab., *5*:438, 1984.

Bettman, A. G.: The rationale of the tannic acid–silver nitrate treatment of burns. J.A.M.A., *108*:1490, 1937.

Blair, V., and Byars, L.: Treatment of wounds resulting from deep burns. J.A.M.A., *110*:1802, 1938.

Bondoc, C. C., Quinby, W. C., and Burke, J. F.: Primary surgical management of the deeply burned hand in children. J. Pediatr. Surg., *11*:335, 1976.

Boswick, J. A.: Rehabilitation of the burned hand. Clin. Orthop., *104*:162, 1974.

Braithwaite, F.: Treatment of dorsal burns of the hand. Br. J. Plast. Surg., *2*:21, 1949.

Brown, H. C.: Current concepts of burn pathology and mechanisms of deformity in the burned hand. Orthop. Clin. North Am., *4*:987, 1973.

Brown, J. B.: The repair of surface defects of the hand. Ann. Surg., *107*:952, 1938.

Brown, J. B.: Surface defects of the hand. Am. J. Surg., *46*:690, 1939.

Bunyan, J.: Envelope method of treating burns. Rec. R. Soc. Med., *34*:65, 1941.

Burke, J. F., Bondoc, C. C., Quinby, W. C., Jr., and Remensynder, J. P.: Primary surgical management of the deeply burned hands. J. Trauma, *16*:593, 1976.

Cannon, B., and Zuidema, G.: Care and treatment of the burned hand. Clin. Orthop., *15*:111, 1959.

Coan, G.: Ferric chloride coagulation in treatment of burns. Surg. Gynecol. Obstet., *61*:687, 1935.

Cohen, S. M.: Experience in the treatment of war burns. Br. Med. J., *2*:251, 1940a.

Cohen S. M.: The treatment of burns, tannic acid versus saline. Br. Med. J., *2*:754, 1940b.

Cope, O, Langohr, J., Moore, F. D., and Webster, R. C.: Expeditious care of full thickness burn wounds by surgical excision and grafting. Ann. Surg., *125*:1, 1947.

Edstrom, L., Robson, M. C., Macchiauerna, J. R., and Scala, A. D.: Management of deep partial thickness dorsal hand burns: study of operative vs. nonoperative therapy. Orthop. Rev., *8*:27, 1979.

Fissette, J., Onkelinx, A., and Fandi, N.: Carpal and Guyon tunnel syndrome in burns at the wrist. J. Hand Surg., *6*:13, 1981.

Gant, T. D.: The early enzymatic debridement and grafting of deep dermal burns to the hand. Plast. Reconstr. Surg., *66*:185, 1980.

Greeley, P. A.: The plaster repair of cutaneous injuries of the hand. Ind. Med., *9*:300, 1940.

Hooker, D. H., and Lam, C.: Absorption of sulfanilamide from burned surfaces. Surgery, *9*:534, 1941.

Huang, T., Larson, D., and Lewis, S.: Burned hands. Plast. Reconstr. Surg., *56*:21, 1975.

Hunt, J., and Sato, R.: Early excision of full thickness hand and digit burns: factors affecting morbidity. J. Trauma, *22*:414, 1982.

Janzekovic, Z.: A new concept. Early excision and immediate grafting burns. J. Trauma, *10*:1103, 1970.

Labandter, H., Kaplan, I., and Shavitt, C.: Burns of the dorsum of the hand. Br. J. Plast. Surg., *29*:352, 1976.

Levine, B. A., Sorinek, K., Peterson, H., and Pruitt, B. A.: Efficacy of tangential excision and immediate autografting of deep second degree burns of the hand. J. Trauma, *19*:670, 1979.

Magliacani, G., Bormioli, M., and Cerutti, V.: Late results following treatment of deep burns of the hand. Scand. J. Plast. Reconstr. Surg., *13*:137, 1979.

Mason, M. L.: Plastic surgery and repair. Ind. Med., *10*:49, 1941.

McIndoe, A. H.: The burned hand. Med. Press Circ., *211*:57, 1944.

Moncrief, J. A., Switzer, W. E., and Rose, L. R.: Primary excision and grafting in the treatment of third-degree burns of the dorsum of the hand. Plast. Reconstr. Surg., *33*:305, 1964.

Moyer, C. A., Brentano, L., Gravens, D. L., Margraf, H. W., and Monafo, W. W., Jr.: Treatment of large human burns with 0.5% silver nitrate solution. Arch. Surg., *90*:812, 1965.

Peacock, E. E., Jr., Madden, J. W., and Trier, W. C.: Some studies on the treatment of burned hands. Ann. Surg., *171*:903, 1970.

Ross, J. A., and Hulbert, K. F.: Treatment of burns by siver nitrate–tannic acid and gentian violet. Br. Med. J., *2*:702, 1940.

Ross, J. A., and Hulbert, K. F.: Treatment of 100 war wounds and burns. Br. Med. J., *1*:618, 1941.

Ross, W. P.: The treatment of recent burns of the hand. Br. J. Plast. Surg., *2*:233, 1950.

Roulston, T. J.: Closed plaster treatment of burns of the extremities. Br. Med. J., *2*:611, 1941.

Salisbury, R. E., Loveless, S., Silverstein, P., Wilmore, D. W., Moylan, J. A., and Pruitt, B. A.: Postburn edema of the upper extremity. J. Trauma, *13*:857, 1973.

Salisbury, R. E., McKeel, D., and Mason, A. D.: Ischemic necrosis of the small muscles of the hand after thermal injury. Bone Joint Surg.., *56A*:1701, 1974.

Salisbury, R. E., Taylor, J. W., and Levine, N. S.: Evaluation of digital escharotomy in burned hands. Plast. Reconstr. Surg., *58*:440, 1976.

Salisbury, R., and Wright, P.: Evaluation of early excision of dorsal burns of the hand. Plast. Reconstr. Surg., *69*:670, 1982.

Sherman, W.: The paraffin wax or closed method of treatment of burns. Surg. Gynecol. Obstet., *26*:450, 1918.

Smith, J. W.: Burned hands in children. Am. J. Surg., *112*:58, 1966.

Storch, M., Dolich, B., and Stein, J.: Impending ischemic contracture in the burned hand and upper extremity. Bull. Hosp. Joint Dis., *37*:63, 1976.

Trueta, J.: Principles and Management of War Surgery. London, Hamish, H., & Heinemann, Ltd., 1946.

Wakely, C.: The treatment of war burns. Surgery, *10*:208, 1941.

Whitson, T. C., and Allen, B. D.: Management of the burned hand. J. Trauma, *11*:606, 1971.

Henry W. Neale

Electrical Injuries of the Hand and Upper Extremity

Electricity was first introduced for commercial use in 1849, but the first reported fatality occurred in 1879 when a carpenter from Lyons, France was killed by a 250 volt alternating current source while working on a generator (Arturson and Hedlund, 1984). This initial case essentially established a pattern of injury that is maintained today. Fortunately, electrical burn injuries are uncommon, making up only 3 to 5 per cent of admissions to major burn units. Most of these injuries are work related and the victims are almost exclusively male. Nonindustrial injuries are usually related to erecting television or radio antennas or to children playing with faulty electrical wiring. Since most of the injuries are work related, the hands and upper extremity are usually the entrance site because of the initial contact, and the legs and feet are the exit, or grounding point.

Electrical injuries vary from a relatively harmless shock requiring no treatment to major life-threatening injuries with loss of extremities, long-term sequelae, and sometimes death. The major electrical injuries involve tissue destruction beyond skin and subcutaneous tissue into nerve, muscle, and bone to varying degrees. The present management of these patients remains difficult and in some cases controversial despite major advancements in the care of burn victims.

ELECTRICAL PHYSIOLOGY

Electrical burn injuries occur with the passage of electrons or current through tissue. Some controversy persists as to whether the resultant damage is secondary to the direct effect of current flow or to the head produced by this flow. The current flow (I) is dependent on two factors, the voltage (V) and the resistance (R). They are related by Ohm's law: $I = V/R$.

Voltage represents the amount of electromotive force, or push, behind the electrons. Jellinek (1931) showed that a voltage source as low as 40 volts can be fatal if applied under appropriate conditions. Voltage is supplied either as a constant source, i.e., direct current, or a cyclic source such as alternating current. Alternating current is more dangerous than direct and may induce cardiac ventricular fibrillation and tachycardia with subsequent arrest. Common household electric current at 110 to 120 volts and 60 Hz may be dangerous from a cardiac standpoint. By convention, high tension injuries are usually defined as voltage levels of 1000 volts or greater. Since current flow is directly propor-

$$\text{Least} \xleftarrow{\hspace{1cm}} \frac{\text{Tissue resistance to current damage}}{\text{Nerve, vessel, muscle, skin, tendon, fat, bone}} \xrightarrow{\hspace{1cm}} \text{Greatest}$$

tional to voltage (Ohm's law), the higher the voltage, the greater is the tissue destruction and sequelae in electrical injuries. Death from electrical injury may occur at much lower levels with little tissue changes because of cardiac arrhythmias and/or respiratory arrest induced by passage of the current through the brain stem.

Resistance is that quality of a material which resists the flow of electrons. In uniform, nonbiologic conductors such as copper or silver, this is a relative constant and predictable factor. However, in biologic materials, resistance varies widely from tissue to tissue, influenced by a host of factors including skin thickness, moisture, vascularity, breaks in skin continuity, and type of contact with the skin.

The generally accepted ranking of resistance of electrical injuries in tissue is that from least to greatest (see above).

Specific values are impossible to interpret as all values are relative and dependent on a number of factors. However, a few generalities can be stated. Chapuis (1919–1920) showed that skin has an average resistance of approximately 4000 ohms/sq cm and the hand about 40,000 ohms/sq cm. The dry, hard, calloused hands of a laborer may even approach a resistance of 2,000,000 ohms/sq cm. Critchley (1934) demonstrated that resistance can be reduced by approximately 10 to 12 times where moisture or perspiration is present. It then becomes clear that an individual's make-up may determine whether he sustains a minor shock or a fatal encounter. Once current flow is established, the electrical energy views the limb, the trunk, and the rest of the human body as a volume conductor. The current fans out and flows through the entire cross section of the limb. This important physiologic concept of current density, measured in amps per square centimeter, determines the heat and damage produced by an electrical injury (Sances and associates, 1981). Anatomically, the current density is concentrated at both the entrance and exit sites, and thus the most clinical damage is seen here also. Additionally, as current flows through the hand, wrist, and forearm there is a relatively high degree of concentration of current, and greater tissue destruction can be noted at these sites. As the current passes through the large cross sectional areas of the trunk and thigh, the current density is diminished and often little tissue damage is noted. However, as the current flows down the leg, its density increases as it approaches the relatively small cross sectional area of the ankle and foot, and more tissue destruction is noted. This is confirmed in the author's clinical experience, since the most tissue-destructive effects in the upper extremity are seen at the entry site, and in the lower leg through the exit sites.

ELECTRICAL PATHOPHYSIOLOGY

Early research efforts in electrical injuries showed two theories available to explain the tissue destruction that occurred. The first theory held that injury was produced by the actual flow of electrons through the cell membrane causing changes, subsequent cell injury, and death. The second theory proposed that tissue injury occurred secondary to the thermal injury that accompanied current flow. Joule's law states that P = power or heat = I^2R. Heat is produced at the time of current flow, and subsequent studies have shown that most electrical injuries were due to the heat produced and its multiple effects. There is evidence from Skoog's work (1970) that tissue damage may occur without heat production. In his experiments Skoog applied current through intact sciatic nerves of rats and cats and showed that the effects of heat were negated by immersing the nerve in cool electrolyte solution. He found that changes were induced in the peripheral nerves, which resulted in an increased threshold and prolonged latency. In a significant study in 1928, Jaffe attempted to explain the empirical observation that vascular injury was associated with electrical burns, by applying current to isolated segments of femoral arteries. It was noted that no damage occurred in the vessels when blood flow was maintained; however, when blood flow was interrupted during the passage of current, significant structural alterations occurred. The pathologic findings in these vessels were duplicated by the application of a wire heated and flamed. It is now generally accepted that the destruction seen with electrical burn injuries is primarily due to the production of heat from current flow. Joule's law determines how this heat is produced.

Nerve, with its relatively low tissue resistance, carries the greatest amount of current and therefore generates the largest amount of heat. Blood vessels carry the next greatest current flow and produce a great deal of heat energy. The latter are extremely heat sensitive, and it is here that most clinical pathologic conditions and subsequent injuries occur through thrombosis of nutrient vessels. Bone, with its high current resistance, was believed for years to be the source of deep tissue destruction from heat, but one recalls that its high resistance means little current flow with little heat generation. Studies by Hunt (1976) and others have shown that bone eventually reached the temperature of the limb in electrical injuries but did not exceed the temperature of the surrounding tissues.

There remains some controversy regarding the pathologic changes of electrical injuries and their subsequent course. It has been proposed that progressive tissue destruction occurs perhaps secondary to "heat" generated by bone. The management of electrical injuries is sometimes difficult and frustrating in that the wound appears to undergo continuing changes with further tissue loss often for weeks after the acute injury. Even prostaglandins have been proposed as a cause of the progression of tissue loss (Robson, Murphy, and Hegger, 1984).

In 1974 Hunt and associates clarified much of this tissue. They performed a series of arteriograms of extremities in victims of acute electrical burns in an attempt to delineate the exact level of tissue destruction, and made a number of interesting findings. With complete vascular occlusion there was massive tissue destruction, which was found significantly proximal to the point of complete occlusion. Areas of "pruning" and partial occlusion were noted that led to the presence of apparent "skip" areas. In areas of decreased nutrient muscular branches, the muscle tissue on surgical exploration was found to be pale and irreversibly damaged, despite evidence of bleeding when cut. It was thought that the progressive muscle necrosis seen with electrical injuries was not actually progressive, but rather the normal evolution of irreversible muscle injury that occurred with the initial vascular insult. The arteriographic findings are often subtle, consisting of decreased nutrient vessels, beading, narrowing, and irregularity, and their pathologic significance in terms of muscle injury is usually grossly underestimated. The findings of this clinical experience were further refined and reinforced in a controlled laboratory experience (Hunt, 1976).

MECHANISM OF INJURY

Electrical injuries have been likened to crush injuries because of the massive tissue destruction and the complex nature of involvement (Artz, 1974). A flame burn may be sustained by the electrical flash from arcing, which may ignite the victim's clothing, adding routine thermal injury to the complex problems. If contact with an electrical source establishing grounding is present, heat induces tissue damage from current flow, as previously discussed. A phenomenon frequently observed with high tension injury (>1000 volts) is arcing across flexor surfaces (Fig. 130–1). Approximately 10,000 volts are required to jump a gap of 1 cm, but once established, this arc may be for greater distances. Arc injuries are particularly devastating because they are capable of generating temperatures in the range of 3000° to 5000°C. At this temperature, soft tissue and bone are vaporized. The usual anatomic site of arcing is between the hand and wrist, and from the

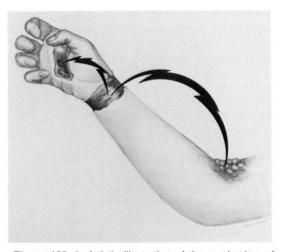

Figure 130–1. Artist's illustration of the mechanism of arc electrical injury of the palm to the wrist to the antecubital area after grabbing a high tension line. The clinical example in Figure 130–2A illustrates this process.

forearm across the elbow to the upper arm (Fig. 130–1).

The extent of electrical injury is dependent on numerous factors such as the type of current, voltage, the path of flow through the victim, and resistance, especially at the entrance site. The current flow at the initiation of electrical injury is often high but then precipitously falls at the time of arcing. With arcing vaporization and charring of the tissue, there is a rise in resistance that prevents further current flow.

As long as current flow is established, heat is generated in the limb, primarily in the nerves, blood vessels, and muscles. Blood vessels are especially susceptible to heat and can easily thrombose. Bone eventually attains a uniform temperature, but not as rapidly as the soft tissues (Hunt, 1976).

ASSESSMENT

Because electrical injuries can occur from any number of mechanisms, a thorough history must be obtained. One should elicit from the victim, the family, or the emergency medical team any available information regarding the source of the electricity, contact point, type of grounding, voltage, duration of contact, presence of moisture, loss of consciousness, occurrence of fall at the time of injury, and any emergency or resuscitation measures undertaken at the scene of the accident. It is especially important to know the amount of voltage because, in general, the higher the voltage, the greater is the degree of tissue destruction, associated injuries, and sequelae.

A complete physical assessment must be performed, since most injuries are work related and associated with muscle tetany. The victim is often hurled away from the contact point, adding the possibility of blunt trauma and head and long bone injuries. Respiratory and cardiac disorders and arrests, compressions to the vertebral bodies, and extremity fractures secondary to tetany must be evaluated. In assessing the upper extremity electrical injury, one should note the presence or absence of swelling, tense skin, pain on passive extension of the digits, numbness, absence of pulses, distal cyanosis or poor capillary refill, fixed contractures, or charred appearance.

The initial appearance of the electrical injury often belies the extent of tissue destruc-tion beneath. This underestimation is usually made by the patient, the family, and even the attending physician. Typically, one realizes only the "tip of the iceberg" on the initial assessment of the electrical injury, and the true extent of devitalized tissue is apparent only weeks later. In cases of more severe injuries, the primary physician should stress the uncertainty of outcome to the patient and family rather than make optimistic promises as to salvage or loss of injured extremities. The extent of damage from electrical injuries is almost always greater than one's first impression.

TREATMENT

Early Management

FLUID RESUSCITATION AND MONITORING

In contrast to common thermal burn injuries, the total body surface area involved in electrical injuries has little relationship to the required fluid replacement. Baxter (1970) and others laid down general guidelines and formulas for fluid replacement. The vascular pathology associated with these injuries extends the tissue loss far beyond the apparent cutaneous limits of the involvement, often involving the entire extremity in a fourth degree manner with extensive muscle damage. At a minimum, the patient will require 4 ml/kg of Ringer's lactate per percentage of burn as recommended by the Parkland Formula. It is impossible to predict accurately the total fluid resuscitation requirement necessary in electrical injuries. The patient should be carefully monitored and subsequent fluid should be administered to maintain a urine diuresis of 50 to 100 ml per hour, as measured by Foley catheter. This is especially important, as electrical injuries release a large amount of myoglobin into the bloodstream. Depending on the patient's cardiac status, fluid requirement may necessitate the insertion of a central venous line or Swan-Ganz catheter to resuscitate the patient adequately and monitor the cardiovascular status. A high rate of urine output should be maintained as long as the urine contains pigment. In a badly damaged extremity, it is not uncommon for fluid replacement to exceed 6 to 8 liters in 24 hours. Acidosis is a common constituent in major burn injuries and is more threatening in electrical injuries because of the extensive tissue devitalization. The pH should be monitored by serial arterial blood gases and corrected by administration of sodium bicarbonate when indicated.

The problem of myoglobinuria in electrical injuries can be serious and must be addressed. Butler and Gant (1977) and Rouse and Dimick (1978) report the incidence of acute renal failure in patients with electrical injuries as varying from 1.5 to 7.5 per cent. The low flow status associated with a large chromatin load secondary to tissue destruction can rapidly lead to renal impairment from precipitation of the pigments in the renal tubules. The complication can be successfully avoided by maintaining an adequate diuresis and alkalinization of the urine. Mannitol, an osmotic diuretic, has been especially effective in promoting and maintaining an adequate urine flow when administered with concomitant intravenous replacement of fluid. Initially, 25 gm followed by 5 to 10 gm per hour may be given in conjunction with adequate fluid replacement. Serum electrolytes and renal function studies should be frequently monitored during the fluid resuscitation period.

ASSOCIATED INJURIES

Fractures and dislocations can be associated with electrical injuries. During the initial insult the victim is sometimes thrown or falls from a height, sustaining a fracture. An alternating current electrical injury causes a tetanizing effect, and this sudden, mass contracture of muscle can lead to fractures and dislocations. A careful, thorough examination of all extremities and the spine should be undertaken and appropriate x-ray studies obtained. In the unconscious patient care should be taken to protect and stabilize the cervical spine. X-ray examination of both the skull and spine should be performed to rule out any occult injury. It is important to remember to obtain x-ray films of the involved hand and upper extremity that incurs the electrical injury.

Electrical current that flows through the heart can cause ventricular fibrillation and cardiac standstill. Alternating current of 40 to 100 cycles per second and as little as 80 to 100 milliamp flow can lead to fibrillation. Since ventricular fibrillation is the leading cause of sudden death following electrical injury, an electrocardiogram should be obtained and the patient monitored after such an injury. Approximately 40 per cent of patients exhibit some form of abnormality including ST-T irregularities, intraventricular block, supraventricular extrasystoles, ventricular systole, and atrial fibrillation. Enzymatic serum levels are not particularly helpful in the overall management because a large amount of cellular enzymes are released into the bloodstream in electrical injuries along with the extensive muscle destruction.

Additional associated injuries include direct neuronal damage to the brain, spinal cord, and peripheral nerves. The electrically injured victim may appear neurologically intact initially, only to demonstrate ascending and progressive neurologic damage several days later. Even more disturbing are reports of neurologic injury appearing several months after the accident. Patients sustaining significant electrical injury should undergo early and periodic neurologic evaluations.

Visceral damage from electrical injuries ranges from simple ileus to slough of the entire abdominal wall, with necrosis of numerous intra-abdominal organs and Curling's stress ulcer. Special examinations of the abdomen should be undertaken if the electric current path involves the abdominal cavity, even though there may be no gross evidence of entrance or exit wounds.

DIAGNOSIS

Electrical injuries often appear deep, diffuse, and spotty in nature and at one time were thought to undergo progressive de nouveau necrosis. Hunt's studies (1976) showed that these changes occur acutely and are only the natural progression of the initial injury. Although this knowledge is helpful, the clinical judgment involved in determining which areas are viable remains a perplexing problem. In attempting to further define the territory of tissue loss, Hunt in 1976 performed arteriography acutely on electrically injured victims. These studies, while important in defining limits of vascular pathology, were not practical or accurate enough to aid surgical debridement beyond standard clinical means. The vascular nature of these wounds led to further investigations attempting to determine viability on the basis of muscle perfusion. Because the contrast dye of an arteriogram induces an osmotic diuresis that can result in hypovolemia, this procedure should be performed when indicated only after the patient has been adequately resuscitated.

Technetium-99m stannous pyrophosphate is an isotope used extensively to detect areas of muscle necrosis (Hunt and associates, 1979). Damaged skeletal myocytes preferentially take up this isotope. Clinical trials utilizing this isotope unfortunately proved it to be too sensitive a method for the detection of myonecrosis. Muscle groups with as little as 20 per cent necrosis and potential recovery were interpreted as positive on scan. However, Holliman and associates (1982) reported the isotope as a helpful adjunct in determining the extent of muscle injury after the initial fasciotomy in severely damaged limbs. Xenon-133 has been used in a wash-out technique to determine the level of muscle-blood flow (Clayton and associates, 1977). This method was not sensitive enough to predict tissue viability. In both techniques clinical evaluation of the muscle was required to determine accurately the need for surgical debridement. Intravenous fluorescein has also been of limited value intraoperatively in distinguishing viable from nonviable muscle.

In normal individuals there is a wide range of muscle-blood flow and even the gross presence of distal pulses, either palpable or measured by Doppler, is no guarantee of proximal tissue viability in electrical injuries. In order to refine surgical debridement, attempts have been made to utilize frozen section and permanent section pathologic examination to guide surgical debridement (Quinby and associates, 1978). Again, clinical diagnostic acumen predominates as the major determining factor. Histologic examinations only confirm the pathologic process at hand. At the present time, the patchy, diffuse nature of the disease process defies accurate preoperative assessment, and the surgeon's best diagnostic tool is his own surgical judgment.

INITIAL SURGICAL CARE

It is recommended that patients with electrical injuries, as in all cases of severe tissue destruction, receive tetanus toxoid and, in some cases, hyperimmune globulin. The administration of antibiotic is controversial for complex injuries, but clostridial infection, although rarely reported, is always a possibility. The mainstay of treatment in severe electrical injuries, aggressive surgical debridement, is repeated, and antibiotics are usually administered in the infection phase after the taking of appropriate cultures and sensitivity determination. Once stabilized the injured extremity should be carefully examined, and clothing, restrictive apparel, and jewelry removed. The posture and attitude should be observed, and the extent of cutaneous burns, evidence of arcing, and the presence or absence of pulses should be documented. It is important to remember that the mere presence of a peripheral pulse does not ensure viability of the injured extremity.

Fasciotomy. In view of the extensive neurologic problems that may evolve, a thorough neuromuscular examination of the injured extremity and the entire patient should be performed. Every reasonable attempt should be made to salvage a neurologically intact limb in an electrical injury (Hunt, Sato, and Baxter, 1980). Of the three major nerves of the upper limb, the median usually sustains the greatest loss, while the radial sustains the least (DiVincenti, Moncrief, and Pruitt, 1969). Because of the involvement of all tissues, Artz (1974) compared electrical with crush injuries. As in the latter type, fasciotomy plays a major role in the early management of decompression of extensively damaged tissue. While a simple escharotomy is often adequate for third degree thermal injuries, an extensive and deep fasciotomy is indicated for tense and edematous upper extremity electrical wounds (Fig. 130-2). A thorough, complete release of all involved compartments must be carried out and this usually precludes treatment at the bedside. These procedures are best undertaken in the operating room with proper anesthesia, lighting, instruments, and equipment. As a general rule, fasciotomies should be performed shortly after admission, and initial stabilization ideally within the first six hours. If the patient's condition permits, debridement of grossly devitalized tissue can also be carried out at this time. Fasciotomy is indicated in mummified or charred extremities, for extensive burns, and in the presence of decreased perfusion, deteriorating neurologic status, or marked edema (Fig. 130-3). In marginal cases, wick catheters may be helpful in determining the level of intramuscular pressure, as shown by Saffle, Zeluffe, and Warden in 1980. In equivocal cases, however, one should err on the side of performing a fasciotomy rather than adopting a "wait and

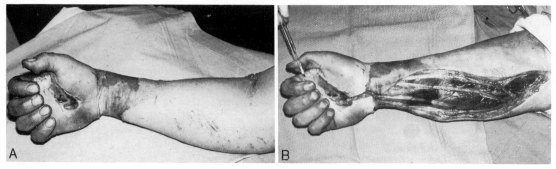

Figure 130–2. *A,* Appearance of a workman's right hand after sustaining high tension, high voltage electrical injury where the exits were the feet and knees. Note the deep fourth degree burn of the palm of the hand and wrist secondary to arcing of the electrical current, and the relatively normal skin of the thenar eminence and volar forearm. The hand was clenched and the wrist flexed as a result of tetanic contraction. *B,* Appearance of the same subject six hours later after "lazy-S" fasciotomy, which was extended into the palm to release the carpal tunnel. Note the marked bulging of the muscle with skip areas of black necrosis. The extent of nerve and vascular damage after the fasciotomy was equivocal, and three days later the patient underwent a below the elbow amputation and secondary wound closure with split-thickness skin graft.

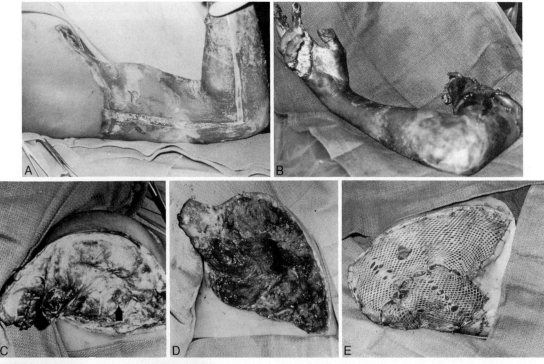

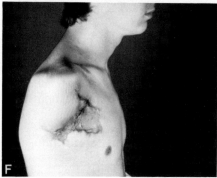

Figure 130–3. *A,* Right arm of a 16 year old boy who sustained a 12,000 volt high tension electrical injury to his hand, forearm, and arm with the mummified, charred right extremity extending into the axilla. *B,* After an early fasciotomy, amputation of the right arm at the high humeral level was performed three days after admission, to prevent sepsis. *C,* Appearance of the right shoulder with a short humeral bone stump protruding, and appearance of the soft tissue wound with extensive necrosis persisting. The dark arrow points to suture ligated axillary vessels. This wound required four additional aggressive surgical debridements. *D,* Healthy appearance of the wound following disarticulation at the shoulder, excision of all devitalized muscle, and more proximal ligation of the thrombosed axillary artery to avoid delayed hemorrhage. *E,* Appearance of the wound after coverage with nonexpanded mesh graft for wound closure. This wound could have been covered with a latissimus dorsi musculocutaneous flap, but there was thrombosis of the thoracodorsal vessel upon exploration. *F,* Appearance of right shoulder disarticulation after the skin graft and wound edges had contracted. This was three months after the initial injury and the patient was awaiting fitting of a shoulder disarticular limb prosthesis.

see" attitude. In fasciotomies all compartments should be released and (just as important) explored for viability. It should be remembered that viable muscle may overlie deep necrotic structures in electrical injuries. When the hand is involved, the "lazy-S" fasciotomy incisions should be carried across the wrist as in a formal carpal tunnel release (Fig. 130–2).

When the neurologic evaluation for possible median and ulnar nerve compression at the carpal level is equivocal, electromyography performed at the bedside may help decide the status of early neural decompression. The goals of the surgeon caring for electrical injuries of the upper extremity should be (1) adequate decompression; (2) aggressive and thorough removal of all devitalized tissue; (3) preservation of important functional structures such as nerves, tendons, vessels, and joints; and (4) safe but rapid wound closure. To expedite this end, attempts have been made to establish the limits and extent of debridement by the use of arteriography, scanning, and pathologic tissue examination, but in general these have been unsuccessful. Hunt (1976) demonstrated in electrical injuries that muscle, while appearing pale and noncontractile, actually bled when cut and later proved to be nonviable. The extent of surgical debridement often mandates clinical judgment at the operating table, and even under direct examination the amount of tissue to sacrifice is a difficult decision. Although amputation is rarely indicated during the initial debridement, it may be required in a highly unstable patient. A "medical amputation" of the affected extremity may be performed with a tourniquet and by packing the extremity in ice until the patient's overall condition permits formal amputation.

After fasciotomy and initial debridement, the wound should be carefully dressed in a topical antibiotic. A number of antibiotics especially designed for burn care are available, such as silver sulfadiazine (Silvadene), mafenide (Sulfamylon), and silver nitrate. In view of the deep nature of electrical injuries, Baxter (1970) and others recommended Sulfamylon as the primary drug of choice; it penetrates tissues to a greater degree than other topical agents, but its use is complicated by pain on application and occasional hypochloremia and acidosis. Following initial debridement and dressing, the hand should be carefully splinted, since the goal is to pre-

serve motion and hand function. The optimal hand posture is in the "safe" position with the wrist in 30 degrees of extension, the metacarpophalangeal joints in 70 degrees of flexion, the proximal interphalangeal joints in extension, and the thumb in full palmar abduction. This position places all ligaments in full stretch and prevents shortening during the acute coverage phase. Plans should be made to involve a hand therapist early in the course of treatment to preserve and maximize function of the injured extremity.

If the patient's general condition permits, he should be returned to the operating room every other day for additional clinical evaluation and debridement of all devitalized tissues. Even in electrical injuries restricted to the upper extremity, numerous procedures may eventually be required to obtain satisfactory debridement and coverage (Fig. 130–3). Holliman and associates (1982) reported an average of 7.8 surgical procedures per patient. Vital structures that are viable but exposed because of debridement of overlying necrotic tissue should be kept moist with Vaseline, or preferably dressed with a temporary biologic dressing as a homograft or heterograft. The filmy peritenon or epineurial protective covering over tendons and nerves should be kept intact if viable. If exposed nerve or tendon is not grossly necrotic and septic, it may be possible to preserve and later cover these structures. Such treatment may allow some nerve regeneration and useful tendon glide without muscle unit shortening, as is seen with tendon debridement. Fasciotomy incisions may be closed by delayed primary closure following resolution of edema, or by skin grafting if swelling persists. Exposed muscle bellies usually are easily covered with split-thickness skin grafts. An attempt should be made after debridement to obtain rapid, durable coverage to permit early motion and primary healing and subsequent reconstructive procedures. Electrical wounds of the upper extremity are complex and their multiple areas of partial devitalization lead to extensive scarring, which is only further promoted if these wounds are allowed to heal by secondary intention.

Nerves, Tendons, Bones, Joints, Vessels. Nerves, tendons, bone, and joints require thick vascular and durable coverage. Tendons and joints especially need well-padded coverage under which to glide and move.

Initial coverage efforts should take into account further reconstructive procedures such as tendon, nerve, and bone grafts. In some cases, acute coverage can be obtained with split-thickness skin grafting, acknowledging that this will be replaced at a later date with flap coverage when the patient is in a more stable condition. Some authors have recommended that exposed intact bone, lacking periosteal coverage, be left in situ to act as a bone graft provided it is clean and not infected (Luce and Gottlieb, 1984). Although this approach has been successful for exposed calvarium following electrical injuries, relatively early flap coverage is mandatory. Because of the heavily contaminated burn wound, compound fractures should be reduced and stabilized by skeletal fixation rather than by open plating and screws, in order to reduce the risk of future osteomyelitis or sepsis (Salisbury and Dingeldein, 1982a).

After extensive surgical debridement, major vessels may be thrombosed, subjecting them to secondary thrombosis and infection through exposure. Wang and associates (1982, 1984) reported successful attempts to salvage extremities with severe electrical injuries by vascular thrombosis at the wrist level, using interpositional vein grafts. Although these heroic efforts are sometimes successful, the results are often complicated by secondary infection, exposure, or even hemorrhage. If this very early and aggressive course of treatment is chosen, debridement must be extremely thorough, the wound must be free of infection, and immediate flap coverage is necessary.

Later Management

WOUND COVERAGE (See also Chap. 132)

After all the devitalized tissues of the electrical injuries of the extremity have been excised, all viable tissues have been preserved, and the immediate threat of infection is past, vital structures such as nerves, tendons, vessels, and bone often need flap coverage. Local or adjacent flaps, e.g., cross finger flaps, are ideal coverage for small but important structures such as flexor tendons and digital nerves (Figs. 130–4, 130–5). In limited areas of the hand and forearm, local rotation muscle flaps may be utilized, but infrequently, since they require further sacrifice of already jeopardized muscle.

For larger defects a number of options are available to provide soft tissue flap coverage. Since the early 1970's the mainstay of coverage has been the groin flap, as first described by MacGregor and Jackson (1972) (Fig. 130–6). One of the main problems in using this flap has been the dependent position in which it places the injured hand for several weeks. This immobilization may lead to edema, swelling, and further fibrosis in an

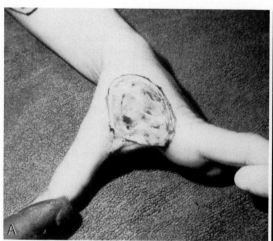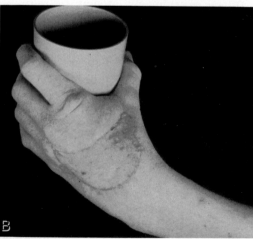

Figure 130–4. *A,* Appearance of a full-thickness electrical burn of the dorsum of the first web along with a thermal flame burn of the volar forearm in a teenager who had sustained a medium volt injury. Both areas underwent full-thickness excision of the necrotic tissue two days after admission. *B,* Appearance of an adequate first web reconstructed with a distally based flap from the dorsum of the hand, with the donor site covered by a split-thickness skin graft. Because of the importance of the first web, a local flap was the first choice of soft tissue coverage in this area.

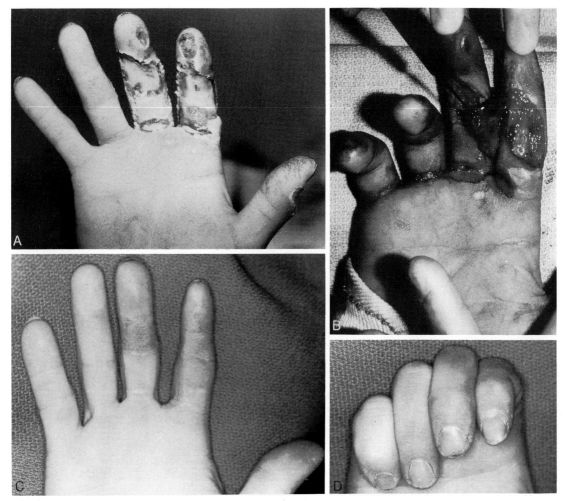

Figure 130–5. *A,* Volar appearance of the right hand shortly after a roofer sustained a 7,200 volt injury after placing an aluminum ladder against a high tension wire. Note the full-thickness burn of the volar aspect of the index and middle fingers. *B,* Appearance one week later with debridement of the volar aspect of the index finger and exposure of the flexor tendons. A cross finger flap from the dorsum of the middle phalanx of the middle finger has been raised and turned for coverage of the exposed flexor tendon. The wound of the middle finger was debrided and covered with a thick split-thickness skin graft. *C, D,* Full extension and almost complete full flexion of the fingers at the seven year follow-up.

already compromised extremity. In addition, it may make necessary hand therapy more difficult. There often is extensive loss of tissue, and the groin flap may prove to be inadequate in size. In these situations, larger defects may require coverage by an abdominal flap. Basing the pedical flap inferiorly may aid in its venous and lymphatic drainage and hopefully decrease resulting swelling. Again, as in groin flaps, the hand is placed in a somewhat dependent position and carries with it its attendant problems. Use of the pectoralis major island flap has also been reported to cover upper extremity electrical injuries; this flap produces less dependent edema (Luce and Gottlieb, 1982).

Bearing in mind that all the aforementioned flaps are biologically parasitic in nature (depending on the recipient bed for their blood supply), musculocutaneous flaps with their inherent blood supply appear to be ideal for partially devascularized electrical injuries of the upper extremity. These flaps, requiring their vascular pedicle base to be kept intact, are uncommonly used in upper extremity trauma. However, in extensive injuries from the elbow to the axilla, the latissimus dorsi musculocutaneous flap, with its inherent broad vascularized muscle, often provides excellent coverage for an area badly in need of a new blood supply (Lai, Milroy, and Pennington, 1982). If the injury extends into the

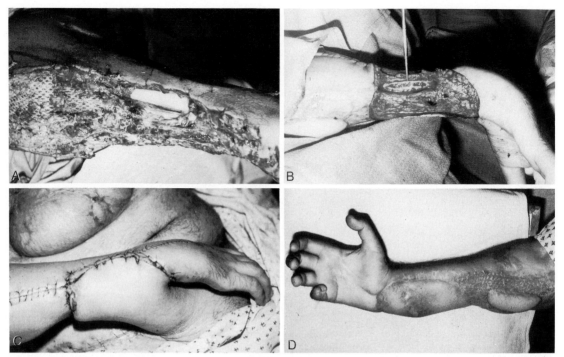

Figure 130–6. *A,* Appearance of the ulnar aspect of the right forearm in a 45 year old man who had sustained an 8,000 volt electrical injury. The wound has been debrided and the proximal portion skin grafted. Bone in the mid-distal ulnar area remains exposed. The patient also sustained severe abdominal wall injuries. *B,* Six weeks after injury the exposed cortex of the ulna has been debrided, ready to receive a soft tissue flap for coverage. (The instrument points to the distal ulna.) *C,* Groin flap applied for soft tissue coverage of the exposed ulna. (Note the abdominal wall hernia in the upper portion of the photograph following a split-thickness skin graft after debridement of the necrotic abdominal wall.) *D,* Appearance six months later of groin flap to the ulnar aspect of the distal forearm.

axilla, care should be taken to verify that the vascular pedicle to the latissimus dorsi muscle was not damaged by the original injury (see Fig. 130–3). Free tissue transfers may occasionally be used for early coverage in electrical injuries of the upper extremity, but are rarely indicated and may even be in jeopardy in view of the vascular nature of the injury.

AMPUTATIONS AND PROSTHETICS

Although rarely indicated in the initial treatment of an injured extremity, amputations are often performed later in the patient's first hospitalization to avoid sepsis or when a firm decision can be carefully made regarding viability. Salisbury and associates (1973) and Hunt (1976) reported a 37 per cent and 46 per cent amputation rate, respectively, for upper extremity electrical injuries. An understanding of neural pathophysiology with its low resistance in electrical injuries can aid the surgeon in his ultimate decision

regarding the value of saving an extremity. Without functional musculature and especially lacking protective sensation, a viable extremity may represent a burden to the patient. In the face of a salvaged electrically injured limb that is not neurologically intact, the surgeon's mental, clinical, and emotional investment in the patient's injury may need to be reevaluated. At times the decision to amputate is difficult for the primary surgeon to make unilaterally after numerous operations have been undertaken to preserve the limb. A consultation with another experienced hand surgeon without personal involvement in the case may be helpful. In view of the major recent advances in prosthetic limbs, the surgeon must always keep in mind that the remaining extremity, with the prospective reconstructive results, must function and be of as much benefit to the patient as an artificial prosthesis.

Acknowledgement: The author would like to thank Dr. David A. Billmire for his assistance in completion of this work.

REFERENCES

Apfelberg, D. B., Masters, F. W., and Robinson, D. W.: Pathophysiology and treatment of lightning injuries. J. Trauma, *14*:453, 1974.

Arturson, G., and Hedlund, A.: Primary treatment of 50 patients with high-tension electrical injuries: I. Fluid resuscitation. Scand. J. Plast. Reconstr. Surg., *18*:111, 1984.

Artz, C. P.: Changing concepts of electrical injury. Am. J. Surg., *128*:600, 1974.

Baxter, C. R.: Present concepts in the management of major electrical injury. Surg. Clin. North Am., *50*:1401, 1970.

Billmire, D. A., Neale, H. W., and Stern, P. J.: Acute management of severe hand injuries. *In* Symposium on Wound Management. Surg. Clin. North Am., *64*:683, 1984.

Boswick, J. A., Jr.: The management of fresh burns of the hand and deformities resulting from burn injuries. Clin. Plast. Surg., *1*:621, 1974.

Buchanan, D. L., Erk, Y., and Spira, M.: Electric current arterial injury: a laboratory model. Plast. Reconstr. Surg., *72*:199, 1983.

Burke, J. F., Quinby, W. C., Jr., Bondoc, C., McLaughlin, E., and Trelstad, R. L.: Patterns of high tension electrical injury in children and adolescents and their management. Am. J. Surg., *133*:492, 1977.

Butler, E. D., and Gant, T. D.: Electrical injuries, with special reference to the upper extremities. A review of 182 cases. Am. J. Surg., *134*:95, 1977.

Chapuis, P.: Le danger des courants electriques industriels et domestiques de faible tension. Paris Theses, 1919–1920, Paris.

Christensen, J. A., Sherman, R. T., Balis, G. A., and Wuamett, J. D.: Delayed neurologic injury secondary to high-voltage current, with recovery. J. Trauma, *20*:166, 1980.

Clayton, J. M., Hayes, A. C., Hammel, J., Boyd, W. C., Hartford, C. E., and Barnes, R. W.: Xenon-133 determination of muscle blood flow in electrical injury. J. Trauma, *17*:293, 1977.

Critchley, M.: Neurological effects of lightning and of electricity. Lancet, *1*:68, 1934.

DiVincenti, F. C., Moncrief, J. A., and Pruitt, B. A.: Electrical injuries: a review of 65 cases. J. Trauma, *9*:497, 1969.

Esses, S. I., and Peters, W. J.: Electrical burns: pathophysiology and complications. Can. J. Surg., *24*:11, 1981.

Farrell, D. F., and Starr, A.: Delayed neurological sequelae of electrical injuries. Neurology, *18*:601, 1968.

Francis, D. A., and Heron, J. R.: Progressive muscular atrophy and posterior dislocation of the humerus following electric shock. Postgrad. Med. J., *60*:143, 1984.

Holbrook, L. A., Beach, F. X. M., and Silver, J. R.: Delayed myelopathy: a rare complication of severe electrical burns. Br. Med. J., *4*:659, 1970.

Holliman, J. C., Saffle, J. R., Kravitz, M., and Warden, G. D.: Early surgical decompression in the management of electrical injury. Am. J. Surg., *144*:733, 1982.

Huang, T. T., Larson, D. L., and Lewis, S. R.: Burned hands. Plast. Reconstr. Surg., *56*:21, 1975.

Hunt, J. L.: Electrical injuries of the upper extremity. Major Probl. Clin. Surg., *19*:72, 1976.

Hunt, J. L., Lewis, S., Parkey, R., and Baxter, C.: The use of technetium-99m stannous pyrophosphate scintigraphy to identify muscle damage in acute electric burns. J. Trauma, *19*:409, 1979.

Hunt, J. L., Mason, A. D., Jr., Masterson, T. S., and Pruitt, B. A., Jr.: The pathophysiology of acute electrical injuries. J. Trauma, *16*:335, 1976.

Hunt, J. L., McManus, W. F., Haney, W. P., and Pruitt, B. A., Jr.: Vascular lesions in acute electric injuries. J. Trauma, *14*:461, 1974.

Hunt, J. L., Sato, R. M., and Baxter, C. R.: Acute electric burns: current diagnostic and therapeutic approaches to management. Arch. Surg., *115*:434, 1980.

Jaffe, R. H.: Electropathology: a review of the pathologic changes produced by electrical currents. Arch. Pathol., *5*:837, 1928.

Jaffe, R. H., Willis, D., and Bachem, A.: The effect of electric currents on the arteries. Arch. Pathol., 7:244, 1929.

Jellinek, S.: Der Elektrische Unfall. 3rd Ed. Leipzig & Vienna, Franz Deuticke, 1931.

Kay, N. R. M., and Boswick, J. A., Jr.: The management of electrical injuries of the extremities. Surg. Clin. North Am., *53*:1459, 1973.

Lai, M. F., Milroy, B. C., and Pennington, D. G.: Shoulder defect cover with functional restoration using the latissimus dorsi myocutaneous flap: a case report. Br. J. Plast. Surg., *35*:140, 1982.

Lazarus, H. M., and Hutto, W.: Electric burns and frostbite: patterns of vascular injury. J. Trauma, *22*:581, 1982.

Levine, N. S., Atkins, A., McKeel, D. W., Peck, S. D., and Pruitt, B. A., Jr.: Spinal cord injury following electrical accidents: case reports. J. Trauma, *15*:459, 1975.

Lewis, G. K.: Electrical burns of the upper extremities. J. Bone Joint Surg., *40A*:27, 1958.

Luce, E. A., and Gottlieb, S. E.: "True" high-tension electrical injuries. Ann. Plast. Surg., *12*:321, 1984.

Luce, E. A., and Gottlieb, S. F.: The pectoralis major island flap for coverage in the upper extremity. J. Hand Surg., *7*:156, 1982.

Lynch, J. B., and Lewis, S. R.: Management of electrical injuries. South. Med. J., *64*:97, 1971.

MacGregor, I. A., and Jackson, I. T.: The groin flap. Br. J. Plast. Surg., *25*:3, 1972.

Mann, R. J., and Wallquist, J. M.: Early decompression fasciotomy in the treatment of high-voltage electrical burns of the extremities. South. Med. J., *68*:1103, 1975.

Masters, F. W., Robinson, D. W., Ketchum, L. D.: Management of electrical burns. *In* Symposium on the Treatment of Burns. St. Louis, C. V. Mosby Company, pp. 82–92.

McCormack, R. M.: Problems in the treatment of burnt hands. Clin. Plast. Surg., *3*:77, 1976.

Muir, I. F. K.: The treatment of electrical burns. Br. J. Plast. Surg., *10*:292, 1958.

Neale, H. W.: Problem burns and their treatment. *In* Hummel, R. P. (Ed.): Clinical Burn Therapy. Littleton, MA, P. S. G. Publishing Company, 1982, pp. 239–278.

Newsome, T. W., Curreri, P. W., and Eurenius, K.: Visceral injuries. Arch. Surg., *105*:494, 1972.

Peterson, R. A.: Electrical burns of the hand; treatment by early excision. J. Bone Joint Surg., *48A*:407, 1966.

Poticha, S. M., Bell, J. L., and Mehn, W. H.: Electrical injuries with special reference to the hand. Arch. Surg., *85*:852, 1962.

Pruitt, B. A., Jr.: Complications of thermal injury. Clin. Plast. Surg., *1*:667, 1974.

Quinby, W. C., Jr., Burke, J. F., Trelstad, R. L., and Caulfield, J.: The use of microscopy as a guide to primary excision of high-tension electrical burns. J. Trauma, *18*:423, 1978.

Robinson, D. W., Masters, F. W., and Forrest, W. J.:

Electrical burns: a review and analysis of 33 cases. Surgery, 57:385, 1965.

Robson, M. C., Murphy, R. C., and Heggers, J. P.: A new explanation for the progressive tissue loss in electrical injuries. Plast. Reconstr. Surg., 73:431, 1984.

Rouse, R. G., and Dimick, A. R.: The treatment of electrical injury compared to burn injury: a review of pathophysiology and comparison of patient management protocols. J. Trauma, 18:43, 1978.

Saffle, J. R., Zeluff, G. R., and Warden, G. D.: Intramuscular pressure in the burned arm: measurement and response to escharotomy. Am. J. Surg., 140:825, 1980.

Salisbury, R. E., Hunt, J. L., Warden, G. D., and Pruitt, B.: Management of electrical injuries of the upper extremity. Plast. Reconstr. Surg., 51:648, 1973.

Salisbury, R. E., and Dingeldein, G. P.: Peripheral nerve complications following burn injury. Clin. Orthop., 163:92, 1982a.

Salisbury, R. E., and Dingeldein, G. P.: The burned hand and upper extremity. In Green, D. P. (Ed.): Operative Hand Surgery. New York, Churchill Livingstone, 1982b, pp. 1523–1552.

Salisbury, R. E., and Pruitt, B. A.: Burns of the Upper Extremity. Philadelphia, W. B. Saunders Company, 1976.

Sances, A., Myklebust, J. B., Larson, S. J., Darin, J. C., Swiontek, T., et al.: Experimental electrical injury studies. J. Trauma, 21:589, 1981

Skoog, T.: Electrical injuries. J. Trauma, 17:487, 1970.

Steiner, A. K., Allgower, M., Matter, R., Meine, J., Hunter, W., and Perren, S. M.: Circulatory changes after local tissue destruction by electric heat. J. Surg. Res., 1:23, 1971.

Sturim, H. S.: The treatment of electrical injuries. J. Trauma, 11:959, 1971.

Sullivan, W. G., Scott, F. A., and Boswick, J. A., Jr.: Rehabilitation following electrical injury to the upper extremity. Ann. Plast. Surg., 7:347, 1981.

Thompson, J. C., and Ashwal, S.: Electrical injuries in children. Am. J. Dis. Child., 137:231, 1983.

Tyler, G.: Treatment of special burns. In Hummel, R. P. (Ed.): Clinical Burn Therapy. Littleton, MA, P.S.G. Publishing Company, 1982, pp. 193–238.

Wang, X., Liu, H., Sang, H., Jai, S., and Cheng, X.: Early vascular grafting to prevent upper extremity necrosis after electrical burns. Clin. Med. J., 97:53, 1984.

Wang, X., Wei, J., Sung, Y., Li, Y., Wang, N., et al.: Early vascular grafting to prevent upper extremity necrosis after electrical burns. Burns, 8:303, 1982.

Weeks, A. W., Alexander, L., and Dennis, R. M.: The distribution of electric current in the animal body: an experimental investigation of 60 cycle alternating current. J. Indust. Hyg. Toxicol., 21:517, 1939.

Wilkinson, C., and Wood, M.: High voltage electric injury. Am. J. Surg., 136:693, 1978.

Williams, D. B., and Karl, R. C.: Intestinal injury associated with low-voltage electrocution. J. Trauma, 21:246, 1981.

Yang, Z. N., Shih, H., Chao, L., and Shih, T.: Free transplantation of sub-axillary lateral thoraco-dorsal flap in burn surgery. Burns, 10:164, 1983/1984.

Yost, J. W., and Holmes, F. F: Myoglobinuria following lightning stroke. J.A.M.A., 228:1147, 1974.

James F. Murray

Cold, Chemical, and Irradiation Injuries

COLD INJURIES
  Chilblain
  Frostbite

CHEMICAL INJURIES
  Acid Burns
  Alkali Burns
  Phosphorus Burns
  Chemical Injection Injury

IRRADIATION INJURIES
  Acute Injuries
  Chronic Injuries

In the practice of most surgeons, cold, chemical, and irradiation injuries are common afflictions of the hand. This chapter is a merger of the author's personal experience and a condensation of the extensive literature. Primarily, these injuries are not surgical problems. The emphasis, therefore, is on their proper early management based on the pathophysiology of the lesions so that reconstructive or ablative surgery can be avoided.

COLD INJURIES

Cold injuries in civilian life are not common, even though most people live north of latitude 40 and are exposed to below freezing environmental temperatures. An average of only eight cases a year are admitted to the hospitals of Saskatoon, Canada, which service about one-half million people who, during the winter months, endure a mean low tempera-

ture of $-24°C$ (Miller and Chasmar, 1980). The experience of one individual treating civilians who have this injury is not extensive, and designated treatment centers with appropriate facilities and experienced staff are the ideal for urban areas. Most patients with significant cold injuries have both upper and lower limbs involved and require hospital admission.

Chilblain

Chilblain is a nonfreezing injury of the skin of the hands, feet, and legs. It is seen most often in children and young women after exposure to damp, above freezing cold. This type of climate is prevalent in parts of the British Isles in winter. In the acute case, the patient has burning pain, sometimes with itching, of red or reddish cyanotic skin. There is no tissue loss, but ulceration can occur in chronic chilblain as well as sensitivity to cold and hyperhydrosis. Aside from local measures to relieve discomfort, there is no specific treatment, but the afflicted areas must be protected from damp cold with dry, warm clothing.

Frostbite

Frostbite is an injury that results from exposure to cold temperatures that are low enough to cause ice crystal formation in the tissues. A benign, superficial, and rapidly healing frostbite can occur on the face, nose, and ears, but serious injuries that result in tissue loss primarily involve the extremities. When a person is exposed to a temperature of $-6.5°C$ or below for an hour or more, there will consistently be a frostbite injury with tissue loss (Knize and associates, 1969).

In addition to temperature, other important environmental conditions affect the rate and extent of tissue freezing (Boswick, 1976).

Wind Velocity. High winds rapidly dissipate radiant body heat, and this cooling by convection augments the rate of local and general body cooling (Mills, 1973).

Moisture. Wet clothing transmits body heat by conduction and in the presence of wind further increases the convection heat loss.

Contact with Cold Objects. Such contact, especially with metal, rapidly transfers heat from the body to the environment.

Altitude. The lower atmosphere oxygen level at high altitudes aggravates the insult because there is reduced oxygenation of the tissues.

Although the environment determines the amount of tissue freezing, certain features about the patient affect the severity of the injury.

Mental State. An altered mental state is commonly associated with frostbite injuries. The patient is rendered incapable of either recognizing the cold environment or taking protective measures to avoid injury. Excess alcohol consumption is usually responsible. In one series it involved 80 per cent of patients admitted to the hospital (Boswick, 1976). Psychoses, senility and confusion in the elderly, and other mental aberrations have the same effect.

Susceptibility to Cold. A previous frostbite injury renders a person susceptible to tissue damage from a repeat cold exposure. Local adaptation of the hands to cold is seen in people living in cold climates or working in a cold environment (Nelms, 1972). Dark-skinned individuals exhibit faster hand cooling on exposure and are at greater risk of cold injury (Whayne and DeBakey, 1958; Nelms, 1972).

Mobility. The heat generated by the body from exercise exerts a powerful protective influence against cooling of the hands and extremities. Immobilization has the opposite effect.

PHYSIOLOGY OF FROSTBITE INJURY

The hands go through three physiologic phases leading to the development of a frost-bite injury. The initial vascular response to cold is followed by two phases that determine the extent of cellular death: ice crystal formation and the vascular response to thawing.

Vascular Response to Cold. Cooling of the hands when the body is in a positive thermoregulatory state results in local vasoconstriction. This is followed by vasodilatation and a sensation of tingling, the Lewis-Hunting reaction, or cold-induced vasodilatation. Local injury occurs when the body core temperature is threatened. Holm and Vanggaard (1974) described the important role played by the extremities (which make up more than 50 per cent of the total body surface) in the regulation of body temperature. High blood flow in digits in a warm environment is due to the many arteriovenous anastomoses from arteries to superficial veins. It is because of this vascular arrangement that the digits are warmer than more proximal parts of the limbs on exposure to cold, provided that the individual is in positive heat balance. However, when the core temperature is threatened, the extensive heat-losing area of the limbs is minimized by closing of the peripheral arteriovenous anastomoses. The decrease in blood flow is so drastic that the rate of fall of the local temperature is similar to that seen after an arterial occlusion under the same environmental conditions (Vanggaard, 1969). Frostbite occurs when the local temperature drops below the freezing point of tissue $(-2°C)$, and ice crystals form in the extracellular spaces.

Tissue Response to Ice Crystals. The ultimate mechanism of tissue injury from freezing is unknown, but it appears that the extracellular ice crystals do not cause enough mechanical injury to the cells to cause their death. They affect cells by reducing the amount of extracellular water and thereby making them hypertonic. This creates an osmotic gradient that results in a shift of water from cells into the interstitial spaces. Continuation of the frozen state propagates the process and produces cellular dehydration and concentration of solutes, damages cell membranes, and possibly leads to cellular death (Meryman, 1957; Mills, 1973).

Vascular Response to Thawing. Immediately after thawing, circulation through frozen tissue resumes, but within minutes vascular stasis develops. Aggregations of platelets, clumped erythrocytes, and fibrin start to plug capillaries and venules, and microthrombi progress in retrograde fashion into the arterioles. Complete irreversible stasis occurs within two hours or less, with edema and extravasation into perivascular spaces (Lange and Boyd, 1945; Quintanella, Krusen, and Essex, 1947). Assays of blister fluid suggest that the release of thromboxane and prostaglandins at the site of injury may play a role in causing vascular thrombosis and progressive dermal ischemia (Robson and Heggers, 1981).

CLINICAL PRESENTATION

The frozen hand has a cadaveric appearance. It may be white, yellowish or grayish white, or a mottled bluish white. Even areas of relatively shallow freezing are cold, hard, and insensitive. With the hand in the frozen state and soon after thawing, it is impossible to predict the extent and depth of the injury.

With thawing, the hand becomes flushed and swollen. Sensation returns for a time until blisters appear after an hour or more. In many patients, the hands have thawed at room temperature by the time they are first seen and the injury can appear quite benign, with only slight swelling of the fingers (Fig. 131–1A). Significant edema and blister formation may not occur for two or three days (Fig. 131–1B). Blisters filled with clear fluid are usually associated with more superficial injuries, whereas blood-filled, dark, hemorrhagic blisters are an ominous sign of damage to deeper tissues. As they dry up from fluid absorption, rupture, or debridement, the areas of deep dermal damage develop a black eschar (Fig. 131–1C). This often separates in three to four weeks to uncover a healthy epithelized surface, whereas avascular fingertips that do not survive shrivel into dry gangrene (Fig. 131–1D). Digits that remain cold

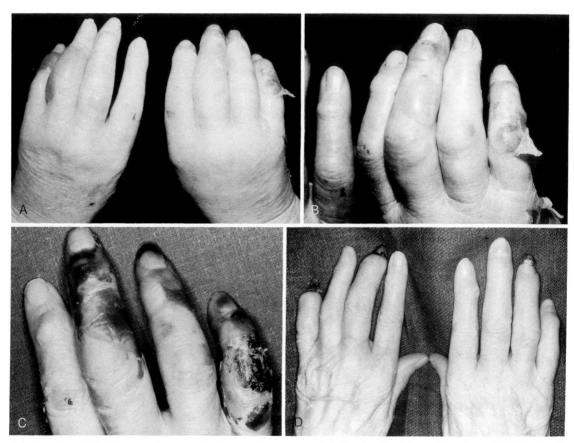

Figure 131–1. *A,* A 72 year old woman 24 hours after exposure to below freezing temperatures for an indefinite length of time. Room temperature thawing has occurred and the injury appears to be minimal. *B,* The right hand after 48 hours with increased swelling and blister formation. *C,* Eschars covering areas of dermal injury with dry gangrene appearing at the distal nail bed of the ring finger. *D,* Eight weeks after injury all eschars have separated and the tips of three fingers have progressed to dry gangrene.

and cyanotic and that have minimal or absent swelling rapidly become mummified (Fig. 131–2A).

Page and Robertson (1983) related the level of early skin changes in the fingers to the eventual level of amputation. One-third of those with changes to the proximal interphalangeal joint ended up with amputations at the distal joint or beyond. When early changes extended to the metacarpophalangeal joint, three-quarters of them were amputated at the proximal interphalangeal joint or base of the finger. The shorter, more easily protected thumb usually escaped injury.

Associated Skeletal Injuries. In addition to the obvious soft tissue injury, freezing may cause damage to the bones and joints of the hand.

Demineralization. Moderate to severe demineralization is seen in 50 per cent of cases (Tishler, 1972). It appears four to ten weeks after injury and may persist for many months. While it is usually more marked in cases with a lot of soft tissue damage, it can occur when the cold injury is relatively minor (Carrera and associates, 1981).

Epiphyseal Injuries. Frostbite in the presence of growing epiphyseal cartilage results in its abnormal growth and premature fusion. The effect is malformed phalanges and joint changes that mainly involve the distal, and occasionally the proximal, interphalangeal joints. Direct cellular injury to the chondrocytes, along with small vessel damage, is probably responsible. Dull, aching pain in the distal and proximal interphalangeal joints several months after a cold exposure may be the presenting symptom, and the parents may never have recognized a frostbite injury (Hakstian, 1972). Later on, there is angulation and stubbiness of the ends of the fingers. The middle finger is less frequently involved because of its relatively protected position, and the epiphysis of the thumb is rarely damaged.

Late Bone and Joint Changes. These may appear months to years after frostbite. Areas of increased density, thought to represent infarcts, may occur in the tops of the terminal phalanges, and punched-out zones in the juxta-articular bone can develop along with radiologic evidence of osteoarthritis (Fig. 131–3).

TREATMENT

The Frozen Hand. Treatment of the frozen hand has gone through the gamut of slow thawing by immersion in baths filled with ice and snow, slow rewarming in baths with

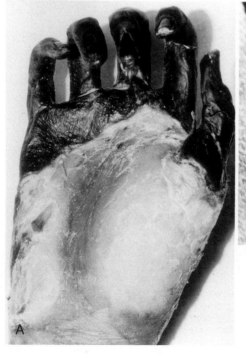
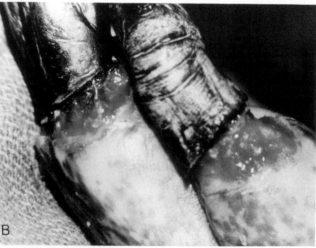

Figure 131–2. *A,* All digits are mummified following a severe frostbite injury. Both hands and both feet are often involved in injuries of this severity. *B,* Demarcation has started between the viable and nonviable tissue after three weeks.

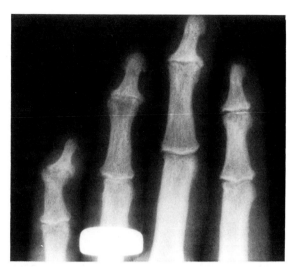

Figure 131–3. Late bone and joint changes in one hand many years after a frostbite injury. The opposite hand was normal.

temperatures increasing from 10° to 40°C over 30 minutes, and rapid rewarming in baths between 38° and 42°C. Experiments with rapid rewarming produced impressive results (Fuhrman and Crismon, 1947) and today this is widely regarded as the method of choice for clinical use (Mills, 1973). It appears to diminish the dangerous period of high extracellular hypertonicity in frozen tissues. Rapid thawing is painful, and sedatives should be given, intravenously if necessary. The frozen white digits become flushed as they thaw, and once this has extended to the ends of all the digits warming is discontinued. Sensation returns until muted by blister formation. Rapid rewarming must be performed only for those patients who are seen with their hands in the frozen state. It is of no benefit to hands that have already thawed, and may indeed be harmful.

The Thawed Hand. The goal of treatment is to salvage all possible lengths and function of the digits. Antitetanus prophylaxis is administered on admission to the hospital, and systemic antibiotics are indicated, especially while edema persists.

Local Care. The hand should be kept exposed, in a sterile environment. Blisters are barriers to infection and ideally should be kept intact, but if already ruptured or broken accidentally, the blistered skin should be trimmed to avoid maceration. Involved areas are gently cleansed at least twice daily with a mild disinfectant solution. Enveloping the hands in occlusive bags with silver sulfadiazine salt (Flamazine) has been advocated as a useful method for preventing infection, and at the same time allowing regular physiotherapy and free active movement of the digits while they are bathed in the antibacterial cream (Page and Robertson, 1983). The wrists should be held in slight dorsiflexion with a light splint that permits free digit movement, and the fingers regularly moved both actively and passively through their maximal range.

Ancillary Measures. Many forms of treatment have been advocated for this injury. For the most part, they reflect the era of their introduction into the armamentarium of measures to promote the blood supply and oxygenation of vascularly "threatened" tissues. Their value is usually demonstrated in controlled freezing and thawing experiments, but clinical benefit has been equivocal. The greatest obstacle to a comparative analysis of frostbite therapy is the impossibility of making a quantitative assessment of the extent of the injury before instituting therapy. No method or set of criteria exists for evaluating the injury prior to thawing.

Heparin was considered a rational method for preventing microthrombi after thawing (Lange and Boyd, 1945), but its value has never been established in patients. Low molecular weight dextran has more antisludging effect than heparin (Weatherley-White, Paton, and Sjöstrom, 1965), but the clinical benefits are uncertain, probably because many patients are seen after thawing has occurred and microthrombi have already formed. Both heparin and dextran carry some risk of gastrointestinal complications in the alcoholic patient with this injury (Page and Robertson, 1983).

Hyperbaric oxygen, at one time considered the saviour of all anoxic tissue, has not been widely adopted for frostbite injury.

Regional sympathectomy by surgery (Shumacker and Kilman, 1964) and intra-arterial injection of sympathetic blocking drugs (Snider and Porter, 1975) have been used to promote limb vasodilatation. In a clinical study, Mills (1973) found that surgical sympathectomy decreased pain, producing a more rapid resolution of infection and a more rapid demarcation of dead tissues. The latter may be a result of increased vascular shunting, which would have an adverse effect on tissue survival, and indeed sympathectomy was found to have no effect on preserving tissues.

The demonstration of thromboxane and prostaglandin in frostbite blisters suggests that they play a role in the pathogenesis of the local injury (Robson and Heggers, 1981). *Aloe vera* as a specific inhibitor of thromboxane is applied to debrided blisters, and aspirin or indomethacin given as a systemic antiprostaglandin. McCauley and associates (1983) consider this "rational" treatment of frostbite.

Role of Surgery. Surgery is restricted to the amputation of nonviable parts of digits. The problem is one of timing rather than technique. Although soft tissue and bone scintiscanning demonstrate the level of viable tissue within five days of injury (Miller and Chasmar, 1980), the decision regarding the timing of surgical debridement is still a clinical one. There is no urgency about removing mummified fingertips that are painless, do not interfere with active movement of joints, and are progressively shrinking and uncovering viable tissue (see Fig. 131–1*D*), unless the patient is a wage earner. There is nothing to be gained by delaying amputation of gangrenous fingers that have started to separate from viable tissues (see Fig. 131–2*B*). They are removed in guillotine fashion at the level of demarcation. Bone is trimmed back until it is deep to a cuff of granulation tissue. Ideally, the wounds should be left open, or at most dressed with a thin free skin graft. Wound contraction draws in the surrounding viable tissues. Maximal length is preserved and in many cases secondary revisions are not needed.

CHEMICAL INJURIES

Contact with irritant chemicals is an ever-present source of injury in an industrialized society. More than 25,000 products capable of causing serious chemical injuries are presently marketed for use in the home, agriculture, and industry. As an exposed part of the body, and the part handling these noxious materials, the hands and upper limbs are the most frequently injured sites, and indeed suffer chemical burns as often as all other sites combined (Curreri, Asch, and Pruitt, 1970).

CHARACTERISTICS OF CHEMICAL BURNS

The potential for a noxious chemical to cause injury depends on its concentration and reactivity as well as the volume involved and the method and duration of its contact. Such agents all cause cell injury, but by means of different types of chemical reactions. Generally speaking, acids produce a coagulative necrosis, alkalies are liquefactive, and vesicants cause an ischemic and anoxic necrosis that follows the edema produced by the liberation of histamine and serotonin (Jelenko, 1947). Although the insult of a thermal burn is momentary, the tissue damage from a chemical agent continues until it is washed off or neutralized, or until its toxicity is exhausted by reaction with the tissues.

An important feature of some chemicals is their systemic toxicity. Oxalic and hydrofluoric acid and phosphorus burns can cause hypercalcemia. Liver and/or kidney damage can occur with tannic, formic, and picric acids and phosphorus injury (Ben-Hur, 1972). Inhalation injuries may follow exposure to strong acids or ammonia, especially when it occurs in a closed environment.

FIRST AID TREATMENT

The importance of immediate and continuous irrigation of the great majority of chemical burns cannot be overstressed. Tap water is usually only seconds away, and hand and forearm injuries are especially easy to irrigate. Constant water flow will dissipate any heat of dilution that is produced. This simple action is the most important step toward minimizing the morbidity of a chemical burn injury, as demonstrated in the series reported by Leonard, Scheulen, and Munster (1982). They found that the incidence of full-thickness burns was five times greater among patients who did not receive irrigation within ten minutes of chemical contact.

The only exceptions to the need for water irrigation are rare injuries from elemental sodium, potassium, or lithium. These are substances that ignite spontaneously when exposed to water (Jelenko, 1974; Polakoff, 1986).

Acid Burns

Most acid burns are very painful and the patient may require a considerable amount of sedative. The appearance varies from the erythema of a superficial injury to a yellowish gray or black eschar with the leather-like quality of a deep burn. Experimentally, the effect of irrigation of acid burns occurs in the first ten minutes (Gruber, Laub, and Vistnes, 1975). The most commonly used antidote, in addition to irrigation, is a dilute solution of sodium bicarbonate. Following the primary first aid measures, the local wound care is similar to that for a thermal burn. Wounds that are obviously full-thickness injuries should be surgically excised and skin grafted.

HYDROFLUORIC ACID BURNS

Burns caused by hydrofluoric (HF) acid require special attention. This is a very corrosive, inorganic acid of elemental fluorine that is used in the manufacturing of many products, including plastics, and for glazing pottery and removing rust (Dibbell and associates, 1970; Hentz, 1985). Burns can occur through small perforations in work gloves, accidental splashing, or failure of the worker to recognize the virulence of the benign-looking, watery-like solution of acid.

There are two mechanisms of injury. The immediate one is due to the high tissue hydrogen ion concentration that occurs in all acid burns and produces a typical caustic skin injury that alters the skin's normal protective barrier. The damage is minimized by prompt water irrigation. The second mechanism is more subtle and more serious: soluble free fluoride ions penetrate the damaged skin and cause a liquefaction necrosis of the soft tissues, decalcification of bone, and local dehydration. The extent and seriousness of the injury depends on the concentration of the acid and the extent and duration of contact. With weaker solutions, symptoms may not appear for several hours; in the early stages of injury from more concentrated solutions, the local clinical changes do not always reflect the gravity of the injury, and the excruciating pain may be dismissed as a sign of a low pain threshold in the patient (Fig. 131–4). The process of destruction can go on for many hours or even days, with extensive damage and systemic toxic effects if treatment is delayed (Fig. 131–5A, B).

TREATMENT

In addition to prompt water irrigation, fingernails should be trimmed so that acid is not trapped beneath them, and measures must be taken to inactivate the toxic free fluoride ions and change them into an insoluble salt.

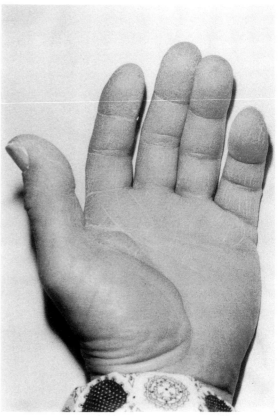

Figure 131–4. Hydrofluoric acid burn of the distal pulp of the fingers. In spite of the benign clinical appearance, the patient had marked pain that responded dramatically to calcium gluconate injection of the involved sites.

Topical Applications. Many topical applications have been proposed, but only calcium gluconate burn gel reduced the hydrofluoric acid burn size in an experimental study on rats. No effect was seen from others that have been recommended, including benzalkenium chloride (Zephiran), vitamins A and D ointment, aloe gel, or magnesium ointment (Bracken and associates, 1985). Clinically the prompt topical application and massage of a 10 per cent calcium gluconate gel into the involved skin will control the pain and the progress of the less severe injuries (Wetherhold and Shepard, 1965; Wale, 1986).

Local Injection. The injection of 10 per cent calcium gluconate solution into the area of injury is presently the most widely used method to abort the progress of the injury, relieve pain, and prevent systemic fluoride poisoning (Bunt, 1964; Dibbell and associates, 1970; Iverson, Laub, and Madison, 1971; Kleinert and Bronson, 1976; Koehnlein and Achinger, 1982). Multiple injections of 0.1 to

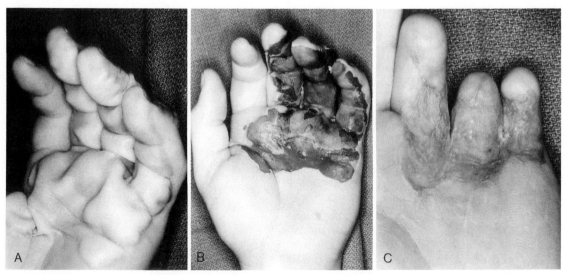

Figure 131–5. *A,* An untreated, severe hydrofluoric acid burn 12 hours after injury. *B,* Extensive full-thickness skin loss and distal gangrene of the ulnar three fingers. *C,* After amputation and skin grafts.

0.2 ml are given through a 30 gauge needle without anesthesia. Relief of pain is dramatic and this is the indicator for the number and frequency of injections. Edematous pulp tissue of the digits must be injected cautiously, with minimal amounts of the drug, to avoid vascular embarrassment in these "closed" spaces (Wale, 1986). It has been shown experimentally that magnesium salts cause less local irritation than calcium salts (Harris, Ranack, and Bregman, 1981).

Intra-arterial Injection. Intra-arterial infusion of calcium gluconate has been introduced to treat hydrofluoric acid burns in the limbs (Koehnlein and Achinger, 1982). The method has been enthusiastically endorsed as a valuable adjunct to treatment of this injury (Pegg, Sin, and Gillet, 1985; Vance and associates, 1986). The technique is described by Vance. Once the arterial catheter is properly located, a dilute solution of calcium gluconate or calcium chloride (10 ml of a 10 per cent solution mixed with 40 to 50 ml of 5 per cent dextrose) is infused with a pump apparatus over four hours. The catheter is left in place for a four hour period of observation, and the treatment is repeated until the patient is painfree for four hours.

Calcium is made readily available for locally absorbed fluoride ions by this method; it gives immediate relief of pain, stops the systemic effects of hydrofluoric acid burns, and eliminates the need for local painful injections in an already painful area. In severe injuries, it provides much more calcium to the fluoride-impregnated tissues.

Alkali Burns

Alkalies are the most common chemicals around the home. They are the active component in products used for unblocking drains and cleaning ovens, and in garden lime, fertilizers, and cement (Wale, 1986). As a rule, alkalies produce less immediate damage than acids, but ultimately cause more tissue destruction. They liquefy tissue and allow for deeper penetration. The initial reaction in a lye burn is saponification of tissue fats, which results in death of the fat cells. Unattached alkali molecules are then free to penetrate and cause further injury (Orcutt and Pruitt, 1976; Stewart, 1985; Polakoff, 1986). This is why the pH changes in the subcutaneous tissue beneath an alkali injury are much greater and more prolonged than in an acid burn, and the irrigation of these injuries should continue for at least an hour (Gruber, Laub, and Vistnes, 1975). Many alkali burns initially are superficial and appear quite benign, but if left untreated they can progress to a full-thickness injury.

After irrigation, the injuries that appear partial thickness are treated by an occlusive dressing and periodic observation. Topical mafenide acetate (Sulfamylon) has been recommended not only for its bacteriostatic effect, but also because it combines with any active lye in the wound to form sodium acetate and sulphamyelon radicals that are innocuous. The sulfate radicals of gentamicin, on the other hand, produce an exothermic reaction and can cause further injury (Orcutt and Pruitt, 1976).

Obvious full-thickness injury should be treated by early excision and skin grafting.

CEMENT BURNS

Wet cement is caustic, with a pH as high as 12.9, and can cause a full-thickness alkali burn. Such injuries usually occur in amateur cement workers who handle, kneel in, or walk barefoot in wet cement (Fig. 131–6). Typically, the symptoms of pain and burning do not appear until several hours after exposure (Peters, 1984; McGeown, 1984; Wilson and Davidson, 1985). Prolonged irrigation of the area is essential, and early excision and grafting should be carried out in deep partial-thickness or full-thickness injuries.

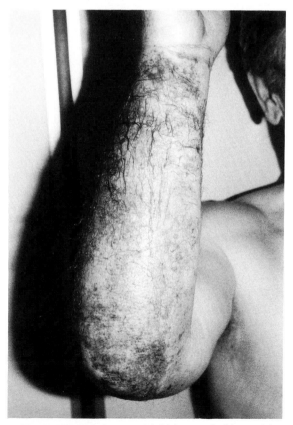

Figure 131–6. A deep partial-thickness alkali burn of the forearm from exposure to wet cement.

PLASTER OF PARIS

Surgeons must be aware of the burns that can be caused by the exothermic reaction of wet plaster of paris (calcium sulfate), which is used for casts and splints, and should take measures to protect patients against such injuries (Kaplan, 1981; Hedeboe and associates, 1982).

Phosphorus Burns

Although phosphorus burns are more common in military personnel, they do occur in civilians, usually from the phosphorus in fireworks, insecticides, rodent poisons, and fertilizers. Phosphorus ignites spontaneously when exposed to air and is rapidly oxidized to phosphorus pentoxide. It is extinguished by water, but may reignite upon drying. Particles of phosphorus embedded in skin continue to burn in an exothermic oxidation reaction that continues until they are debrided, neutralized, or completely oxidized (Curreri, Asch, and Pruitt, 1970). Emergency treatment consists of copious water irrigation and debridement of visible particles. The wound should be briefly washed with 1 per cent copper sulfate to form black cupric phosphide and facilitate the removal of phosphorus particles. Copper sulfate is not a form of treatment and should be washed off to prevent copper toxicity after all particles have been removed.

Chemical Injection Injuries

The interstitial injection of irritating chemicals or medications is almost always caused by their extravasation during intravenous administration. The great majority of cases, therefore, occur in the upper limb between the antecubital fossa and dorsum of the hand (Upton, Mulliken, and Murray 1979; Larsen, 1985). The result of extravasation is an inflammatory reaction that can progress to tissue death, slough, and ulceration, depending on the amount, concentration, and toxicity of the injected material. Although this is a common occurrence in patients on prolonged intravenous therapy, most cases are recognized promptly and result in nothing more than a temporary localized erythema. Major injuries are those that require surgical debridement and repair, or even amputation. Many of these occur when patients are unable to communicate the discomfort of extravasation because of age (the very young or the elderly), anesthesia, or a comatose state, or because they are still being resuscitated (Upton, Mulliken, and Murray, 1979; MacCara, 1983). Major injuries have become more prevalent with the widespread use of vesicant antineoplastic drugs.

DRUGS CAUSING EXTRAVASATION INJURIES

Upton, Mulliken, and Murray (1979) and MacCara (1983) classified the drugs that most often cause extravasation injuries on the basis of their mode of tissue damage.

Osmotically Active Agents. Hypertonic solutions containing cations such as calcium and potassium in ionized form cause an osmotic imbalance across the cell membrane, disruption of cell transport mechanisms, and cell death from intracellular fluid imbibition. Solutions of urea are nonmetabolic and nonelectrolyte, and draw fluid from the cells, resulting in cell dehydration. In this group of osmotically active agents are solutions of calcium gluconate, potassium and calcium chloride, Renografin-60 (used for radiographic examination), intravenous solutions of 30 per cent urea and 10 per cent dextrose, and hypertonic parenteral nutrition solutions.

Ischemia-Inducing Agents. The catecholamines and vasopressin cause injury by local ischemia. Epinephrine, norepinephrine, metaraminol, dopamine, and dobutamine have all been reported to cause tissue slough as a result of ischemic necrosis after their extravasation.

Agents Causing Direct Cellular Toxicity. Most major extravasation injuries are due to the direct toxic effect of the extravasated drugs on living cells in the area. At present, the most common and often the most perplexing to treat are those involving vesicant antineoplastic drugs. Others in this group are sodium bicarbonate, sodium thiopental (Pentothal), digoxin, diazepam, nafcillin, and tetracycline.

Contributing to the degree of tissue damage are the mechanical compression caused by the extravasated fluid and secondary wound infection (Upton, Mulliken, and Murray, 1979). Three pharmacologic classes of vesicant antitumor drugs are in general use

(Dorr and Ignoffo, 1984). The intercalating antibiotics include the anthracyclines, doxorubicin hydrochloride (Adriamycin), and daunorubicin. Alkylating agents include mechlorethamine (nitrogen mustard) and mitomycin and the vinca alkaloids vinblastine, vincristine, and vindesine. Special attention must be paid to doxorubicin, which is the most commonly used antitumor drug and consequently is involved in most extravasation injuries (Larsen, 1985). Over the past several years, no drug has been the subject of more clinical reports and experimental studies concerning its extravasation into tissues (Rudolph, Stein, and Patillo, 1976; Reilly, Neifeld, and Rosenberg, 1977; Bowers and Lynch, 1978; Larsen, 1982, 1985; Linder, Upton, and Osteen, 1983; Cohen, Manganaro, and Bezzozo, 1983; Loth and Eversmann, 1986).

Doxorubicin was isolated from cultures of a mutant of *Streptomyces peucetius,* and since 1967 has become the mainstay drug in the treatment of breast, prostate, bladder, and lung cancers, lymphomas, and many sarcomas (Rothberg, Place, and Shteir, 1974). When extravasated it has a direct cellular toxic effect by combining with the DNA cycle to inhibit nucleic acid synthesis (Mamakos, 1984). The clinical result is a painful subcutaneous reaction. The cytotoxic effect is perpetuated by the release of the doxorubicin-DNA complex from dead cells, making it available to viable cells (Zweig and associates, 1979). The local reaction therefore spreads into a progressively enlarging area of ulceration surrounded by a zone of indurated inflammation (Fig. 131–7). The continuation of tumor therapy with doxorubicin has been reported to increase the rate and extent of tissue necrosis at a site of extravasation, or to cause a breakdown in a previously healed area (Donaldson, Glick, and Wilbur, 1974; Cohen, Dibella, and Michelak, 1975; Mamakos, 1984). However, this so-called "recall phenomenon" has not been observed by others who routinely continued drug therapy within a week of the extravasation incident (Reilly Neifeld, and Rosenberg, 1977; Larsen, 1982, 1985).

CLINICAL FEATURES

The location of the extravasation plays a significant role in the degree of morbidity. The most common site for complex injuries is

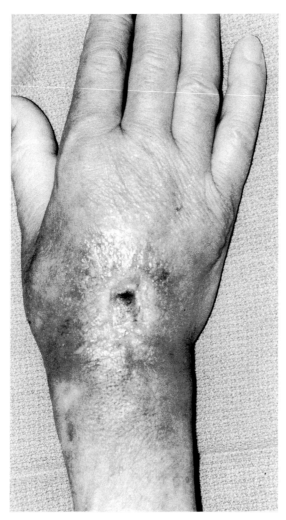

Figure 131-7. A common site for doxorubicin (Adriamycin) extravasation. The ulcer is surrounded by a painful area of rubor and induration.

the dorsum of the hand (Upton, Mulliken, and Murray, 1979), where loose thin skin and subcutaneous tissues lie directly on the extensor tendons, and the extrinsic muscle compartments can easily become involved. Pain, local redness or discoloration, and swelling around the intravenous site signal an extravasation into the tissues. Osmotically active and cationic solutions in the tissues are the most unpredictable from the viewpoint of estimating the ultimate extent of tissue death. The presence of epidermal blisters is invariably an indication of full-thickness rather than partial-thickness skin loss. Demarcation of the nonviable tissues is usually evident within a week with these solutions, whereas doxorubicin extravasation may

smolder for a longer time before an ulcer develops in the spreading, inflamed, indurated, and painful soft tissue mass.

PREVENTION

"Expert intravenous technique still represents the most important controllable factor which can reduce the incidence of extravasation injuries" (Dorr, 1985). Trained personnel with proficient technique, the ability to recognize an extravasation, and knowledge of the protocol to be followed when it occurs not only reduce the incidence but minimize the injury. Individual institutions must prepare their own guidelines for extravasation injuries from the available literature (Upton, Mulliken, and Murray, 1979; Jameson and O'Donnel, 1983; Bacovsky, 1986; Wolfe and Linkewich, 1987). Venous access ports, although not totally without risk, are an important advance in technology for the delivery of cancer chemotherapy to patients who have limited vascular access because of inadequate peripheral veins.

TREATMENT

Primary Treatment. Documentation of the circumstances of the incident, and if possible an estimate by the person attending of the volume extravasated, can help to predict the extent of the injury. There is a lack of consistency in the various local measures advocated.

Removal of Intravenous Line. Prompt removal would seem to be an obvious measure, but some authors recommend that it be left in place and an attempt made to withdraw extravasated solution—surely a futile gesture—and use the line to inject an antidote that "may" be of value (Reilly, Neifeld, and Rosenberg, 1977).

Cold Applications. The vasoconstriction created by cold application to the area is intended to keep the extravasated drug in the area. It is the only local treatment used by Larsen (1985) for all antitumor drug extravasations. Experimentally, cold appears to have a direct effect on doxorubicin that decreases its toxicity, but cold was also shown to increase the toxicity of the vinca alkaloids (Dorr, 1985). Cold has been applied for 15 minutes four times daily for three days (Larsen, 1985). Jameson and O'Donnel (1983) are much more aggressive and apply cold for 50 minutes of each hour during the first 24 to 36 hours.

Warm Applications. Ignoffo and Friedman (1980) recommend warm to hot compresses to the area of extravasation, to provide vasodilatation and increase fluid absorption and thereby reduce the extravasated drug concentration. There is some rationale for this when hyaluronidase is being used to promote drug dispersion (see below), but Dorr (1985) observed that heat consistently increased the toxicity of doxorubicin.

Antidotes. Some medications are recognized as being useful as an antidote for certain extravasations.

HYALURONIDASE (WYDASE). This enzyme destroys tissue "cement" and thereby reduces injury after extravasation by allowing rapid diffusion of the irritant fluids. It is advocated for extravasation of solutions of 10 per cent dextrose, calcium, and potassium, aminophylline, nafcillin, radiocontrast media, and parenteral nutritional solutions (Zenck, 1981). Experimentally it is beneficial for extravasations of the vinca alkaloids (Dorr, 1985).

PHENTOLAMINE (REGITINE). As an alpha blocking agent, this is the usual antidote for extravasations of vasopressors.

SODIUM THIOSULFATE. The prompt injection of 1/6 M sodium thiosulfate significantly reduces the skin ulceration caused by nitrogen mustard.

TOPICAL DIMETHYL SULFOXIDE (DMSO). In 90 per cent alpha-tocopherol succinate, this may be of some benefit after doxorubicin extravasation (Loth and Eversmann, 1986).

CORTICOSTEROIDS. Injection of either dexamethasone or hydrocortisone has been the most consistently reported antidote for antitumor drug extravasation. The addition of sodium bicarbonate is reputed to augment its effect. Experimental studies by Cohen (1979), Dorr (1985), and Loth and Eversmann (1986) cast considerable doubt on the efficacy of corticosteroids, and Jackson and Robinson (1976) have shown that sodium bicarbonate is potentially harmful.

General Measures. The involved limb should be kept elevated to promote free venous and fluid drainage. The area of extravasation should be left open if possible or covered with a light dressing that can be easily removed for frequent inspection. A light splint should be made to hold the wrist in about 30 degrees of dorsiflexion, permit the fingers to fall into full flexion at the metacarpophalangeal joints, and allow the fingers free active and passive movement. These measures should be taken regularly under the guidance of a therapist.

ROLE OF SURGERY

Inclusion of a surgeon on the "treatment team" for acute extravasation injuries, especially those involving vesicant antitumor drugs, would be of benefit to the patient and a learning experience for surgeons, physicians, pharmacists, and intravenous personnel. There is a striking difference in the experience of Larsen (1985), who started patients promptly on conservative treatments after antitumor drug extravasation, and that of Linder, Upton, and Osteen (1983), who saw their patients in consultation from six days to nine weeks (usually three to five weeks) after the incident. In Larsen's series, 89 per cent of 119 acute extravasation injuries healed uneventfully after nothing more than cold applications. Linder, Upton, and Osteen state that "very few of these lesions will heal spontaneously," and over a three year period only four extravasations treated nonsurgically formed excessive scar tissue. The latter is the experience of most surgeons, who for the most part see only those injuries that fail to heal. Surgeons involved in all cases from the day of injury would develop an appreciation of the conservative measures that are useful and the clinical course of the many extravasation injuries that do heal. Just as important, physicians and others would appreciate the many benefits of early surgical treatment of injuries unlikely to heal. Finally, the patients would be subject to a much shorter sentence of pain, surgical procedures, and hospitalization. With extravasation of antitumor drugs, Larsen feels that the only indication for surgery is local pain that is persisting or increasing a week after the injury. This represents early excision as distinct from immediate excision of the area.

Early aggressive surgery is indicated for massive extravasations when there is any suggestion of arterial compromise, muscle compartment syndrome, or rapidly spreading skin necrosis.

Patients with well-demarcated areas of slough should have a generous debridement carried out under the antibiotic cover. Repair should be done by primary or delayed grafting when the wound is ready. The simplest method is the one of choice, and multistage flap procedures are seldom necessary.

The surgical problems with established doxorubicin ulcerations have been alluded to and are extensively reported (Fig. 131–8). Excision must be radical, including a margin of normal skin and subcutaneous tissue and extending to healthy tissue on the deep surface. Involved fascia and tendons may have to be sacrificed. Since doxorubicin is fluorescent, ultraviolet light has been used to identify infiltrated areas, and fluorescein injection to distinguish viable tissue (Cohen, Manganaro, and Bezzozo, 1983). Local muscle flaps in the forearm may be indicated to protect major nerves and vessels before covering with a free graft. A biologic dressing and delayed grafting can be useful at the initial stage to "test" the receptivity of the bed for a definitive free skin graft.

IRRADIATION INJURIES

The harmful effects of ionizing radiation on living tissues were recognized within a year of the discovery of x-rays by Wilhelm Roentgen in 1895 (Daniel, 1896). However, this was a new type of injury! There had never been a noxious agent that could not be seen or felt, nor one with such delayed effects. It took more than half a century to create a general awareness of the long-term irreversible damage that occurred from repeated small doses or a large single dose of radiation (Barnett, 1979). Repeated exposure to low doses was particularly prevalent among physicians, dentists, veterinarians, and x-ray technicians, and because they handled radiation sources or manipulated parts of the patient being examined, their hands were the parts most often afflicted (Fig. 131–9). The hands were involved in 90 per cent of cases of radiodermatitis in physicians (Leddy and Rigos, 1949); among dentists, the fingers they used to hold intraoral x-ray films were the usual site (Hoffmesiter, Macomber, and Wang, 1969). Many patients suffered radiodermatitis from prolonged treatment of benign conditions (Cannon, Randolph, and Murray, 1959). Excessive single dose injuries were less common, but occurred to both patient and doctor as a result of the fluoroscopic search for a foreign body (Wright, 1978). Severe burns to the hands from an unshielded fluoroscope terminated the career of a surgical resident (Smith, 1973). He became a successful anesthetist! These types of injuries were mainly blameable on a casual or careless attitude to radiation exposure. With time and the development and widespread use of powerful radiation sources, there has grown a general awareness of the hazards. Injuries from "medical misadventures" are now rare.

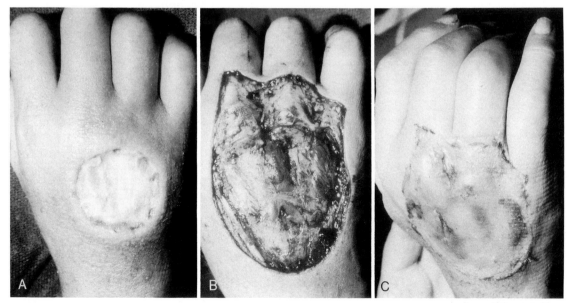

Figure 131–8. *A*, A failed free graft after local excision of a doxorubicin ulcer. *B*, A more extensive excision with sacrifice of extensor tendons. *C*, Satisfactory take of a free graft.

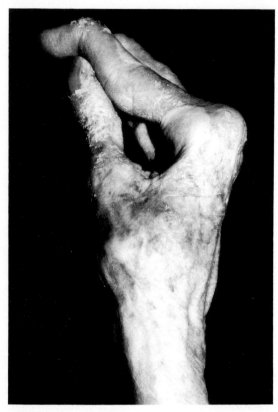

Figure 131–9. Extensive radiation damage of the hand of a 75 year old patient who had worked for 35 years as an x-ray technician. In addition to the marked atrophy and scaling of the skin, fibrosis of intrinsic muscles has produced a marked intrinsic plus deformity.

Very few major industries today do not use radioactive materials. In addition to the more widely known uses for electric power, heat, transportation, and weaponry, such materials are used for such mundane manufacturing processes as detecting wear on piston rings, testing the efficiency of detergent washing machines, and adjusting rollers to control the thickness of paper (Holly and Beck, 1980). When local radiation injuries occur in industry, they are usually due to an inadvertent exposure to radioisotopic sources or commercial irradiators such as cobalt-60, iridium-192, and x-ray generators used in laboratory analysis and research. About 85 per cent of cases involve the hands, and most are caused by malfunction or improper operation of industrial gamma ray radiographic units (Lushbraugh and associates, 1980; Saenger and associates, 1980). The incidence of these injuries is very low in relation to the widespread use of these materials.

IONIZING RADIATION

Ionization of cells is a transitory disruption of the normally stable chemical system of the cell caused by excessive radiant energy. This disruption lasts for an estimated 10^{-8} seconds and results in cell damage. How this damage occurs is still a matter for conjecture, but it is thought to be primarily the result of altered DNA metabolism and destruction of associated enzymes (Shearin, 1980). The ionization may be caused by one of two types of concentrated radiation energy that have similar cumulative effects on tissues.

1. Particular or corpuscular radiation consists of subatomic particles that travel at speeds that depend on their mass and energy. Radium, uranium, and cobalt-60 release energy spontaneously and give off relatively large positively charged alpha particles and small negatively charged beta particles. Extra energy to these can be generated by machines that deliver less than 1 million volts to particles (orthovoltage) or more than 1 million volts (supervoltage). Beta particles ionize cells to only a few millimeters in the skin unless they are part of a high energy electron beam as produced by the betatron, cyclotron, or linear accelerator with their several million electron volts (mev).

2. Electromagnetic radiation is a wave type of energy that includes the spectrum of long wavelength radio waves through progressively decreasing wavelengths of visible and ultraviolet light, grenz rays, x-rays, and gamma rays. All travel at the speed of light and the energy depends on their wavelength. Only those with shorter wavelengths are capable of ionizing molecules by the liberation of photoelectrons. The rad is the unit of measurement most commonly used to include the energy absorbed from the ionizing particles per unit mass of irradiated tissue. It is calculated from the known energy source, the distance to the tissue, and the type of tissue irradiated. One rad represents 100 ergs absorbed per gram of irradiated tissue.

The amount of damage from radiation depends on the energy (degree of penetration of the tissue), dose, and dose rate. Particulate radiation with energy of less than 10 mev and the long wavelength grenz or "soft" x-rays have low tissue penetration and have an effect only on skin. Supervoltage x-rays with short wavelength and high energy spare skin at the point of entry and exert their ionizing effect on deeper tissues. In the hands, clearly, the deeper tissues may be the skin on the surface opposite to that of entry.

Most industrial accidents to the hands involve very high dose rates (500 to 100,000 rads), usually delivered for less than one minute, but occasionally up to several hours. The effect is an early extensive local damage to skin, muscle, bone, and blood vessels, and necrosis occurs within weeks. When the dose and dose rates are lower, there is a latent period of months or years before a gradual obliterative endarteritis produces chronic ischemia, fibrosis, and atrophy (Barnett, 1979).

Acute Injuries

Saenger and associates (1980) use a clinical classification based on the severity of the acute injury.

Type I. Erythema only. This is comparable with the first degree thermal burn, but the symptoms and redness appear much later. After a brief exposure to a few hundred rads, the sensation of warmth or itching of the hand may appear during the first day or two. Erythema may not appear for two or three weeks. The only skin damage is superficial scaling when the erythema fades.

Type II. Transepidermal injury, or partial-thickness skin damage equivalent to a second degree thermal burn. This results after a brief exposure of 1000 to 2000 rads. Early itching and pain is followed by erythema, and blisters form within a week or two, leaving painful superficial ulcers. Healing occurs after a few weeks, but the new skin is thin and tenuous and ultimately resembles that of chronic radiation exposure.

Type III. Dermoradionecrosis. This is full-thickness skin loss that occurs after exposure to doses in excess of 2000 rads. The actual dose of radiation that is totally incompatible with tissue viability in a composite organ such as the hand is not known (Krizek and Ariyan, 1973). Erythema, swelling, vesicles, joint stiffness, severe pain, and skin changes similar to those of a full-thickness thermal or chemical burn may appear within hours, or after two or three days. This is followed by sloughing of the skin and varying amounts of deeper tissues. Injuries of this severity have occurred in individuals who handled fresh fission product materials and after accidental exposure to the direct beam of an electron accelerator. In these patients with local injuries to the hands, there rarely are systemic manifestations or the laboratory findings associated with acute radiation syndrome from total body radiation (Saenger and associates, 1980). Serial blood counts and chromosome analysis of blood lymphocytes are useful indicators of whole body radiation.

HISTOPATHOLOGY

The more quickly a given radiation dose is administered, the greater are the biologic effects (Barnett, 1979). The early effects of radiation are the result of an acute cell injury that is not specific, but rather resembles those of other cytotoxic agents (Watson, 1980). Cell nuclei are shrunken, there is both intra- and extracellular edema, and inflammatory cells infiltrate the dermis, the epidermis, and areas of necrosis. Blood vessels are dilated and show endothelial proliferation and thrombosis that creates secondary ischemic changes (Warren, 1943; Lever and Schaumburg-Lever, 1983).

TREATMENT

Dosimetry studies by a radiation physicist should be carried out in all cases to provide an estimate of the dosage and the extent of tissue damage that may be expected.

No treatment is needed for Type I injuries. Type II injuries may require sedatives for relief of pain, and light dressings to the involved area of the hand may be indicated to protect blisters and cover superficial ulcerations. Troublesome secondary skin changes may eventually need the same surgical treatment as that for some chronic injuries.

The clinical course of Type III injuries is much more prolonged than that of full-thickness thermal burns, and is accompanied by pain that may require large doses of narcotics (Smith, 1973). During the early weeks, it is usually impossible to predict accurately the extent of tissue loss, and consequently there is never a case for early excision and grafting (Fryer and Brown, 1962; Brown and Fryer, 1965). During this phase, it is important to minimize swelling, to try to preserve maximal joint movement, and to prevent joint contracture. To achieve this, the hands must be elevated and the joints put through their maximal range of active and passive movements at regular, frequent intervals. Resting splints must be used between exercise sessions to hold the wrist in slight dorsiflexion, the metacarpophalangeal joints in full flexion, and the interphalangeal joints close to full extension. The thumb must be in palmar abduction.

When the depth of necrosis becomes obvious, debridement is performed to a healthy bleeding surface. An intermediate-thickness free skin graft provides a satisfactory cover for most cases (Fryer and Brown, 1962; Krizek and Ariyan, 1973). A pedicle flap must be used when nerve, tendon, bone, or joint is exposed or when secondary repair of these structures is planned (Krizek and Ariyan, 1973). Occasionally, a flap may be needed to replace an unstable free graft. Free neurovascular island flaps may have an appropriate role in secondary reconstructive surgery following these injuries (May and associates, 1977; Stern, 1980; Stern, Kreilein, and Kleinert, 1983).

There have been rare cases of such massive destruction that amputation of the hand is necessary (Lanzl, Rosenfeld, and Tarlov, 1967; Ciano and associates, 1981). Even in these cases, a period of observation is essential to determine the appropriate level of amputation, and it also allows the patient to appreciate the necessity for such radical measures.

Chronic Injuries

Chronic injuries constitute the late changes that occur in the skin and subcutaneous and deeper tissues of the hand after excessive radiation that has occurred in one of the following ways: (1) a single dose injury that has healed (Type II acute injury) but develops subsequent skin changes; (2) repeated exposure of significant doses that in many cases have been administered for therapeutic reasons (Fig. 131–10*A, B*); and (3) repeated long-term exposure to low doses, usually encountered in people who have ignored protective measures while using radiation equipment (see Fig. 131–9) or in the unfortunate patient who has been given long-term low-dose therapy for a benign condition (Fig. 131–11*A*).

CLINICAL FEATURES

Changes may appear after a few months, but more often it will be many years after radiation exposure. Initially, the skin be-

comes thin and atrophic, with superficial scaling and hyperkeratosis. Scattered areas of pigmentation may develop on the dorsum of the hands and digits, as well as loss of hair. The palmar skin atrophies and loses its dermal ridges. In time, areas of telangiectasia and slow-healing superficial ulcers may develop. Chronic ulcers with bone exposed suggest a radionecrosis of bone or a malignant change in the ulcer. There is progressive atrophy and fibrosis of the subcutaneous tissues, which contributes to joint stiffness in the digits.

It is a strange paradox that radiation used in the therapy for cancer causes changes in the skin that make it prone to this disease. Malignant changes occur in 20 to 30 per cent of patients with chronic radiodermatitis after an average latent period of 28 years (Cannon, Randolph, and Murray, 1959). Epidermoid carcinoma is the usual malignancy in the hand, although basal cell tumors can occur.

HISTOPATHOLOGY

The epidermis shows changes similar to those of solar keratoses that are caused by solar radiant energy. There is a combination of atrophy, hyperkeratosis, acanthosis, and irregular downgrowths around telangiectatic vessels. The cell nuclei may be atypical, and it is from the epidermal cells that are altered and anaplastic that invasive squamous cell carcinoma develops. Sweat glands are usually present, but hair follicles and sebaceous glands disappear.

The dermis shows changes that are more specific for radiodermatitis. Collagen bundles are swollen and strain irregularly, and new collagen with few cells is present. Blood vessels show telangiectasia near the epidermis, and in the deeper dermis they have varying degrees of thickening of the wall and occlusion of the lumen. Ulceration is often associated with complete obliteration of the deeper vessels.

TREATMENT

All patients with radiodermatitis of the hand must be made aware of the fact that they have a premalignant condition, and should know the signs of malignant change. Persistent scaling, active hyperkeratoses, and recurrent or spreading ulceration should be promptly reported. Many patients require no

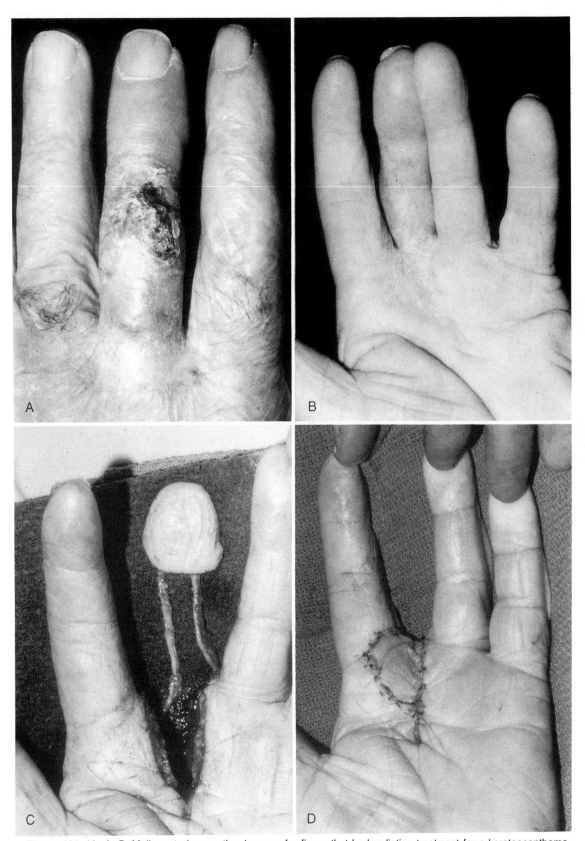

Figure 131–10. *A, B,* Malignant ulcer on the dorsum of a finger that had radiation treatment for a keratoacanthoma. The palmar surface shows loss of normal skin ridges and creases, ecchymosis, and pulp atrophy. *C, D,* Ray deletion with a neurovascular island flap of healthy pulp to cover an involved area in the palm.

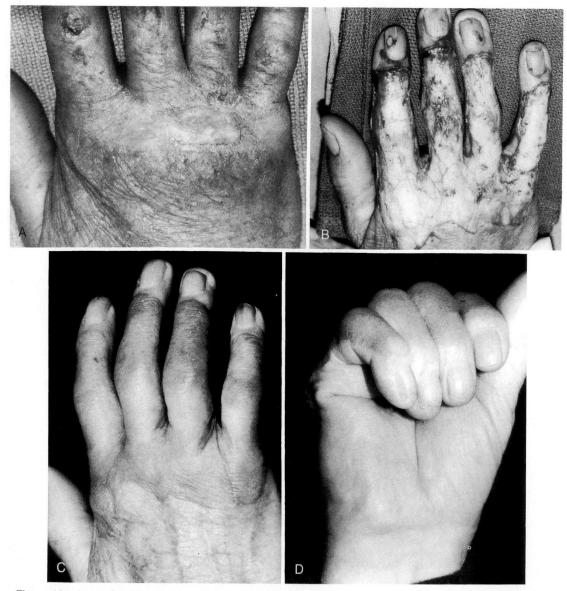

Figure 131–11. *A,* Chronic radiodermatitis with joint stiffness, 25 years after radiation treatments for a benign skin condition. *B,* Radical excision of the involved skin. *C, D,* Intermediate-thickness skin graft with good flexion restored.

treatment except skin care and alertness for signs of change.

Surgical treatment should be tailored to the patient and should depend on the extent of the injury, the degree of disability, and the individual's general health and age. Many local areas of suspicious malignant change can be excised and skin grafted under local anesthesia. More extensive involvement on the dorsum of the hand that is a source of chronic irritation, joint stiffness, and enough problems to interfere with function should be considered for a radical excision and resurfacing with a moderately thick free skin graft (Fig. 131–11*B* to *D*). Painful or extensively involved single digits are often best amputated.

Most malignancies in irradiated skin can be eradicated by surgical excision and free skin grafts. Neglected tumors that invade deep fascial layers require radical excision that requires sacrifice of function in the interests of tumor eradication.

REFERENCES

Allen, W. R.: Ignorance, experimentation, tragedy. Radiation injury to the hand. J. Kansas Med. Soc., *67*:447, 1967.

Bacovsky, R.: Antineoplastic extravasation: prevention and treatment. Can. J. of Hosp. Pharm., *39*:27, 1986.

Bardychev, M. S., Yu, A., Kim, V. D., and Petrik, V. D.: The use of autologous split skin flaps in treatment of delayed radiation injuries of the skin. Acta Chir. Plast., *22*:73, 1980.

Barnett, M. H.: The biological effect of ionizing radiation. Conn. Med., *43*:75, 1979.

Ben-Hur, H.: Phosphorus burns: a pathophysiological study. Br. J. Plast. Surg., *25*:238, 1972.

Blunt, C. P.: Treatment of hydrochloric acid skin burns by injection of calcium gluconate. Ind. Med. Surg., *33*:869, 1964.

Boswick, J. A.: Cold injuries. Major Probl. Clin. Surg. *19*:96, 1976.

Bowers, D. G., Jr., and Lynch, J. B.: Adriamycin extravasation. Plast. Reconstr. Surg., *61*:86, 1978.

Bracken, M., Cuppage, F., McLaury, R. L., Kerwin, C., and Klaassen, C. B.: Comparative effectiveness of topical treatment of hydrofluoric acid burns. J. Occup. Med., *27*:733, 1985.

Brown, J. B., and Fryer, M. P.: High energy electron injury from accelerator machines (cathode rays). Radiation burns of chest wall and neck: a 17 year followup of atomic burns. Ann. Surg., *162*:426, 1965.

Brown, J. B., McDowell, F., and Fryer, M. P.: Surgical treatment of radiation burns. Surg. Gynecol. Obstet., *88*:609, 1949.

Cannon, B., Randolph, J. B., and Murray, J. E.: Malignant radiation for benign conditions. N. Engl. J. Med., *260*:197, 1959.

Carrera, G. F., Kozin, F., Flaherty, L., and McCarty, D.

J.: Radiographic changes in the hands following childhood frostbite injury. Skeletal Radiol. *6*:33, 1981.

Ciano, M., Burlin, J. R., Pardoe, R., Mills, R. L., and Hentz, V. R.: High frequency electromagnetic radiation injury to the upper extremities. Local and systemic effects. Ann. Plast. Surg., *7*:128, 1981.

Cohen, F. J., Manganaro, J., and Bezzozo, R. C.; Identification of involved tissue during surgical treatment of doxorubicin-induced extravasation necrosis. J. Hand Surg., *8*:43, 1983.

Cohen, M. H.: Amelioration of Adriamycin skin necrosis: an experimental study. Cancer Treat. Rep., *63*:1003, 1979.

Cohen, S. C., Dibella, N. J., and Michelak, J. C.: Recall injury from Adriamycin. Ann. Intern. Med., *83*:232, 1975.

Curreri, P. W., Asch, M. J., and Pruitt, B. A., Jr.: The treatment of chemical burns: specialized diagnostic, therapeutic and prognostic considerations. J. Trauma, *10*:634, 1970.

Daniel, J.: The X rays. New Science, *3*:562, 1986.

Dibbell, D. G., Iverson, E. R., Wallace, J., Laub, D. R., and Mitchell, S. M.: Hydrofluoric acid burns of the hand. J. Bone Joint Surg., *52A*:931, 1970.

Donaldson, S. S., Glick, J. M., and Wilbur, J. R.: Adriamycin activating a recall phenomenon after radiation therapy. Ann. Intern. Med., *81*:407, 1974.

Dorr, R. T.: What is the appropriate management of tissue extravasation by antitumor agents (discussion). Plast. Reconstr. Surg., *75*:403, 1985.

Dorr, R. T.: Chemotherapy extravasation. Highlights on Antineoplastic Drugs, May–June, 1984.

Fryer, M. P., and Brown, J. B.: Repair of atomic, cathode ray, cyclotron and x-ray burns of the hand. Long-term followup examinations and microscopic studies. Am. J. Surg., *103*:688, 1962.

Fuhrman, F. A., and Crismon, J. M.: Studies on gangrene following cold injury. J. Clin. Invest., *26*:476, 1947.

Gruber, R. P., Laub, D. R., and Vistnes, L. M.: The effect of hydrotherapy on the clinical course and pH of experimental cutaneous chemical burns. Plast. Reconstr. Surg., *55*:200, 1975.

Hakstian, R. W.: Cold-induced digital epiphyseal necrosis in childhood (symmetrical focal ischaemic necrosis). Can. J. Surg., *15*:168, 1972.

Harris J. C., Ramack, B. H., and Bregman, D. J.: Comparative efficacy of injectable calcium and magnesium salts in the therapy of hydrofluoric acid burns. Clin. Toxicol., *18*:1027, 1981.

Hedeboe, J., Larsen, F. M., Lucht, U., and Christensen, S. T.: Heat generation in plaster of Paris and resulting hand burns. Burns, *9*:46, 1982.

Hentz, V. R.: Burns of the hand, thermal, chemical, and electrical. Emerg. Med. Clin. North Am., *3*:391, 1985.

Hoffmeister, F. S., Macomber, W. B., and Wang, M. K.H.: Radiation in dentistry—surgical comments. J. Am. Dent. Assoc., *78*:511, 1969.

Holly, F. E., and Beck, W. L.: Dosimetry studies for an industrial radiography accident. *In* Hubner, K. F., and Fry, S. A. (Eds.): The Medical Basis for Radiation Accident Preparedness. New York, Elsevier-North-Holland, 1980, pp. 265–277.

Holm, P. C. A., and Vanggaard, L.: Frostbite. Plast. Reconstr. Surg., *54*:544, 1974.

Ignoffo R. J., and Friedman M. A.: Therapy of local toxicities caused by extravasation of cancer chemotherapeutic drugs. Cancer Treat. Rev., *7*:17, 1980.

Iverson, R. E., Laub, D. R., and Madison, M. S.: Hydrofluoric acid burns. Plast. Reconstr. Surg., *48*:107, 1971.

Jackson, I. T., and Robinson, D. W.: Severe tissue damage following accidental subcutaneous infusion of bicarbonate solution. Scott. Med. J., *21*:200, 1976.

Jameson, J., and O'Donnel, J.: Guidelines for extravasation of intravenous drugs. Infusion, 7:157, 1983.

Jelenko, C, III: Chemicals that "burn." J. Trauma, *14*:65, 1974.

Kaplan, S. S.: Burns following application of plastic splint dressings. J. Bone Joint Surg., *63A*:670, 1981.

Kleinert, H. E., and Bronson, J. L.: Hydrofluoric acid burns of the hand. Med. Times, *104*:75, 1976.

Knize, D. M., Weatherly-White, R. C. A., Paton, B. C., and Owens, J. C.: Prognostic factors in the management of frostbite. J. Trauma, *9*:74, 1969.

Knowlton, M. P., Leifer, E., Hogness, J. R., Hempelman, L. H., Blaney, L. F., et al.: Beta ray burns of human skin. J.A.M.A., *141*:239, 1949.

Koehnlein, H. E., and Achinger, R.: A new method of treatment of hydrofluoric acid burns of the extremities. Chir. Plast., *6*:297, 1982.

Koehnlein, H. E., Merkle, P., and Springorum, H. W.: Hydrogen fluoride burns, experiments and treatment. Surg. Forum, *24*:50, 1973.

Krizek, T. J., and Ariyan, S.: Severe acute radiation injuries of the hand. Report of two cases. Plast. Reconstr. Surg., *51*:14, 1973.

Lange, K., and Boyd, L. J.: The functional pathology of experimental frostbite and prevention of subsequent gangrene. Surg. Gynecol., Obstet., *80*:346, 1945.

Lanzl, L. H., Rosenfeld, M. L., and Tarlov, A. R.: Injury due to accidental high dose exposure to 10 mev electrons. Health Phys., *13*:241, 1967.

Larsen, D. L.: Treatment of tissue extravasation by antitumor agents. Cancer, *49*:1796, 1982.

Larsen, D. L.: What is the appropriate management of tissue extravasation by antitumor agents? Plast. Reconstr. Surg., *75*:397, 1985.

Laughlin, R. A., Landeen, J. M., and Habel, M. B.: The management of inadvertent subcutaneous Adriamycin infiltration. Am. J. Surg., *137*:409, 1979.

Leddy, E. T., and Rigos, F. J.: Radiodermatitis among physicians. Am. J. Roentgenol., *45*:696, 1949.

Leonard, L. G., Scheulen, J. J., and Munster, A. M.: Chemical burns: effect of prompt first aid. J. Trauma, *22*:420, 1982.

Lever, W. F., and Schaumburg-Lever, G.: Histopathology of the skin. 6th Ed. Philadelphia, J. B. Lippincott Company, 1983, p. 214.

Linder, R. M., Upton, J., and Osteen, R.: Management of extensive doxorubicin hydrochloride extravasation injuries. J. Hand Surg., *8*:22, 1983.

Loth, T. S., and Eversmann, W. W., Jr.: Treatment methods for extravasation of chemotherapeutic agents: a comparative study. J. Hand Surg., *11A*:388, 1986.

Lushbaugh, C. C., Fry, S. A., Hubner, K. F., and Ricks, R. C.: Total body irradiation. A historical review and follow. *In* Hubner, K. F., and Fry, S. A. (Eds.): The Medical Basis for Radiation Accident Preparedness. New York, Elsevier-North-Holland, 1980, pp. 3–15.

MacCara, M. E.: Extravasation: a hazard of intravenous therapy. Drug. Intell. Clin. Pharm., *17*:713, 1983.

Mamakos, M. S.: Recall phenomenon or severe skin and muscle necrosis following Adriamycin extravasation in the hand. Int. Surg., *69*:73, 1984.

May, J. W., Jr., Chait, L. A., Cohen, B. E., and O'Brien, B. M.: Free neurovascular flap from the first web of the foot in hand reconstruction. J. Hand Surg., *2*:387, 1977.

McCauley, R. L., Hing, D. M., Robson, M. C., and Heggers, J. P.: Frostbite injuries: a rational approach based on the pathophysiology. J. Trauma, *22*:143, 1983.

McGeown, G.: Cement burns of the hands. Contact Dermatitis, *10*:246, 1984.

Meryman, H. T.: Tissue freezing and local cold injury. Physiol. Rev., *36*:233, 1957.

Miller, B. J., and Chasmar, L. R.: Frostbite in Saskatoon: a review of ten winters. Can. J. Surg., *23*:423, 1980.

Mills, W. J., Jr.: Frostbite: A discussion of the problem and a review of an Alaskan experience. Alaska Med., *15*:27, 1973.

Nelms, J. D.: Adaptation to cold and cold injury. J. R. Nav. Med. Serv., *58*:189, 1972.

Orcutt, T. J., and Pruitt, B. A.: Chemical injuries of the upper extremity. Major Probl. Clin. Surg., *9*:84, 1976.

Orr, K. O., and Faines, D. C.: Cold injuries in Korea during the winter of 1950–51. Medicine, *31*:177, 1952.

Page, R. E., and Robertson, G. A.: Management of the frostbitten hand. Hand, *15*:185, 1983.

Pegg, S. P., Siu, S., and Gillett, G.: Intra-arterial infusions in the treatment of hydrofluoric acid burns. Burns, *11*:440, 1985.

Peters, W. J.: Alkali burns from wet cement. Can. Med. Assoc. J., *130*:902, 1984.

Polakoff, P. L. Treating chemical skin burns varies between acids and alkalies. Occup. Health Saf., *55*:24, 1986.

Purdue, G. F., Lewis, S. A., and Hunt, J. L.: Pyrophosphate scanning in early forstbite injury. Am. Surg., *49*:619, 1983.

Quintanella, R. F., Krusen, H., and Essex, H. E.: Studies on frostbite with special reference to treatment and the effect on minute blood vessels. Am. J. Physiol., *149*:149, 1947.

Reilly, J. J., Neifeld, J. P., and Rosenberg, S. A.: Clinical course and management of accidental Adriamycin extravasation. Cancer, *40*:2053, 1977.

Robson, M. C., and Heggers, J. P.: Evaluation of hand frostbite blister fluid as a clue to pathogenesis. J. Hand Surg., *6*:43, 1981.

Rothberg, H., Place, C. H., and Shteir, O.: Adriamycin toxicity: an unusual melanotic reaction. Part I. Cancer Chemother., *58*:749, 1974.

Rudolph, R., Stein, R. S., and Patillo, R. A.: Skin ulcers due to Adriamycin. Cancer, *38*:1087, 1976.

Saenger, E. L., Kereiakes, J. G., Wald, N., and Thoma, G. E.: Clinical course and dosimetry of acute hand injuries to industrial radiographers from multicurie sealed gamma sources. *In* Hubner, K. F., and Fry, S. A. (Eds.): The Medical Basis for Radiation Accident Preparedness. New York, Elsevier-North-Holland, 1980, pp. 169–78.

Shearin, J. C., Jr.: Acute x-ray exposure of the distal phalanx of the fingers. *In* Hubner, K. F., and Fry, S. A. (Eds.): The Medical Basis for Radiation Accident Preparedness. New York, Elsevier-North-Holland, 1980, pp. 247–55.

Shumacker, H. B., Jr., and Kilman, J. W.: Sympathectomy in the treatment of frostbite. Arch. Surg., *89*:575, 1964.

Smith, S. M.: Subjective experiences during a 32 year period after resurfacing of hands for severe and acute radiation burns. Plast. Reconstr. Surg., *51*:23, 1973.

Snider, R. L., and Porter, J. M.: Treatment of experimental frostbite with intra-arterial sympathetic blocking drugs. Surgery, *77*:557, 1975.

Stern, P. J.: Surgical approaches to radiation injuries of

the hand. *In* Hubner, K. F., and Fry, S. A. (Eds.): The Medical Basis for Radiation Accident Preparedness. New York, Elsevier-North-Holland, 1980, pp. 257–63.

Stern, P. J., Kreilein, J. B., and Kleinert, H. E.: Neurovascular cutaneous flaps for the management of radiation-induced fingertip dermal necrosis. J. Hand Surg., *8*:88, 1983.

Stewart, C. E.: Chemical skin burns. Am. Fam. Physician, *31*:149, 1985.

Tishler, J. M.: The soft tissue and bone changes in frostbite injuries. Diagn. Radiol., 102:511, 1972.

Upton, J., Mulliken, J. B., and Murray, J. E.: Major intravenous extravasation injuries. Am. J. Surg., *137*:497, 1979.

Vance, M. V., Curry, S. C., Kunkel, D. B., Ryan, P. J., and Ruggeri, S. B.: Digital hydrofluoric acid burns: treatment with intra-arterial calcium infusion. Ann. Emerg. Med., *15*:890, 1986.

Vanggaard, L.: Arteriovenous anastomosis in temperature regulation. Acta Physiol. Scand., *76*:13a, 1969.

Wale, R.: Chemical burns: First aid and prevention. Aust. Fam. Physician, *15*:425, 1986.

Warren, S.: Effects of radiation on normal tissue. XIII. Effects on the skin. Arch. Pathol., *35*:340, 1943.

Watson, G. M.: The nature of radiation injury. Pathology, *12*:155, 1980.

Weatherley-White, R. C., Paton, B. C., and Sjöstrom, B.: Experimental studies in cold injury. III. Observations on the treatment of frostbite. Plast. Reconstr. Surg., *36*:10, 1965.

Wetherhold, J. M., and Shepard, F. P.: Treatment of hydrofluoric acid burns. J. Occup. Med., 7:193, 1965.

Whayne, T. F., and DeBakey, M. F.: Cold injury, ground type. Washington, DC, U. S. Government Printing Office, 1958.

Wilson, G. A., Sanger, R. G., and Boswick, J. A.: Accidental hydrofluoric acid burns of the hand. J. Am. Dent. Assoc. *99*:57, 1979.

Wilson, G. R., and Davidson P. M.: Full-thickness burns from ready-mix cement. Burns, *12*:139, 1985.

Wolfe, C. A., and Linkewich, J. A.: Preparation of guidelines for the avoidance and treatment of extravasation of antineoplastic drugs. Hosp. Pharm., *22*:125, 1987.

Wright, R. W.: A fluoroscopic burn to a patient's right hand sustained in removing a sewing needle—a 22 year follow-up. Clin. Radiol., *29*:347, 1978.

Zenck, K.: Management of intravenous extravasations. Infusion, *5*:77, 1981.

Zweig, J. I., Kabakow, B., Wallach, R. C., Valencic, M., and Zalusky, R.: Rational effective medical treatment of skin ulcers due to Adriamycin. Cancer Treat. Rep., *63*:2101, 1979.

Matthias B. Donelan

Reconstruction of the Burned Hand and Upper Extremity

HISTORY

The reconstruction of postburn deformities of the hand began to be recognized as a special problem after the extensive experience with hand burns accumulated during the Second World War. Great progress was made during this period in the fundamental understanding of the burn wound and its impact on the function of the hand (see Chapter 129). The long-standing debate between the relative merits of splinting and immobilization versus

early motion began to be resolved in favor of early motion (Braithwaite, 1949). Early closure of the burn wound with skin grafting was recognized as playing a vital role in minimizing edema, and decreasing the chronic inflammation and resulting fibrosis that led to contractures of joints and adhesion of tendons. It became clear that the expeditious provision of durable and elastic skin coverage to the dorsum of the hand was essential to preserve function in the deep, otherwise uninjured parts. In order to facilitate rapid wound healing, Webster and Rowland (1946) proposed a two-stage method for treating dorsal hand burns. They recommended "temporary" skin grafting using "patch" grafts to close the acute wound, followed by elective excision of the skin graft and scar and definitive closure with either thick split-thickness grafts or skin flaps. In the case of full-thickness burns, Cope and associates (1947) pointed out the advantages of early, direct surgical excision to eliminate the development of infection and to minimize scarring and disability. The importance of providing sufficient dorsal skin replacement in order to prevent the development of late contractures was emphasized. Converse (1945) recommended elective total replacement of the skin of the dorsum using a large-sized dermatome to provide a single sheet of skin graft large enough to restore normal flexion and function to the hand. Improved dermatomes greatly facilitated the ability to obtain large, thick split-thickness grafts.

Shaw and Payne (1946) noted that the repair of surface defects of the upper extremity required a complete knowledge of the anatomy and function of the whole hand. The development of hand centers by the military concentrated the experience of hand and upper extremity reconstruction. This led to more sophisticated concepts and the evolution of improved reconstructive techniques. Better understanding of the problems of postburn dorsal scarring, and more reliable techniques of skin grafting, decreased the indications for the use of pedicle flaps in postburn reconstruction of the hand (Farmer and Woolhouse, 1945). Skin grafts were recognized as superior to flaps for replacing dorsal skin on the hand whenever possible (Brown and McDowell, 1958). A general consensus emerged that the use of flaps should be reserved for cases in which complex reconstruction was later required, such as tendon grafting and joint reconstruction. The major emphasis in the literature was placed on the most frequently encountered problem of dorsal hand burns and the resultant secondary deformities. The less common, and often more vexing, problems of severe volar burns and postburn amputations received considerably less attention. There was little discussion of the late esthetic deformities accompanying virtually all burn hand injuries.

GENERAL PRINCIPLES

Burn injuries to the hand and upper extremity result in an enormous spectrum of deformities ranging from the slightly unesthetic to complete loss of the part. Complicating matters even further is the fact that burns to the hand, particularly if severe, are frequently accompanied by burns to other areas of the body. At the U.S. Army Institute of Surgical Research, Brooke Army Medical Center, 75 per cent of burn patients sustained burns of the hand, and 80 per cent of the hand injuries were bilateral (Moncrief, 1958). This association with other, often extensive injuries may impact on the need and timing for reconstruction. It also may severely compromise reconstructive options available because of injury to potential donor sites. The reconstruction of postburn hand deformities, therefore, must always be placed in the overall context of total patient care.

Thermal injuries are characterized by varying degrees of damage to the skin and underlying structures, depending on the temperature and type of heat source, the duration of exposure, and the area over which the heat is transferred. The extent of damage is ordinarily dictated by the severity of the initial injury. However, improper care during the acute phase can result in secondary deformities that would otherwise be preventable. For example, a full-thickness burn of the dorsum, when appropriately treated by early primary excision and grafting, can give a result such as shown in Figure 132–1. On the other hand, a full-thickness burn of the hand incorrectly diagnosed as second degree and allowed to heal over the course of many months by secondary intention can result in the type of deformity shown in Figure 132–2. A clear understanding of the role of wound healing and contraction is necessary in order to make sense of the myriad deformities encountered.

Because the fundamental acute problem is that of loss of skin, it is usually necessary for the purposes of reconstructive surgery to add skin in the form of a graft when dealing with post-burn deformities. Z-plasties and other local flap procedures often do not provide enough tissue and have a higher rate of complications when performed in the context of scar and increased tension. However, there are frequent exceptions to this general rule. One of the fascinations of postburn reconstruction lies in the great variety of deformities seen. Each case must be carefully evaluated in the context of total patient care, and only then can the best individual procedure or treatment plan be chosen.

In the vast majority of patients the initial thermal injury is limited to the skin alone; the underlying tendons and joints are usually spared. Prolonged wound healing with its attendant edema, infection, fibrosis, and immobilization can lead to secondary joint contractures, rupture of extensor tendon mechanisms, and adhesion of gliding tissues. In general, however, it is remarkable how often the deeper structures are spared, particularly in children.

Electrical burns to the hand and upper extremity represent a separate class of injuries. The flash burns from arcing, and the flame burns resulting from ignition of clothing during electrical trauma, give the same pattern of superficial injury seen in thermal burns from other causes. High voltage electrical injuries involving the passage of current through deeper structures result in a completely different pattern of tissue damage and type of secondary deformity (Artz, 1967), and will be discussed independently.

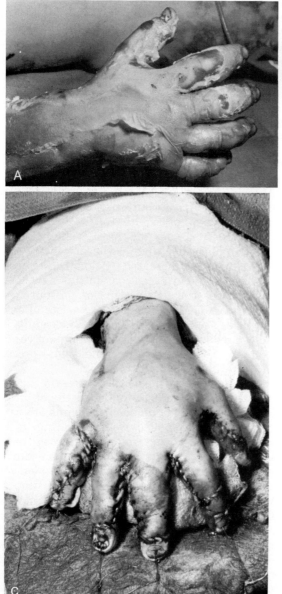

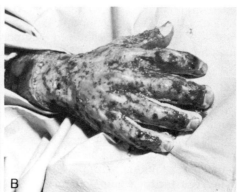

Figure 132–1. Full-thickness burn of the dorsum of the hand treated by excision and grafting. *A,* Acute full-thickness injury. *B,* Excision to the dorsal veins and peritenon. *C,* Resurfacing with thick split-thickness skin grafts.

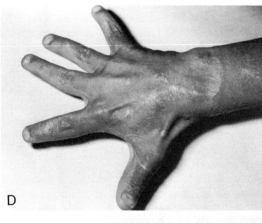

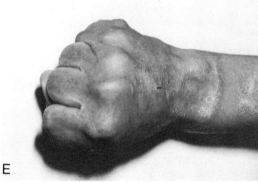

Figure 132–1 *Continued D, E,* Nine years after excision and graft. Full extension and flexion with a good esthetic appearance.

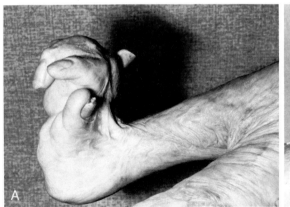

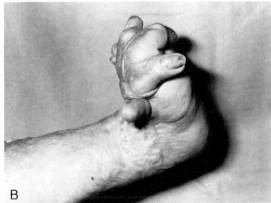

Figure 132–2. Dorsal hand burn with severe hypertrophic scarring and joint deformity after prolonged healing by contraction and epithelization. *A,* Radial view. *B,* Ulnar view.

Postburn hand deformities can be confusing to analyze because the acute injuries vary so widely, previous treatment has often been less than optimal, and there frequently are multiple problems in each hand. For purposes of discussion and treatment, it has been helpful to divide these deformities into three general categories, all of which can be present in a single hand: soft tissue deformities either dorsal or volar; joint deformities with or without tendon injury; and amputations. Some very severe injuries that result in complex deformities include all the above, plus tendon and even bone defects, but fortunately these are rare. In addition, because the hands, along with the face, are always exposed to view, their appearance is important and often of concern to the patient. Esthetic considerations should be taken into account whenever possible in caring for postburn hand deformities.

SOFT TISSUE DEFORMITIES

Web Space Contractures and Postburn Syndactyly

A normal web space is composed of dorsal skin sloping in a gentle fashion from a dorsal-proximal location between the metacarpal heads to a volar-distal location halfway between the metacarpophalangeal joint and the proximal interphalangeal joint. With dorsal hand burns, this normal anatomy is frequently altered. Scars or skin graft suture lines can bridge across the natural concavity between the metacarpal heads, creating bands. Dorsal web scars can be pulled distally by contraction, producing an unsightly dorsal hooding. In mild cases, function is rarely affected. The most appropriate treatment is some form of local tissue rearrangement with either a traditional Z-plasty or a double-opposing Z-plasty (Shaw, Richey, and Nahigian, 1973). Alexander, MacMillan, and Martel (1982) described a V-M plasty that gave good results in 24 cases of mild web space contracture. Excellent results can be obtained and skin grafting is rarely required (Fig. 132–3).

True postburn syndactyly with varying degrees of fusion of the fingers and complete obliteration of the web space is a more complex problem. This usually results from dorsal hand burns that extend beyond the web space and heal over a prolonged period. It is often associated with hypertrophic scarring. In the most severe cases in which the scarring extends onto the dorsum of the fingers, the volar skin is pulled dorsally, and fusion of the soft tissues of the digits occurs (Fig. 132–4). Abduction may be severely limited. The importance of preventing this deformity by early management techniques has been emphasized throughout the literature (Krizek, Robson, and Flagg, 1974; Quan and associates, 1981).

When there is a true postburn syndactyly, as in congenital syndactyly, there is by definition an inadequate amount of local tissue, and it is always necessary to add skin in the form of a graft in order to obtain a satisfactory release. Unlike a congenital syndactyly, however, the dorsal skin between the fused fingers is not normal: it is always either hypertrophic scar or healed skin graft, or both. Many types of local flaps, with or without additional skin grafts, have been proposed to correct postburn syndactyly. Tanzer (1948) rotated a pedicle flap from the side of an adjacent finger combined with a free graft. Adamson and associates (1968) described the use of two small web space flaps combined with a thick split-thickness skin graft. Krizek, Robson, and Flagg (1974) preferred to use local flaps for the correction of burn syndactyly in most patients. McDougal, Wray, and Weeks (1976) described an extension of Tanzer's concept, which they called the "lateral volar flap"; this technique required a skin graft to the flap donor site. Browne, Teague, and Snyder (1978) suggested a modification of the quadrilateral flap described by Bauer, Tondra, and Trusler (1956) for correction of congenital syndactyly. They believed that this created a softer web space with a rectangular shape. Salisbury and Bevin (1981) recommended a modification of the dorsal flap, which they called the "hourglass" technique. All these procedures have their adherents and may be beneficial in selected mild to moderate cases. The use of damaged local tissue as a flap, however, particularly when a skin graft must be utilized anyway, seems to add little in terms of improved function or esthetics, but it does increase the risk, because any flap raised in this tissue has a compromised blood supply and may lead to complications (Fig. 132–5). For this reason, a simpler, more straightforward approach to this deformity may be in-

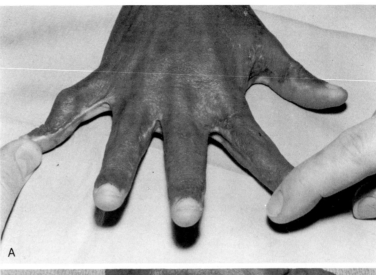

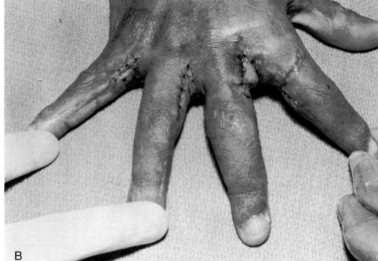

Figure 132–3. *A,* Interdigital web space contractures after dorsal excision and graft. *B,* After standard Z-plasty revision. *C,* Close-up of the web space shows elimination of the band with restoration of normal contour.

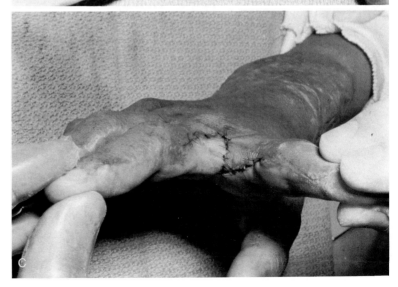

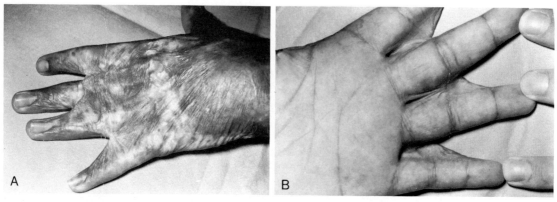

Figure 132–4. Severe postburn syndactyly. *A,* Dorsal view showing fusion of digits beyond the proximal interphalangeal joints. *B,* Volar view showing dorsal displacement of palmar skin with soft tissue fusion to the level of the proximal interphalangeal joints.

dicated in many cases, particularly when severe. Preoperative markings are made (Fig. 132–6) identifying the metacarpal heads, the proximal interphalangeal joints, and the proposed location of the volar edge of the web space. Careful release is then carried out preserving the normal gentle slope of the web space and incorporating darts at the dorsal and volar ends of the release. The extent of the soft tissue deficit in a true postburn syndactyly is often remarkable. A thick split-thickness skin graft is then used to cover the defect, and is sutured into place with a bolster dressing. A full-thickness skin graft can be used if desired and available, and may offer the advantage of less postoperative contraction. Postoperative management consists of pressure garments and web space conformers (Krizek, Robson, and Flagg, 1974; Rousso and Wexler, 1980). Avoiding the use of local flaps

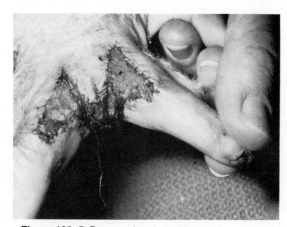

Figure 132–5. Burn syndactyly repair with a dorsal quadrilateral flap. Necrosis of the distal half of the flap.

in the correction of postburn syndactyly has several advantages. It obviates the problem of flap necrosis. Simple release and grafting allows the simultaneous correction of multiple webs because it does not compromise the blood supply of adjacent fingers as can local flaps. Finally, an adequate release can always be carried out without local tissue constraints. Skin grafts can provide a satisfactory result from both a functional and an esthetic standpoint (Fig. 132–7).

Dorsal Contractures and Hypertrophic Scars

Dorsal contractures are the most common problem encountered after hand burns. Gillies and Cuthbert (1943) referred to it as "the invisible skin loss" after burns on the dorsum. Hypertrophic scarring of the dorsum also frequently occurs despite continuing emphasis on splinting and physical therapy, early excision and grafting when indicated, and prolonged pressure and therapy after the acute period. The reasons are numerous. Some second degree burns that heal in gratifying fashion without skin grafting can insidiously develop hypertrophic scarring and contracture over subsequent months if not carefully followed. Deep second degree burns that should be excised and grafted are incorrectly diagnosed and allowed to heal over a prolonged period, with resultant hypertrophy. Sometimes, despite the best of intentions by the treating physicians, other aspects of the patient's injuries take precedence and proper

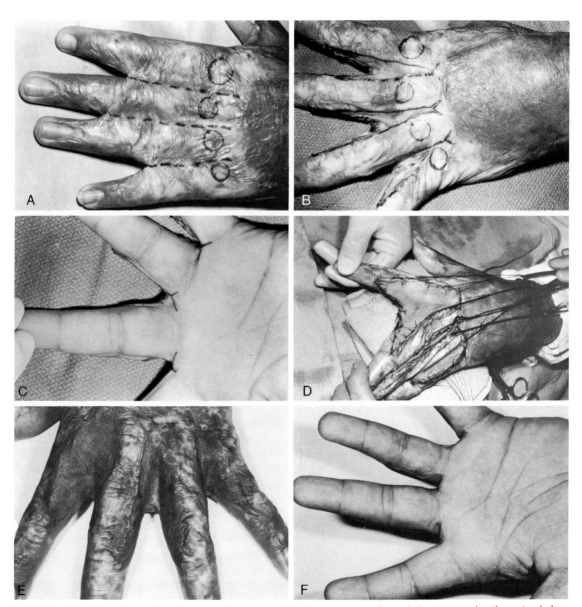

Figure 132–6. *A,* Preoperative markings as outlined in the text. *B,* Release is carried out preserving the natural slope of the web space. *C,* Darts at the palmar extent of the incision to prevent contracture. *D,* The amount of skin required to resurface the web space can be extensive. *E,* Postoperative appearance, dorsal view. *F,* Postoperative volar view.

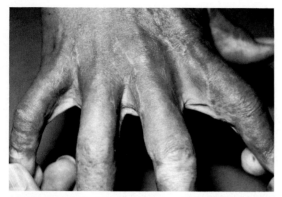

Figure 132–7. Correction of postburn syndactyly with simple release and skin grafting of the web spaces can give a good result functionally and cosmetically. This patient had a simultaneous release and graft of the second, third, and fourth web spaces.

management of the hand burn is not possible during the acute period. Tangential excision of second degree burns or complete excision of full-thickness burns with immediate skin grafting may have decreased the incidence of this complication, although this remains controversial (Rousso and Wexler, 1980; Salisbury and Wright, 1982). Additionally, some patients are noncompliant for various reasons and refuse postacute programs designed to minimize hypertrophy and contraction (Larson and associates, 1971). In the most severe cases of contracture and hypertrophy the hand assumes the "postburn claw deformity" (Fig. 132–8) (McCormack, 1971). There is hyperextension at the metacarpophalangeal joints and flexion at the proximal interphalangeal joints. There is limitation of abduction of the digits and flattening of the normal transverse metacarpal arch. The dorsal scar-

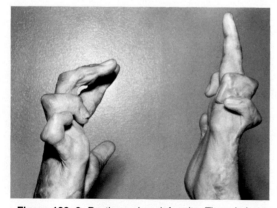

Figure 132–8. Postburn claw deformity. There is hyperextension at the metacarpophalangeal joints and flexion at the proximal interphalangeal joints.

ring over the first web space leads to a thumb adduction contracture, and there is frequently ulnar deviation of the fifth digit resulting from longitudinal scarring along the ulnar aspect of the dorsum (Peterson and Elton, 1976).

When a patient develops dorsal contractures in the early postacute period, initial treatment should be conservative with pressure, splinting, and physical therapy. The timing of surgical intervention should be determined on an individual basis rather than by a mandatory or arbitrary period of nonsurgical treatment. When it becomes clear that physical therapy has plateaued or there is actual loss of function, surgery should be considered. Timely release of dorsal soft tissue contractures can greatly improve the effect of physical therapy and may prevent the development of permanent joint contractures.

Incisional release and grafting is usually preferable to excision and grafting, particularly if the dorsal scarring is fresh and hyperemic (Rousso and Wexler, 1980). This decreases the complexity and potential morbidity of the surgery, and decreasing tension on the residual scar can favorably influence its maturation, with softening and shrinkage over time. It also minimizes the requirement of a skin graft donor site. A transverse release should be carried out just proximal to the metacarpophalangeal joints. Dissection must be careful to preserve adequate vascularized soft tissue over the dorsal hood of the joint and ensure satisfactory skin graft survival. The lateral extent of the releasing incisions should be beyond the axis of metacarpophalangeal joint motion and ended with a Y or "fishtail" to allow maximal release. The metacarpophalangeal joint can be fixed in full flexion with Kirschner wires. This has been a very useful adjunctive technique with few, if any, complications (Jackson and Brown, 1970; Jackson, 1981). Correction of the frequently associated interdigital syndactyly is not possible at the same time because the digits cannot be simultaneously abducted while they are flexed as a result of collateral ligament tension.

In long-standing contractures when the metacarpophalangeal joints have been in extension for considerable time, it is occasionally necessary in adults to carry out a simultaneous release of the collateral ligaments (see Chap. 114). This problem is uncommon in children. Despite long-standing contractures at the metacarpophalangeal joint level, it is very unusual for there to be shortening of the extensor tendons. Tendon surgery is therefore rarely required and the indications for the use of flap tissue for dorsal hand resurfacing are infrequent.

In patients with massive diffuse hypertrophic scarring, complete excision of the scar, preserving the dorsal veins and paratenon, followed by skin graft resurfacing, is indicated (Fig. 132–9). From an esthetic standpoint this is unquestionably superior. This operation is extensive, however, and can be technically more difficult than excision and grafting during the acute period (Salisbury and Dingeldein, 1982). As in cases of early excision and grafting, care must be taken to place darts in the web spaces and along the lateral margins of the skin grafts to avoid pernicious scars and unsightly webbing (Cannon and May, 1982). Excellent esthetic and functional results can be obtained in selected cases.

Because of the exposed nature of the dorsum of the hand, unfavorable scarring can create a conspicuous deformity even when there is no functional deficit. Meshed skin grafts result in permanently abnormal skin texture that does not improve significantly with time. The choice of meshed grafts for dorsal resurfacing during the care of acute hand burns should be carefully weighed against this long-term disadvantage. Focal hypertropic and linear scars of an unfavorable nature can be excised or revised, using local plastic manipulations with good effect. More extensive areas of hypertrophic or ridged scars can be improved by a local excision and grafting, or tangential excision to the dermal plane and thin overgrafting (Peacock, 1988).

First Web Space Adduction Contractures

Adduction contractures of the first web space frequently occur after hand burns. They differ from the web contractures arising between the digits. True syndactyly rarely occurs except when there is partial amputation of the digits and thumb. These contractures can usually be divided into one of three general categories: (1) extensive dorsal scarring with essentially complete sparing of the palmar skin; (2) a linear contracture along the

leading edge of the web space, usually seen after primary excision of the dorsum and skin grafting; (3) contraction of both the dorsal and palmar skin of the web space.

When the contracture involves both the palmar and dorsal skin, a release and skin graft are required (Fig. 132–10). In severe cases there may be an associated tightness of the underlying adductor pollicis and first dorsal interosseous. Care must be taken to avoid excessive division of the origin or insertion of these muscles during the release, otherwise hand function may be significantly weakened. When a satisfactory release is compromised by tightness of the intrinsics, a staged approach can be considered as an alternative to dividing the origin or insertion of the muscles. An initial release and graft can be carried out followed by intensive physical therapy. After six months or longer, a subsequent release and additional grafting can give further improvement. Injury must be avoided to the neurovascular bundles and even the motor branch of the median nerve when releases are carried back to the proximal palm. When there is hyperextension of the metacarpophalangeal joint of the thumb, the releasing incision should be carried dorsally over the metacarpophalangeal joint to allow correction of this deformity. The resulting defect is resurfaced with thick split-thickness skin grafts. In the most extensive cases of contracture when there is damage to deep structures and there is a need for later reconstruction, such as an adductor transfer, flap coverage of the web space may be indicated.

When the contracture is primarily limited to the leading edge of the web space, correction should be carried out whenever possible by a double-opposing Z-plasty with a Y-V advancement, the "five-flap Z-plasty" (Hirshowitz, Karev, and Rousso, 1975; Rousso and Wexler, 1980). A large single Z-plasty should be avoided in this circumstance, since it necessarily transposes dorsal skin graft or scar onto the palm and palmar skin to the dorsum. This creates a conspicuous pigmentary abnormality. In addition, a single large Z-plasty creates an acute angle that is unnatural in the first web space, and there may be difficulty with the blood supply to the large dorsal flap when it is composed of skin graft or scar. The five-flap Z-plasty has the distinct advantages of small flaps with a better blood supply and less abnormal translocation of dorsal and volar skin, and it creates a more natural U-

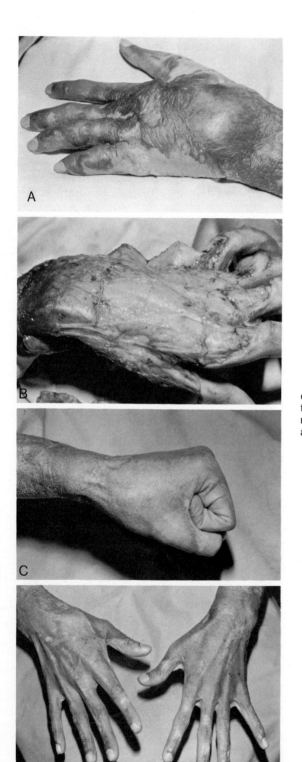

Figure 132–9. *A,* Severe postburn hypertrophic scarring of the dorsum. *B,* Excision of hypertrophic scar, preserving the dorsal veins and peritenon. Note the darts on the ulnar margin. *C, D,* Postoperative result with good function and appearance.

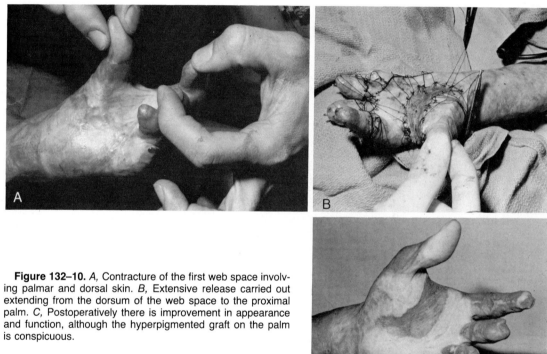

Figure 132–10. *A,* Contracture of the first web space involving palmar and dorsal skin. *B,* Extensive release carried out extending from the dorsum of the web space to the proximal palm. *C,* Postoperatively there is improvement in appearance and function, although the hyperpigmented graft on the palm is conspicuous.

shaped curve to the first web space (Fig. 132–11).

When the first web space contracture is solely the result of dorsal scarring, release or excision of the dorsal scar and replacement with a thick split-thickness skin graft is the best treatment. It is desirable to avoid carrying the release and graft onto the palmar skin, because the hyperpigmentation of the skin graft on the palm leads to a significant esthetic deformity.

Volar Contractures

Volar contractures of the fingers and palm are less frequently seen than dorsal contrac-tures. Because of the thick, specialized nature of palmar skin, full-thickness injuries are rarely encountered except in unusually se-vere cases, or with focal contact burns. For this reason, palmar burns should rarely be excised and grafted. Sensation is always bet-ter in the palmar skin than it would be in grafts, and the residual volar skin is still fixed to the underlying fibrous septa; it there-fore provides a better tactile and grasping surface. Many palmar burns that heal spon-taneously during the acute period, however, go on to develop significant contractures. These should always be treated by incision and grafting rather than excision.

Releasing incisions should be placed so that the usefulness of residual palmar skin is

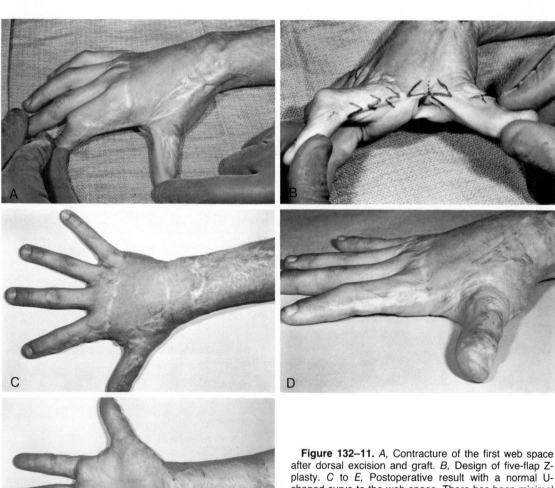

Figure 132–11. *A,* Contracture of the first web space after dorsal excision and graft. *B,* Design of five-flap Z-plasty. *C* to *E,* Postoperative result with a normal U-shaped curve to the web space. There has been minimal displacement of palmar skin to the dorsum. There is no dorsal skin on the palm.

maximized. Opinions vary as to the preferred type of skin graft to use on the palm. Thin split grafts lead to extensive contracture and should be avoided (Jackson, 1981). Some authors have advocated full-thickness grafts believing them to be more durable and to result in fewer recurrent contractures (Huang, Larson, and Lewis, 1975; Parks, Evans, and Larson, 1978; Beasley, 1981). In many patients with extensive burns in other locations, full-thickness donor sites may not be available or may be better utilized for other areas of reconstruction such as the face. Other authors have found no significant functional difference between thick split-thickness grafts and full-thickness grafts (Alexander and associates, 1981). Pensler and associates (1988) considered that split grafts give a superior result cosmetically with less hyperpigmentation. For mild to moderate contractures and for optimal esthetic results, split-thickness skin grafts from the plantar arch of the foot provide the best match in color and texture (Fig. 132–12).

JOINT DEFORMITIES

Proximal Interphalangeal Joints

The proximal interphalangeal joint is the most frequently injured deep structure in the hand after thermal injury (Peterson and Elton, 1976). The overlying dorsal skin is thin and there is very little intervening subcutaneous tissue. The extent of the acute injury to the central slip and extensor mechanism is difficult to ascertain. In cooperative patients who have full-thickness burns to the dorsum of the fingers, proximal interphalangeal joint function often is initially normal. It is intriguing to consider whether this could be maintained if vascularized soft tissue coverage could be provided at that point. Such intervention is rarely possible, however, and acute therapy is usually limited to maintaining the proximal interphalangeal joint in extension through splinting or K-wire fixation to minimize tension on the central slip and transverse retinacular ligaments, and

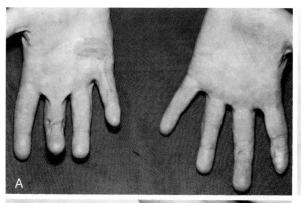
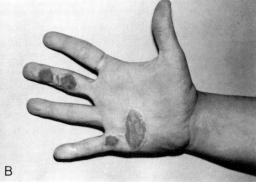
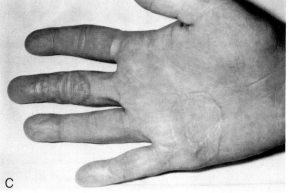

Figure 132–12. *A,* Contracture of the right palm involving the middle and fifth fingers. *B,* After release and split-thickness skin grafting with hyperpigmentation of the grafts. *C,* After excision of pigmented grafts and replacement with split-thickness grafts from the plantar arch.

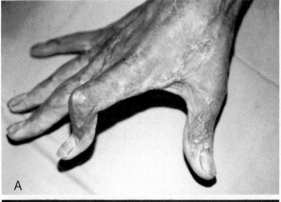

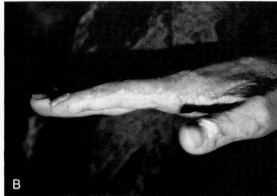

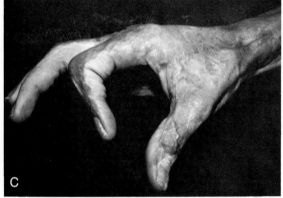

Figure 132–13. *A,* Postburn boutonnière deformity of the index finger. *B, C,* After extensor tendon repair with full extension and 90 degrees of flexion.

attempting to obtain wound closure as expeditiously as possible. In some patients this is successful and proximal interphalangeal joint function remains normal. Some patients develop an early postburn boutonnière deformity that responds well to simple splinting (Maisels, 1965; Larson and associates, 1970). In others the central slip ruptures or is weakened through ischemia or sepsis, leading to a flexion contracture without associated hyperextension at the distal interphalangeal joint. Presumably the integrity of the transverse retinacular ligament is maintained through scar or adhesion and the lateral bands do not sublux. In a third group of patients the central slip ruptures or is weakened, the transverse ligaments give way, and volar subluxation of the lateral bands occurs, leading to the classic postburn boutonnière deformity (Fig. 132–13*A*).

Reconstruction of the proximal interphalangeal joint extensor mechanism in the context of a postburn boutonnière deformity is difficult and rarely successful (Elliott, 1971). Salisbury and Dingeldein (1982) stated that it was appropriately undertaken in only a

few cases. There are several reasons why the results of proximal interphalangeal extensor tendon reconstruction are usually disappointing. This region of the finger is most complex anatomically and physiologically, and the delicate gliding mechanism of extension at that level is easily upset (Tubiana, 1968). The overlying soft tissues in the case of a burn boutonnière deformity are usually poor and there has often been damage to the articular surface of the joint because of a chronic open wound. There is fibrosis and scarring of other joint structures that preclude a delicate and sophisticated reconstruction. Only in selected patients in whom the dorsal tissues are of reasonable quality, the articular surfaces are undamaged, and full passive range of motion is restored through physical therapy should reconstruction be attempted. The method of choice is that described by Elliott (1971) and in selected patients it can give satisfactory results (Fig. 132–13*B, C*).

In the vast majority of patients with disruption of the extensor mechanism at the PIP joint, the most appropriate therapy is arthrodesis (see Chap. 106). In pediatric patients in whom the epiphysis remains open and growth potential exists, arthrodesis should be delayed until the epiphyses have closed. Some authors have been more enthusiastic about the reconstructive potential of hands with postburn boutonnière deformity (Maisels, 1965; Larson and associates, 1970).

Distal Interphalangeal Joints

Mallet finger injuries are commonly seen after burns. Open wounds over the distal interphalangeal joint can lead to rupture or weakening of the extensor tendon with the development of a flexion deformity. This is sometimes associated with hyperextension at the proximal interphalangeal joint, the "swan-neck" deformity (see Chap. 102). Often there is little residual motion in these joints because of destruction of the articular surface during the acute injury. When reconstruction is desired by the patient, arthrodesis is the method of choice (see Chap. 106).

Metacarpophalangeal Joints

Hyperextension of the metacarpophalangeal joints secondary to dorsal hand contractures is the most frequent deformity encountered in this joint after hand burns. After thermal injury it is unusual for there to be damage to the deep tendon and joint structures without severe injury to the distal digital ray. Correction of the hyperextension can usually be accomplished by simple release of the overlying scar contracture. Care must be taken over the joint to preserve the paratenon and other filmy vascularized tissue, in order to provide an adequate bed for skin grafting. With care, this can almost always be achieved, particularly in children. When there has been contraction of the collateral ligaments of the joint, capsulotomy must be carried out simultaneously. Postoperatively, the metacarpophalangeal joint should be held in flexion for two to three weeks with a K-wire, and aggressive physical therapy and splinting then instituted. When the joint contracture is severe and extensive dissection has been carried out, there may be inadequate soft tissue to support a skin graft. In these unusual cases, flap coverage of the dorsum of the hand is indicated.

NAIL DEFORMITIES

Partial or complete loss of fingernails after burn injury is not unusual. The other most common deformity encountered is abnormal growth of the nails secondary to an alteration in the normal anatomy of the nail bed (Zook, 1981). Contraction of the dorsal soft tissues of the digit proximal to the eponychium causes eversion of the nail fold. This deformity in itself is unsightly. The peeling back of the dorsal roof of the fold eliminates its contribution to nail growth and there is grooving, loss of surface shine, and sometimes even arching of the nail. Therapy is directed toward restoration of the normal nail fold relationships, if possible. Reconstruction of the eponychium with local flaps has been described (Barfod, 1972). Hayes (1974) recommended reconstruction in burns with a distally based flap. Ngim and Soin (1986) described a proximally based transposition flap for correction of postburn nail fold retraction. Improvement can also be obtained by releasing the contracted tissues proximal to the eponychium and allowing the thickened eponychium to slide distally, recreating the fold. The proximal defect is skin grafted (Alsbjorn, Metz, and Ebbehoj, 1985). After the contracture has been released, the thickness of the eponychium subsides and improvement can be obtained (Fig. 132–14).

AMPUTATIONS

After the most severe thermal injuries there is mummification of the digits, and amputation is eventually necessary (Fig. 132–15). This most commonly occurs in concentric fashion from distal to proximal, so that when the digital amputation level is at the proximal interphalangeal joint, only the thumbtip is lost. When the fingers are amputated at or just beyond the metacarpophalangeal joints, the thumb metacarpal and the base of the proximal phalanx are usually preserved, creating either a "mitten hand" or a hand with complete adactyly. In these cases a useful reconstructive procedure is pollicization of the index metacarpal ray (May and associates, 1984; Ward, Pensler, and Parry, 1985). This combines the benefits of first web space deepening and thumb metacarpal lengthening, and has been effective in restoring single hand prehension, particularly

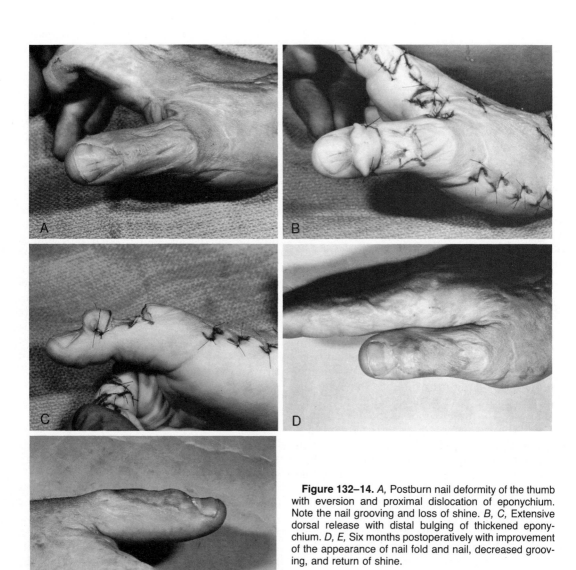

Figure 132–14. *A,* Postburn nail deformity of the thumb with eversion and proximal dislocation of eponychium. Note the nail grooving and loss of shine. *B, C,* Extensive dorsal release with distal bulging of thickened eponychium. *D, E,* Six months postoperatively with improvement of the appearance of nail fold and nail, decreased grooving, and return of shine.

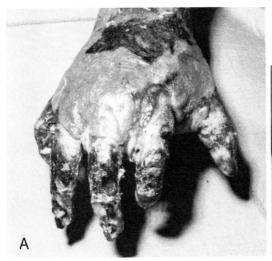

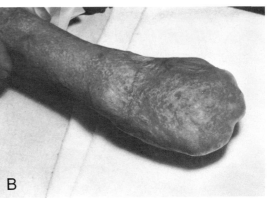

Figure 132–15. *A, B,* Fourth degree burn of the digits leading to mummification and eventual amputation.

in children (Fig. 132–16). Care must be taken to avoid weakening the adductor pollicis muscle by releasing its origin or insertion in order to deepen the web space, because this provides the power for key pinch. This operation is usually a better alternative than amputation and a prothesis (Beasely, 1981), especially in a case of bilateral postburn adactyly. When the metacarpal remnants are less than complete or there has been destruction of the epiphyses in children, this can be combined with a secondary metacarpal lengthening to improve grasping function (Matev, 1979).

Sometimes when there is apparent digital amputation, the phalanges may be hidden and malpositioned because of scar contracture (Fig. 132–17). Radiographic examination of these hands is essential. Often a remarkable degree of improvement can be obtained by careful, straightforward releases and skin grafting. The residual soft tissues, as long as they are carefully preserved during dissection, are remarkably receptive of split-thickness grafts. If the scarring is severe, particularly in the area of the first web space, and further complex reconstruction is anticipated (e.g., an index metacarpal pollicization or tendon grafting), considerations should be given at the time of initial release to the use of a flap for at least partial resurfacing of key areas.

COMPLEX DEFORMITIES

Some digits are so extensively damaged by burn injury that reasonable reconstruction is

not possible. In addition, a stiff, malpositioned, and painful or tender digit, particularly on the ulnar border of the hand, may detract from function and appearance. In such cases, amputation may be the best option (Peacock, 1977; Rousso and Wexler, 1980). Consideration should always be given to the use of the vascularized soft tissue from the digit as a filleted finger flap to aid in other local reconstruction.

ELBOW CONTRACTURES

Flexion contractures are the most common elbow deformity and are usually limited to overlying soft tissue scar and contracted skin grafts. Mild cases may respond to splinting and pressure. Patients may actually have a full range of motion but present with a pterygium of soft tissue arching across the antecubital space when the elbow is in full extension. Treatment is usually uncomplicated and consists of incisional release and grafting, or the use of local flaps or Z-plasties when available. It is rare for the deeper structures to limit extension, but if this is found to be the case, complex muscle-tendon and joint releasing procedures are to be avoided except as a last resort. The best approach is to release as much as possible by freeing the soft tissues alone, and then to carry out an adequate wound closure with grafts or flaps. Postoperative physical therapy and splinting often restore normal length and range of motion. Occasionally, subsequent releases may be necessary (Beasley, 1977).

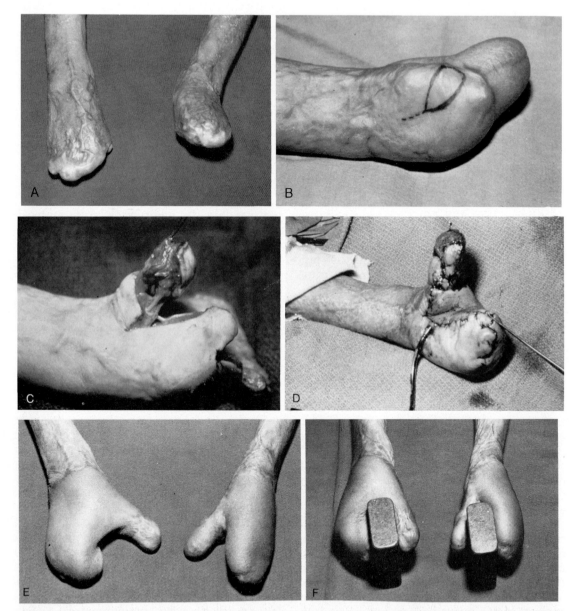

Figure 132–16. *A,* Bilateral postburn adactyly. After the creation of groin flaps for dorsal resurfacing, index metacarpal pollicization was carried out. *B,* The palmar skin island is marked. *C,* The metacarpal is transferred on its neurovascular bundle. *D,* The web space is lined with the thinned groin flap. *E, F,* Postoperative result with a lengthened thumb metacarpal and deepened first web space. Bilateral single hand prehension has been accomplished.

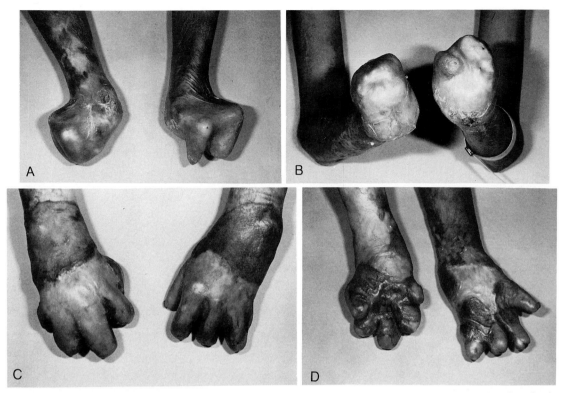

Figure 132–17. *A, B,* Severe bilateral hand burns with apparent digital amputation. *C, D,* Five months after simple release and graft of the left hand, and two months after release and graft of the right hand. Proximal phalanges are present. The metacarpophalangeal joints are intact and the thenar muscles are functional. Further reconstruction should restore single hand prehension bilaterally.

The choice of whether to use a skin graft or local flaps for the releasing procedure is usually straightforward and dictated by local conditions. When the burn extends across the entire antecubital space, there is no tissue available for flaps or Z-plasties. A transverse release should be performed from axis of rotation to axis of rotation of the joint and Y-extensions placed at the end of the releasing incision. A thick split-thickness skin graft is then used to resurface the area. When there is sparing of local tissues in the area of the antecubital space, Z-plasties and flaps can be used to good effect and the need for skin grafting obviated.

Care must be taken when releasing and grafting in this area to avoid creating an iatrogenic contour deformity. In the patient shown in Figure 132–18, the contracture was quite superficial, and the release to fascia with skin grafting created a deformity that was more ojectionable than the original pterygium of scar.

Extension contractures of the elbow are unusual following burns unless there is heterotopic ossification. When they are encountered, release of the tight dorsal skin, combined with excision of the customary chronic open wound and resurfacing with a thick split-thickness graft, is effective. When the bed after release is unsatisfactory or complex reconstructive surgery on the elbow joint is anticipated, flap coverage should be provided (Beasley, 1977). Flap selection must be individualized, but the groin flap has proved useful in this area (McGregor and Jackson, 1972); it is usually available in all but the largest body surface area burns.

AXILLARY CONTRACTURES

Axillary contractures are commonly encountered and are more difficult to treat then flexion contractures at the elbow. The normal resting position of the axilla is in the contracted position, unlike the elbow, where the position of the joint at rest is in maximal extension. Therefore, whenever skin grafts are used for an axillary release, postoperative

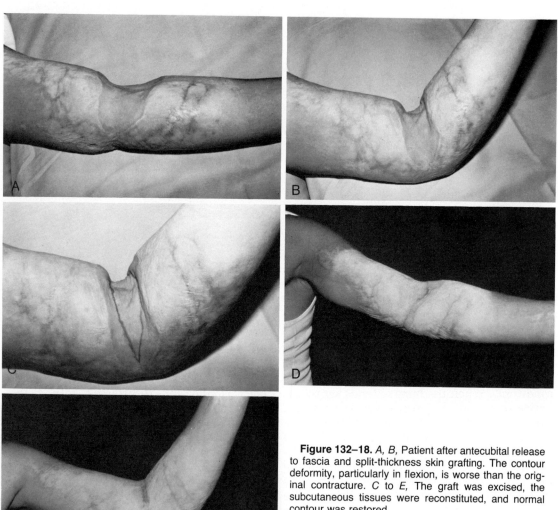

Figure 132–18. *A, B,* Patient after antecubital release to fascia and split-thickness skin grafting. The contour deformity, particularly in flexion, is worse than the original contracture. *C* to *E,* The graft was excised, the subcutaneous tissues were reconstituted, and normal contour was restored.

management is complicated by the need for prolonged splinting in abduction and intense and faithful physical therapy. In addition, release and grafting of the axilla is often complicated by the presence of hair-bearing skin that must be maintained in its location at the apex. If this is allowed to migrate onto the upper arm or lateral aspect of the chest, an unsightly deformity results. For all these reasons, it is advantageous to correct axillary contractures by rearranging the local tissues whenever possible.

There are generally three different types of axillary contractures. After the most severe burns to this region there is full-thickness loss of skin over a wide area with a resultant tight contracture, sometimes causing adherence of the upper arm to the lateral chest wall (Fig. 132–19). Treatment of this deformity requires release of the contracture in the midaxis of the axilla. The release should be carried to the axis of rotation of the shoulder joint both anteriorly and posteriorly, and the incision should be ended with a "fishtail" or Y to provide the maximal possible amount of skin graft. The size of the resultant defect and the amount of skin required to resurface it is often surprising, even to an experienced surgeon. The graft should be sutured into place and a tie-over bolster dressing utilized. Postoperatively, pressure garments and splinting in abduction are required for at least six months to obtain the best possible results. Even with a satisfactory release, good graft "take," and careful postoperative management, further releases are not infrequently required in these patients.

The second type of axillary contracture is that in which there is sparing of the skin at the apex with preservation of axillary hair. In these patients a double release should be carried out with two separate incisions, one proximal and one distal to the unburned skin (Peterson and Elton, 1976). This allows the hair-bearing area to remain in its normal location and prevents migration to the upper arm or lateral chest. It is particularly important to be aware of this problem when treating prepubescent children.

In the third type of axillary contracture there is significant sparing of axillary, thoracic, and/or upper arm skin. This group includes contractures of the posterior axilla, contractures of the anterior axilla and chest, and all more linear types of scars. Not infrequently, irregular but essentially continuous scars extend from the lateral thoracic wall through the axilla onto the arm and to the wrist. In many of these patients, judicious rearrangement of the soft tissues with local flaps and Z-plasties can be extremely effective (Fig. 132–20). Care must be taken when raising flaps in skin grafted and scarred areas. Because of the vertical nature of the blood supply from the deep tissue in these areas and the absence of an adequate subdermal plexus, vascularity is marginal. There can be a high rate of complications when such tissues are used as random flaps. A helpful technique for Z-plasties is to limit the dissection in the scarred tissue to a release. The flap from the adjacent undamaged tissue is then transposed as a "half Z-plasty."

Opinions vary as to the merits of excisional release compared with incisional release for the treatment of burn contractures (Bunnell and Boyes, 1970; Beasley, 1977; Peacock, 1977; Rousso and Wexler, 1980). As a general rule, it seems better to incise scars whenever possible; this approach decreases the requirement for skin graft coverage. After release and grafting, with the decrease of tension and redistribution of contractile forces, remodeling of the remaining local scar often leads to a favorable long-term result both functionally and cosmetically. When there are open wounds in the area, as is often the case with hypertrophic scar under tension, they should be excised as part of the release. Also, if there is marked focal hypertrophy of scar so that it is unreasonable to expect remodeling to be effective, this should be excised. Usually, however, simple incision and grafting are most appropriate.

HETEROTOPIC OSSIFICATION

Heterotopic periarticular ossification is an infrequent complication after thermal injury. The elbow is the joint most often involved (Pruitt, 1974). The next most common locations are the shoulder and the hip (Evans, 1966), and the condition has been reported to occur in the interosseous membrane between the radius and the ulna. The cause is unclear, but it is different from the intra-articular bony ankylosis associated with septic arthritis following burns (Jackson, 1980). There is no correlation between burn size and the development of this condition, but it does appear to be related to the depth of the burn,

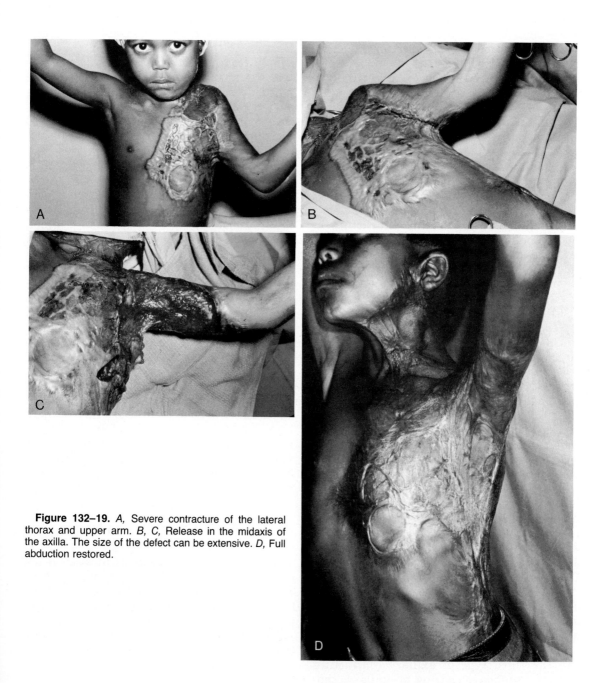

Figure 132–19. *A,* Severe contracture of the lateral thorax and upper arm. *B, C,* Release in the midaxis of the axilla. The size of the defect can be extensive. *D,* Full abduction restored.

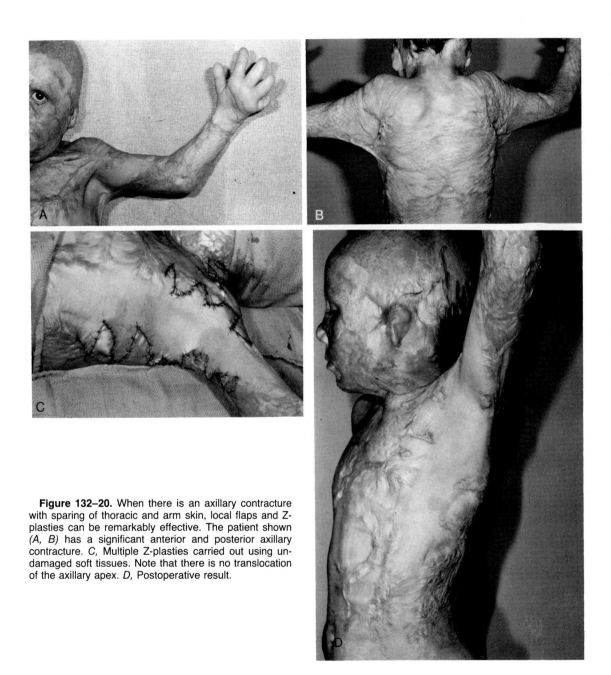

Figure 132–20. When there is an axillary contracture with sparing of thoracic and arm skin, local flaps and Z-plasties can be remarkably effective. The patient shown *(A, B)* has a significant anterior and posterior axillary contracture. *C,* Multiple Z-plasties carried out using un-damaged soft tissues. Note that there is no translocation of the axillary apex. *D,* Postoperative result.

occurring more frequently in patients with third degree injuries (Munster and associates, 1972). The incidence has been variously reported in the literature from 0.1 per cent (Jackson, 1980) to as high as 11.2 per cent (Munster and associates, 1972). Munster and associates performed a prospective study of 88 patients with major burns. Eighteen limbs developed heterotopic ossification with some loss of range of motion at the elbow joint and radiographic evidence of calcification. Spontaneous resolution of the calcification, with return to normal range of motion, occurred in 13 of 18 limbs. Five patients (3.2 per cent) remained clinically symptomatic and required surgical intervention. Large retrospective series of hospitalized burn patients have reported occurrence rates of 2 (Evans, 1966) to 3.3 per cent (Kolar and Vrabec, 1959). It is likely that this range represents the true incidence of clinically significant cases. Many other patients probably develop subclinical calcification, which eventually resolves without specific treatment.

The earliest clinical sign is a loss of active range of motion at the elbow joint. This may precede the development of changes seen radiographically (Munster and associates, 1972). The calcification appears on radiographs as a fluffy shadow posterior to the elbow joint, and gradually spreads to the medial epicondyle of the humerus, to the humeral shaft, and sometimes to the lateral epicondyle (Fig. 132–21). In most patients the calcification resorbs with restoration of a normal range of motion. The role of physical therapy in this process is unclear. Some authors believe that overaggressive therapy may actually cause injury and increase the degree of calcification (Heslop, 1982). In a minority of patients the calcification develops into mature bone and can progress to complete ankylosis.

Surgical excision should be performed through a posterior curvilinear incision as suggested by Evans (1966), modifying it to avoid old scars and grafts as much as possible (Hoffer, Brody, and Ferlic, 1978). The heterotopic bone can be found in the soft tissues surrounding the joint (pericapsular), within the capsule and ligaments (periarticular), or as an actual bone bridge across the posterior aspect of the joint. The ulnar nerve may be completely encased in bone in the cubital canal and must be carefully protected as the bone is resected. Anterior transposition of the ulnar nerve has been recommended by most authors (Evans, 1966; Peterson and Elton, 1976; Hoffer, Brody, and Ferlic, 1978).

ELECTRICAL BURNS

The etiology and pathogenesis of electrical injury is completely different from that of thermal burns, and the deformities resulting from electrical trauma tend to be quite different from those that follow thermal burns. The amount of damage to the skin and subcutaneous tissues is often limited, but there may be extensive destruction of deeper structures such as muscle, tendon, vessels, and nerves secondary to the passage of electrical current (Peterson, 1966). The key to acute management of electrical injuries to the upper extremity is to have a high index of suspicion regarding potential damage to deeper structures even at a distance from the point of contact. Early exploration and debridement must be carried out with removal of all necrotic tissue to prevent the development of sepsis. Because the cutaneous injury is often limited, escharotomy is rarely indicated. As a result of muscle damage, edema in subfascial compartments is common. Pulses should be carefully monitored and fasciotomies performed immediately upon suspicion of a compartment syndrome (see Chap. 120). Carpal tunnel release to minimize compression of the median nerve at the wrist is usually indicated at the time of exploration and debridement.

The hands and upper extremities are the areas of the body most frequently involved in electrical burn trauma (Marshall and Fisher, 1977). Skoog (1970) reported a 75 per cent incidence of upper extremity involvement in 141 patients with electrical injuries. Davies (1959) reported hand injuries in 65 of 70 patients with burns caused by electricity. The hand itself is probably the most frequent point of contact with the source of electric current, and often suffers a massive focal injury (Fig. 132–22). The resultant secondary deformities are more often similar to those after a gunshot wound or a crush injury than to those following thermal burns (Artz, 1967). The incidence of amputation after electrical injury to the upper extremity is high, either because of acute massive destruction at the point of contact, or secondary to devitalization and progressive sepsis as a result of injury to the deeper structures. Salisbury and Pruitt

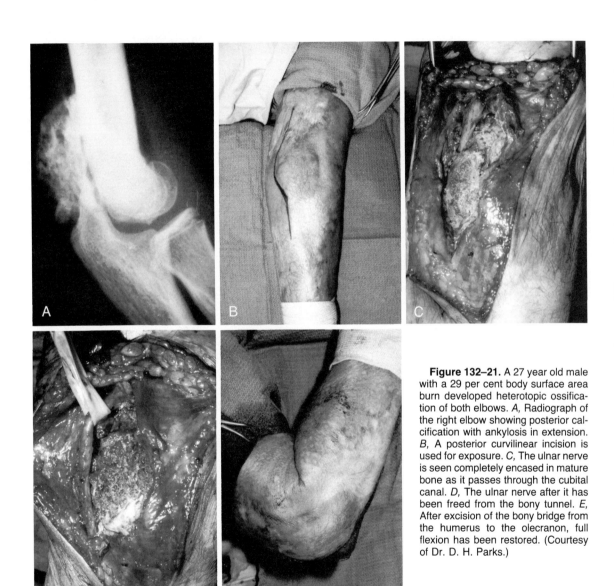

Figure 132–21. A 27 year old male with a 29 per cent body surface area burn developed heterotopic ossification of both elbows. *A,* Radiograph of the right elbow showing posterior calcification with ankylosis in extension. *B,* A posterior curvilinear incision is used for exposure. *C,* The ulnar nerve is seen completely encased in mature bone as it passes through the cubital canal. *D,* The ulnar nerve after it has been freed from the bony tunnel. *E,* After excision of the bony bridge from the humerus to the olecranon, full flexion has been restored. (Courtesy of Dr. D. H. Parks.)

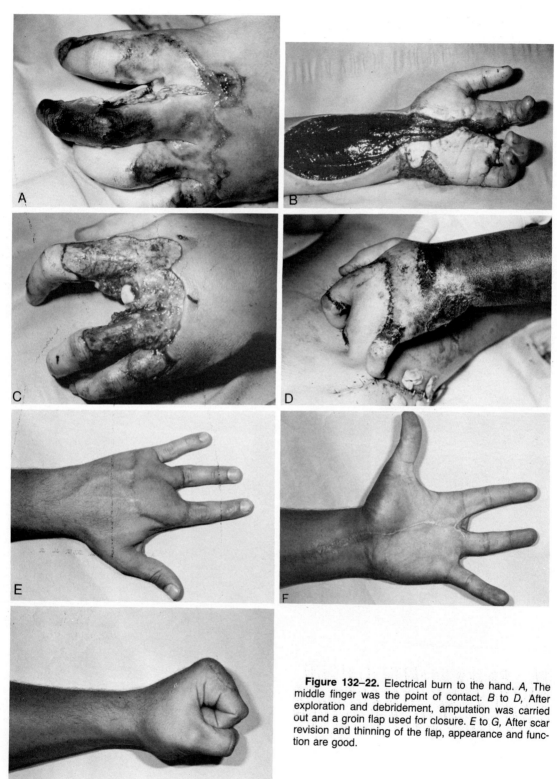

Figure 132–22. Electrical burn to the hand. *A,* The middle finger was the point of contact. *B* to *D,* After exploration and debridement, amputation was carried out and a groin flap used for closure. *E* to *G,* After scar revision and thinning of the flap, appearance and function are good.

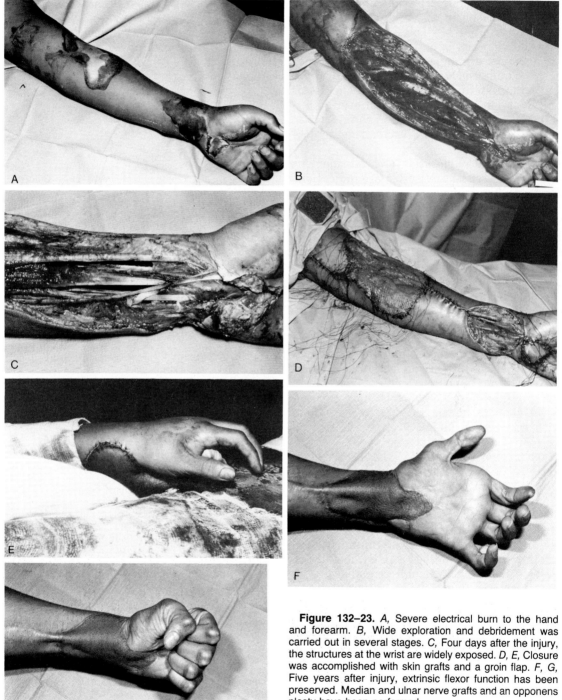

Figure 132–23. *A,* Severe electrical burn to the hand and forearm. *B,* Wide exploration and debridement was carried out in several stages. *C,* Four days after the injury, the structures at the wrist are widely exposed. *D, E,* Closure was accomplished with skin grafts and a groin flap. *F, G,* Five years after injury, extrinsic flexor function has been preserved. Median and ulnar nerve grafts and an opponens plasty have been performed.

(1976) reported a 43 per cent incidence of amputation in 85 patients with electrical injury to the upper extremities. Burke and associates (1977) described 11 upper extremity amputations in 29 children and adolescents after high tension electrical trauma. The vast majority of patients sustaining electrical injury are males either in adolescence or young adulthood. The adolescents are typically injured through inquisitive behavior or while attempting to impress their peer groups (Burke and associates, 1977). The injuries in adult males are almost exclusively in job-related accidents.

After initial exploration and debridement of necrotic tissues, there often are indications for acute flap resurfacing in electrical burns to the upper extremity (Fig. 132–23). This is very different from the situation following thermal burns. Debridement often leaves marginally vascularized nerves, arteries, and tendons exposed at the wrist. Attempts to close these defects with skin grafts usually are only partially successful and can lead to further necrosis and severe contractures. Provision of early flap coverage to these injuries may prevent further damage to the exposed structures and can facilitate later reconstructive surgery, which frequently involves tendon grafting, tendon transfers, and nerve repairs. The best management for exposed flexor tendons at the wrist is flap coverage with adequate drainage even if viability is unclear. Debridement of the tendons results in permanent shortening of the forearm motor units, which significantly compromises later reconstructive potential. After adequate drainage, even if there is partial necrosis of the tendons under the flap, healing eventually occurs, with preservation of the normal muscle-tendon relationships. Similarly, the median and ulnar nerves usually should not be debrided. Even though damage to the nerves may be more extensive than appears upon clinical examination, maintaining the nerve in continuity decreases the resultant gap that must be bridged by nerve grafts during later reconstructive surgery. The groin flap has been a workhorse for acute resurfacing of wrist and forearm defects following electrical burns (May and associates, 1988). Because of the protected location of the donor site, it is almost always available except in the most massive total body injuries. The blood supply is robust, and the long pedicle allows for convenient positioning of the extremity even in patients with multiple trauma. Free flaps have been proposed for acute wound coverage of burn patients (Sharzer and O'Brien, 1975). Because of the frequency of associated proximal vascular lesions in acute electrical injuries (Hunt and Pruitt, 1974), free flaps probably are rarely indicated in this context except in the most unusual circumstances.

REFERENCES

Adamson, J. E., Crawford, H. H., Horton, C. F., and Brown, L. M.: Treatment of dorsal burn adduction contracture of the hand. Plast. Reconstr. Surg., 42:355, 1968.

Alexander, J. W., MacMillan, B. G., and Martel, L.: Correction of post-burn syndactyly: an analysis of children with introduction of the VM-plasty and postoperative pressure inserts. Plast. Reconstr. Surg., 70:345, 1982.

Alexander, J. W., MacMillan, B. G., Martel, L., and Krummel, R.: Surgical correction of postburn flexion contractures of the fingers in children. Plast. Reconstr. Surg., 68:218, 1981.

Alsbjorn, B. F., Metz, P., and Ebbehoj, J.: Nailfold retraction due to burn wound contracture: a surgical procedure. Burns, 11:166, 1985.

Artz, C. P.: Electrical injury simulates crush injury. Surg. Gynecol. Obstet., 125:1316, 1967.

Barfod, B.: Reconstruction of the nail fold. Hand, 4:85, 1972.

Bauer, T. B., Tondra, J. M., and Trusler, H. M.: Technical modification in repair of syndactyly. Plast. Reconstr. Surg., 17:385, 1956.

Beasley, R. W.: Burns of the axilla and elbow. In Converse, J. M. (Ed.): Reconstructive Plastic Surgery. 2nd Ed. Philadelphia W. B. Saunders Company, 1977, p. 3391.

Beasley, R. W.: Secondary repair of burned hands. Clin. Plast. Surg., 8:141, 1981.

Braithwaite, F.: Treatment of dorsal burns of the hand. Br. J. Plast. Surg., 2:21, 1949.

Brown, J. B., Cannon, B., Graham, W. C., Lischer, C. E., Scarborough, C. P., et al.: Direct flap repair of defects of the arm and hand. Ann. Surg., 122:706, 1945.

Brown, J. B., and McDowell, F.: Skin Grafting, 3rd Ed. Philadelphia, J. B. Lippincott Company, 1958, p. 138.

Browne, E. Z., Teague, M. A., and Snyder, C. C.: Burn syndactyly. Plast. Reconstr. Surg., 62:92, 1978.

Bunnell, S., and Boyes, J. H.: Surgery of the Hand. 2nd Ed. Philadelphia, J. B. Lippincott Company, 1970, p. 170.

Burke, J. F., Quinby, W. C., Bondoc, C., McLaughlin, E., and Trelstad, R. L.: Patterns of high tension electrical injury in children and adolescents and their management. Am. J. Surg., 133:492, 1977.

Butler, E. D., and Gant, T. D.: Electrical injuries, with special reference to the upper extremities. Am. J. Surg., 134:95, 1977.

Cannon, B., and May, J. W.: Skin contractures of the hand. In Flynn, J. E. (Ed.): Hand Surgery. 3rd Ed. Baltimore, William & Wilkins Company, 1982.

Converse, J. M.: Skin graft of dorsum of hand. Ann. Surg., *121*:172, 1945.

Cope, O., Langohr, J. L., Moore, F. D., and Webster, R. C.: Expeditious care of full-thickness burn wounds by surgical excision and grafting. Ann. Surg., *125*:1, 1947.

Curtis, R. M.: Capsulectomy of the interphalangeal joints of the fingers. J. Bone Joint Surg., *36A*:1219, 1954.

Davies, M. R.: Burns caused by electricity. A review of 70 cases. Br. J. Plast. Surg., *11*:288, 1959.

Elliott, R. A.: Boutonnière Deformity. *In* Symposium on the Hand. St. Louis, C. V. Mosby Company, 1971, p. 42.

Evans, E. B.: Orthopaedic measures in the treatment of severe burns. J. Bone Joint Surg., *48A*:643, 1966.

Farmer, A. W., and Woolhouse, F. M.: Resurfacing of dorsum of the hand following burns. Ann. Surg., *122*:39, 1945.

Gillies, H. D., and Cuthbert, J. B.: Plastic surgery of burns of the hand. Med. Annu., *61*:259, 1943.

Hayes, C. W.: One-stage nailfold reconstruction. Hand, *6*:74, 1974.

Heslop, J. H.: Heterotopic periarticular ossification in burns. Burns, *8*:436, 1982.

Hirshowitz, R., Karev, A., and Rousso, M.: Combined double Z-plasty and Y-V advancement for thumb web contracture. Hand, *7*:291, 1975.

Hoffer, M., Brody, G., and Ferlic, F.: Excision of heterotopic ossification about elbows in patients with thermal injury. J. Trauma, *18*:667, 1978.

Huang, T. T., Larson, D. L., and Lewis, S. R.: Burned hands. Plast. Reconstr. Surg., *56*:21, 1975.

Hunt, J. L., and Pruitt, B. A.: Vascular lesions in acute electrical injuries. J. Trauma, *14*:461, 1974.

Jackson, D. M.: Destructive burns: some orthopedic complications. Burns, *7*:105, 1980.

Jackson, I. T.: Discussion. Plast. Reconstr. Surg., *68*:225, 1981.

Jackson, I. T., and Brown, G. E. D.: A method of treating chronic flexion contractures of the fingers. Br. J. Plast. Surg., *23*:373, 1970.

Kolar, J., and Vrabec, R.: Periarticular soft-tissue changes as a late consequence of burns. J. Bone Joint Surg., *41A*:103, 1959.

Krizek, T. J., Robson, M. C., and Flagg, S. V.: Management of burn syndactyly. J. Trauma, *14*:587, 1974.

Larson, D. L., Abston, S., Evans, E. B., Dobrkovsky, M., and Linares, H. A.: Techniques for decreasing scar formation and contractures in the burned patient. J. Trauma, *11*:807, 1971.

Larson, D. L., Wofford, B. H., Evans, E. B., and Lewis, S. R.: Repair of the boutonnière deformity of the burned hand. J. Trauma, *10*:481, 1970.

Maisels, D. O.: The middle slip or boutonnière deformity in burned hands. Br. J. Plast. Surg., *18*:117, 1965.

Marshall, K. A., and Fisher, J. A.: Salvage and reconstruction of electrical hand injuries. Am. J. Surg., *134*:385, 1977.

Matev, I. B.: Thumb reconstruction in children through metacarpal lengthening. Plast. Reconstr. Surg., *64*:665, 1979.

May, J. W., Jr., Donelan, M. B., Toth, B. A., and Wall, J.: Thumb reconstruction in the burned hand by advancement pollicization of the second ray remnant. J. Hand Surg., *9A*:484, 1984.

May, J. W., Jr., Quimby, W. C., Donelan, M. B., and Bondoc, C. C.: Early use of the groin flap in high tension electrical wounds of the forearm and hand. Proc. ABA (abstract 158), 1988.

McCormack, R. M.: Principles of treatment and reconstruction of the burned hand and fingers. *In* Symposium on the Hand. St. Louis, C. V. Mosby Company, 1971, p. 42.

McDougal, B., Wray, R. C., and Weeks, P. M.: Lateral volar finger flap for the treatment of burn syndactyly. Plast. Reconstr. Surg., *57*:167, 1976.

McGregor, I. A., and Jackson, I. T.: The groin flap. Br. J. Plast. Surg., *25*:3, 1972.

Moncrief, J. A.: Third degree burns of the hand. Am. J. Surg., *96*:535, 1958.

Munster, A. M., Bruck, H. M., Johns, L. A., Von Prince, K., Kirkman, E. M., and Remig, R. L.: Heterotopic calcification following burns: a prospective study. J. Trauma, *12*:1071, 1972.

Ngim, R. C., and Soin, K.: Post-burn nailfold retraction: a reconstructive technique. J. Hand Surg., *11B*:385, 1986.

Parks, D. H., Evans, E. B., and Larson, D. L.: Prevention and correction of deformity after severe burns. Surg. Clin. North Am., *58*:1279, 1978.

Peacock, E. E.: The burned upper extremity. *In* Converse, J. M. (Ed.): Reconstructive Plastic Surgery. 2nd Ed. Philadelphia, W. B. Saunders Company, 1977, p. 3368.

Peacock, E. E.: Discussion. Plast. Reconstr. Surg., *81*:44, 1988.

Peacock, E. E., Madden, J. W., and Trier, W. C.: Some studies on the treatment of burned hands. Ann. Surg., *171*:903, 1970.

Pensler, J. M., Steward, R., Lewis, S. R., and Herndon, D. N.: Reconstruction of the burned palm: full-thickness versus split-thickness skin grafts—long-term followup. Plast. Reconstr. Surg., *81*:46, 1988.

Peterson, H. C., and Elton, R.: Reconstruction of the thermally injured upper extremity. Major Probl. Clin. Surg., *19*:148, 1976.

Peterson, R. A.: Electrical burns of the hand; treatment by early excision. J. Bone Joint Surg., *48A*:107, 1966.

Pruitt, B. A.: Complications of thermal injury. Clin. Plast. Surg., *1*:667, 1974.

Quan, P. E., Bieringer, R., Alston, D. W., and Curreri, P. W.: Control of scar tissue in the finger webspaces by use of graded pressure inserts. J. Burn Care Rehabil., *2*:27, 1981.

Rousso, M., and Wexler, M. R.: Management of the burned hand. *In* Goldwyn, R. M. (Ed.): Long-term Results in Plastic and Reconstructive Surgery. Boston, Little, Brown & Company, 1980.

Salisbury, R. E., and Bevin, A. G.: Atlas of Reconstructive Burn Surgery. Philadelphia, W. B. Saunders Company, 1981.

Salisbury, R. E., and Dingeldein, G. P.: The burned hand and upper extremity. *In* Green, D. P. (Ed.): Operative Hand Surgery. New York, Churchill Livingstone, 1982.

Salisbury, R. E., Hunt, J. L., Glenn, D. W., and Pruitt, B. A.: Management of electrical burns of the upper extremity. Plast. Reconstr. Surg., *51*:648, 1973.

Salisbury, R. E., Pruitt, B. A.: Burns of the Upper Extremity. Philadelphia, W. B. Saunders Company, 1976, pp. 72–83.

Salisbury, R. E., and Wright, P.: Evaluation of early excision of dorsal burns of the hand. Plast. Reconstr. Surg., *69*:670, 1982.

Sharzer, L. R., and O'Brien, M. C.: Clinical application of free flap transfer in the burn patient. J. Trauma, *15*:767, 1975.

Shaw, D. T., Li, C. S., Richey, D. G., and Nahigian, S.

H.: Interdigital butterfly flap in the hand (the double-opposing Z-plasty). J. Bone Joint Surg., 55A:1677, 1973.

Shaw, D. T., and Payne, R. L.: Repair of surface defects of the upper extremity. Ann. Surg., 123:705, 1946.

Skoog, T.: Electrical injuries. J. Trauma, 10:816, 1970.

Tanzer, R. C.: Correction of interdigital burn contractures of the hand. Plast. Reconstr. Surg., 3:434, 1948a.

Tanzer, R. C.: Reconstruction of the burned hand. N. Engl. J. Med., 238:687, 1948b.

Tubiana, R.: Surgical repair of the extensor apparatus of the fingers. Surg. Clin. North Am., 48:1015, 1968.

Ward, J. W., Pensler, J. M., and Parry, S. W.: Pollicization for thumb reconstruction in severe pediatric hand burns. Plast. Reconstr. Surg., 76:927, 1985.

Webster, G. V., and Rowland, W. D.: Skin-grafting the burned dorsum of the hand. Ann. Surg., 124:449, 1946.

Zook, E. G.: The perionychium: anatomy, physiology, and care of injuries. Clin. Plast. Surg., 8:21, 1981.

Stephan Ariyan

Benign and Malignant Soft Tissue Tumors of the Hand

TUMORS ARISING FROM SKIN
  Benign
    Actinic keratosis
    Inclusion cyst
    Knuckle pad
    Keratoacanthoma
  Malignant
    Bowen's disease
    Squamous cell carcinoma
    Basal cell carcinoma
    Malignant melanoma
    Sweat gland carcinoma

TUMORS OF CONNECTIVE TISSUES
  Benign
    Ganglion
    Extensor sheath cyst
    Mucous cyst
    Giant cell tumor
    Fibroma
    Pyogenic granuloma
    Lipoma
    Fibrous histiocytoma
  Malignant
    Sarcomas

TUMORS OF VASCULAR TISSUE
    Hemangioma
    Malformations
    Arteriovenous fistulas
    Glomus tumors
    Malignant vascular tumors

TUMORS OF NEURAL TISSUE
    Neuromas
    Neurilemomas
    Neurofibromas
    Malignant schwannoma

Soft tissue tumors of the hand are quite common, and this chapter covers the subject of tumors in the descriptive sense: "masses." They are essentially nonmalignant, and while a few are benign neoplasms, most are non-neoplastic and are derived from local structures. Metastatic tumors also are rare, but must be considered in the differential diagnosis and the surgeon dealing with pathology of the hand must be aware of them.

Although diagnostic tests such as soft tissue x-rays, angiography, electromyography, and hematologic studies may be helpful, the vast majority of the lesions can be diagnosed after careful questioning of the patient and a thorough examination of the hand. The treatment is based on the functional limitations caused by the lesion, the symptoms present, and the needs of the patient. It is important to take time to explain to the patient the diagnosis of the lesion, the implications and prognosis of the entity, and the benefits anticipated by the planned treatment.

Almost all of these lesions require surgery. This necessitates a bloodless field and the use of a pneumatic tourniquet to remove the lesion completely, adequately, and expeditiously with little damage to neurovascular structures. The surgical procedure can be performed under a choice of anesthetic techniques (general, axillary block, intravenous block, or digital block), and the selection should be based on the particular requirements of the patient and of the lesion to be removed or repaired.

Although the incidence of soft tissue tumors of the hand varies among several reports (Leung, 1981; Posch, 1982; Johnson, Kilgore, and Newmeyer, 1985), 85 to 90 per cent of these tumors are represented by the

Table 133–1. Five Most Common Soft Tissue Tumors of the Hand

	Reported Incidence	Compiled Cases from Series	Percentage of Total
1. Ganglion	(61%–72%)	1837	63%
2. Giant cell tumor	(3%–11%)	270	9%
3. Inclusion cyst	(4%–14%)	160	6%
4. Vascular malformation	(2%–6%)	149	4%
5. Fibroma	(1%–1.4%)	39	1%
All other benign lesions		395	14%
All malignant lesions		52	2%
Total:		2902	

From a compilation of 2902 reported cases (Leung, 1981; Posch, 1982; Johnson, Kilgore, and Newmeyer, 1985.

five most common types (Table 133–1). In spite of the fact that malignant soft tissue tumors represent less than 2 per cent of all the lesions seen, they are by far the most important, and the hand surgeon needs to be familiar with their diagnosis, treatment, and prognosis.

An important question arises regarding what a surgeon should do if a mass is encountered during the operation that is different from what had been expected. Under these circumstances the decision is based on whether the surgeon has the assistance of pathologists skilled at reliable diagnoses by frozen section specimens. For example, a mass that is determined to be a nerve tumor is most likely a neurilemoma. This benign tumor should be easily dissected from its capsule without requiring any significant sharp dissection. If, however, it is densely adherent, a frozen section examination of a biopsy is not helpful unless it is examined by an experienced neuropathologist.

Inevitably, malignant tumors require extensive surgical procedures, some of which lead to significant disability. Therefore, it is usually best to wait for the permanent sections to determine the correct histologic diagnosis, evaluate the risks, consult the radiotherapists and chemotherapists regarding the prognosis with multimodality treatment, and present the appropriate recommendations to the patient, citing the alternatives and the risks involved. The choice between an incisional or an excisional biopsy can be made according to the size of the tumor mass. This should be done with the least amount of dissection or disruption of anatomic planes, to avoid local dissemination, and the wound should then be closed to await the final diagnosis.

If the diagnosis reveals a malignant tumor metastasis to the hand, it may also determine the site of the primary tumor. The most common tumors to metastasize to the bones of the hand are those of the lung, breast, and gastrointestinal tract, followed by the thyroid and kidney. In these circumstances, the extent of the primary tumor or its management may help determine the extent of surgical

Table 133–2. Distribution of Soft Tissue Tumors

	Benign	Malignant
I. Skin	Warts Actinic keratosis Inclusion cyst Knuckle pads Keratoacanthoma	Bowen's disease Squamous cell carcinoma Basel cell carcinoma Malignant melanoma Sweat gland carcinoma
II. Connective tissue	Ganglion Mucous cyst Giant cell tumor Fibroma Pyogenic granuloma Lipoma Fibrous histiocytoma	Malignant fibrous histiocytoma Dermatofibrosarcoma protuberans Malignant synovioma Liposarcoma Rhabdomyosarcoma
III. Vascular tissue	Hemangioma Vascular malformation Lymphatic malformation A-V fistula Glomus tumor	Hemangioendothelioma Hemangiopericytoma Hemangiosarcoma Kaposi's sarcoma Lymphangiosarcoma
IV. Neural tissue	Neuroma Neurofibroma Neurilemoma	Malignant schwannoma

treatment required for the metastasis to the hand. Finally, the decision whether to use exsanguination and a tourniquet can be made prognostically. The risks involved in dislodging tumor cells and forcing them to disseminate through the circulation are not significant, because in the author's opinion, all tumors are shedding cells through the circulation repeatedly. The use of the tourniquet in melanomas of the extremity and in otherwise unsuspected malignancies has not justified any concern about these risks. On the contrary, the use of a bloodless field permits a clearer evaluation of the extent of the tumor or adjacent tissue involvement in deciding the extent of resection that is necessary.

This chapter reviews the soft tissue tumors of the hand in terms not of their order of prevalence, but of their distribution among the various tissues in which they arise (Table 133–2). It is true that some lesions may arise from more than one anatomic area, but each lesion is discussed according to the location within which it is most often found.

TUMORS ARISING FROM SKIN

Benign

Although warts may be the most common benign lesion of the hand, patients with warts are not often referred to the hand surgeon. These lesions are induced by a papovavirus and usually resolve spontaneously after a time (Sanders and Stretcher, 1976). Although

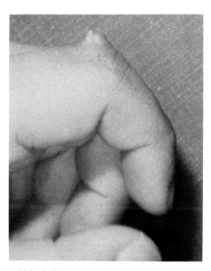

Figure 133–1. Warts on the hands are usually sessile and occur more commonly on the fingers than on the back of the hand.

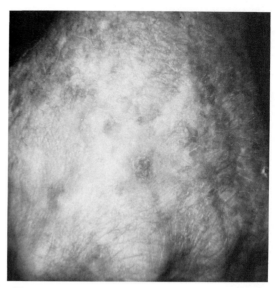

Figure 133–2. Actinic keratosis occurs more commonly on the dorsum of the hand where the skin is exposed to the effects of the sun.

verruca vulgaris, the most commonly seen wart, occurs most often in the early teens, it may arise at any age. It is easily recognized (Fig. 133–1), but its greatest significance is that more serious conditions such as deep fungal infection or carcinomas may occasionally be mistaken for warts.

ACTINIC KERATOSIS

Actinic keratoses are superficial dry lesions on the dorsum of the hands of patients in the older age groups (Fig. 133–2). They are often seen among sailors, farmers, and golfers who have been exposed to the drying and damaging effects of exposure to the weather and the sun. Keratoses can also be found on the skin of patients who have had long-term chemical exposure to arsenicals. Both types of these lesions need to be watched for possible malignant changes, and any suspicious lesions should simply be excised.

INCLUSION CYST

These common benign growths are most often seen on the volar aspects of the fingers or on the palm. They normally occur in tailors, seamstresses, industrial workers, and carpenters who are subject to repeated minor traumas to the hand. The pathogenesis of these cysts is believed to be a puncture wound that penetrates the skin and implants epithelial cells deep into the soft tissues. These

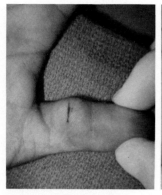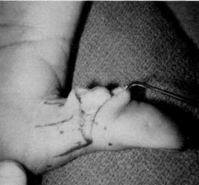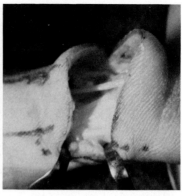

Figure 133–3. An inclusion cyst on the volar aspect of the thumb. The mass had continued to grow for months before the patient requested removal. The cyst was easily enucleated from the adjacent digital nerves. (From Ariyan, S.: The Hand Book. Baltimore, Williams & Wilkins Company, 1983.)

most often form a small epithelial cyst that then causes an inflammatory response and gets absorbed. Occasionally, the cyst persists and continues to produce the cheesy keratin that accumulates and causes it to enlarge (Fig. 133–3). These cysts are best treated by excision if small, or enucleation of the intact larger masses under tourniquet control. The epithelial lining of the cyst must be completely removed to avoid recurrence.

KNUCKLE PADS

Thickening of the skin, dermis, and subcutaneous tissues is seen over the interphalangeal (IP) or metacarpophalangeal (MP) joints of patients with Dupuytren's disease (Fig. 133–4) or rheumatoid arthritis. These

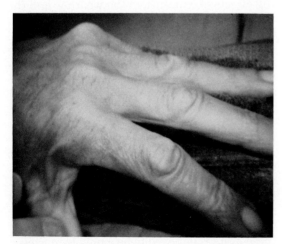

Figure 133–4. Prominent proximal interphalangeal joint knuckle pads in a patient with Dupuytren's disease.

nodules in the skin are usually asymptomatic, and their removal is normally for cosmetic reasons rather than for functional problems. In patients with rheumatoid arthritis, the removal of these lesions may lead to postoperative hematomas and problems in wound healing that arise from the steroid treatment these patients may recieve.

KERATOACANTHOMA

Keratoacanthoma is an umbilicated lesion that grows on the surface of the skin without any history of previous trauma (Fig. 133–5). Although most commonly found on the face, the lesion does occur on the dorsum of the hand and is difficult to differentiate from squamous cell carcinoma. Much has been written about this lesion, some authors placing it "somewhere between benign and malignant," but it is indeed benign.

It is differentiated from squamous cell carcinoma by a history of very rapid onset, usually two to six weeks; in cases when the diagnosis is suspected and the patient is watched, the lesion usually begins to regress over the following four to six weeks. Histologically, however, the lesion has characteristics very similar to those of squamous cell carcinoma, and often the pathologist has difficulty differentiating between the two; both lesions may also have pseudoepitheliomatous hyperplasia at the borders.

Typically, keratoacanthoma has a keratin plug in the center that can easily be removed, leaving a bloodless crater with heaped-up margins. The common squamous cell carci-

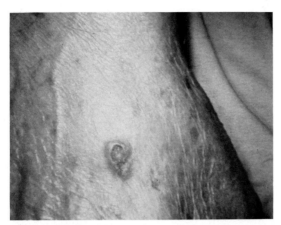

Figure 133–5. Keratoacanthoma of the dorsum of the hand with a three-week history of sudden growth. The central keratin plug has been moved to illustrate the crater.

noma, on the other hand, has an adherent central portion. Whenever there is doubt (and this is often), the lesion should be excised in the manner of a squamous carcinoma (Cohen and associates, 1972).

Malignant

Malignant tumors of the hand are rare, but when they occur they are much more likely to be primary soft tissue tumors than metastatic lesions to the hand. Skin cancers lead the list of these malignant tumors, and squamous carcinoma is by far the most common skin tumor, accounting for about 90 per cent of these lesions (Butler and associates, 1960; Haber, Alter, and Wheelock, 1965).

The frequent occurrence of skin cancers on the dorsum of the hand has led to the acceptance of chronic exposure to sunlight as an etiologic factor. The association of a greater incidence of melanomas as the population gets closer to the equator has provided circumstantial evidence that sunlight is also an etiologic factor in this group of malignancies. Chronic exposure to chemicals (arsenic) and radiation, infections, and scars have also played an important role in the etiology of skin cancers. Before the correlation with exposure to x-ray beams had been appreciated, many patients with skin cancers of the hand were dentists, physicians, and x-ray technicians who had chronic exposure to radiation; in the series of Butler and associates (1960), this history was given in 53 of 90 patients with squamous cell carcinoma.

There is also evidence that cancer may develop as a result of deficiencies in the patient's immune surveillance system. In patients who are chronically immunosuppressed because they have received allograft kidney transplants, there is a 20- to 50-fold increase in the incidence of malignant disease. A review of the Transplant Registry in the United States by Penn and Starzl (1972) revealed an incidence of 6 per cent among 286 organ recipients, and this was subsequently verified by a prospective study of the Scandia Transplant Programme of Denmark (Birkeland, Kempy, and Hauge, 1975). Among these transplant recipients, the most common malignancies have been lymphomas (the risk being 25 times that in the normal population), followed by skin tumors (the risk being four times that in the normal population). Keratoacanthomas have also been reported among patients who have been immunosuppressed for kidney transplants (Walder, Robertson, and Jeremy, 1971; Jacobsson, Linell, and Rausing, 1974). However, since squamous cell carcinoma is more prevalent in this group, and since the differentiation between the two lesions is difficult even by histopathology, further data are required to substantiate this finding.

BOWEN'S DISEASE

Bowen's disease is an intraepidermal squamous cell carcinoma (or in situ carcinoma) that was believed by Bowen (1912) to lead ultimately to invasive squamous cell carcinoma. Since Bowen's subsequent report (1920) of the development of an intestinal carcinoma in one of his patients, there have been numerous reports of the association of intra-abdominal malignancies in patients with Bowen's disease. However, a true causal relationship does not exist, and the only conclusion is that systemic cancer is associated more frequently in this group of patients than in a control group of patients in the same age group but without Bowen's disease (Hugo and Conway, 1967).

The lesion presents as a flat, crusty, or scaly lesion, usually on the dorsal surface of the hand (Fig. 133–6). Because it is an early development of a malignancy, the aim of therapy is to eliminate the lesion. While this lesion has been successfully treated with topical fluorouracil (Klein and associates, 1971), the standard treatment is surgical excision of the entire lesion.

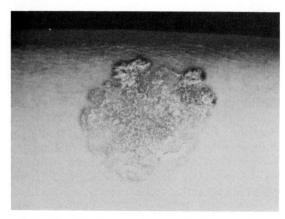

Figure 133–6. Bowen's disease with the typical, thin, scale, cigarette paper appearance in the upper half and hyperkeratosis in the lower half of the lesion.

SQUAMOUS CELL CARCINOMA

In contrast to the head and neck area where basal cell carcinoma (BCC) is more common than squamous cell carcinoma (SCC), the latter represents the significant majority of cases in the hand, accounting for 90 per cent of the 104 cases of Butler and associates (1960), and 76 per cent of the 67 cases of Bean and associates (1984).

The lesion is usually a dry keratinaceous lesion (Fig. 133–7) or an ulcerated lesion. It usually is freely mobile and not deeply invading local structures. Treatment by total ex-

cision of the lesion and primary closure or a small skin graft is successful in preventing local recurrences in the significant majority of cases.

As mentioned above, there is a frequent association with previous exposure to chronic radiation or open wounds, and to immunosuppression for renal transplants (Bean and associates, 1984). Since dermatologists are still using ionizing radiation to treat benign skin disorders, radiation-induced carcinomas still develop among these patients (Bunkis, Mehrhof, and Stayman, 1981). The association between chronic open wounds and the subsequent development of squamous cell carcinoma (Marjolin's ulcer) is well known (Mason, 1937). In a similar fashion, the chronic wounds of epidermolysis bullosa have been known to transform into aggressive squamous cell carcinomas (Crikelair and associates, 1970; Gipson, 1975) that have required extremity amputation for control of the disease (Fig. 133–8).

Another rare but aggressive squamous cell carcinoma is that which occurs in the nail bed. These subungual carcinomas are slow growing and are often misdiagnosed as fungal diseases. By the time the diagnosis is made, the lesion has grown more extensive and may already invade the distal phalanx (Hazelrigg and Renne, 1982). In such cases the phalanx or finger should be amputated, depending on the extent of the invasion (Carroll, 1976).

With regard to lymph node metastases, there is a great disparity between squamous cell carcinoma of the hand and that elsewhere on the trunk and face. In general, squamous cell carcinoma of the skin rarely metastasizes to regional lumph nodes; the incidence is reported as between 0.1 (Katz, Urback, and Lilienfeld, 1957) and 3 per cent (Lund, 1965).

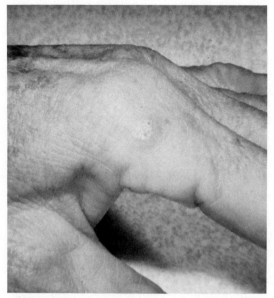

Figure 133–7. Squamous cell carcinoma with a dry thick scale over the surface of the lesion.

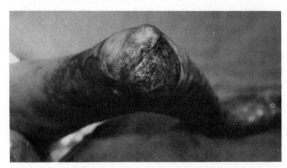

Figure 133–8. Malignant transformation after repeated injury and healing of epidermolysis bullosum, resulting in a squamous cell carcinoma in the ulcerated wounds. (Courtesy of Dr. C. B. Cuono.)

On the other hand, the incidence of lymph node metastases from squamous cell carcinoma of the hand is reported to be 5 to 15 per cent in some series (Haber, Alter, and Wheelock, 1965; Forsythe and associates, Bean and associate, 1984), while there were no metastases in Carroll's (1976) series of 27 cases. These risks are still too low to recommend prophylactic lymphadenectomy (Kendall, Robinson, and Master, 1969); this operation is reserved only for patients who have persistent palpable axillary lymph nodes (indeed, epitrochlear lymph nodes metastases are truly rare; this author has never seen one and is not aware of any documented by other hand surgeons). Lymph node metastases are usually seen in patients who have the most aggressive form of squamous cell carcinoma related to burns, chronic ulcers, or arsenical dermatoses (Lund, 1965; Bean and associates, 1984).

BASAL CELL CARCINOMA

Basal cell carcinoma (BCC) is less common than the squamous variety and is nonaggressive. It appears as a heaped-up lesion with pearly borders, usually with ulceration in the center (Fig. 133–9). It rarely metastasizes to lymph nodes, the incidence being reported as only 0.1 per cent (Domarus and Stevens,

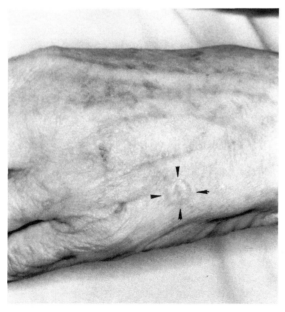

Figure 133–9. Basal cell carcinoma with the heaped-up "pearly" borders to the lesions.

1984). Treatment involves excision of the tumor and primary closure, or coverage with a skin graft if necessary.

Occasionally a basal cell carcinoma may occur in the nail bed and present clinically as a paronychia or fungal infection (Alpert, Zak, and Werthamer, 1972). If the diagnosis is recognized early, the tumor may be excised and the nail bed covered with a skin graft. Otherwise, further growth may require amputation of the distal phalanx.

MALIGNANT MELANOMA

Melanoma is considered by some to be an uncommon tumor of the hand, accounting for less than 2 per cent of the tumors in reported series (Butler and associates, 1960; Haber, Alter, and Wheelock, 1965; Kendall, Robinson, and Masters, 1969; Johnson, Kilgore, and Mewmeyer, 1985). This is misleading because patients often are not referred to the hand surgeon, but to a surgeon with a decided interest and expertise in the management of this specific malignancy. In reported series of melanomas, 14 to 19 per cent of the primary melanomas in the United States and Australia were found to be located in the upper extremity (Balch and associates, 1981, 1982).

Three different classifications are employed for malignant melanoma: a clinical staging system, a morphologic classification, and a microscopic classification. Each of these was established to provide prognostic guidelines for the treating physician, and to permit a logical approach to treatment planning based on this prognosis.

Clinical Staging. This is the earliest classification that has been used and is based on the localization or spread of the disease. Stage I melanoma is the designation related to patients who have a primary melanoma, but who have no clinical symptoms or signs of spread of the tumor to regional lymph nodes or distant sites. Overall, the disease-free survival of stage I melanoma is substantially better than that of the higher stages, and is usually reported to be about 80 per cent at five years (Goldsmith, Shah, and Kim, 1970). A special category of this limited disease is that employed by the M.D. Anderson Hospital in which the primary melanoma is associated with extensions of lesions or "satellite lesions" within several centimeters from the primary tumor (Sugarbacker and McBride, 1976). Such satellite lesions confer an ominous prognosis.

Table 133–3. Significance of Nodal Metastases (1483 Patients)

Clinical Stage		5 Year Cure Rate	
		(In-Group)	*Overall*
I. (707 patients) No RND—411			
RND—296	negative nodes—246	(85%)	78%
	positive nodes—50	(48%)	
II. (537 patients) No RND—56			
RND—481	negative nodes—75	(64%)	40%
	positive nodes—406	(38%)	

RND = regional node dissection.

Modified from Goldsmith, H. S., Shah, J. P., and Kim, D. H.: Prognostic significance of lymph node dissection in the treatment of malignant melanoma. Cancer, *26*:606, 1970.

Stage II melanoma is associated with clinically palpable regional draining lymph nodes. In general, these patients have microscopic spread of tumor that can be confirmed by histologic examination of these nodes in 80 per cent of cases. Although the five year survival rate is about 40 per cent, the prognosis in stage II melanoma has been shown to be associated with the number of lymph nodes involved (Balch and associates, 1981), as well as with the clinically inapparent, but histologically detected, disease in lymph nodes (Table 133–3).

Stage III melanoma is seen in a heterogeneous group of patients with distant metastases, and is generally thought to be fatal. However, melanoma metastatic to the skin and subcutaneous tissues has a better prognosis than metastases to the liver or multiple viscera (Amer, Al-Sarraf, and Vaitkevicius, 1979).

Morphologic Classification. Melanoma has been categorized morphologically into four types: superficial spreading, nodular, lentigo maligna, and acral lentiginous (Fig. 133–10). The differentiation of these various types provides a prognostic assessment based on the clinical appearance of the melanoma (Clark and associates, 1969; McGovern and associates, 1973).

Superficial spreading melanoma represents a lesion that is growing in the radial phase (or growing in the horizontal plane) and will convert into the vertical growth phase over a period of years.

Nodular melanoma appears to evolve into the vertical phase in the early course of the disease, and become invasive into the dermis from the outset. It has been found to have a poorer prognosis than superficial spreading melanoma.

Lentigo maligna melanoma is differentiated from the preceding two morphologic types by its development within a Hutchinson's freckle (lentigo maligna). It occurs in older patients on sun-exposed surfaces of the skin of the face, neck and hands. This melanoma was previously believed to have a better prognosis than the other two types, but has now been shown to have the same prognosis as superficial spreading melanoma for comparable depths of histologic invasion (Koh and associates, 1984) (see below).

Acral lentiginous melanoma represents a fourth and relatively recent addition to the morphologic classification. These melanomas are typified as macular lesions occurring on the palms of the hands, on the soles of the feet, or in subungual areas of the fingers and toes (Taylor and South, 1980). This variant probably represents the most common melanoma among black patients (Alpert, Zak, and Werthamer, 1972). The prognosis for acral lentiginous melanoma is the worst of all the variants, generally in the range of 10 to 20 per cent five year survivals (Coleman and associates, 1980; Feibleman, Stoll, and Maize, 1980).

Histologic Classification. The depth of invasion of the melanoma into the dermis and subcutaneous layer has been recognized as the most powerful determinant of the prognosis for melanoma. The earliest correlation of prognosis with depth was reported by Mehnert and Heard in 1965. Four years later, Clark and associates (1969) described a system for determining levels according to the depth of invasion of the primary melanoma into the dermis (Fig. 133–11):

Level I: (In situ melanoma) limited to the epidermis.

Level II: Invading the papillary dermis.

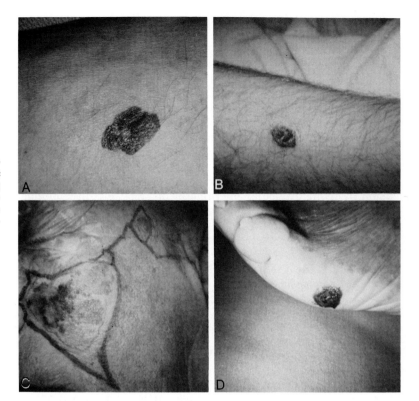

Figure 133–10. Malignant melanoma of the various morphologic types. *A,* Superficial spreading melanoma. *B,* Nodular melanoma. *C,* Lentigo maligna melanoma. *D,* Acral lentiginous melanoma.

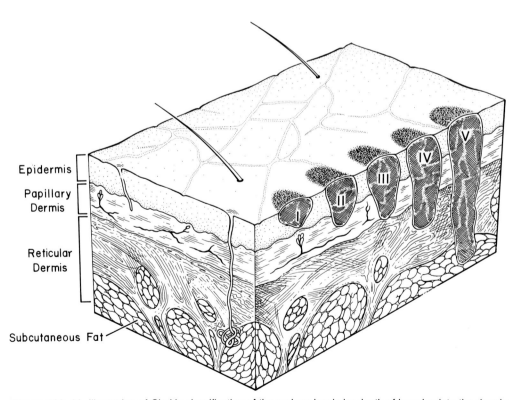

Figure 133–11. Illustration of Clark's classification of the various levels by depth of invasion into the dermis.

Level III: Invading the papillary dermis and expanding to the interface of the papillary-reticular dermis.

Level IV: Invading the reticular dermis, without invasion of the subcutaneous fat.

Level V: Invading the subcutaneous fat or any associated subdermal tissue.

The assessment of melanoma by Clark's level of invasion has now given way to the simpler and more easily reproducible system of microstaging. Breslow (1970) first reported this system for determining the depth of invasion by using an ocular micrometer on the microscopes to measure the tumor thickness to the deepest tumor cells of the primary lesion. The Breslow system has been shown in various studies employing sophisticated multivariate analyses to employ the most powerful prognostic evaluators available for stages I and II melanoma (Balch and associates, 1978).

Surgical Treatment. The purpose of wide excision of a melanoma is to decrease the incidence of local recurrence. Whereas primary melanomas of the trunk and some areas of the extremities may be excised with more liberal margins and still be closed easily, melanomas of the hand and forearm need to be considered with more forethought because of the extent of disability or cosmetic deformity.

It has been generally accepted that lesions less than 0.76 mm thick are uniformly curable and can be treated by a local excision with 1 to 2 cm of adjacent normal skin. Melanomas 0.76 mm or thicker require a wide local excision. The issue has been raised in the literature of how wide to resect (Day and associates, 1982), although the trials needed to prove that narrower margins do not compromise cure have yet to be completed (Ariyan and Kirkwood, 1982). A World Health Organization (WHO) retrospective study evaluating 693 patients with clinical stage I melanoma found a minimal distance for borders of excision more frequently in the case of excisions of the head and neck and the extremities, while most excisions on the tunk had 4 cm margins or more. The study also found that although resection margins did not influence survival, the curability decreased with increasing thickness of the tumor (Cascinelli and associates, 1980). Indeed, for melanomas with more than 2 mm of invasion, retrospective data suggest that the use of margins under 2 cm may well compromise cure (Roses and associates, 1983). It is not possible to draw conclusions from earlier studies on the width of excision (all of which have been retrospective), but it is hoped that these questions will be answered by the current WHO prospective randomized trial evaluating whether or not narrower margins of excision may be considered for thin cutaneous lesions less than 2.0 mm deep (Cascinelli and Vaglini).

Therefore, when an excision of melanoma of the hand or upper extremity is expected to result in deformity or disability, the more conservative approach should be considered, selecting only those patients who will need more extensive resections if and when a recurrence develops. Thin melanomas of the fingertips can be treated with excision of the lesion, and reconstruction with volar advancement flaps (Fig. 133–12). Lesions thicker than 0.76 mm should be treated by interphalangeal joint amputation or ray amputation, depending on the degree of confidence in excising adjacent normal tissue with the selected procedure.

Melanomas of the nail bed are more diffi-

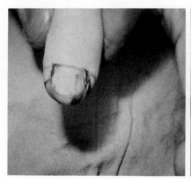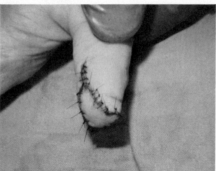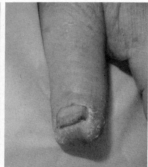

Figure 133–12. A thin melanoma excised from a thumb and resurfaced with an Atasoy advancement flap.

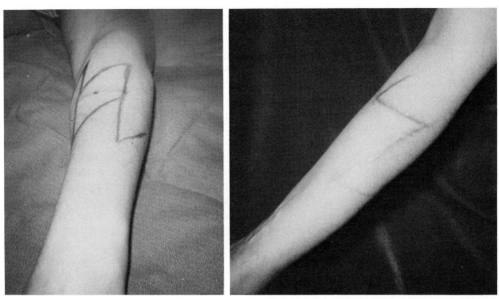

Figure 133–13. A melanoma that was widely excised resulted in a large wound that was covered with a double-Z rhomboid flap.

cult to evaluate because there is a paucity of dermis and subcutaneous fat. Although there are acral lentiginous melanomas growing in the radial phase, as in lentigo maligna melanoma, they are far more aggressive, frequently metastasize, and have a low cure rate. Since the nail bed is so thin, the procedure for a diagnostic biopsy in a suspected lesion should include removal of the nail, excision of the nail bed, and coverage of the wound with a skin graft. If this diagnosis is confirmed, a wider excision needs to be performed. Unless there is evidence of more extensive spread, an amputation of the distal phalanx should suffice. If there is a suggestion of more proximal inflammation or edema, the entire digit should be removed.

Melanomas of the dorsum of the hand, forearm, or arm may be treated by wide local excision. These wounds have traditionally been covered with split-thickness skin grafts. However, coverage of these wide excisions at various sites with local flaps in 85 consecutive patients (34 of whom had melanomas on extremities) were found to be successful for local control (Cuono and Ariyan, 1985). In addition, these patients were free of classic contour defects, were permitted earlier mobilization, and had shorter hospital stays than patients treated with skin grafts (Fig. 133–13).

Lymphadenectomy. The decision whether to perform a cervical lymphadenectomy requires further consideration. There is uniform agreement among surgeons regarding complete axillary lymphadenectomy for patients with clinically palpable (metastases suspected or proved) axillary nodes (clinical stage II). In the clinically negative axilla (clinical stage I), however, the advantage of delaying the lymphadenectomy until the development of subsequent axillary metastases is that only those patients with demonstrable nodal spread will undergo this major operation.

A review of several series of melanomas demonstrates that patients with *intermediate-thickness* melanomas (0.76 mm to 4.0 mm) have up to a 60 per cent risk of lymph node metastases (Balch and associates, 1978; Roses and associates, 1982). Therefore, prophylactic lymphadenectomy has the advantage of providing definitive treatment to these patients at a relatively early period, when there would be the least tumor burden in the lymph nodes of patients subsequently found to have micrometastases. Contrary to this opinion, a randomized trial of stage I melanomas of the upper and lower extremities by the W.H.O. concluded that a delayed lymphadenectomy was as effective as an immediate prophylactic lymphadenectomy (Veronesi and associates, 1977). However, the criticism of this study was that a significant majority of the patients were women (who are well known to have better survival rates with melanomas), and many patients included in the study had thin lesions. Indeed, there were subgroups of patients in this study with 1.6 mm to 4.5 mm melanoma thickness who did better with immediate prophylactic lymph node dissections (78.5 per cent versus 69.7 per cent).

An analysis of other series from the United States and Australia has shown that an elective lymph node dissection was most significant for benefit in patients with melanomas of 1.5 mm to 3.0 mm thickness (Balch and associates, 1979; Milton and associates, 1982). The survival benefit for patients with 0.76 mm to 1.5 mm melanomas was less significant, and primarily limited to male patients (Balch and associates, 1982). Accordingly, the decision to perform a prophylactic lymphadenectomy in this latter group of patients would have to be individualized on the basis of the anatomic site of the primary tumor ulceration, and the morbidity of the added procedure. However, it is important to remember that there is no place for simple excision of the involved palpable nodes alone, because of the likelihood of additional lymph nodes harboring metastatic tumor cells. The only accepted procedure is a total axillary lymphadenectomy.

If the melanoma is found to metastasize to the lung, brain, or liver and these metastases are found to be single and small, surgical removal of the solitary metastasis may be worthwhile. However, multiple metastases generally require chemotherapy. Patients with local recurrences or in-transit metastases along the upper extremity may be treated by regional isolation-perfusion of the extremity with high doses of a chemotherapeutic agent.

It should be noted that, while there has been some emphasis by some surgeons (Krementz and Ryan, 1972; McBride, Sugarbaker, and Hickey, 1975; Stehlin and associates, 1975; Sugarbaker and McBride, 1976) to perform prophylactic isolation-perfusion of the extremities with L-phenylalanine mustard (L-PAM) to reduce the risk of recurrences in patients at high risk, there has been no valid evidence that this alters the survival rates. Although it seems to provide local control of the disease, the complication and toxicity from this drug has been significant (McBride and Clark, 1971; Krementz and Ryan, 1972). On the other hand, Ariyan, Mitchell, and Kirkwood (1984) have been treating in-transit metastases of the extremities with isola-

tion-perfusion of that extremity with dacarbazine (DTIC), which has been shown to eradicate the lesions in some patients and which has a hepatic and systemic toxicity far less than that following perfusion with L-PAM.

SWEAT GLAND CARCINOMA

Sweat gland tumors are very rare epidermal growths, and essentially all of those found on the hand are from eccrine glands rather than apocrine glands. An excellent review of this rare tumor was written by Yaremchuk and associates (1984) when they reported two cases of the malignant variant. These authors report that the incidence of sweat gland tumors is less than 0.05 per cent of pathology specimens, and about 90 per cent of these are benign. The benign lesions can be treated by local excision, while the malignant variants need to be differentiated into low grade and high grade. Low grade tumors need to be treated with wide local excision, and high grade tumors should be considered for wide local excision and elective lymphadenectomy. Experience with these two cases of rare malignant tumors reinforces the inadvisability of merely observing patients with these tumors rather than excising the tumors.

TUMORS OF CONNECTIVE TISSUES

Benign

The vast majority of the masses of the hand are caused by growths within the soft tissue structures. Hematomas, infections, and soft tissue swelling are excluded from the present discussion, which is limited to discrete masses that occur in the hand.

GANGLION

By far the most common tumors of the hand are ganglia and other mucous cysts. A ganglion appears insiduously and grows under some tension, so that pressure on this mass does not result in collapse or decompression. In a review of several series, McEvedy (1962) found that a ganglion is most commonly located on the dorsum of the wrist (61 per cent), its location on the radial volar aspect being

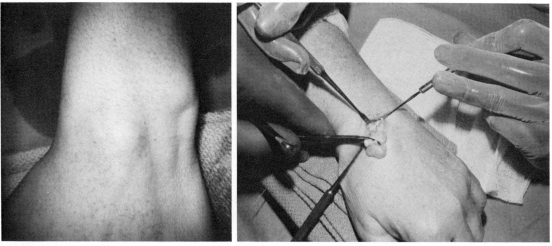

Figure 133–14. The dorsal wrist ganglion usually presents between the tendons of the extensor pollicis longus and the common extensors to the finger.

next most common (13 per cent); a ganglion cyst can also be found to arise from the flexor sheath (9 per cent), usually at the metacarpophalangeal flexion crease at the base of the fingers (Figs. 133–14 to 133–16). Another location is the distal interphalangeal joint, where it appears as a mucous cyst of the dorsum of the finger.

Several theories have been proposed regarding the development of ganglia, including synovial degeneration, connective tissue proliferation, synovial herniation, or development from synovial rests. However, in a series of arthrograms performed on 59 pa-

tients with dorsal and volar wrist ganglia, Andren and Eiken (1971) found direct communication between the wrist joint and a ganglion in 23 of 27 volar ganglia, and 14 of 32 dorsal ganglia; in another nine dorsal ganglia, part of the duct was visualized. Angelides and Wallace (1976) reported their observation on 500 dorsal wrist ganglia, including intraoperative examination and recording of anatomic findings of 65 specimens in which all cases were found to be connected to the scapholunate joint. These authors found by serial sections of complete specimens that the cysts are not lined by endothelium,

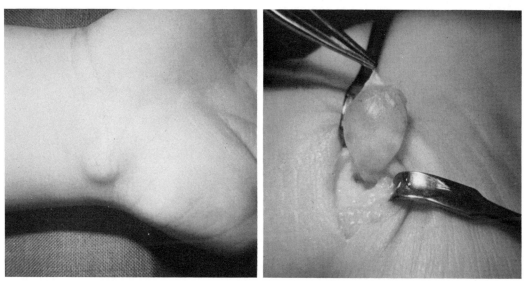

Figure 133–15. The ganglia on the volar aspect of the wrist are located on the radial side, commonly between the artery and the flexor carpi radialis.

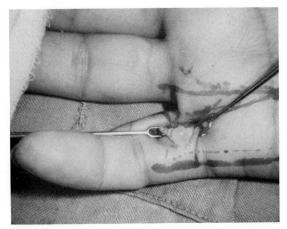

Figure 133–16. Ganglia of the flexor sheath are located most commonly at the base of the finger.

but by fibrous tissue. In addition, there were smaller cysts closer to the attachment to the scapholunate ligament. These smaller cysts were not isolated structures, but were found to communicate with the main cyst and each other, suggesting that they were "ducts" and not cysts. Angelides and Wallace (1976) suggest, therefore, that the ganglion communicates with the scapholunate joint through tortuous ducts consisting of communicating "cysts." Pressure on these cysts causes collapse of the communicating ductlike structures and prevents decompression. This in effect leads to a one-way valve that allows for the one-way flow of synovial fluid into the large cyst.

Linscheid and associates (1972) showed the stress placed on the scaphoid and its ligamentous structures, which lends support to the observation of the scapholunate joint as a pump for the source of joint fluid into the cyst.

Although the ganglion fluid is similar to synovial fluid, the mucous content is much greater. The fluid in the joint space is a mixture of mucin and a dialysate of serum. As this fluid is aspirated from a joint space, the synovial fluid reforms rapidly, but it is of a lower viscosity until the mucin is added more slowly later (McEvedy, 1962). Andren and Eiken (1971) proposed that the thick contents of the ganglion cyst are probably the synovial fluid of the joint space in which the dialysate is being reabsorbed from the cyst, leaving the thicker mucin behind.

The dorsal wrist ganglion is most commonly located on the wrist between the tendons of the extensor pollicis longus and the extensor digitorum communis (Fig. 133–14).

The volar wrist ganglion is usually found on the radial aspect of the wrist in close proximity to the tendon of the flexor carpi radialis and the radial artery (Fig. 133–15). The treatment of ganglia has included splinting, bursting the cyst by external pressure, or needle aspiration. These are usually unsuccessful. However, the definitive treatment remains the surgical excision of the ganglion, including identification and removal of the stalk communicating with the joint space.

A transverse skin incision along a wrist crease gives exposure to these tendons, which are dissected free from the cyst and retracted. The cyst needs to be gently separated from the adjacent structures, taking care not to thin out the fibrous tissue lining, lest the mucous material leak out and decompress the cyst. A decompressed cyst is more difficult to remove completely. On the basis of the previous studies noted above, the joint capsules should be incised in a wrist ganglion, and the cyst should be excised together with a portion of the connective tissue of the joint capsule.

Ganglia of the flexor sheath usually present at the base of the finger, in the area of the entrance of the tendon sheath (Figure 133–16). These are removed through a skin incision directly over the cyst, followed by excision of the cyst together with a portion of the attached flexor sheath.

The recurrence rate of ganglia in a review of series is 3 to 50 per cent (McEvedy, 1962). This incidence was reported by Angelides and Wallace (1976) to be less than 1 per cent if the stalk is dissected down to the joint space and the joint connective tissue is excised with the stalk. In addition, the wrist must be immobilized for seven to ten days to allow the joint ligaments to heal with little stress on the operated joint articulation.

EXTENSOR SHEATH CYST

These are cysts on the dorsum of the wrist that arise from and are attached to the tendon synovia (Fig. 133–17) (Newmeyer, Kilgore, and Graham, 1974). They must be distinguished from dorsal wrist ganglia. On clinical evaluation, the dorsal wrist ganglion does not change shape with flexion or extension of the fingers. On the other hand, with excursion of the extensor tendons, an extensor sheath cyst flattens and broadens on finger flexion, and shortens and becomes more prominent on full extension. This cyst changes shape with the

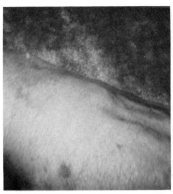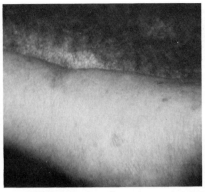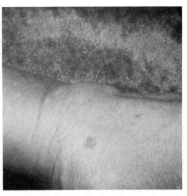

Figure 133–17. Extensor sheath cysts *(left)* flatten when the extensor tendons move distally on flexion *(center)*, and become more prominent when the tendons move proximally on extension *(right)*. (From Ariyan, S.: The Hand Book. Baltimore, Williams & Wilkins, 1983.)

tendon extension because it is attached to the synovium of the extensor tendons.

MUCOUS CYST

This cyst is a dorsal ganglion of the distal interphalangeal joint (Fig. 133–18). Kleinert and associates (1972) reported preoperative radiographic evidence of osteoarthritis in 64 per cent of the 36 patients in their series, and intraoperatively found a definite pedicle between the cyst and the interphalangeal joint. This communication of mucous cysts was verified by Newmeyer, Kilgore, and Graham (1974) with interphalangeal joint injections of methylene blue, which then entered the cyst and stained the contents. Eaton, Dobranski, and Littler (1972) found that these cysts are associated with Heberden's nodes of degenerative arthritis, and believe that it is this marginal osteophyte of the joint that causes the irritation of the synovial tissue to form the cyst.

These cysts develop on the dorsum of the finger and cause pressure over the germinal matrix of the nail. As a result of this pressure, the nail that is formed grows with a definite groove at the location of the cyst. This grooving often appears before any clinical evidence of the cyst mass, and is a heralding sign of a mucous cyst.

Numerous treatments have been recommended for mucous cysts beside excision, including incision and drainage, injection with steroids, injection with a variety of sclerosing agents, freezing with CO_2, and radiation therapy. However, the single long-term evaluation (up to 20 years) of various treatments of mucous cysts by Dodge and associates (1984) demonstrated the lowest recurrence rate (16 per cent) among patients treated with excision of the cyst, an arthrotomy of the distal interphalangeal joint, and removal of any protruding osteophytes or proliferative synovium. Aspiration or drainage of the cysts had a 25 per cent recurrence rate, while those

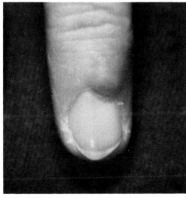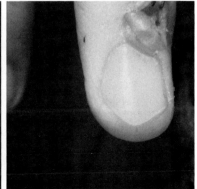

Figure 133–18. Mucous cysts usually develop at the DIP joint, pressing at the nail germinal matrix and causing a grooving of the nail at that location.

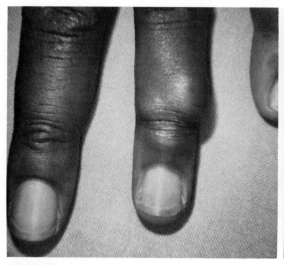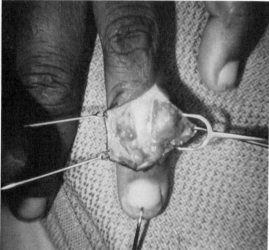

Figure 133–19. Giant cell tumors appear as multilobulated, firm, fibrous masses that are gray to yellow in color. (From Ariyan, S.: The Hand Book. Baltimore, Williams & Wilkins Company, 1983.)

that were not treated persisted in 40 per cent of cases.

GIANT CELL TUMOR

This tumor is a painless, slow-growing mass in the digit or hand and is the second most common tumor of the hand (Fig. 133–19). The name is derived from the histologic identification of multinucleated giant cells, mononuclear histiocytes, fibroblasts, and synovial cells (Carstens, 1978). Grossly the tumor is composed of an encapsulated material resembling a xanthoma. It has a fibrous consistency and a yellow or yellowish-brown color.

The etiology of the giant cell tumor is not known. However, it is known to develop from the tendon sheath of fingers, or the collateral ligament or synovial tissue of a joint. This tumor is not invasive, but grows insidiously through tissue planes and small openings in anatomic structures. It can therefore be dissected by meticulous separation from the adjacent structures. Care must be taken because the growth around the adjacent anatomic structures leads it to entanglement among nerves and vessels.

Since giant cell tumors are encapsulated, treatment involves meticulous dissection for complete removal of the entire multilobulated mass under tourniquet control. Recurrence rates of up to 50 per cent have been reported (Wright, 1951), but meticulous dissection and complete removal should decrease these to

less than 10 per cent (Moore, Weiland, and Curtis, 1984; Savage and Mustafa, 1984).

FIBROMA

Fibromas are rare tumors of the hand that can occur on the palmar aspect, as well as on the volar or dorsal aspects of fingers. The etiology is unknown. Clinically, these lesions need to be differentiated from inclusion cysts or neurogenic tumors. They usually appear as a single mass that can be easily treated by surgical excision.

A unique type of fibroma is that first reported by Reye in 1965 as digital fibromas in six children, in the tissues of whom he found cytoplasmic inclusion bodies. There currently are fewer than 100 cases reported in the literature. This entity, which has come to be called recurring digital fibrous tumors (RDFT) of childhood, has been found to appear either congenitally or in the first few months of life. These tumors are limited essentially to the fingers (Fig. 133–20) and toes, and according to the review of the literature by Beckett and Jacobs (1977), more than 60 per cent have recurred after surgical excision. However, some cases of regression have been reported when the lesions were left alone (Bloem, Vuzevski, and Huffstadt, 1974). The epidermis is not involved; the tumor, which is limited to the dermis, is composed of fibroblasts containing the characteristic inclusion bodies reported by Reye (1965). The significance of these inclusion bodies has been dif-

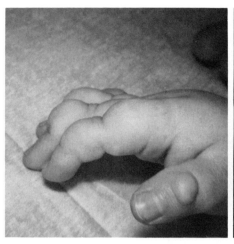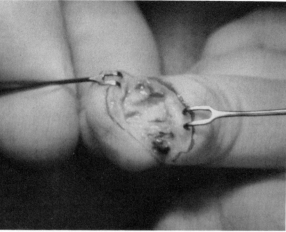

Figure 133–20. Fibromas of infancy present as masses in the dermis of the distal portions of the fingers, but may also include the palm.

ficult to determine and some interpreted them to mean that a virus was the causative agent. However, examinations by electron microscopy have revealed that these cells are myofibroblasts, and that the inclusion bodies are contractile protein and may represent normal contraction of actin filaments (Mortimer and Gibson, 1982; Iwasaki and associates, 1983).

Fibromas, therefore, are benign tumors that need not be removed unless they grow large enough to be a cosmetic deformity or to affect function. If they need to be removed, they should be excised completely. Digital fibrous tumors in children and infants should be treated conservatively with observation. If removal is indicated, surgical excision must be complete, and the possibility of recurrence must be considered.

PYOGENIC GRANULOMA

A pyogenic granuloma is a hypertrophic growth of granulation tissue as a result of a break in the skin. This benign tumor is composed of capillary buds, fibroblasts, and collagen. It usually grows rapidly after the initial injury, but the injury itself may not be remembered by the patient. The tumor is usually pedunculated (Fig. 133–21) but may also be sessile; it bleeds easily when rubbed with dry gauze. The treatment is to cauterize the lesion if it is small. If it persists or it grows, surgical excision may be required.

LIPOMA

This is a benign tumor similar to a lipoma elsewhere in the body. It seldom causes significant symptoms. However, when lipomas are large, they may pose difficulty in the use of the hand. Care must be taken in the surgical removal of the lipoma to prevent injury to vital anatomic structures (Fig. 133–22). It must always be done with tourniquet control.

Figure 133–21. Pyogenic granuloma is a friable soft tumor that may be sessile or pedunculated, and may appear on the volar or dorsal surfaces of the fingers or the hand.

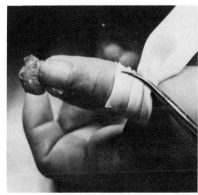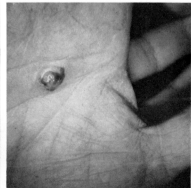

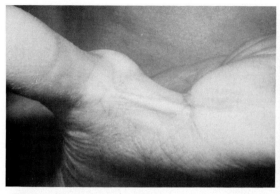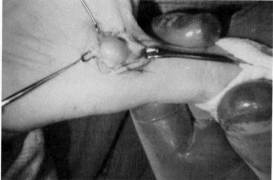

Figure 133–22. A lipoma appears similar to an inclusion cyst but is softer, and the skin moves freely over the mass.

FIBROUS HISTIOCYTOMA

Fibrous histiocytoma is a term applied fairly widely to a group of benign and malignant lesions that have grown from cells of histiocytic origin as classified by Stout and Lattes (1976). The benign form of this lesion is seen in giant cell tumors of the tendon sheath, fibrous xanthomas, and dermatofibromas; the malignant forms include dermatofibrosarcoma protuberans and malignant fibrous histiocytomas (Fu and associates, 1975).

In a series report of 200 cases from the Armed Forces Institution of Pathology, Weiss and Enzinger (1978) reported that 49 per cent of cases were located on the lower extremity, while 19 per cent were on the upper extremity. Histologically, these malignant fibrous histiocytomas (MFH) were in various forms: (1) in the *storiform pattern*, the MFH had spindle cells arranged in short fascicles in a cartwheel-like pattern, closely resembling dermatofibrosarcoma protuberans, but differing by the presence of large round histiocytes; (2) in the *pleomorphic pattern*, which is far more common for MFH, the cells are in a more haphazard or random fashion; and (3) in the *fascicular pattern*, which accounted for only 10 per cent of cases, the cells were lined up together in linear fascicles. These authors thought that the prognosis of the MFH was most reliably based on the depth of the initial tumor; if the tumor has borderline histological features, it is probably best regarded as potentially malignant (Weiss and Enzinger, 1978).

Dermatofibrosarcoma protuberans is a lesion of the dermis and can be treated with wide local excision. If this lesion recurs, it does so locally and should be reexcised (Fu and associates, 1975; Wirman, Sherman, and Sullivan, 1981). *Malignant fibrous histiocytoma* may be localized to the dermis alone, may occur in the subcutaneous tissue alone, or may begin in the dermis and grow deeper into the supporting structures.

The treatment of these lesions should be wide local excision. Amputation should not be considered unless the tumor has grown extensively or invaded adjacent structures deeply, as it sometimes may; lymph node dissections are not indicated unless they are clinically palpable (Weiss and Enzinger, 1978).

Malignant

SARCOMAS

Rhabdomyosarcoma of the hand is a rare tumor, although it is becoming more recognized as a soft tissue sarcoma in children and young adults. The decision to amputate or to excise the tumor while preserving functional parts of the hand requires judgment. However, amputation should be considered for recurrent tumors, tumors that exhibit deep invasion, or tumors that do not permit local resection. Chemotherapy should be considered for these patients, since the dissemination is often blood-borne.

Malignant synovioma, or synovial sarcoma, is a rare tumor, even though it may be among the more common soft tissue sarcomas of the hands and feet. This tumor may arise from the joint capsule, bursa, or tendon sheath (Fig. 133–23). An evaluation of this tumor by electron microscopy revealed that it is "bi-

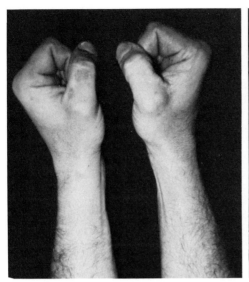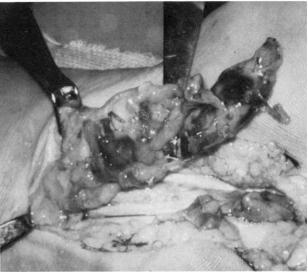

Figure 133–23. A synovioma of the volar wrist with a multilobulated mass attached to the flexor tendon.

phasic," i.e., it contains epithelial-like and fibrosarcoma-like elements (Dische, Darby, and Howard, 1978).

Another variant of this has been reported by several authors as *epithelioid sarcoma*, which involves the skin of the palm or of the fingers (Goodwin and Salama, 1982; Tsur and Lipsker, 1982; Archer, Brown, and Fitton, 1984). Hoopes, Graham, and Shack (1985) reviewed 115 cases (including three of their own) and found that the uniform experience of most authors was that this tumor was aggressive, with local recurrences in 50 to 92 per cent, lymph node involvement in 10 to 50 per cent, and metastases in 30 to 46 per cent. Because of the aggressive nature of this tumor, the treatment must also be aggressive, with wide local excision, and consideration of amputation in confirmed cases. The data are not sufficient to permit any recommendation for elective lymphadenectomy as opposed to observation for clinical involvement of the lymph nodes and subsequent therapeutic lymphadenectomy.

TUMORS OF VASCULAR TISSUE

Tumors of the blood and lymphatic vessels are not uncommon in the hand. In large series of hand tumors, vascular tumors accounted for 2.2 to 6.8 per cent of cases (Butler and associates, 1960; Haber, Alter, and Wheelock,

1965; Leung, 1981; Johnson, Kilgore, and Newmeyer, 1985). There are a variety of types of vascular tumors, but there is no uniformity of opinion regarding their classification. Virchow (1863) considered hemangiomas to be vascular tumors and classified them as simplex, cavernosum, and racemosum. Stout and Lattes (1976) listed a variety of congenital and acquired lesions and preferred to classify them on the basis of microscopic appearance. Morris and Owsley (1975) classified them simply as involuting or noninvoluting types; the involuting hemangiomas were divided into superficial, deep, or a combination of both.

A classification was proposed by Mulliken and Glowacki (1982) that is oriented to the endothelial cells and the clinical behavior of these lesions. According to this classification, vascular lesions are either *hemangiomas* or *malformations* (Table 133–4). Hemangiomas are limited to lesions that make their appearance in late fetal or early neonatal life, grow rapidly for six to eight months, and usually undergo regression to a variable extent. During the proliferating phase, the endothelium of hemangiomas shows hyperplasia and incorporate ^{3}H-thymidine; during the involuting phase they demonstrate fibrosis and fat deposition, and low or absent uptake of ^{3}H-thymidine by the endothelial cells.

Vascular malformations, on the other hand, are recognized at birth, grow only commen-

Table 133–4. Classification and Features of Vascular Malformations

	Hemangiomas	Malformations
Components	Capillary	Capillary Venous Arterial Lymphatic Fistulas
Clinical Features	Rapid early growth Slow involution	Growth commensurate with growth of child
Histologic Features	Endothelial cell proliferation	Normal endothelial cell activity

Modified from Mulliken, J. B., and Glowacki, J.: Hemangiomas and vascular malformations in infants and children: a classification based on endothelial characteristics. Plast. Reconstr. Surg., 69:412, 1982.

surately with the child, and do not show evidence of regression. None of these lesions show increased endothelial uptake of ³H-thymidine, reflecting normal endothelial mitotic activity. Although most of the malformations are the venous type, they may have any combination of lymphatic, arterial, or capillary components, with or without fistulas. The port-wine stains are classified as malformations that consist mostly of venule-like channels in the dermis. The lymphatic malformations may shrink, but do not show histologic evidence of involution or regression; therefore, they should be said to undergo resolution or deflation. According to this classification system, the diagnosis can usually be made accurately by history taking and physical examination.

HEMANGIOMAS

Hemangiomas of a localized character are present in the skin and are readily diagnosed (Fig. 133–24). They are usually asymptomatic and are most often treated for cosmetic appearance. Because of their rapid growth, the more extensive lesions cause apprehension in the patient's parents, who must be reassured about the ultimate regression. These lesions may be treated by compressive dressings or custom-fitted gauntlets to induce regression (Smith, Miller, and Shochat, 1976). Prednisone may be given for four to eight weeks to diminish the lesion (Zarem and Edgerton, 1967). However, the lesion should not be injected with sclerosing agents, freezed with dry ice, or treated with radiation

therapy, since all of these lead to significant scarring and late sequelae.

MALFORMATIONS

Vascular malformations of the venous, arterial, or mixed type may require excision to remove the tumor mass. If this procedure is chosen, it should be performed with tourniquet control, but without complete exsanguination of the extremity before the tourniquet is inflated, in order to permit some blood to remain in the vessels so that the lesion may be identified and removed as completely as possible (Fig. 133–25). It is not uncommon for these lesions to grow back to their previous size, because some vessels may have been left behind that then permit the flow to increase into the remaining lesion. Also, some of these lesions may grow into the muscles of the hand and forearm, and care must be taken to preserve all vital adjacent structures.

ARTERIOVENOUS FISTULAS

Arteriovenous (AV) fistulas may be due to congenital abnormalities, or may be secondary to trauma. Congenital arteriovenous fistulas may be localized to a finger or may be more generalized to a hand. They are always associated with dilated veins. There may be chronic ulceration of a wound from a trivial injury that will not heal until the fistula is excised or closed. The finger or hand may become hypertrophied or increase in size if

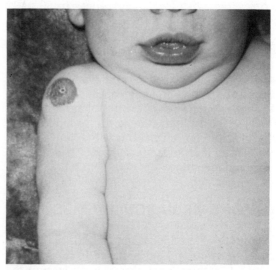

Figure 133–24. A capillary hemangioma of the upper arm in an infant with a history of rapid growth over several months.

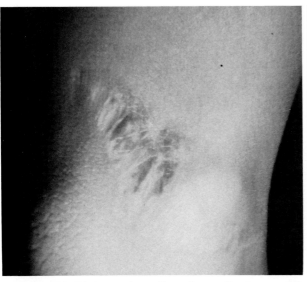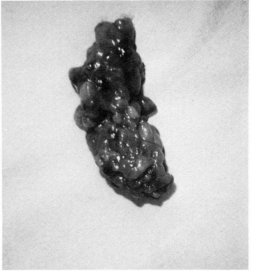

Figure 133–25. A vascular malformation on the dorsum of the wrist had a mass that could be palpated deep to the skin; it consisted of arterial and venous components. (From Ariyan, S.: The Hand Book. Baltimore, Williams & Wilkins Company, 1983.)

the epiphyses are still open and a significant shunt persists (Fig. 133–26).

In cases of extensive arteriovenous fistulas, an arteriogram is essential to delineate the extent of the malformation. Under these circumstances, the surgery must be performed with the intention of closing or excising as many of these fistulas as possible without compromising the circulation to the finger or the hand. It may be possible to reduce the shunting sufficiently to permit healing of the

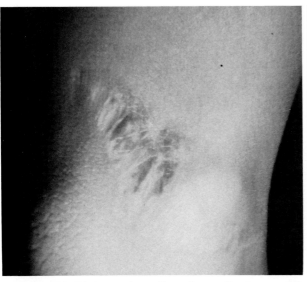

Figure 133–26. Congenital arteriovenous malformation of the ulnar aspect of the hand, resulting in enlargement of that portion of the hand and of the little finger.

ulcer or a skin graft, before the shunting resumes again. The arteriovenous fistula may be so extensive as to persist or recur after surgery.

An arteriovenous fistula may also be due to an injury that damages the vessels and leads to this abnormal vascular communication. There is usually a discrete history of an injury with a lag period before the mass is visible (Fig. 133–27). An arteriogram can delineate the extent of involvement, and determine whether a large vessel is involved. This lesion needs to be explored in the operating room with magnification (either operating loops or microscope) to identify the vessels and communications. Again, the extremity should not be completely exsanguinated, in order to permit some blood to remain in the vessels to assist identification.

Lymphatic malformations do occur in the hand, but are rare. They may be localized to a finger or may involve the whole hand (Fig. 133–28). Most appear soon after birth, although some have a history of being slight until adolescence or adulthood before becoming more prominent. There is no effective treatment for these lesions. They may be surgically removed to decrease the extent of involvement, but these procedures lead to unsightly scars. Occasionally the involved hand or foot may be associated with a constricting band that needs to be released with a Z-plasty.

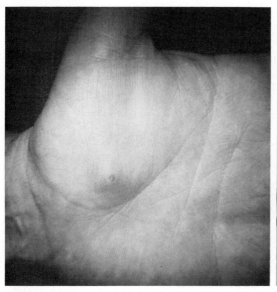
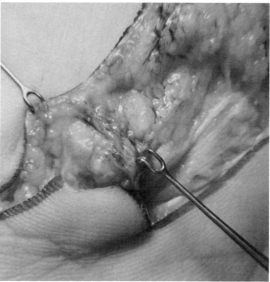

Figure 133–27. Traumatic arteriovenous (AV) malformation from a puncture wound had resulted in this painful mass several weeks after the injury. Under loupe magnification, the AV fistula was identified and resected. (From Ariyan, S.: The Hand Book. Baltimore, Williams & Wilkins Company, 1983.)

GLOMUS TUMOR

This is a rare benign tumor of the normal glomus, which is a neuromyoarterial canal system called the Sucquet-Hoyer canal. Patients report cold intolerance, and a positive nail–ice cube test is often diagnostic. The most detailed report of the glomus apparatus was made by Popoff (1934); he described an afferent arteriole, an anastomotic vessel, a primary collecting vein, an intraglomular reticulum, and a capsule. The function of the glomus appears to be to regulate local blood pressure and to regulate local heat by blood flow. The etiology of its development is unknown, although some patients associate the development with an injury to the area. In a series of sections of toes and fingers in a young adult, Popoff (1934) found 64 glomera, about one-third of which were beneath the nail bed. Clinically, more than one-half of these tumors occur under the nail bed (Carroll and Berman, 1972; Carlstedt and Lugnegard, 1983). The diagnosis is suspected by a history of excruciating pain with mechanical stimulation or cold stimulation of the tumor. Occasionally the tumor may be seen by a blue discoloration under the nail or the skin. Treatment consists of surgical excision of the lesion under tourniquet control and magnification for complete removal of the lesion, which is easily shelled out.

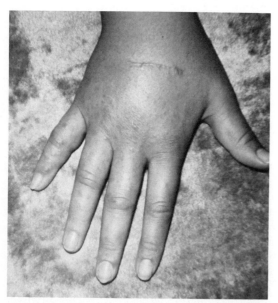

Figure 133–28. Lymphatic malformation is soft and feels cystic to examination, but shows no pitting edema. (From Ariyan, S.: The Hand Book. Baltimore, Williams & Wilkins Company, 1983.)

MALIGNANT VASCULAR TUMORS

These malignant tumors are extremely rare in the hand and upper extremities. They are named after the cells from which they originate: hemangioendothelioma develops from endothelial cells, hemangiopericytoma arises from the pericytes on the external surface of capillaries, Kaposi's sarcoma is a mixture of vascular tumor and fibrosarcoma, and lymphangiosarcoma is a sarcoma in which lymph vessels predominate.

Hemangioendothelioma and hemangiopericytoma are tumors of the individual vascular cells alone, while hemangiosarcoma also involves the endothelial cells and fibroblastic connective tissues. Hemangioendotheliomas and hemangiopericytomas can be slow growing or may grow rapidly and metastasize; their clinical behavior cannot be predicted by the histologic appearance. They should be treated by wide local resections if on the hand, and amputation if the phalanges are involved. Hemangiosarcomas, on the other hand, are more aggressive and metastasize early. The lesions on the hand should be treated by wide local excision, and radiation therapy should be considered as a postoperative adjuvant treatment.

TUMORS OF NEURAL TISSUE

Tumors of nerve tissue may be the common neuromas following injury, neurofibromas of von Recklinghausen's disease, neurilemomas, or the rare malignant schwannomas.

NEUROMAS

Neuromas are probably the most common tumors of nerve tissues, most of which remain undiagnosed because they are asymptomatic. Occasionally, however, a nerve is crushed, cut, or amputated and this leads to a painful mass of regenerated axons. The neuromas at the end of cut digital nerves in amputation stumps can be removed, but may recur. It may be more meaningful to transpose the nerve to a more protected site after the neuroma is excised, such as translocation to the dorsum of the phalangeal stump. A neuroma in continuity may develop after a partial laceration or a crush injury of a major nerve. If these are to be resected, they need to be performed with magnification by a microscope or operating loops. In this way, the neuroma can be removed with the least damage to the adjacent intact fascicles.

NEURILEMOMAS

Neurilemomas, or schwannomas, are tumors consisting of the cells of the nerve sheaths, or the Schwann cells (Phalen, 1976). Thorsrud (1960) reviewed over 450 cases and classified these lesions by the histologic cell types. There are two tumor cell types: the Antoni A areas are composed of long, slender cells arranged in a palisading fashion as seen by their nuclei; the Antoni B areas are composed of loose cells with small, round nuclei and show areas of cystic degeneration. According to Thorsrud, neurilemomas made up one group that was predominantly of Antoni B cells and he called type I, while the more common group of tumors were made up pre-

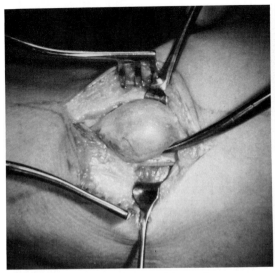
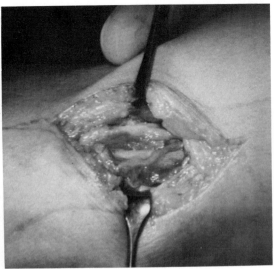

Figure 133–29. A neurilemoma of the median nerve can usually be easily dissected out of the median nerve, preserving the fascicles. (From Ariyan, S.: The Hand Book. Baltimore, Williams & Wilkins Company, 1983.)

dominantly of Antoni A cells, which he called type II; the remainder were composed of both types, which he called type III.

These tumors usually result in round or fusiform masses in connection with small nerves, or within the sheath of large nerves (Fig. 133–29). These are benign tumors and are asymptomatic in general. They are removed by meticulous dissection from the remainder of nerve, preserving the fascicles to which they are attached.

NEUROFIBROMAS

Neurofibromas are thickenings of the nerve sheath elements between the individual nerve fibrils, resulting in a tortuosity of these peripheral nerves (Fig. 133–30). This tortuosity is a result of extensive involvement at several points along the nerve, and the tumors are called plexiform neuromas. These tumors are often associated with overgrowth of the involved finger (macrodactyly) or of the hand (Barsky, 1967). The tumors may be removed and the digit made narrower for cosmetic appearance. The tumors are centrally located with the nerve fibers travelling through the tumor mass, making it more difficult to remove the tumor and sparing nerve fibers. Tumors of larger nerves can be removed with the microscope, and the nerve repaired with primary repair or fascicular interposition nerve grafts. It has been re-

ported that 13 per cent of patients with neurofibromatosis of von Recklinghausen's disease develop malignant transformation of these tumors (Hosoi, 1931).

MALIGNANT SCHWANNOMA

Malignant schwannoma is an uncommon variant of the benign neurilemomas. These malignant cells grow in whorls resembling a fibrosarcoma, which Thorsrud further classified into types IV, V, and VI. Type IV are "low grade" malignancies, with a scarcity of cells but abundant intercellular substance, and a mortality rate of 5 per cent. Type V are "medium grade" malignancies with a moderate amount of cells and intercellular substance, and a 20 per cent mortality. Type VI are "high grade" malignancies that show densely packed cells with minimal intercellular substance, and a 40 per cent mortality.

Only 13 per cent of patients with von Reckinghausen's disease are known to develop malignant schwannomas, but one-half of the malignant schwannomas are found in patients with this disorder. These tumors grow along the nerve trunks, invading adjacent structures or metastasizing to distant organs. If malignancy is suspected because of adherence to or invasion of adjacent structures, a biopsy should be performed. If the malignancy is diagnosed, the tumors should be widely excised for several inches from the

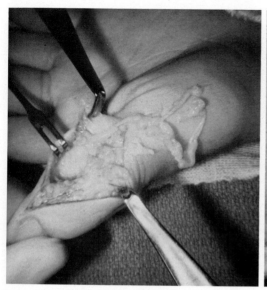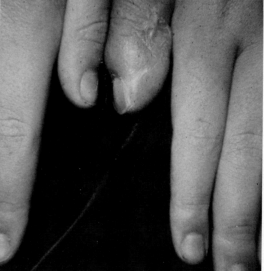

Figure 133–30. Multiple neurofibromas of von Recklinghausen's disease may lead to gigantism of a digit or a hand.

tumor. If adjacent tissue invasion is prominent, an amputation may be indicated. The prognosis for these malignant tumors is not good (Thorsrud, 1931; Seddon, 1972).

REFERENCES

Alpert, L. I., Zak, F. G., and Werthamer, S.: Subungual basal cell epithelioma. Arch. Dermatol., 106:599, 1972.

Amer, M. H., Al-Sarraf, M., and Vaitkevicius, V. K.: Clinical presentation, natural history and prognostic factors in advanced malignant melanoma. Surg. Gynecol. Obstet., 149:687, 1979.

Andren, L., and Eiken, O.: Arthrographic studies of wrist ganglions. J. Bone Joint Surg., 52A:299, 1971.

Angelides, A. C., and Wallace, P. F.: The dorsal ganglion of the wrist: its pathogenesis, gross and microscopic anatomy, and surgical treatment. J. Hand Surg., 1:228, 1976.

Archer, I. A., Brown, R. B., and Fitton, J. M.: Epithelioid sarcoma in the hand. J. Hand Surg., 9B:207, 1984.

Ariyan, S., and Kirkwood, J. M.: Malignant melanoma margins. N. Engl. J. Med., 307:439, 1982.

Ariyan, S., Mitchell, M. S., and Kirkwood, J. M.: Regional isolated perfusion of high risk melanoma of the extremities with imidazole carboxamide. Surg. Gynecol. Obstet., 158:238, 1984.

Balch, C. M., Murad, T. M., Soong, S. J., Ingalls, A. L., Halpern, N. B., and Maddox, W. A.: A multifactorial analysis of melanoma: prognostic histopathological features comparing Clark's and Breslow's staging methods. Ann. Surg., 188:732, 1978.

Balch, C. M., Soong, S. J., Milton, G. W., Shaw, H. M., McGovern, V. J., et al.: A comparison of prognostic factors and surgical results in 1,786 patients with localized (stage I) melanoma treated in Alabama, USA and New South Wales, Australia. Ann. Surg., 196:677, 1982.

Balch, C. M., Soong, S. J., Murad, T. M., Ingalls, A. L., and Maddox, W. A.: A multifactorial analysis of melanoma: II. Prognostic factors in patients with stage I (localized) melanoma. Surgery, 86:343, 1979.

Balch, C. M., Soong, S. J., Murad, T. M., Ingalls, A. L., and Maddox, W. A.: A multifactorial analysis of melanoma. III. Prognostic factors in melanoma patients with lymph node metastases. Ann. Surg., 193:377, 1981.

Barsky, A. J.: Macrodactyly. J. Bone Joint Surg., 49A:1255, 1967.

Bean, D. J., Rees, R. S., O'Leary, P., and Lynch, J. B.: Carcinoma of the hand: a 20-year experience. South. Med. J., 77:998, 1984.

Beckett, J. H., and Jacobs, A. H.: Recurring digital fibrous tumors of childhood: a review. Pediatrics, 59:401, 1977.

Birkeland, S. A., Kempy, E., and Hauge, M.: Renal transplantation and cancer. The Scandia Transplant Material. Tissue Antigens, 6:28, 1975.

Bloem, J. J., Vuzevski, V. D., and Huffstadt, A. J. C.: Recurring digital fibroma of infancy. J. Bone Joint Surg., 56B:746, 1974.

Bowen, J. T.: Precancerous dermatoses: a study of two cases of chronic atypical epithelial proliferation. J. Cutan. Dis., 30:241, 1912.

Bowen, J. T.: Precancerous dermatoses: the further course of two cases previously described. Arch. Dermatol. Syph., 1:23, 1920.

Breslow, A.: Thickness, cross-sectional areas and depth of invasion in the prognosis of cutaneous melanoma. Ann. Surg., 172:902, 1970.

Bunkis, J., Mehrhof, A. I., and Stayman, J. W.: Radiation-induced carcinoma of the hand. J. Hand Surg., 6:384, 1981.

Butler, E. D., Hammil, J. P., Seipel, R. S., and De-Lorimier, A. A.: Tumors of the hand. A ten-year survey and report of 437 cases. Am. J. Surg., 100:293, 1960.

Carlstedt, T., and Lugnegard, H.: Glomus tumor in the hand. A clinical and morphologic study. Acta Orthop. Scand., 54:296, 1983.

Carroll, R. E.: Squamous cell carcinoma of the nailbed. J. Hand Surg., 1:92, 1976.

Carroll, R. E., and Berman, A. T.: Glomus tumors of the hand. J. Bone Joint Surg., 54:691, 1972.

Carstens, H. B.: Giant cell tumors of the tendon sheath. Arch. Pathol. Lab. Med., 102:99, 1978.

Cascinelli, N., and Vaglini, M.: Evaluation of optimal margins of resection in cutaneous malignant melanoma thinner than 2 mm. WHO Clinical Trial No. 10.

Cascinelli, N., Van der Esch, E. P., Breslow, A., Morabito, A., and Bufalino, R.: Stage I melanoma of the skin: the problem of resection margin. Eur. J. Cancer, 16:1079, 1980.

Clark, W. H., From, L., Bernardino, E. A., and Mihm, M. C.: The histogenesis and biologic behavior of primary human malignant melanomas of the skin. Cancer Res., 29:705, 1969.

Cohen, N., Plaschkes, Y., Pevzner, S., and Loewenthal, M.: Review of 57 cases of keratoacanthoma. Plast. Reconstr. Surg., 49:138, 1972.

Coleman, W. P., Loria, P. R., Reed, R. J., and Krementz, E. T.: Acral lentiginous melanoma. Arch. Dermatol., 116:773, 1980.

Crikelair, G. F., Hoehn, R. J., Domonkos, A. N., and Binkert, B.: Skin homografts in epidermolysis bullosa dystrophica. Plast. Reconstr. Surg., 46:89, 1970.

Cuono, C. B., and Ariyan, S.: Versatility and safety of flap coverage for wide excision of cutaneous melanoma. Plast. Reconstr. Surg., 76:281, 1985.

Day, C. L., Mihm, M. C., Sobert, A. J., Fitzpatrick, T. D., and Malt, R. A.: Narrower margins for clinical stage I malignant melanoma. N. Engl. J. Med., 306:479, 1982.

Dische, F. E., Darby, A. J., and Howard, E. R.: Malignant synovioma: electron microscopical findings in three patients and review of the literature. J. Pathol., 124:149, 1978.

Dodge, L. D., Brown, R. L., Niebauer, J. J., and McCarroll, H. R.: The treatment of mucous cysts: long-term follow-up in sixty-two cases. J. Hand Surg., 9A:901, 1984.

Domarus, H. V., and Stevens, P. J.: Metastatic basal cell carcinoma. J. Am. Acad. Dermatol., 10:1043, 1984.

Eaton, R. G., Dobranski, A. I., and Littler, J. W.: Marginal osteophyte excision in the treatment of mucous cysts. J. Bone Joint Surg., 54A:909, 1972.

Feibleman, C. E., Stoll, H., and Maize, J. C.: Melanomas of the palm, sole, and nailbed. A clinicopathologic study. Cancer, 46:2492, 1980.

Forsythe, R. L., Bajaj, P., Engeron, O., and Shadid, E. A.: The treatment of squamous cell carcinoma of the hand. Hand, 10:104, 1978.

Fu, Y. S., Gabbiani, G., Kaye, G. I., and Lattes, R.: Malignant soft tissue tumors of probable histiocytic origin (malignant fibrous histiocytomas): general considerations and electron microscope and tissue culture studies. Cancer, 35:176, 1975.

Gipson, M.: Squamous cell carcinoma in epidermolysis bullosa dystrophica. Hand, 7:179, 1975.

Goldsmith, H. S., Shah, J. P., and Kim, D. H.: Prognostic significance of lymph node dissection in the treatment of malignant melanoma. Cancer, 26:606, 1970.

Goodwin, D. R. A., and Salama, R.: Synovial sarcoma of the finger. Hand, 14:198, 1982.

Haber, M. H., Alter, A. H., and Wheelock, M. C.: Tumors of the hand. Surg. Gynecol. Obstet., 121:1073, 1965.

Hazelrigg, D. E., and Renne, J. W.: Squamous cell carcinoma of the nailbed. J. Dermatol. Surg. Oncol., 8:200, 1982.

Hoopes, J. E., Graham, W. P., and Shack, R. B.: Epithelioid sarcoma of the upper extremity. Plast. Reconstr. Surg., 75:810, 1985.

Hosoi, K.: Multiple neurofibromatosis (von Recklinghausen's disease). Arch. Surg., 22:258, 1931.

Hugo, N. E., and Conway, H.: Bowen's disease: its malignant potential and relationship to systemic cancer. Plast. Reconstr. Surg., 39:190, 1967.

Iwasaki, H., Kikuchi, M., Ohtsuki, I., Enjoji, M., Suenaga, N., and Mori, R.: Infantile digital fibromastosis. Identification of active filaments in cytoplasmic inclusions by heavy meromyosin binding. Cancer, 52:1653, 1983.

Jacobsson, S., Linell, F., and Rausing, A.: Florid keratoacanthomas in a kidney transplant recipient. Scand. J. Plast. Reconstr. Surg., 8:243, 1974.

Johnson, J., Kilgore, E., and Newmeyer, W.: Tumorous lesions of the hand. J. Hand Surg., 10:284, 1985.

Katz, A. D., Urbach, F., and Lilienfeld, A. M.: The frequency and risk of metastases in squamous cell carcinoma of the skin. Cancer, 10:1162, 1957.

Kendall, T. E., Robinson, D. W., and Masters, F. W.: Primary malignant tumors of the hand. Plast. Reconstr. Surg., 44:37, 1969.

Klein, E., Stoll, H. L., Milgrom, H., Helm, F., and Walker, M. J.: Tumors of the skin. XII. Topical fluorouracil for epidermal neoplasms. J. Surg. Oncol., 3:331, 1971.

Kleinert, H. E., Katz, J. E., Fishman, J. H., and McCraw, L. H.: Etiology and treatment of the so-called mucous cyst of the finger. J. Bone Joint Surg., 54A:1455, 1972.

Koh, H. K., Michalik, E., Sobert, A. J., Lew, R. A., Day, C. L., et al.: Lentigomaligna melanoma has no better prognosis than other types of melanoma. J. Clin. Oncol., 2:994, 1984.

Krementz, E. J., and Ryan, R. F.: Chemotherapy of melanoma of the extremities by perfusion; fourteen years' clinical experience. Ann. Surg., 175:900, 1972.

Leung, P. C.: Tumors of the hand. Hand, 12:169, 1981.

Linscheid, R. L., Dobyns, J. H., Beabout, J. W., and Bryan, R. S.: Traumatic instability of the wrist: diagnosis, classification, and pathomechanics. J. Bone Joint Surg., 54A:1612, 1972.

Lund, H. Z.: How often does squamous cell carcinoma of the skin metastasize? Arch. Dermatol., 92:635, 1965.

Mason, M. L.: Tumors of the hand. Surg. Gynecol. Obstet., 64:129, 1937.

McBride, C. M., and Clark, R. L.: Experience with L-phenylalanine mustard dihydrochloride in isolation-perfusion of extremities for malignant melanoma. Cancer, 28:1293, 1971.

McBride, C. M., Sugarbaker, E. V., and Hickey, R. C.: Prophylactic isolation-perfusion as the primary therapy for invasive malignant melanoma of the limbs. Ann. Surg., 182:316, 1975.

McDowell, C. L., and Henceforth, W. D.: Malignant fibrous histiocytoma of the hand: a case report. J. Hand Surg., 2:297, 1977.

McEvedy, B. V.: Simple ganglion. Br. J. Surg., 49:585, 1962.

McGovern, V. J., Mihm, M. C., Bailly, C., et al.: The classification of malignant melanoma and its histologic reporting. Cancer, 32:1446, 1973.

Mehnert, J. H., and Heard, J. L.: Staging of malignant melanomas by depth of invasion. A proposed index to prognosis. Am. J. Surg., 110:168, 1965.

Milton, G. W., Shaw, H. M., McCarthy, W. H., Pearson, L., Balch, C. M., and Soong, S. J.: Prophylactic lymph node dissection in clinical stage I cutaneous malignant melanoma: results of surgical treatment in 1,319 patients. Br. J. Surg., 69:108, 1982.

Moore, J. R., Weiland, A. J., and Curtis, R. M.: Localized nodular tenosynovitis: experience with 115 cases. J. Hand Surg., 9A:412, 1984.

Morris, W. J., and Owsley, J. Q.: Plastic surgery. In Dunphy, J. E., and Way, L. W. (Eds.): Current Surgical Diagnosis and Treatment. 2nd Ed. Los Altos, Lange Publishing, 1975.

Mortimer, G., and Gibson, A. A. M.: Recurring digital fibroma. J. Clin. Pathol., 35:849, 1982.

Mulliken, J. B., and Glowacki, J.: Hemangiomas and vascular malformations in infants and children: a classification based on endothelial characteristics. Plast. Reconstr. Surg., 69:412, 1982.

Newmeyer, W. L., Kilgore, E. S., and Graham, W. P.: Mucous cysts: the dorsal interphalangeal joint ganglion. Plast Reconstr. Surg., 53:313, 1974.

Penn, I., and Starzl, T. E.: Malignant tumors arising in immunosuppressed organ transplant recipients. Transplantation, 14:407, 1972.

Phalen, G. S.: Neurilemomas of the forearm and hand. Clin. Orthop., 114:219, 1976.

Popoff, N. W.: The digital vascular system with reference to the state of the glomus in inflammation, arteriosclerotic gangrene, thromboangiitis obliterans and supernumerary digits in man. Arch. Pathol., 18:294, 1934.

Posch, J. L.: Soft tissue tumors of the hand. In Flynn, J. E. (Ed.): Hand Surgery. 3rd Ed. Baltimore, Williams & Wilkins Company, 1982, p. 877.

Reye, R. D. K.: Recurring digital fibrous tumors of childhood. Arch. Pathol., 80:228, 1965.

Roses, D. F., Harris, M. N., Hidalgo, D., Valensi, Q. J., and Dubin, N.: Primary melanoma thickness correlated with regional lymph node metastases. Arch. Surg., 117:921, 1982.

Roses, D. F., Harris, M. N., Rigel, D., Carrey, Z., Friedman, R., and Kopf, A. W.: Local and in-transit metastases following definitive excision for primary cutaneous malignant melanoma. Ann. Surg., 198:65, 1983.

Sanders, B. B., and Stretcher, G. S.: Warts. Diagnosis and treatment. J.A.M.A., 235:2859, 1976.

Savage, R. C., and Mustafa, E. B.: Giant cell tumor of tendon sheath (localized nodular tenosynovitis). Ann. Plast. Surg., 13:205, 1984.

Seddon, H. J.: Surgical Disorders of Peripheral Nerves. Baltimore, Williams & Wilkins Company, 1972.

Smith, R. L., Miller, S. H., and Shochat, S.: Compression treatment of hemangiomas. Plast. Reconstr. Surg., 58:573, 1976.

Stehlin, J. S., Giovanella, B. C., DeIpolyi, P. D., et al.: Results of hyperthermia perfusion for melanoma of the extremities. Surg. Gynecol. Obstet., *140*:339, 1975.

Stout, A. P., and Lattes, R.: Tumor of the soft tissues. *In* Atlas of Tumor Pathology. 2nd series. Washington, DC, Armed Forces Institute of Pathology, 1976.

Sugarbaker, E. V., and McBride, C. M.: Survival and regional disease control after isolation-perfusion for invasive stage I melanoma of the extremities. Cancer, *37*:188, 1976.

Taylor, D. R., and South, D. A.: Acral lentiginous melanoma. Cutis, *26*:35, 1980.

Taylor, H. B., and Helwig, E. B.: Dermatofibrosarcoma protuberans. A study of 115 cases. Cancer, *15*:717, 1962.

Thorsrud, G.: Neurinoma. Acta Chir. Scand. (Suppl.), *252*:16, 1960.

Tsur, H., and Lipsker, E.: Epithelioid sarcoma of the hand. Ann. Plast. Surg., *8*:420, 1982.

Veronesi, U., Adamus, J., Bandiera, D. C., et al.: Inefficacy of immediate node dissection in stage I melanoma of the limbs. N. Engl. J. Med., *197*:627, 1977.

Virchow, R.: Angiome. *In* Die Krankhaften Geschwulste. Vol. 3. Berlin, August Hirschwald, 1863, p. 806.

Walder, B. K., Robertson, M. R., and Jeremy, D.: Skin cancer and immunosuppression. Lancet, *2*:1282, 1971.

Weiss, S. W., and Enzinger, F. M.: Malignant fibrous histiocytoma. An analysis of two cases. Cancer, *41*:2250, 1978.

Wirman, J. A., Sherman, S., and Sullivan, M. R.: Dermatofibrosarcoma protuberans arising on the hand. Hand, *13*:187, 1981.

Wright, C. J. E.: Benign giant cell synovioma. Br. J. Surg., *38*:257, 1951.

Yaremchuk, M. J., Elias, L. S., Graham, R. R., and Wilgis, E. F. S.: Sweat gland carcinoma of the hand: two cases of malignant eccrine spiradenoma. J. Hand Surg., *9A*:910, 1984.

Zarem, H. A., and Edgerton, M. T.: Induced resolution of cavernous hemangiomas following prednisolone therapy. Plast. Reconstr. Surg., *39*:76, 1967.

Richard J. Smith

Benign and Malignant Bone Tumors of the Hand

Most hand surgery is reconstructive surgery, the goal being to restore form and function. Most tumor surgery is destructive. Thus, the reconstructive surgeon may have to assume the role of an ablative surgeon when treating aggressive or malignant tumors of the hand. For a surgeon who is accustomed to spending hours repairing small vessels, nerves, and tendons, tumor surgery requires a most difficult and unpleasant change in thoughts and attitudes. However, these changes are necessary if the patient is to be treated appropriately.

Tumor surgery of the hand has as its goals the diagnosis and treatment of the tumor and, when possible, restoration of function. After many benign tumors are removed, no reconstructive procedures are needed. Diagnosis,

treatment, and reconstruction are often achieved at the same operation. In treating malignant tumors of the hand, however, three or more operations may be needed, since surgery for diagnosis, treatment, and reconstruction may require separate stages. In addition, many patients with malignant tumors may require radiotherapy or chemotherapy before or after tumor excision.

If it is the reconstructive surgeon who is to treat a patient with a bone tumor, the patient will benefit by the ability of the surgeon to perform local or remote pedicle flaps, grafts, and free tissue transfers. However, the reconstructive surgeon must be cognizant of the priorities of tumor surgery, and should assume the role of reconstructive surgeon only after the diagnosis has been made and the tumor appropriately treated. Only then should the surgeon's skills be used to restore maximal form and function to the operated hand.

PREOPERATIVE EVALUATION

Most bone tumors of the hand can be diagnosed by history, physical examination, routine x-rays, and laboratory studies (Jaffe, 1958; Dahlin, 1978; Mirra, 1980). Infections, collagen disease, gout, and hyperparathyroidism are only a few of the many conditions that may cause bone changes that masquerade as neoplasms (Fig. 134–1). The clinical examination of the patient should not be restricted to the symptomatic limb. The patient must be questioned carefully about other sites of potential bone or joint lesions, and the physical examination must include at a very minimum inspection and palpation

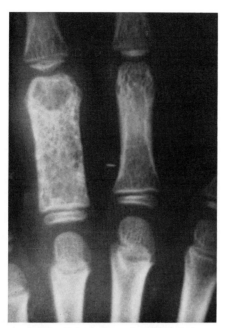

Figure 134–1. Tuberculous dactylitis of the proximal phalanx of this child's finger has radiologic features similar to those of a tumor. The correct diagnosis was suspected because of abnormal chest radiographs and abnormal laboratory findings.

of both upper limbs, including the axillae. Usually the true nature of the lesion can be suspected if the surgeon obtains a detailed case history. Whereas the symptoms of most bone neoplasms develop slowly, bone infection develops more suddenly. Whereas most tumors continue to enlarge, inflammatory and metabolic diseases may have periods of remission and exacerbation. On physical examination, most bone tumors feel firm and have little or no apparent increased heat. They usually are relatively nontender. Inflammatory conditions of bone, however, are often hot, red, and exquisitely tender to touch.

At a minimum, laboratory tests should include complete blood count and differential analysis, sedimentation rate, serum uric acid, rheumatoid screening tests, acid and alkaline phosphatase, and albumin to globulin ratio (Fig. 134–2). If the results of these tests are within the normal range, it is less likely that the lesion being examined results from infection, gout, collagen disease, metastatic tumor, or metabolic bone disease. It is more probably a primary neoplasm.

Routine radiographic studies should include x-rays of the hand in two or three planes. In addition, anterior-posterior and lateral tomograms often identify with more

precision the extent of the lesion. These films can also locate the sites of pathologic fracture. With larger defects, or if there is a suggestion that the tumor may have broken out of the periosteum, xerography and computerized body tomography (CBT) or magnetic resonance imaging (MRI) may prove helpful (Fig. 134–3). A radioisotope scan with technetium or gallium locates "hot spots" of increased blood supply that deserve further study. Bone scan is particularly useful in evaluating a patient with highly vascular tumors or tumors that tend to be multicentric such as giant cell tumor of bone, enchondroma, or osteochondroma (Peimer and associates, 1980).

If all screening procedures are consistent with the diagnosis of a common benign bone tumor, the surgeon is justified in planning to remove the tumor and to reconstruct the deficit in one stage. However, he must be thoroughly familiar with the gross appearance of the lesion he has diagnosed. Both the surgeon and the patient must be prepared for a change in the treatment plan if the operative findings do not correspond with the preoperative diagnosis. For example, if the preoperative diagnosis of a metacarpal lesion is enchondroma, the surgeon is justified in proceeding with curettage and bone graft if car-

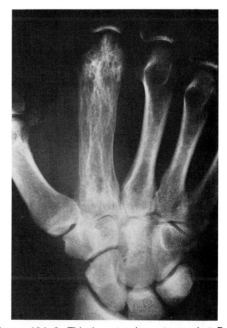

Figure 134–2. This is not a bone tumor, but Paget's disease of bone involving the second metacarpal. An abnormally high alkaline phosphatase is a characteristic of this disease.

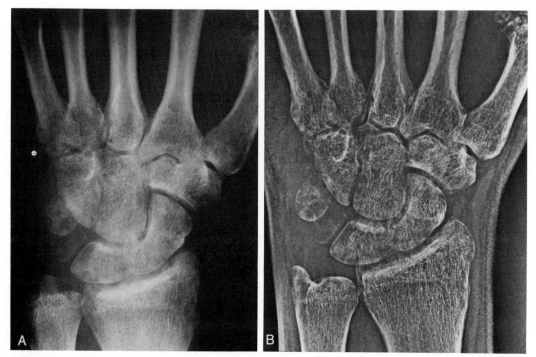

Figure 134–3. *A*, Routine x-ray views have identified an osteolytic lesion of the ulnar side of the wrist. The extent of the lesion is difficult to determine on this view. *B*, Xeroradiography more clearly shows that the lesion is in the triquetrum. Biopsy revealed metastatic renal cell carcinoma to the hand. The primary tumor was excised and the metastatic lesion was irradiated.

tilage is found filling the bone. However, if the tissue within the bone is red and friable, plans must change. The lesion is biopsied and further treatment awaits histologic examination. If the preoperative evaluation suggests that the tumor may be an aggressive or frankly malignant lesion, biopsy must precede excision and reconstruction.

BIOPSY

Needle Biopsy

One way to obtain a biopsy of bone tumor tissue is by means of a closed biopsy with a needle or trephine (Schajowicz and Derqui, 1968; Moore and associates, 1979). Needle biopsy of bone tumors usually must be done under anesthesia and with the help of an image intensifier to guide the needle. If successful, there are many advantages to needle biopsy: (1) skin puncture creates a smaller operative hematoma than with an open biopsy, and thus there is a smaller hematoma reservoir from which the tumor cells may spread through local tissue planes in the days after biopsy and before tumor excision; (2) the small skin wound required for needle biopsy is easily included in the en bloc excision margins at the time of the definitive procedure; (3) there is less likelihood that the patient will suffer pathologic fracture after needle biopsy of bone than after open biopsy because there is a much smaller bone defect; and (4) if radiation therapy is required, it can be started promptly after needle biopsy and need not be delayed to await wound healing.

However, needle biopsy does have disadvantages (Mankin, Lange, and Spanier, 1982): (1) even in the best series, 25 to 33 per cent of needle biopsies have yielded insufficient tissue for diagnosis; and (2) the small tissue sample obtained by needle biopsy can lead to errors in diagnosis and grading of the tumor. These are serious shortcomings that may far outweigh the many advantages of needle biopsy. If needle biopsy of bone tumors is to be performed at all, it is probably most acceptable when the surgeon suspects that the tumor is one with a homogeneous cell type such as multiple myeloma, metastasis, or round cell tumor.

Open Biopsy

Open incisional biopsy of a bone tumor is advisable before definitive treatment is performed if the diagnosis of benign tumor cannot be made with confidence (Simon, 1982). Such would be the case with large bone lesions that do not have the typical calcific stipling of enchondroma, with rapidly expanding lesions, and with lesions that have broken through the bone cortex or caused extensive periosteal elevation. The biopsy should be planned so that adequate tissue can be removed for study with as little contamination of adjacent tissues as possible.

The biopsy incision should permit en bloc excision as a definitive secondary procedure without extending the margins of the incision to include the biopsy-contaminated tissues. Biopsy incisions should be made vertically if there is a possibility that the tumor is aggressive and may require en bloc excision. For example, in treating a bone tumor of the fourth metacarpal, a transverse incision might be considered more esthetic than a vertical one. However, if the tumor proved to be malignant, the entire biopsy wound would be contaminated with tumor cells. In order to perform an adequate en bloc excision it would be necessary to excise three or four rays. If the tumor had been biopsied through a longitudinal incision, definitive en bloc excision would require removing only the fourth ray.

Thus, in planning biopsy of a potentially aggressive tumor, the surgeon should assume the worst. The incision must be adequate for the biopsy, but it should be made within the area that will be excised if the tumor proves to be malignant. An effective way to design biopsy incisions is for the surgeon first to draw on the skin the incision that later will be used to excise the tumor if it proves malignant. This incision should include en bloc excision margins. Next, a longitudinal biopsy incision is planned at least 2 cm from the potential en bloc excision borders; this should ensure safe margins about the biopsy field.

The author prefers to operate in a bloodless field when performing biopsy or excision of any tumor in the forearm or hand, and always uses a padded pneumatic tourniquet just distal to the axilla. Some authors have feared that applying a tourniquet may increase the risk of metastases after biopsy or excision of a malignant tumor. They believe that tumor cells entering the vascular system in the surgical field at the time of the operation will shower the peripheral circulation as soon as the cuff is released. Theoretically, the sudden assault of a large number of tumor cells on the lungs and other tissues might increase the likelihood that the tumor will seed, lodge, and grow in these remote regions. However, no study has ever proved an increased incidence of metastases as a result of the use of a tourniquet; indeed, there is less trauma at the operative site when the tourniquet is used than when it is not. There is less sponging, clamping, and dissection in a dry field than in a bloody one. Thus, fewer cells are dislodged and enter the circulation. For these reasons, there may be less risk of metastasis with a tourniquet than without one.

The author does not exsanguinate the limb by using a compressive bandage before inflating the cuff. To wrap a rubber bandage ("Esmarch" or "Martin") about a tumor or adjacent to it before inflating the cuff is unnecessary and potentially harmful. Tumor cells may have entered the lymphatics adjacent to the lesion. Squeezing these vessels proximally may push the cells into the peripheral circulation far from the area of biopsy or excision. Wrapping a rubber bandage about the bone tumor also may cause a pathologic fracture of the fragile bone and may spill tumor cells throughout the local tissues just as the surgeon is about to make the incision. For biopsy or excision of all potentially aggressive bone lesions, the limb is elevated for three or four minutes to exsanguinate it, and then the tourniquet is inflated. Excellent hemostasis is achieved with safety.

Excisional biopsy is appropriate treatment for small benign bone tumors of the hand such as the typical osteochondroma, osteoid osteoma, or enchondroma. As all tissue is removed with excisional biopsy, the pathologist is assured of having representative tissues for study (Fig. 134–4). For lesions that appear more aggressive, incisional biopsy should be performed. Here, error may occur. If the tissue removed is not from the tumor itself, but rather from the reactive local tissue, necrotic tissue, or normal tissue adjacent to the tumor, the pathologist and the surgeon may be misled. According to a study of 329 patients biopsied for bone tumors, major errors in diagnosis were made in over 18 per cent and nonrepresentative or technically poor biopsies in over 10 per cent (Simon, 1982).

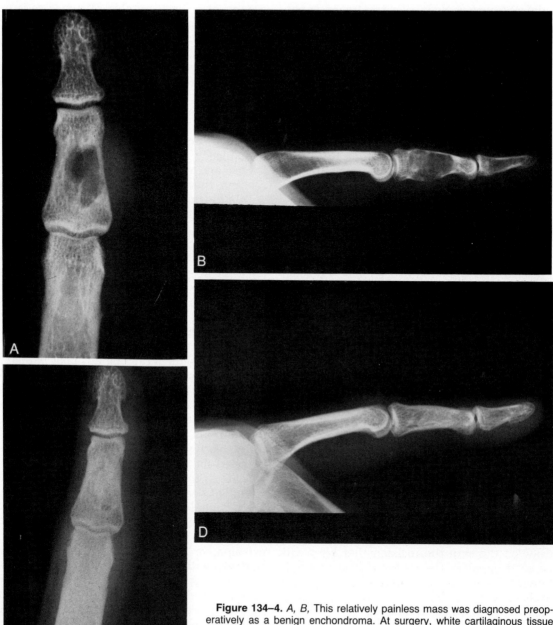

Figure 134–4. *A, B,* This relatively painless mass was diagnosed preoperatively as a benign enchondroma. At surgery, white cartilaginous tissue was found within the phalanx. As the gross findings correlated with the preoperative diagnosis, excisional biopsy (curettage) and bone graft were performed simultaneously. *C, D,* One year later, there is early bone reconstitution.

The least differentiated and least mineralized portion of the tumor is most representative of the lesion. It is from these tissues that the incisional biopsy should be taken. Areas of subperiosteal bone are poor sites for biopsy, as reactive bone from this region may be misinterpreted on histologic examination as osteosarcoma. A benign bone tumor may thus be "overdiagnosed." The surgeon should take care not to rongeur or crush the biopsy tissue when removing it. Crushed tissue is difficult for the pathologist to interpret, since the cell patterns and tissue architecture are disturbed. As much as possible, the biopsy tissue is removed by sharp dissection. Areas of radiated tissue are poor biopsy sites, as radiation causes fibrosis and necrosis and atypism of the tumor cells. As a general rule, the periphery of a malignant tumor is the best area from which to take a tissue specimen. The central region of a large, rapidly growing tumor often has become ischemic and is difficult to diagnose.

The tourniquet should be released before the wound is closed, and hemostasis should be obtained without undue manipulation and sponging of the wound. If necessary, a drain may be used, but it should exit from the wound or just proximal to it. A drain lying in a site remote from the wound may contaminate the entire drain tract with tumor cells and condemn the patient to a wider excision than otherwise would be necessary.

A well-informed and well-prepared pathologist is as important in obtaining an accurate tissue diagnosis as is the technique of biopsy. This requirement does not reflect on the pathologist's competence, but involves his knowledge of the case about which he is to pass judgment. The surgeon should not force the pathologist to evaluate the biopsy as an isolated puzzle, but should personally speak to the pathologist before biopsying a potentially aggressive bone tumor. The pathologist should be made familiar with the patient's history and physical findings, and with all relevant laboratory and radiographic data.

STAGING OF TUMORS

With aggressive bone tumors, the extent of the excision to be performed depends not only on the tumor cell type but also on its *grade,* its *location,* and the presence or absence of *metastases.* Tumor staging categorizes each lesion on the basis of these three factors.

There have been many methods of staging bone tumors. A simple and effective method was introduced by the musculoskeletal tumor committee of the American Academy of Orthopaedic Surgeons (Table 134–1) and has won acceptance as a standard staging system of bone tumors.

Examples of benign bone tumors of the hand (G_0) include enchondroma, osteochondroma, fibrous dysplasia, and osteoid osteoma (Fig. 134–5). Low grade malignant tumors of bone (G_1) include malignant giant cell tumor of bone, chondrosarcoma (low grade), and parosteal osteosarcoma. High grade (G_2) malignant tumors of bone include central osteosarcoma, Ewing's sarcoma, and angiosarcoma.

Regarding location, any tumor that is confined within the medullary cavity of bone is T_1, since it is within one anatomic compartment. A tumor that has broken out of the bone at the site of the pathologic fracture is a T_1 lesion if tumor cells remain in one soft tissue anatomic compartment. If the tumor has contaminated more than one soft tissue compartment, it is T_2. An example of T_2 is a through and through fracture of a malignant

Table 134–1. Staging of Bone Tumors*

1. Histologic Grade (G)

G_0 = benign
G_1 = low grade
G_2 = high grade

Low Grade (G_1)	High Grade (G_2)
Few cells	Many cells
Much stroma	Little stroma
Little necrosis	Much necrosis
Mature	Immature
Mitoses less than 5 to 10 HPF	Mitoses more than 5 to 10 HPF

2. Location of Tumor (T)

T_1 = tumor within one anatomic compartment (bone or soft tissue)
T_2 = tumor in more than one compartment (bone or soft tissue)

3. Presence or Absence of Metastases (M)

M_0 = no metastases
M_1 = with metastases

Staging of Malignant Tumors

Stage	G	T	M
1A	G_1	T_1	M_0
1B	G_1	T_2	M_0
2A	G_2	T_1	M_0
2B	G_2	T_2	M_0
3	any	any	M_1

*Introduced by the American Academy of Orthopaedic Surgeons. (From Enneking, W. F., Spanier, S. S., and Goodman, M. A.: Current concepts review. The surgical staging of musculo-skeletal sarcoma. J. Bone Joint Surg., 62A:1027, 1980.)

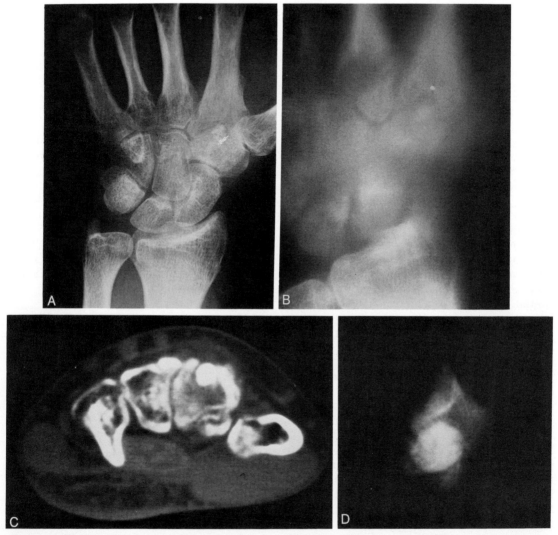

Figure 134–5. This young man had persistent pain at the dorsal radial aspect of his hand. Routine x-ray films suggest a circular lesion at the base of the second metacarpal. *B,* Anteroposterior tomograms show increased density at the distal end of the trapezoid. *C,* With CT scan the lesion stands out "like an electric light bulb." It is at the dorsum of the trapezoid, and is diagnosed as osteoid osteoma. *D,* X-ray film of the excised specimen shows the osteoid osteoma to have been completely removed. All pain was relieved postoperatively.

giant cell tumor of the third metacarpal that contaminates the volar and dorsal compartments of the hand.

A soft tissue sarcoma that has invaded bone is histologically not a "bone tumor" although it may have the radiologic appearance of one. If such a tumor has penetrated bone and exposed both the dorsal and volar compartments of the hand to the tumor, it can be considered T_2. If the soft tissue tumor has invaded only one cortex of bone, has remained on the volar or dorsal side of the hand, has not entered into a synovial sheath, and has not communicated with the opposite side (palmar or dorsal) of the hand through soft tissue extension, it is considered T_1. Thus, although the intramedullary cavity of bone is an anatomic compartment, a tumor is considered T_1 if it remains in one *soft tissue* compartment and one bone "compartment."

TUMOR TREATMENT

Adjuvant Treatment and Informed Consent

Once the diagnosis has been made, the treatment is planned. If the tumor is metastatic to the hand, the principal treatment is directed toward the primary lesion. Metastatic tumors to the hand are most frequently from the lung, kidney, breast, or thyroid. Appropriate diagnostic studies, including radioisotope scanning, chest tomography, and intravenous pyelography, usually identify the location from which the tumor originated. Treatment of the lesion of the hand may be only palliative, since the prognosis for most patients with metastatic lesions to the hand is very grave.

Many primary malignant tumors of the bones of the hand are best treated by a combined program that includes radiation, chemotherapy, and surgery (Morton and associates, 1976). Only rarely will the reconstructive surgeon feel confident in planning this program without appropriate consultation with the oncologist or radiotherapist. Whether nonsurgical treatment should precede or follow surgery—or whether it is even indicated—depends on the stage, the size, and the histologic pattern of the lesion. All persons who participate in the patient's care should agree on the plan before the patient is told of the recommendations and prognosis.

The final decision whether or not to proceed rests with the patient, but it is the surgeon's responsibility to present the patient with both the recommendations and the anticipated results of treatment. If there are any differences of opinion among the consultants, these should be explained to the patient, who should always be offered the option of seeking outside consultation before treatment is begun.

Almost all primary aggressive and malignant tumors of the bones of the hand require excision whether or not adjuvant radiation or chemotherapy is given. Although cryotherapy has been successful in treating some intramedullary bone tumors elsewhere in the body (Marcove and associates, 1973), it is rarely indicated in the hand. The liquid nitrogen used in cryotherapy can cause thermal burns to local tissues.

Surgical Excision of Bone Tumors

Standardized nomenclature has also been developed to describe *surgical margins* of tumor excision (Table 134–2).

Intralesional excision is the appropriate treatment of an enchondroma, because this tumor is benign, nonaggressive, and unlikely to recur after it has been curetted.

Marginal excision is appropriate for an osteochondroma, which is a benign tumor. It may recur if the perichondrium or periosteum at its base is not removed; therefore, excision should include the "pseudocapsule," which is the perichondrium and periosteum overlying the tumor and its base (Figs. 134–6 to 134–8).

Wide excision of an intramedullary lesion involves excising the tumor with a normal cuff of tissue about it. Thus, for a malignant giant cell tumor at the distal end of the radius that has not broken through, the cortex should have a "wide" excision with osteotomy

Table 134–2. Surgical Margins of Tumor Excision

Type of Excision	Method of Excision
Intralesional	Curettage or piecemeal
Marginal	Shelled out in pseudocapsule
Wide	Intracompartmental en bloc with cuff of normal tissue
Radical	Extracompartmental en bloc

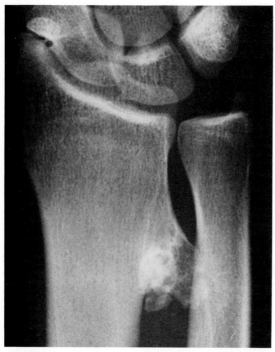

Figure 134–6. Osteochondroma of the distal radius is a benign tumor. It can be cured by marginal excision. The tumor and the periosteum and perichondrium around the tumor are removed.

5 cm proximal to the apparent proximal margin of the lesion, and excision of the entire distal end of the radius (Fig. 134–9). This is an *intracompartmental* excision. The cortex and periosteum about the lesion at the distal radius make up the cuff of normal tissue. Several centimeters of tumor-free medullary cavity (checked by biopsy and frozen section)

distal to the osteotomy is the cuff of normal proximal tissue. Excision of the distal radius would not be considered "radical excision" since the intramedullary compartment was entered.

As another example, for a pathologic fracture through a low grade chondrosarcoma of the first metacarpal, *wide excision* should include removing the metacarpal and a cuff of normal soft tissue at the site of pathologic fracture. Most likely this requires amputation of the entire first ray if tumor tissue lies about the tendon and neurovascular bundle anteriorly. This is an *intracompartmental excision* and *not* radical excision, because the "compartment" of the involved tendon sheath extends to the volar forearm and also includes the flexor tendon of the little finger. These areas have not been excised.

In an en bloc excision, the tumor must not be exposed with the dissection. Normal tissue should be taken with the tumor. The width of normal tissue cuff that should be taken for en bloc excision depends on local anatomic tumor barriers. Bone and interosseous ligament usually effectively block extension of tumor in soft tissue (Figs. 134–10, 134–11). Therefore, bone and interosseous ligament may be excised as the peripheral border of an en bloc excision. For example, if chondrosarcoma of the first metacarpal has broken into the soft tissues and lies adjacent to the radius, the radial cortex should be removed as part of the en bloc excision. A tumor that lies dorsally between the second and third metacarpals should be removed with the interosseous ligament. If there is no anatomic bar-

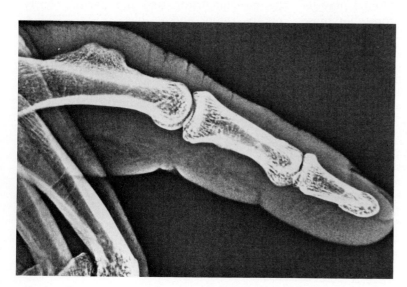

Figure 134–7. A "turret exostosis" of the dorsum of the proximal phalanx is a benign tumor that only requires marginal excision of the lesion and periosteum over it. The dorsal aponeurosis may require shortening.

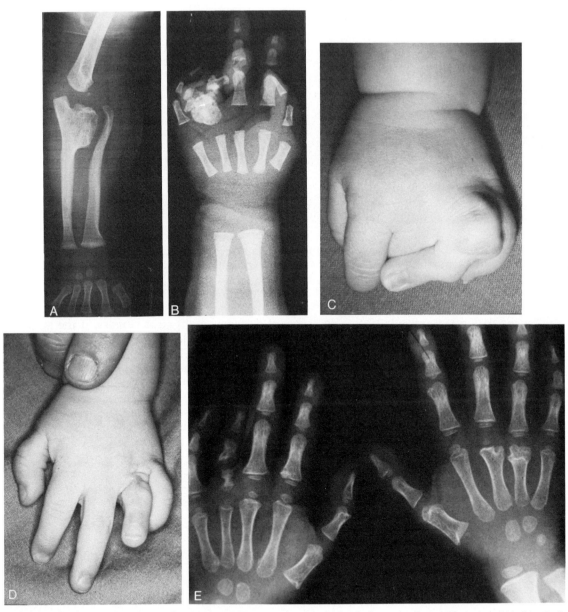

Figure 134–8. Multiple osteocartilagenous exostoses are present in the limbs and spine of this boy and his identical twin brother. *A,* A large exostosis of the proximal ulna displaced and deformed the proximal radius. *B,* At birth the proximal and middle phalanx of the ring finger were almost completely replaced by tumor. *C,* The ring finger was deformed and interfered with motion of the adjacent fingers. *D,* Postoperatively, the ring finger no longer interferes with the function of the adjacent fingers. It will require lengthening and scar revision in the future. *E,* The tumor has not recurred in the operated ring finger. Note the many abnormalities of the other digits due to multiple osteochondromatosis.

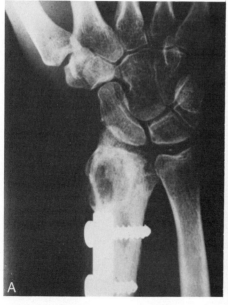
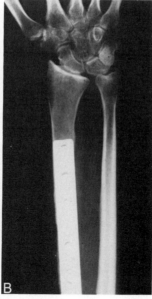

Figure 134–9. *A,* This patient with multicentric giant cell tumor of bone had been treated elsewhere by resection of the radius and its replacement by fibular autograft. There is evidence of tumor in the graft. This raises a question of whether the tumor has been transferred with the graft. *B,* En bloc excision of the graft and its replacement with an allograft restored good wrist function. The author prefers to use an inverted right radial allograft for left radial replacement, and vice versa. In this case, the tumor did not recur again.

rier to tumor extension, a clinically tumor-free margin of 2 cm usually represents a safe border. At all times the tissue at the bed of the excised lesion should be examined by frozen section to see if it is tumor free; if not, higher dissection is required.

In treating aggressive or malignant bone tumors of the hand, a secondary consideration is that of hand function and appearance. The patient's life must not be jeopardized for the sake of leaving a more functional or esthetic hand. However, with many lesions, subtotal amputation or en bloc intracompartmental excision may run no higher risk of tumor

recurrence than total amputation or radial excision. Saving even one or two digits of the hand may permit the patient to continue with an occupation and many activities of daily living, whereas total amputation may not. In the case of malignant tumors, if the surgeon feels that en bloc excision can be performed successfully with safe, tumor-free borders, both surgeon and patient should be prepared to accept that a higher amputation is appropriate. For example, if the surgeon has biopsied a chondrosarcoma of the third metacarpal and planned to perform an en bloc excision of the three central rays, he should

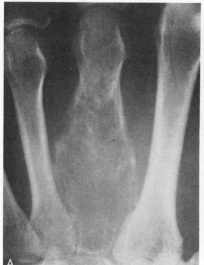
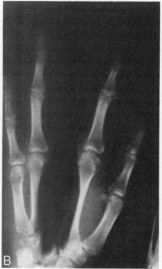
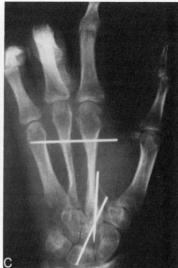

Figure 134–10. *A,* Giant cell tumor of the third metacarpal has broken into the soft tissue of the second and third interspaces. *B,* The third ray is excised with the bordering cortices of the second and fourth metacarpals. *C,* The index ray is transposed to the capitate. Today we would use plate fixation at the metacarpal base.

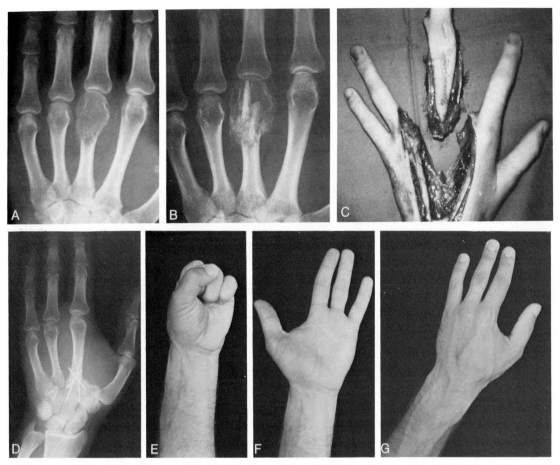

Figure 134–11. *A,* Giant cell tumor of the third metacarpal head. *B,* The patient was treated elsewhere by curettage and bone graft. The tumor recurred. *C,* Wide excision included removing a soft tissue cuff around the bone. The area of previous curettage and graft was considered as potentialy contaminated with tumor. Tumor was not seen during dissection. *D,* The index ray is transposed to the base of the third metacarpal at the time of third ray excision. *E, F, G,* Postoperative function and appearance were good. There was no recurrence.

be prepared to perform a below elbow amputation if the tumor has broken through the cortex and contaminated the carpal canal. The patient and the family should be prepared for this more radical surgery also.

After the tumor has been excised, the wound may be closed by primary suture. When malignant lesions are excised, the biopsy tract and 2 cm borders from this tract also have to be excised. Under some circumstances, soft tissue coverage may become a problem demanding reconstructive techniques.

Radical excision of an intramedullary bone lesion that has not broken through the cortex requires only excision of the bone itself. For example, "radical" excision of a G_2 fibrosarcoma of the fifth metacarpal would involve excision of the entire metacarpal. However, if fibrosarcoma of the distal radius has broken through the cortex anteriorly, it requires excision of all soft tissues in the volar aspect of the forearm and volar aspect of the hand, as well as excision of the entire radius, in order to excise the contaminated compartments. Under these circumstances, the surgeon may well prefer to consider either "wide" excision (en bloc resection of the tumor) or amputation.

RECONSTRUCTIVE SURGERY

Bone

Once the tumor has been excised, the third priority of treatment—reconstruction—begins. After excising a small eccentric benign tumor, little need be done in the form of reconstructive surgery. The skin usually closes easily. If an exostosis has stretched the skin over it, the redundant skin may be excised with elliptic incisions. Occasionally, extrinsic bone tumors of the phalanges may lengthen and thin the dorsal aponeurosis of the finger. If this occurs, the loose tendons may be imbricated to help restore their function.

After benign intramedullary lesions have been excised by curettage, the cortex of the phalanx or metacarpal may be extremely thin and fragile. For this reason, it is often best to fill the defect with bone. The author prefers to use cancellous bone graft from the ilium or distal radius. Cancellous autogenous bone has osteogenic potential, and the curetted bone regains integrity and strength more rapidly than does the bone that is allowed to "fill in" spontaneously. The author applies a protective splint for about three weeks and then advises against using the hand for athletics or heavy activities for an additional two months. At the end of three months, full activities usually may be resumed.

If a metacarpal has been resected, it can be replaced with a metatarsal autograft or allograft (Averill, Smith, and Campbell, 1980; Smith and Koniuch, 1983). The author uses a metatarsal allograft in order to avoid donor site morbidity of shortened and flaccid toe and also a scarred donor site (Fig. 134–12). No clinical signs of allograft rejection have been seen. There have been no infections and no evidence of redness or unusual swelling about the wound after insertion of an allograft to replace the small bones of the hand. If an allograft of appropriate size is selected and if it is stabilized appropriately, good healing and revascularization may be expected. The manner in which the grafts are harvested, tested, and stored have been described (Smith and Koniuch, 1983).

Whether metatarsal autograft or allograft is used, the collateral ligaments should be retained on the donor metatarsal so that they may be sutured to the collateral ligaments of the recipient proximal phalanx. If the metatarsal collateral ligaments have not been preserved, those of the phalanx should be sutured to the metatarsal head. If possible, the volar plate and dorsal capsule are also sutured. The joints are stabilized with Kirschner wires for three weeks while the collateral ligaments heal. It is preferable not to maintain a mobile joint at the base of the metatarsal graft, but rather to arthrodese the metatarsal bone graft to the adjacent carpal

bone. Arthrodesis of the metacarpal base to the carpus is stabilized with a rigid plate so that it is not dependent on Kirschner wire fixation for long periods. With plate fixation, the base of the metatarsal is held solidly during the weeks when the patient and the therapist can try to restore motion at the reconstructed metatarsophalangeal joint.

If the middle or proximal phalanx is removed for an aggressive nonmalignant lesion, it may be replaced by a toe phalanx. After replacement of the middle phalanx, it is best to arthrodese the distal interphalangeal joint and concentrate therapy on attempts to restore motion at the proximal interphalangeal joint. If the proximal phalanx is replaced, attempts should be made to retain motion at both the proximal interphalangeal joint and the metacarpophalangeal joint.

In reconstruction of the wrist after resection of the distal end of the radius for aggressive lesions, there are many alternatives. Some surgeons prefer to replace the distal radius with the proximal end of the fibula. The fibula can be either a free graft or a vascularized tissue transfer. Although some good results have been achieved by fibula transfer, it is not the author's preferred method of treatment. The articular cartilage of the proximal carpal row does not match the size or shape of that of the proximal fibula. Nonetheless, some satisfactory long-range results have been reported after fibula graft to the wrist.

For some patients, arthrodesis of the wrist is a preferred treatment after distal radial resection, since it renders the hand stable and painless. If pronation and supination of the forearm are to be retained, a large bone graft is required to bridge the defect from the carpus to the radial osteotomy site in the distal forearm. This gap may be 6 to 10 cm in length. The graft gradually revascularizes from the proximal end and must be stabilized. Revascularization may take up to four years. For this reason, rigid internal fixation with plate and screws is recommended to bridge the corticocancellous bone graft.

More rapid arthrodesis of the wrist can be achieved if the radius is bypassed and the ulnar head is buried in the carpus (Fig. 134–13). The ulnar head is decorticated and placed in a slot fashioned by osteotomy of the carpus. A heavy Kirschner wire or rigid plate supports the arthrodesis, which is further reinforced with cancellous bone chips. Ulnocarpal arthrodesis causes loss of both wrist motion

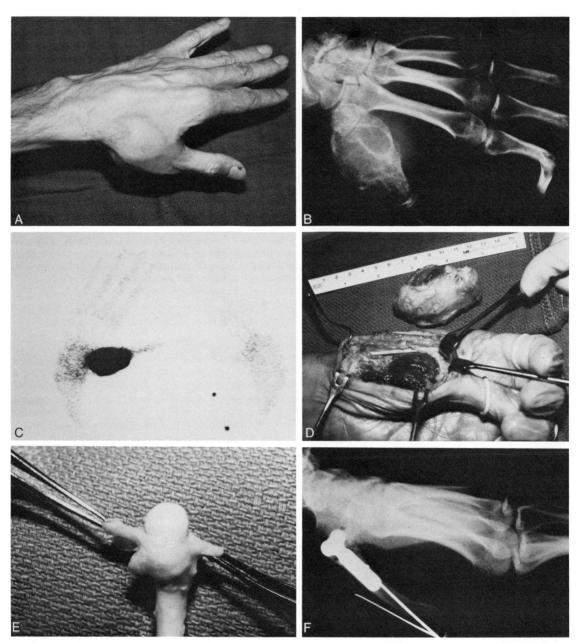

Figure 134–12. A, This man had a slowly growing chondrosarcoma of the first metacarpal. He had been treated elsewhere two years earlier. The metacarpal had been curetted and filled with cancellous bone graft. This is an intralesional excision and is not satisfactory treatment of a malignant tumor, or of an aggressive benign tumor. The tumor recurred. B, X-ray films showed that the entire metacarpal has been replaced by the tumor. The cortex has expanded. There is no evidence of pathologic fracture. C, Technetium bone scan showed no evidence of bony lesions elsewhere. D, The entire metacarpal was removed by radical excision. The scar of the previous surgical excision and a cuff of normal tissue that surrounded the metacarpal were also removed. The bed was biopsied and showed no evidence of tumor. E, An appropriate metatarsal allograft was selected to replace the metacarpal. The collateral ligaments of the allograft were identified and sutured to the collateral ligaments of the recipient at the base of the proximal phalanx. F, The metatarsal allograft was arthrodesed to the trapezium and held with a T-plate. The metacarpophalangeal joint was held with Kirschner wire for four weeks.

Illustration continued on following page

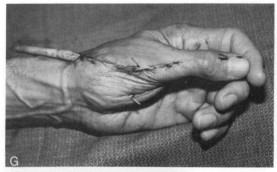
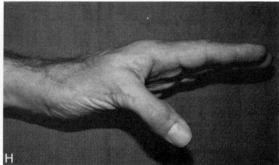

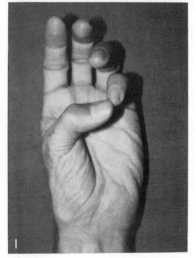

Figure 134–12 *Continued G,* At the end of the operation, the thumb lies in a functional position. The skin was closed easily despite excision of the scar because the allograft was of a smaller diameter than the excised tumor. The drain exited from the proximal end of the wound and was not passed under skin to a remote site. *H, I,* One year later there is good fuction and appearance and no evidence of recurrence.

and forearm rotation, but more rapid healing and an earlier return to more strenuous activities are the rewards. If the patient has good elbow and shoulder motion, ulnocarpal arthrodesis is better than using a large bridge graft.

With most patients the author's preference for reconstructing the wrist after excising the distal radius is to use a radial allograft to bridge the defect (Smith and Mankin, 1977). X-ray films of the patient's wrist should be compared with available distal radial allografts, and an appropriate-sized allograft selected. In order to better stabilize the radiocarpal joint and to decrease the risk of late radiocarpal volar subluxation, the author recommends using a radial allograft from the opposite wrist and rotating it so that the volar side is dorsal. Thus, to replace the right radius, a left radial allograft is selected. Because its distal articular surface normally has a 20 degree volar slope, reversing the graft at the recipient site results in a 20 degree dorsal slope. This increases the stability of the carpus on the allograft because of

the 40 degree correction (from 20 degrees palmar flexion normally, to 20 degrees dorsiflexion with the reversed allograft). The allograft is held to the proximal radius with a compression plate. The wrist capsule is closed both volarly and dorsally by suturing ligaments of the allograft to those of the recipient with 2-0 absorbable sutures. One or two Kirschner wires are placed across the radiocarpal joint for wrist stability.

After the allograft has been inserted and stabilized, the integrity of the radioulnar joint should be checked by fully pronating and supinating the forearm. Operating room x-rays should be taken. If there is marked incongruity, impingement, or crepitation with forearm rotation, the distal ulna should be resected or hemiarthroplasty performed. With hemiarthroplasty the ulnar head is excised, but the ulnar styloid and shaft remain undisturbed.

Postoperatively the Kirschner wires remain in place for six weeks, during which time the wrist is protected with a plaster cast. A protective splint should be used for at least a year thereafter, as the allograft gradually revascularizes.

The results of distal radial allografting are somewhat varied. Most patients do quite well, and up to 60 degrees of painless wrist motion may be anticipated. After four or five years, when revascularization has reached the subchondral bone, many patients show signs of osteoarthritic change or volar subluxation of the carpus. If the patient is relatively asymptomatic, nothing further need be done except for the intermittent use of a wrist splint. For some patients, wrist arthrodesis or silicone arthroplasty at the allograft-carpal juncture may be useful if these late complications develop.

Skin

After resection of aggressive tumors of the hand, it is usually unwise to cover soft tissue defects with remote pedicle flaps. En bloc resection of a tumor with adequate tumor-free margins and biopsy of the remaining border tissues should reduce the risk of tumor cell contamination of the flap to almost zero. However, some risk of local recurrence always remains, and if this happens, amputation can be performed. However, if a presumably tumor-free hand that is still contaminated with aggressive tumor cells is held sutured to the groin, abdomen, chest wall, or opposite arm for several weeks while a remote flap is revascularizing, there is risk that the tumor may contaminate the remote donor site. Free tissue transfers to cover soft tissue defects in the hand do not suffer the risks of contaminating the donor site as do the direct remote pedicle flaps.

After bone tumor excision, most soft tissue defects can be covered with local tissue. For example, en bloc excision of an aggressive metacarpal tumor that has broken into the

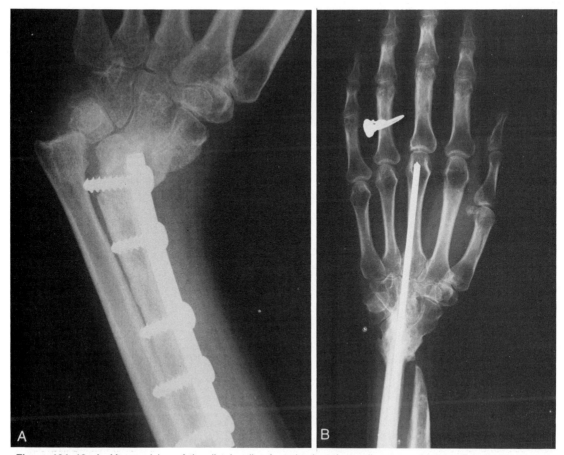

Figure 134–13. A, After excision of the distal radius for a benign giant cell tumor, a bone graft had been inserted. Within three years, the graft had fractured and resorbed and the wrist was unstable. B, A solid arthrodesis was achieved between the ulna and the carpus. Although pronation and supination is lost when the ulna is fused to the carpus, the hand is strong and functions well.

palm may require excision of palmar skin and tendons as well as the metacarpal. This operation leaves a large defect proximally but spares the fingers. In this case, the finger can be filleted and its skin used to provide excellent soft tissue cover in the palm (Fig. 134–14).

Local flaps can be transferred to cover many soft tissue defects in the hand after tumor surgery. The donor site may be covered with a split-thickness skin graft. Neither the gloves nor instruments used to excise the tumor should be within the surgical field where the remote graft or free flaps are being harvested. The surgeon harvesting these grafts should use a separate instrument table to ensure no contamination from the tumor field.

Digital Transposition

Transposition of an adjacent digit immediately after wide excision of an aggressive tumor can achieve two purposes: (1) it closes a large soft tissue defect and (2) it provides better hand function and appearance. For example, if the first ray is excised along with a cuff of surrounding soft tissue for a tumor at the base of the thumb, the defect may measure several centimeters. En bloc excision may have also removed a portion of the base of the second ray in the region of the second metacarpal. By means of an index finger pollicization, the defect is closed and an opposable "thumb" has been constructed.

The method by which pollicization is performed under these circumstances is similar, but not identical, to that of pollicization after traumatic thumb amputation. After tumor excision the soft tissue defect is greater than that of a patient having elective post-trauma thumb reconstruction. The surgeon should not hesitate to use generous quantities of split-thickness skin grafts rather than attempt to modify the resection margins. When resecting first ray to remove a tumor, large

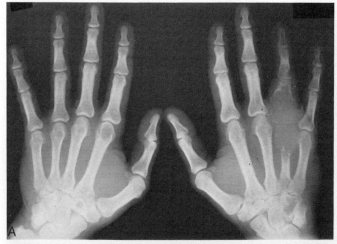

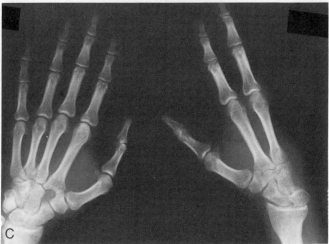

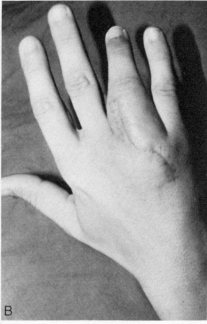

Figure 134–14. *A,* Multicentric giant cell tumor involved the left trapezoid and the right ring finger metacarpal and proximal and middle phalanges, the little finger metacarpal, and the hamate. The ulnar head previously had been excised for giant cell tumor. *B,* The ring finger metacarpal and proximal phalanx were biopsied elsewhere. A smaller incisional biopsy or a needle biopsy would have been preferable. *C,* The fourth and fifth rays were removed from the right hand. The trapezoid was removed from the left hand.

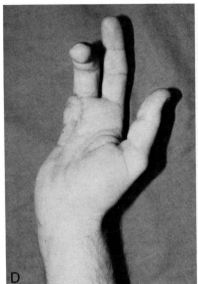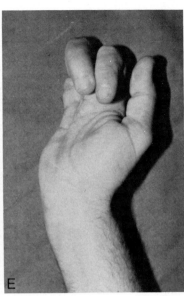

Figure 134–14 *Continued D, E,* The volar skin of the little finger was filleted and used as a local flap to cover soft tissue defect at the ulnar side of the right hand.

portions of the first dorsal interosseous may have to be resected as well. Under these circumstances it is best to place the pollicized index finger in at least 60 degrees of (palmar) abduction and 90 degrees of pronation in order to achieve better grasp. Occasionally a secondary tendon transfer may be required for improved opposition. The Huber transfer of abductor digiti quinti to abductor pollicis brevis is well suited for transfer to a pollicized index finger.

If the third or fourth ray requires ablation because of aggressive tumor, transfer of the adjacent second or fourth ray may fill the defect. Ray resection for tumor usually requires disarticulation at the carpometacarpal joint. Thus, unlike ray transfer for trauma, the metacarpal is not transposed to the base of the recipient metacarpal. If the third ray is deleted, the index metacarpal is arthrodesed to the capitate. With excision of the fourth ray, the fifth metacarpal is arthrodesed to the hamate. Kirschner wires or a small T-plate can be used to hold the transferred ray in place.

Secondary Procedures

Often, reconstruction should not be performed at the time of tumor excision. The surgeon may be well advised to wait until the tissues "settle down" before proceeding with elective reconstructive operations. He may wish to wait until permanent sections of all specimens are thoroughly reviewed and evaluated before transferring remote tissues to the tumor site. In many cases it may be wise to wait six months or more after tumor resection to make certain that there is no recurrence locally and no evidence of distant metastases. If radiation is to be given postoperatively, the viability of tissues with a fragile blood supply may be placed in jeopardy. Therefore, if radiation therapy is planned, the prudent surgeon performs only such reconstructive procedures as are necessary to fill bone and soft tissue defects at the time of tumor excision. Elective procedures should be delayed.

If the central rays have been excised, grasp between the thumb and little finger may be awkward and weak. In the unoperated hand, the thumbtip and little fingertip can readily appose, but after wide excision of the central palmar tumor, there is usually residual stiffness caused by edema and scarring. Transposition of the fifth ray to the position of the fourth ray may improve pinch. Another method of improving grasp is to rotate the fifth metacarpal into supination. The osteotomy is done at the metacarpal neck. The metacarpal is then held in position with rigid internal fixation.

After extensive tumor resection, many patients benefit by the late application of remote pedicle flaps to areas where skin grafts or scars appear unsightly. The risk of spreading tumor to a remote pedicle flap six months after tumor excision is extremely low if there have been no signs of recurrence during that time.

Free tissue transfers to replace absent digits, to fill bony defects, to replace scarred or unsightly skin, or to restore sensibility to a portion of the hand after nerve excision can often restore improved function and appearance to the operated hand. Techniques and indications are similar to those for replacing the traumatic loss of tissues. In patients who have received radiotherapy, however, the surgeon should anticipate increased scarring about the entire area irradiated, including local recipient vessels.

SUMMARY

A bone tumor should not be excised without definite histologic diagnosis unless a presumptive diagnosis is supported by surgical findings. In all other cases, incisional biopsy should precede definitive surgery.

The surgical treatment of aggressive primary bone tumors of the hand should include at least wide excision (en bloc intracompartmental) or radical excision (en bloc extracompartmental).

The extent of surgical excision and the indications for chemotherapy and/or radiotherapy should be determined by the cell type and the size and staging of the tumor. Staging includes consideration of tumor grade, tumor location, and whether or not there have been metastases.

Treatment of tumors metastatic to the hand should be directed principally toward the primary lesion. Treatment of the hand tumor is usually only palliative.

For biopsy or excision of a tumor of the hand, an Esmarch bandage should not be used. After en bloc excision of an aggressive tumor, frozen section of border tissues must confirm the absence of tumor cells. If tumor remains, the choices are excision with wider borders or amputation. The patient should have given consent for amputation before surgery even if wide excision is planned.

Remote flaps to cover soft tissue defects at the time an aggressive tumor is excised should be avoided. Skin grafts, local flaps, or, when necessary, free flaps are preferable. Bone may be replaced by autograft or allograft.

Reconstructive surgery should be performed at the time of tumor excision if only local tissues are used or if reconstruction is necessary to cover soft tissue defects. Complex reconstructive procedures should be delayed at least six months after removal of aggressive tumors of the hand.

When treating aggressive tumors of the hand, the reconstructive surgeon must maintain the following priorities: (1) diagnosis, (2) excision of tumor and appropriate nonsurgical therapy, and (3) reconstruction. Diagnosis and tumor excision must never be compromised for the sake of more effective surgical reconstruction.

REFERENCES

Averill, R. M., Smith, R. J., and Campbell, C. J.: Giant-cell tumors of the bones of the hand. J. Hand Surg., 5:39, 1980.

Dahlin, D. C.: Bone Tumors: General Aspects and Data on 6,221 Cases. 3rd Ed. Springfield, IL, Charles C Thomas, 1978.

Enneking, W. F., Spanier, S. S., and Goodman, M. A.: Current concepts review. The surgical staging of musculo-skeletal sarcoma. J. Bone Joint Surg., 62A:1027, 1980.

Jaffe, H. L.: Tumors and Tumorous Conditions of the Bones and Joints. Philadelphia, Lea & Febiger, 1958.

Mankin, H. J., Lange, T. A., and Spanier, S. S.: The hazards of biopsy in patients with malignant primary bone and soft-tissue tumors. J. Bone Joint Surg., 64A:1121, 1982.

Marcove, R. C., Lyden, J. P., Huvos, A. G., et al.: Giant-cell tumors treated by cryosurgery. A report of 25 cases. J. Bone Joint Surg., 55A:1633, 1973.

Mirra, J. M.: Bone Tumors. Diagnosis and Treatment. Philadelphia, J. B. Lippincott Company, 1980.

Moore, T. M., Meyers, M. H., Patzakis, M. J., Terry, R., and Harvey, J. P., Jr.: Closed biopsy of musculoskeletal lesions. J. Bone Joint Surg., 61A:375, 1979.

Morton, D. L., Eilber, F. R., Townsend, C. M., Jr., et al.: Limb salvage from a multidisciplinary treatment approach for skeletal and soft tissue sarcomas of the extremity. Ann. Surg., 184:268, 1976.

Peimer, C. A., Schiller, A. L., Mankin, H. J., and Smith, R. J.: Multicentric giant-cell tumor of the bone. J. Bone Joint Surg., 62A:652, 1980.

Schajowicz, F., and Derqui, J. C.: Puncture biopsy in lesions of the locomotor system. Review of results of 4,050 cases including 941 vertebral punctures. Cancer, 21:531, 1968.

Simon, M. A.: Current concepts review. Biopsy of musculoskeletal tumors. J. Bone Joint Surg., 64A:1253, 1982.

Smith, R. J., and Koniuch, M. P.: Tumors of the hand. In Evarts, C. M. (Ed.): Surgery of the Musculoskeletal System. New York, Churchill Livingstone, 1983.

Smith, R. J., and Mankin, H. J.: Allograft replacement of distal radius for giant-cell tumor. J. Hand Surg., 2:299, 1977.

135

Mary H. McGrath

Infections of the Hand

HISTORY

Studies in industrialized areas during the first half of the twentieth century showed that disability, deformity, and even death commonly accompanied hand infection. From a 1915 review of industrial insurance claims, it was estimated that 65 per cent of the hand accidents involving disability resulted from minor injuries that had become infected; the remaining 35 per cent included all fractures, lacerations, and crush and other injuries; and an estimated 50 to 75 per cent of hand deformities were the result of infection (Mock, 1915). In 1934, Koch discussed the deadly menace of acute lymphangitis, which had a 28 per cent mortality rate and developed most commonly after a trivial injury to the finger or hand. In 1936, Welch reviewed human bite infections of the hand and found that amputation of a finger was required in 10 per cent of patients treated within 12 hours of injury. When treatment was delayed for one to seven days, 10 per cent died, 30 per cent required amputation, and 30 per cent developed a stiff or flail finger.

In these years before the advent of antibiotics, it was clear that surgical treatment itself could contribute to these grim statistics. To cut into cellulitis or lymphangitis was to introduce the possibility of converting a local infection to septicemia; to enter a tendon sheath mistakenly while draining a subcutaneous abscess could be the cause of unnecessary tendon necrosis. Recognizing these risks, Kanavel became the instigator of a continuing interest in the surgical anatomy of the hand and the differential diagnosis of acute infections of the hand. In the Preface to his 1905 paper on fascial space infections, Kanavel stated his purpose as defining anatomic planes and channels for the localization of pus, and this done, to determine the proper sites for the placement of incisions. His monograph on Infections of the Hand (Kanavel, 1912) was to become a foundation of modern hand surgery and a reference for Koch, who expanded studies in the area of felon and lymphangitis (Koch, 1929, 1934), osteomyelitis (Koch, 1937), and human bite wounds at the flexed metacarpophalangeal joint (Mason and Koch, 1930). The principles of elevation, properly positioned immobilization, hot wet dressings, and judiciously timed and placed hand incisions emerged during these years and became the backbone of treatment in the preantibiotic era.

With the availability of antibiotics, the severity of hand infections and the grave sequelae of chronic osteomyelitis, stiffness, and amputation diminished. Flynn (1982) reported a 75 per cent decrease in the yearly incidence of tenosynovitis at Boston City Hospital by the early 1950's, and Robins' 1952 review of 1000 cases showed the radical improvement penicillin had made in the prognosis for bone, joint, and tendon sheath infections.

Severe hand infections continue to remain relatively uncommon, but the incidence has not changed dramatically since the 1940's. A review comparing 400 cases of hand infection treated in 1947 with a similar number of cases treated in 1974 showed exactly the same number of tenosynovial infections, although pulp, web, and deep palmar space infections decreased (Bell, 1976). It has been suggested that an over-reliance on antibiotics and the emergence of resistant organisms may be contributing factors in maintaining this stable population of patients. Neviaser (1982) pointed out that antibiotics alone are curative in only a small number of hand infections because the compartmentalization of the hand tends to contain the infection in regions poorly accessible to systemic antibiotics.

While it is clear that a large number of patients with hand infections will continue to require surgical treatment, it is curious that the increasingly sophisticated culturing techniques and newer available antibiotics have not had more impact on the overall incidence of serious hand infections. Perhaps the continuing growth in the pool of patients with diminished host resistance plays some role, as evidenced by the reports of uncommon bacterial and fungal infections in diabetic or immunosuppressed patients.

CLASSIFICATION

Establishment of a clinical infection requires a shift in the normal three-way equilibrium between the virulence of the organism, the strength of the patient's natural host defenses, and the characteristic features of the involved tissue. The concept of virulence has changed from old descriptions of "deadly" bacteria, such as plague or typhoid organisms. Now it is seen as the ability of the organism to gain entry, to enter as a larger inoculum, to multiply within the wound, or to resist chemotherapeutic agents. Host defenses include local inflammation and leukocyte migration to the wound edges for opsonization, phagocytosis, and actual killing of the bacteria within the phagocyte. These immunologic defenses can be impaired by several systemic host factors, including old age, diabetes, malnutrition, renal failure, and atherosclerosis. The host defense also can be impaired by conditions at the local level, and thus the involved tissue or location of a wound can become critical determinants of infection risk. Defective blood supply, the presence of devitalized tissue, dead space, hematomas, and foreign bodies clearly promote wound infection. Ischemia, even though transient, may favor tissue necrosis and bacterial growth; devascularized tissue becomes a protected focus because of rapid loss of opsonizing activity from dead space fluid and ineffective penetration of the coagulum by leukocytes and systemic antibiotics.

Etiologic Classification

A survey of the etiology and anatomic classification of hand infections illustrates that almost all hand infections develop after a break in the skin of the hand, and despite the staggering frequency with which this must occur, infections are not common. Moreover, published series reviewing etiology indicate that up to 50 per cent of infections are secondary to the highly virulent human or animal bite, are related to substance injection in drug abuse, or are present in diabetic patients (Table 135–1) (Chuinard and D'Am-

Table 135–1. Etiology of Hand Infections

Author/Date	Number of Patients	Human Bite	Animal Bite	Drug Abuse	Trauma	Diabetes Mellitus	Unknown
McConnell and Neale, 1979	204	24%	10%	10%	35%	7%	13%
Glass, 1982	138	21%	2%	—	67%	7%	9%
Stern and associates, 1983	200	29%	4%	11%	36%	—	20%
Robson, Schmidt, and Heggers, 1983	25	←——— 33% ———→		16.7%	50%	—	0%
Chuinard and D'Ambrosia, 1977	205	29%	—	—	—	—	—

brosia, 1977; McConnell and Neale, 1979; Glass, 1982; Stern and associates, 1983; Robson, Schmidt, and Heggers, 1983).

Anatomic Classification

A review of the incidence of the various types of hand infections shows that cellulitis, lymphangitis, and subcutaneous and nail fold infections make up the large majority of infections treated on an outpatient basis (Nicholls, 1973) and make up over 50 per cent of cases of hand infections requiring hospitalization for treatment (Table 135–2) (McConnell and Neale, 1979; Glass, 1982; Stern and associates, 1983; Palmieri and Schwartz, 1985). From these statistics two conclusions can be drawn. First, a certain proportion of the more superficial "minor" infections progress to major infections requiring hospitalization for parenteral antibiotics or other measures. Second, the bulk of the tendon, bone, and joint infections in the hand are the result of extension from more superficial "minor" infections; e.g., osteomyelitis of the distal phalanx may develop from a pulp space infection.

Analysis of local host tissue factors helps to explain the relatively high risk from these superficial infections. The hand is composed of many spaces or potential spaces that protect neurovascular structures and permit gliding for motion. Rapid extension of infection can occur in these spaces, either by direct extension, as with contiguous osteomyelitis, or by spreading along tendon sheaths, joint spaces, lymphatics, or fascial planes of the hand's spaces and bursae. The second local factor favoring infection is the ease with which these enclosed and septated structures can become ischemic. In the hand, tissue reaction and swelling cause early venous and lymphatic congestion and local arterial insufficiency. Tissue tension becomes critical, as tissue necrosis results from microvascular thrombosis and newly devitalized tissue promotes infection. Elevation of the infected extremity to improve venous return, drainage procedures to decompress the tissue, and the avoidance of constricting dressings are thus all important. An improvement in circulation hastens the resolution of the infection.

ORGANISMS AND ANTIBIOTICS

Before the availability of penicillin, the micro-organism most feared in hand infections was the rapidly spreading beta-hemo-

Table 135–2. Incidence of Various Types of Hand Infections

Author/Date	Number/ Type of Patients	Cellulitis Lymphan- gitis	Subcu- taneous Abscesses	Paronychia, Eponychia, Subungual Infections	Felon	Deep Space Abscesses	Teno- synovitis	Osteo- myelitis	Septic Arthritis
Nicholls, 1973	91 Outpatients	Excluded	34%	45%	11%	2%	0	0	0
McConnell and Neale, 1979	204 Hospitalized	46%	←——— 47% ———→				11%	0	0
Glass, 1982	138 Hospitalized	16%	22%	4%	16%	21%	9%	—	13%
Stern and associates, 1983	200 Hospitalized	Excluded	←——— 76% ———→			1%	10%	6%	6%
Palmieri and Schwartz, 1985	950 Both	←——— 21% ———→		36%	26%	8%	5%	0	0

lytic streptococcus. Because it proved highly vulnerable to antibiotics, its preeminent place was taken by *Staphylococcus aureus*, the most common pathogen isolated in hand infections. Although this was initially sensitive to penicillin, a 1970 review of hand infections indicated that 66 per cent of the community-acquired *S. aureus* had become penicillin resistant (Eaton and Butsch, 1970). Subsequent studies continued to implicate *S. aureus* as a major pathogen in up to 76 per cent of cases (Nicholls, 1973) and its increasing penicillin resistance in 80 or 93 per cent of infections (Chuinard and D'Ambrosia, 1977; McConnell and Neale, 1979). From these findings came the recommendations for a penicillinase-resistant penicillin, such as nafcillin, for the treatment of hand infections. For some ten years or more, a standard empiric antibiotic started while culture results were awaited was nafcillin or a first-generation cephalosporin such as cephalothin or cefazolin (Fitzgerald and associates, 1977; Weckesser, 1980; Peeples, Boswick, and Scott, 1980; Glass, 1982).

With improved culture techniques and an increased awareness of the pathogenicity of anaerobic organisms, a clearer picture of the bacterial spectrum in hand infections began to emerge in the 1980's. Anaerobes had been cultured in as many as 60 per cent of a small series of cases of clenched fist injuries (Goldstein and associates, 1978b). A subsequent prospective study of 200 established hand infections showed that 74 per cent of the patients grew aerobes, most commonly *S. aureus* (35 per cent) and *Streptococcus viridans* (29 per cent), but that 26 per cent of the patients grew anaerobes, most often *Bacteroides melaninogenicus* (10 per cent) and *Peptostreptococcus anaerobius* (6 per cent). There was a strong relationship between human bite wounds and the presence of anaerobes. Over 60 per cent of the patients grew multiple organisms and 95 per cent of the organisms were sensitive to cefamandole, a second-generation broad-spectrum cephalosporin effective against both aerobes and anaerobes (Stern and associates, 1983). A second study appearing at the same time had an even larger proportion of infections due to anaerobes (42 per cent) with 21 per cent of the patients growing *Peptostreptococcus anaerobius*. Of the 58 per cent with aerobic infections, *S. aureus* (21 per cent) and *Streptococcus viridans* (19 per cent) remained the most

common organisms. A mixed flora was cultured in 33 per cent of the patients and cefamandole was efficacious in all but one case (Robson, Schmidt, and Heggers, 1983).

Antimicrobial therapy is regarded generally as a useful adjunct in the treatment of established hand infections, and appropriate antibiotic selection should be based on the results of wound culture and sensitivity testing. Unfortunately the treating surgeon may not have this bacteriologic data at the time antibiotic treatment must be initiated, and it is in this setting that information about the usual causative organisms is helpful. Recent studies suggest that aerobic gram-positive, aerobic gram-negative, and anaerobic organisms in a mixed flora are cultured in a significant number of hand infections, particularly when caused by human bites, and that a broad-spectrum second-generation cephalosporin is a good choice for initial empiric therapy.

Prophylactic Antibiotics

Because of the morbidity associated with infections of the hand, the use of prophylactic antibiotics in the management of simple open hand injuries treated in an emergency room has been investigated. In two series of 368 and 265 patients with hand lacerations, there was no difference in the incidence of infection in the antibiotic and untreated groups, and it was concluded that prophylactic antibiotics are an unnecessary adjunct in the treatment of simple hand lacerations (Roberts and Teddy, 1977; Grossman, Adams, and Kunec, 1981). It might be anticipated that prophylactic antibiotics would have a place in the treatment of mutilating hand injuries, since any partially devitalized tissue remaining after debridement would be particularly susceptible to infection. However, analysis of 120 of these injuries failed to show any benefit from prophylactic antibiotics in preventing infection, although the authors continue to recommend prophylaxis in some cases of mutilating injury, depending on the status of the wound (Fitzgerald and associates, 1977).

High Risk Categories

The frequency of infections, the clinical course, the long-term complications and disability, and the spectrum of organisms are different in three types of hand infection. As seen in Table 135–1, infections in the diabetic, the drug addict, and the bitten hand make up a substantial portion of all hand infections and each has several singular features.

DIABETES MELLITUS

Diabetes is a metabolic disorder that appears to increase susceptibility to infection. There is some evidence that the immunocompetence in diabetic patients under poor metabolic control is impaired, and defects in white cell chemotactic ability and phagocytosis have been identified. The leukocyte dysfunction returns toward normal when the metabolic derangements are corrected and the diabetes is under control.

The course of hand infections in patients with diabetes mellitus is characterized by (1) a longer mean treatment delay of seven to ten days, (2) a need for repeated surgical drainage and debridement procedures, (3) a higher incidence of gram-negative bacilli (30 to 60 per cent) among the causal organisms, (4) a slower resolution of the infection, and (5) a poorer outcome with amputation of a finger in 20 to 50 per cent of patients in different series (Mann and Peacock, 1977; Glass, 1982). This poor prognosis is reflected also in a higher incidence of complications such as a stiff finger (Stern and associates, 1983) and has prompted recommendations for early aggressive treatment, such as appropriate antibiotics to combat mixed pathogens including gram-negative bacilli, and repeated surgical intervention to debride necrotic tissue and limit further spread of the infection (Fig. 135–1). Others have recommended caution in the outpatient management of minor injuries in these patients (McConnell and Neale, 1979) and examination of the blood glucose levels in patients presenting with pulp and deep space infections of the hand, since a high incidence of overt or subclinical diabetes has been diagnosed in patients with severe, deep hand infections (Mandel, 1978).

DRUG ABUSE

Abscesses of the dorsum of the hand and fingers are the most common lesions in drug abusers who are using the veins of the hand or fingers for venous access. Both the intro-

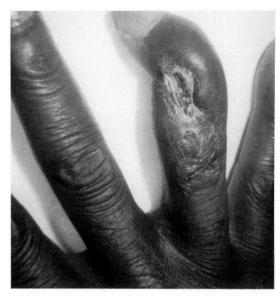

Figure 135–1. Chronic osteomyelitis with ankylosis secondary to septic arthritis following a neglected paronychia in a 59 year old woman with diabetes mellitus.

duction of pathogens and local chemical necrosis from the extravasation of injected materials are responsible for abscesses that may become tense and produce necrosis of the overlying skin (Fig. 135–2). Secondary lymphedema and extensive subcutaneous fibrosis are late sequelae, and infections of the tendon sheath, bone, or joints were diagnosed in about 30 per cent of hand infections in

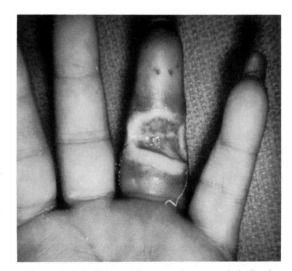

Figure 135–2. Skin and flexor tendon necrosis in the ring finger of a young drug abuser. She developed a volar finger abscess following a subcutaneous drug injection and presented because of concern about palmar erythema and tenderness.

drug addicts in one series (McKay, Pascarelli, and Eaton, 1973).

Early aggressive treatment of these patients with a definitive operative procedure has been stressed because of their poor compliance with long-range, staged treatments (McKay, Pascarelli, and Eaton, 1973). Multiple hospitalizations for repeated infections are characteristic (McConnell and Neale, 1979), as are late presentation for treatment, mixed flora in bacterial isolates, and a relatively low incidence of disabling complications in comparison with diabetic or human bite populations (Stern and associates, 1983).

HUMAN AND ANIMAL BITES

Bite wounds to the hand are responsible for 25 to 30 per cent of infections (Table 135–1), and a laceration over the dorsum of the metacarpophalangeal joint after striking an opponent's teeth with a clenched fist can be found in 87 per cent (Bilos, Kucharchuk, and Metzger, 1978), 86 per cent (Chuinard and D'Ambrosia, 1977), 71 per cent (Peeples, Boswick, and Scott, 1980), 56 per cent (Mann, Hoffeld, and Farmer, 1977), or 50 per cent (Guba, Mulliken, and Hoopes, 1975) of patients with infections due to human bites. Tooth wounds are particularly problematic for three reasons. First, the patient generally does not recognize the severity of the injury and delays presenting for care. Second, the mechanism of injury provides an ideal local environment for implanted organisms, since a tooth easily can penetrate the thin tissue and often the joint capsule over the flexed metacarpophalangeal joint. When the clenched fingers are extended, the extensor tendon and skin shift to seal an inoculated wound with traumatized tissue and rich synovial fluid in an anaerobic environment (Mason and Koch, 1930). These infections spread chiefly in the subcutaneous and subfascial spaces on the dorsum of the hand, but can involve the interosseus and lumbrical sheaths and be carried to the fascial spaces of the palm. Meanwhile, pus accumulating within the metacarpophalangeal joint produces a septic arthritis, which leads to disintegration of the articular cartilage and resorption of subchondral bone (Fig. 135–3). Destruction of the infected joint, osteomyelitis in the adjacent metacarpal, and tenosynovitis are reported in 6 to 30 per cent of cases (Shields and associates, 1975; Guba, Mulliken, and

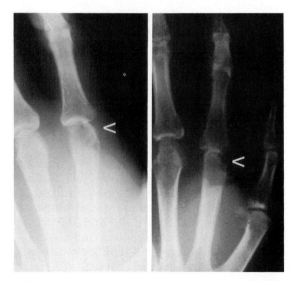

Figure 135–3. Radiographs at 17 days (*left*) and 90 days (*right*) after a human tooth wound to the index metacarpophalangeal joint of a 29 year old man who did not seek medical attention until five days after the injury. The late films show destruction of the joint and adjacent metacarpal (*arrows*) despite treatment for septic arthritis and osteomyelitis.

Hoopes, 1975; Mann, Hoffeld, and Farmer, 1977; Bilos, Kucharchuk, and Metzger, 1978).

In addition to patient delay and the favorable anatomic region for infection, the inoculum delivered to these wounds is particularly virulent. Human saliva may contain more than 10^8 organisms per milliliter (Mann, Hoffeld, and Farmer, 1977) and as many as 42 different species (Shields and associates, 1975). Harmless in the healthy mouth, this flora rapidly causes infection in damaged tissue. Moreover, the oral microorganisms vary with the host's dentition and oral hygiene. In the neglected mouth, the bacterial types are mainly anaerobic and proteolytic. In the well-kept mouth the dominant flora are aerobic or facultatively anaerobic. It has been pointed out that bites by children are numerous but innocuous, and this may be due to the healthier condition of their mouths (Boyce, 1942).

Multiple studies have shown *Streptococcus viridans* to be the single most frequent isolate in bite wounds, and while *Staphylococcus aureus* is identified in only about one-half the wounds, its presence alone or in a mixed flora has been associated with a higher incidence of severe complications. *S. aureus* was cultured in 50 per cent (Mann, Hoffeld, and Farmer, 1977) and 70 per cent (Guba, Mulliken, and Hoopes, 1975) of the hands with tenosynovitis, septic arthritis, or osteomyelitis.

As culture techniques became more sophisticated, an impressive number of anaerobic bacteria were recognized. In 1978, anaerobes were isolated in 50 per cent of human bite and clenched fist wounds and 50 per cent of animal bites in a total of 88 anaerobic strains, mostly various common *Bacteroides* species (Goldstein and associates, 1978a), including *Bacteroides corrodens* (Goldstein and associates, 1978b). This organism was later renamed *Eikenella corrodens* and it became clear that this gram-negative rod was not a strict anaerobe but rather a facultative organism best grown in 10 per cent CO_2 atmosphere and sensitive to penicillin. The presence of *E. corrodens* has been associated with more severe hand infections (Johnson and Pankey, 1976; Bilos, Kucharchuk, and Metzger, 1978; McDonald, 1979; Goldstein, Barones, and Miller, 1983), but its incidence is unclear since some series using appropriate culture techniques have grown the organism only rarely (Glass, 1982; Stern, Staneck and associates, 1983).

In wounds from animal sources, *Pasteurella multocida* is frequently encountered and has been the focus of particular attention in cat bites, where it was cultured in 100 per cent of cases in one series (Peeples, Boswick, and Scott, 1980). Penicillin has been the drug of choice for *P. multocida*. As with human bites, the incidence of anaerobes in animal bites is proving to be as high as 75 per cent of cases (Goldstein, Citron, and Finegold, 1980), and a broad-spectrum antibiotic such as cefamandole is recommended for initial empiric antibiotic therapy (Robson, Schmidt, and Heggers, 1983). No organism has yet been identified in seal bites, which progress to cellulitis and septic arthritis and are treated with tetracycline (Mass, Newmeyer, and Kilgore, 1981).

Delay in the onset of treatment is directly proportional to an unfavorable outcome in hand infections, and it is rare that a bite wound, regardless of whether the joint was penetrated, goes on to serious complications if treated within one day of injury (Mann, Hoffeld, and Farmer, 1977; McConnell and Neale, 1979). Aggressive treatment, including immediate exploration for examination of joint capsule integrity and hospitalization for surgical exploration and irrigation of a violated joint space, has been recommended (Chuinard and D'Ambrosia, 1977), as have immediate tetanus prophylaxis, wound cultures, antibiotics, immobilization and elevation, secondary wound healing, and other general measures (Fig. 135–4).

PRINCIPLES OF TREATMENT

The management of any given hand infection is dictated in part by the anatomic type and the etiology of the infection, but the goal of eliminating infection while preserving and

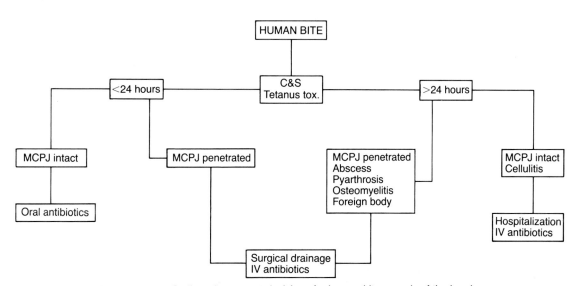

Figure 135–4. Outline of treatment decisions for human bite wounds of the hand.

restoring hand function is universal. Immobilization, elevation, the selective use of surgical drainage and antibiotics, and early rehabilitation are the mainstays of management.

Immobilization and Elevation

The purpose of immobilizing the infected hand is twofold: to prevent the dissemination of infection by muscular action (Kanavel, 1905) and to splint the hand in a moderate intrinsic plus position to help prevent secondary joint contractures (Linscheid and Dobyns, 1975). A bulky or well-padded dressing incorporating plaster should immobilize the hand in the position of "safety," which consists of 30° to 50° of extension at the wrist joint, 50° to 90° flexion of the metacarpophalangeal joints, 0° to 10° flexion at the interphalangeal joints, and the thumb maximally abducted palmar to the line of the index metacarpal. A long arm cast may be needed to keep the arm at rest in children or unreliable adults (Kilgore, 1983), but the dressing must be removable to enable the hand to be inspected at intervals, particularly to monitor swelling.

Elevation of the hand above heart level is critical for gaining control of the edema and swelling that compromise venous return and contribute to early ischemia and late stiffness of the infected hand. Good drainage is obtained in the supine patient with the hand and forearm supported on pillows. Some manufacture a sling with stockinette, pins, and tape for suspension of the arm from a bedside pole (Linscheid and Dobyns, 1975), while others feel that suspension with a noose or sling that may become constricting is not advisable (Carter and Mersheimer, 1970).

Diagnostic Studies

Evaluation of the patient with a hand infection should include a medical history for general health and medication information. A radiograph of the hand will evaluate for osteitis, osteomyelitis, fracture, bone abscess, or the presence of a foreign body—particularly a retained tooth fragment (Smith and Manges, 1937). For those with more severe infections, a blood glucose and complete blood count should be included.

Surgical Management

Surgery may be undertaken for several reasons: (1) therapeutic evacuation of pus, (2) therapeutic relief of tissue tension or decompression to abort a peripheral neuropathy, and (3) diagnostic recovery of an organism in a closed space infection, especially for culture of the responsible organisms when pyarthrosis or osteomyelitis is suspected.

Before the hyperemic infected tissue is incised, the arm is exsanguinated by elevation, not by wrapping, which may dislodge bacteria into proximal vessels and lymphatics. An upper arm tourniquet is inflated for visual control over the placement of incisions. Anesthesia is given proximal to the infected area by local nerve block or general anesthesia.

SURGICAL INCISIONS

There was a tendency in the past to use certain well-defined incisions for access to all hand infections, and this practice may have followed from Kanavel's (1912) rule that incisions should be placed away from tactile surfaces and situated so as to form flaps to shield vital structures, and scar with a minimum of deforming contracture. Later, as massive or life-threatening infections became fewer, more efficient and limited incisions directly over the collection were introduced, as well as catheter placement for continuous postoperative irrigation (Carter, Burman, and Mersheimer, 1966; Bunnell, 1970; Neviaser, 1982).

For drainage of an abscess, the incision is located at the point of maximal tenderness or fluctuance; is made in parallel with the neurovascular structures with gentle, blunt deep dissection; and is kept as limited as is expedient. Debridement of necrotic tissue should be adequate but minimized to avoid damage to the neurovascular bundles or exposure of uninvolved bone, joint, or tendon sheath. Fine plastic catheters can be secured in the wound for several days of postoperative irrigation, or drains and packing for 48 to 72 hours may be chosen to provide wide access for debridement or egress of heavy drainage.

Incisions must run parallel or oblique to flexion creases to avoid secondary scar contractures, and midlateral incisions in the fingers are used for wide exposure (Fig. 135–5). Long, zigzag volar incisions are best avoided in the edematous infected digit since the

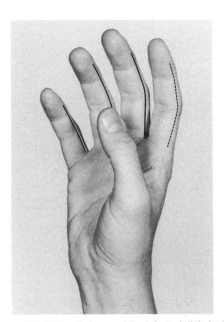

Figure 135–5. For drainage of the infected digit, incisions in the midlateral line of the fingers give good exposure, permit extension, and observe generally accepted guidelines for incision placement.

wounds may be left open, and scarring after healing of these small flaps may be poorer. Incisions for drainage of web spaces may be volar and dorsal longitudinal or straight incisions, or a zigzag in the palm just proximal to the web space (Neviaser, 1982).

Palmar incisions are made parallel with the palmar or thenar creases, and special care must be taken with thenar space abscesses, which may be approached from both palmar and dorsal sides to ensure drainage of pus on both sides of the adductor. Thenar crease incisions must avoid the palmar cutaneous and the motor branches of the median nerve, which lie subcutaneously and subfascially, respectively (Fig. 135–6) (Bunnell, 1970).

Remobilization

Once the hand infection is brought under control and erythema and tenderness have cleared, supervised mobilization can begin despite the presence of open wounds and dressings. Continued splinting may be desirable between exercise sessions. In situations in which signs of inflammation persist despite surgery and appropriate antibiotics, residual infection is suspect and further investigation for a sequestrum, joint infection, or osteomyelitis is indicated.

SUBCUTANEOUS INFECTIONS

Purulent infections of the skin and subcutaneous space account for more than 90 per cent of hand infections, and cellulitis, lymphangitis, and subepidermal and subcutaneous abscesses are the primary superficial soft tissue infections.

Cellulitis

Cellulitis is a nonsuppurative inflammation of the subcutaneous tissue extending along connective tissue planes with widespread swelling, erythema, tenderness, warmth, and throbbing pain without definite localization. Skin blebs and bullae may form in severe infections, and central necrosis with abscess formation and suppuration is seen in later stages. A variety of aerobic and anaerobic organisms produce cellulitis, but the hemolytic streptococcus is classically associated with the rapidly progressive process, erysipelas. Treatment is nonsurgical with elevation, immobilization, and antibiotics. If antibiotic selection is problematic because of an atypical history or presentation, aspiration may yield a pathogen even in the absence of fluctuance. Radiographs are indicated to rule out a foreign body. Incision and drainage are avoided because of their ineffectiveness and

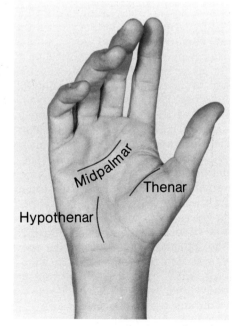

Figure 135–6. Incisions for drainage of an abscess of the midpalmar, thenar, or hypothenar space.

the risk of contamination of deeper tissues, but if the inflammatory swelling fails to subside after 48 to 72 hours of antibiotic therapy, it is suggestive of an abscess or closed space collection that should be sought and drained.

Lymphangitis

Inflammation of the lymphatic pathways usually is visible as erythematous streaking on the volar or dorsal aspect of the arm proximal to a finger or hand infection. Lymphadenitis, or associated swelling of the lymph nodes, generally presents as tenderness and enlargement of the epitrochlear or axillary nodes, and as the lymphangitis worsens, fever and leukocytosis develop. Most patients are hospitalized for strict immobilization, elevation, and empiric parenteral antibiotic therapy as soon as cultures of the primary site of infection are taken. Although lymphangitis was dreaded in the preantibiotic era as the harbinger of systemic sepsis and proximal abscesses, it generally clears rapidly with appropriate antibiotics and is problematic only in patients with chronic lymphedema or the fibrosis caused by chronic drug abuse.

Abscess

An abscess is a localized collection of pus surrounded by an area of inflamed tissue with marked hyperemia and leukocyte infiltration. It may be intraepidermal or subepidermal, impetigo or pyoderma, respectively, or it may present as a furuncle, or boil, which is an abscess in a sweat gland or hair follicle. *Staphylococcus aureus* is the causative organism in all of these, although a mixed flora occasionally is implicated in persons with lowered resistance. Furuncles present on the hair-bearing dorsum of the hand, especially the dorsum of the proximal phalanx, and often enjoy a self-limited course requiring no specific therapy (Fig. 135–7). However, they may progress to a carbuncle, which is a multilocular suppurative extension of a furuncle into the subcutaneous space with multiple heads and draining sinuses. Incision and drainage with appropriate antibiotics are necessary, and because of the large size of the lesion and its tendency to mature slowly to fluctuance, systemic signs of infection are not uncommon.

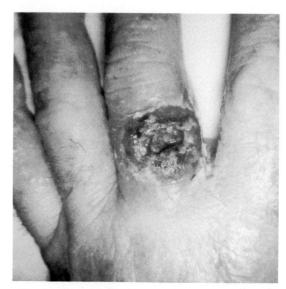

Figure 135–7. Carbuncle, with multiple draining sinuses, in the dorsal hair-bearing area of the hand of a 54 year old man.

Infections in the periungual area appear as abscesses in the soft tissues around the fingernail and tend to be well localized in the thin, nondistensible skin of the nail folds. Their high incidence is related to the frequency of trauma in the fingernail area coupled with repeated or prolonged exposure to moisture and keratolytics. The possibility of the presence of a foreign body should be considered in these infections, but poor nail care habits are implicated more often.

PARONYCHIA

In acute paronychia, inflammation of the radial or ulnar sides of the nail fold produces erythema, swelling, and throbbing pain and may extend into the proximal nail fold as an eponychia. The infection is generally a mixed one with a spectrum of normal skin and gastrointestinal flora. Anaerobes have been identified in about 75 per cent of paronychia in the pediatric age group, in which thumb sucking and nail biting habits are prevalent (Brook, 1981). An occasional early paronychia may be managed with antibiotics alone, although the majority require surgical drainage. For the well-localized abscess, drainage through the rim of the nail fold with the blade held flat against the nail is effective and does not require anesthesia or produce bleeding. Pain relief is dramatic with the evacuation of pus. For the less mature paronychia that is not yet pointing at the margin of the nail fold, a direct stab wound is made at the point of maximal swelling and tenderness, and a small wick is placed to keep the wound open for 24 to 48 hours. The latter procedure requires anesthetic and a tourniquet (Fig. 135–8).

Chronic paronychia are seen in cooks, dishwashers, cleaning people, and others in whom repeated wetting of the hands produces softening and elevation of the nail fold, which becomes erythematous, swollen, tender, and retracted from the nail. The fingernails become scaly and discolored and it is not uncommon to see involvement of multiple digits. A chronic process that may persist for months or years with repeated episodes of inflammation and incomplete resolution, the chronic paronychia grows yeast; causative agents may include fungi as well as bacteria and *Candida albicans* in symbiotic balance with lower bowel organisms (Barlow and associates, 1970). Treatment requires avoidance of moisture and trauma, and packing of the nail fold with antifungal agents such as nystatin cream.

SUBUNGUAL ABSCESS AND SUBEPONYCHIAL ABSCESS

A subungual abscess occurs between the nail and the nail bed. It is drained without a skin incision by removing the base of the fingernail and leaving a wick or small pack beneath the nail fold for 24 to 48 hours to ensure drainage.

Subeponychial or apical abscesses occur deep to the nail bed in the subcutaneous tissue lying between the nail bed and the distal phalanx. These are due more commonly to puncture wounds and can be drained through the fingernail.

Pyogenic Granuloma

A pyogenic granuloma is a projection of granulation tissue, or "proud flesh," from a

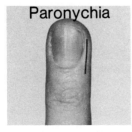

Figure 135–8. Incision for drainage of a paronychia involving the lateral nail fold. The incision should be beveled slightly away from the nail matrix.

wound that is kept moist and has a low grade bacterial infection. Foreign bodies are present in a high proportion of these infections, and pyogenic granuloma occurs with higher frequency in the diabetic population. Treatment includes leveling or excising the granulation tissue, cauterization of the base for hemostasis, and topical antibacterial dressings. Systemic antibiotics are not necessary. Recurrence of a pyogenic granuloma should prompt cultures and biopsy to rule out an unusual fungal infection or malignant growth (Fig. 135–9).

DEEP SPACE INFECTIONS

Felon

The word felon is derived from the Middle English "feloun" meaning suppurative sore. A subcutaneous infection of the pulp space of the distal phalanx of a digit, the felon is considered a closed space infection of the multiple compartments created by fibrous septa passing vertically in the distal fat pad between the skin and the periosteum. The characteristic symptoms of a felon are throbbing pain, swelling, erythema, and tenderness. There may be a history of a penetrating injury and the course is rapid and severe. Contained by the unyielding skin of the fingertip, the infection creates tension with microvascular compromise, necrosis, and abscess formation. The abscess may "point" in the center of the pulp space and decompress spontaneously, with slough of necrotic skin over the pulp space. It also may produce osteitis or osteomyelitis of the distal phalanx or even sequestration of the diaphysis of the phalanx. Rupture into the distal interphalangeal joint with septic arthritis can occur, or extension into the distal end of the flexor tendon sheath, producing tenosynovitis (Fig. 135–10) (Bolton, Fowler, and Jepson, 1949; Lowden, 1951).

A very early felon may be treated with antibiotics alone, but surgical drainage is required for later lesions to interrupt the cycle of inflammatory-ischemic events. A variety of incisions have been considered in the effort to ensure drainage of the septated spaces and avoid scar placement on a tactile surface, loss of sensibility, or invasion of the tendon sheath. A fishmouth or horseshoe incision curving around the fingertip at the fat pad–nail bed junction was discarded early on

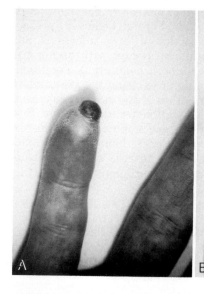
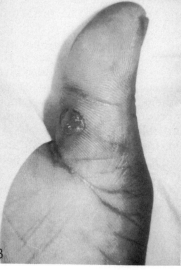

Figure 135–9. *A,* Pyogenic granuloma in the tip of the little finger of a 30 year old man who kept a minor laceration covered continuously with ointment and dressing. *B,* Pyogenic granuloma appearing 18 days after a superficial wound to the thumb of a diabetic 60 year old man.

because of resultant anesthesia of the tip (Koch, 1929). Through and through incisions and hockey stick or J-shaped incisions occasionally are needed for severe problems, but most felons can be drained through a single straight lateral or volar incision (Fig. 135–11). A liberal incision placed just dorsal to the midlateral aspect of the finger, directed volarly, and crossing the midline will open the entire anterior closed space in diffuse felons. A midvolar longitudinal incision of the fat pad obviates potential problems with skin slough over an ischemic pulp that is undermined from the side (Kilgore, Brown, and Newmeyer, 1975), but the midvolar incision places a scar over the pinch surface of the digit and it may be best reserved for

felons that are localizing anteriorly. Once the felon is incised, a pack or wick may be left in the wound, and frequent warm soaks are begun to promote drainage.

Thenar Space Infection

A potential space lying deep to the flexor tendons, the thenar space occupies the area of the thenar eminence, and abuts the adductor pollicis dorsally and the index flexor tendon sheath and first lumbrical anteriorly (Fig. 135–12). Infections may follow puncture wounds, local subcutaneous abscesses, acute suppurative tenosynovitis of the index finger or thumb, or extension from an adjacent bursa or space. Symptoms of a thenar space infection include pain, swelling, tension, and tenderness in the thenar area. The first web

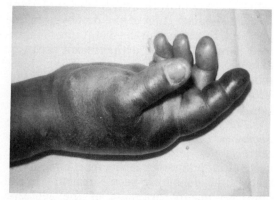

Figure 135–10. The swelling and tissue tension accompanying a neglected felon has progressed to vascular compromise of the index finger in this 20 year old man. Despite aggressive drainage procedures, amputation and later ray resection of the digit were necessary.

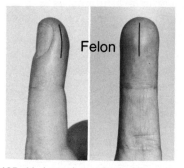

Felon

Figure 135–11. Lateral or volar incisions may be used for drainage of a felon.

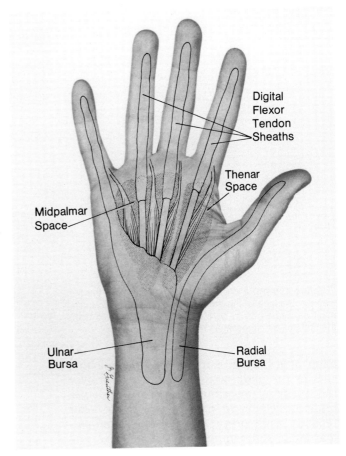

Figure 135–12. The relationship of the thenar and midpalmar fascial spaces of the hand to the synovial sheaths of the ulnar bursa and radial bursa in the palm and the fibrous sheaths of the flexor tendons in the digits.

space becomes involved as the infection passes around the lateral edge of the adductor pollicis, forcing the thumb into abduction and presenting as a web space abscess pointing in the center of the dorsal thumb web (Fig. 135–13).

A thenar space infection can be drained through a dorsal longitudinal incision along the radial margin of the first dorsal interosseus in parallel with the index metacarpal. Since the pus lies volar to the adductor or upon both the volar and dorsal surfaces of the muscle, blunt dissection must be continued in front as well as behind the adductor. A second volar incision in the thenar crease may be necessary, and if the abscess is pointing over the thenar musculature, it should be drained in that area. The palmar cutaneous and motor branches of the median nerve must be borne in mind with anterior incisions (Bunnell, 1970). Drains are placed or soft catheters may be secured in the wounds for intermittent or continuous postoperative irrigation with sterile saline for 24 to 48 hours.

Midpalmar Space Infection

Bounded by the flexor tendons and lumbricals anteriorly and the metacarpals and interosei dorsally, the midpalmar space contacts the proximal ends of the long, ring, and little flexor tendon sheaths and their associated lumbricals. Thus, the midpalmar space abscess can be produced by ruptures of a suppurative tenosynovitis of the long, ring, or little fingers; by extension of a distal palmar infection along one of the lumbrical canals; or by direct penetrating injury (Fig. 135–14). Pain and tenderness develop in the midpalm, but the unyielding palmar fascia limits swelling; although the concavity of the central palm may be obliterated, the fullness does not attain the dramatic proportions of the thenar abscess. Owing to the direction of lymphatic flow, swelling is maximal in the loose areolar tissue on the dorsum of the hand (Fig. 135–15).

The midpalmar space may be drained through a transverse incision in the distal

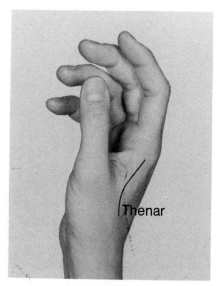

Figure 135–13. A dorsal longitudinal incision in the first web for drainage of the thenar space infection. Dissection must be carried down between the adductor pollicis and the first dorsal interosseous muscle.

palm or a slightly curved longitudinal incision in the more proximal palm placed over the point of maximal tenderness. Gentle blunt dissection in parallel with the flexor tendons, while preserving the superficial palmar arch and common digital arteries and nerves, opens the space, and drains or irrigating catheters are left postoperatively in the depths of the abscess cavity.

Web Space Abscess

Infection of the web between any of the digits can be caused by puncture wounds, or

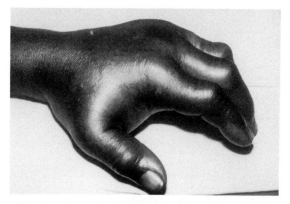

Figure 135–15. The impressive dorsal swelling associated with the midpalmar space infection shown in Figure 135–14.

by extension from a subcutaneous abscess on the proximal part of a finger or from an infected callus over the metacarpal head. Web space and distal palmar infections have a tendency to erode through the palmar fascia, producing a secondary abscess on the dorsum of the hand. Termed a collar button abscess, these dumbbell-shaped infections generally point in the looser tissue on the dorsal side, and recognition of the volar component may require a high index of suspicion (Fig. 135–16).

The web space abscess is drained through a dorsal longitudinal incision between the fingers and a volar curved or zigzag incision extending from just proximal to the margin of the web to the distal palmar crease. Communication is established between the two incisions, and drains or irrigating catheters

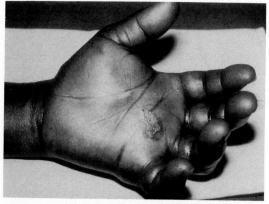

Figure 135–14. A midpalmar abscess presenting several days after a penetrating wound to the distal palm. Despite the posture and appearance of the ring finger, the flexor sheath of the ring finger was not involved.

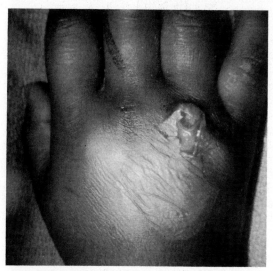

Figure 135–16. A collar button abscess of the distal palm that has drained spontaneously on the dorsum of the hand.

are used postoperatively until drainage ceases (Fig. 135–17).

Other Infections

Hypothenar Space. Kanavel described the hypothenar space, a potential space among the intermuscular septa of the isolated hypothenar musculature. Infection can result from penetrating injury, and abscesses are drained through an incision at the point of maximal tenderness (Kanavel, 1905).

Radial and Ulnar Bursae. The radial bursa is the proximal half of the sheath of the flexor pollicis longus tendon and extends proximally to a point several centimeters above the volar wrist crease. The ulnar bursa is the expansion of the flexor tendon sheath of the little finger to envelop the index, long, and ring finger flexors in the midpalm, and it also extends to a point several centimeters proximal to the volar wrist crease. A suppurative tenosynovitis of the thumb or little finger involves the radial or ulnar bursa, respectively, and in the substantial number of patients in whom these bursae communicate, a "horseshoe" abscess presents with infection traveling from the distal thumb to the distal little finger across the wrist (see Fig. 135–12).

Drainage of an ulnar bursal infection requires an incision along the radial border of the hypothenar eminence to gain access to the flexor tendon sheath of the little finger, and a second incision proximal to the wrist along the ulnar side of the forearm at the dorsal margin of the flexor carpi ulnaris. To protect the dorsal branch of the ulnar nerve, blunt dissection deep to the ulnar artery and nerve is used to expose the bursa, which lies between the flexor tendons superficially and the pronator quadratus on the dorsal side. Drains can be introduced or through and through catheter irrigation can be established (Fig. 135–17).

The radial bursa is opened distally with a thenar crease incision, and proximally with an incision along the border of the radius or medial to the flexor carpi radialis. If a "horseshoe" abscess is present, a combined approach to both bursae is necessary.

Parona's Space. The potential space between the flexor pollicis longus tendon, the flexor digitorum profundus tendons, and the pronator quadratus muscle in the forearm is the subtendinous space of the wrist, or Parona's space. Extension of a radial or ulnar bursitis can infect this space. It is drained through the same ulnar forearm incision as is the ulnar bursa, again protecting the ulnar artery and nerve, and the dorsal branch of the ulnar nerve. Drains or irrigating catheters are used postoperatively.

FASCIAL INFECTIONS

Necrotizing fasciitis is an acute, life-threatening infection of the superficial fascia and subcutaneous tissue caused by a variety of aerobic and anaerobic bacteria. Necrotizing fasciitis of the upper extremity occurs in an indigent population and is associated with street drug and alcohol abuse (Schecter and associates, 1982).

The clinical process at first appears to be a low grade cellulitis, but fulminant infection develops rapidly in the subcutaneous fascia, which may become liquefied with accompanying fat necrosis, thrombosis of subcutaneous vessels, and occasional myositis and myonecrosis. As the blood supply to the skin is compromised, cutaneous erythema and edema progress to cyanosis, bullae, and gangrene. Cutaneous gangrene is associated with fever, shock, and a higher mortality rate.

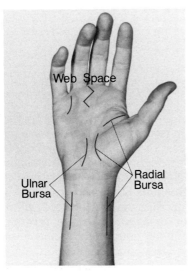

Figure 135–17. The web space abscess may be drained through a curved longitudinal or zigzag volar incision; this may be combined with a dorsal longitudinal incision placed just proximal to the web space. Drainage of an ulnar bursal infection or infection of the radial bursa requires incisions into the palm and distal forearm.

Since skin anesthesia occurs as the subcutaneous gangrene spreads, an acutely ill patient with extensive painless cellulitis or cutaneous gangrene should undergo surgical debridement for diagnosis and treatment. Adequate debridement of necrotizing fasciitis entails resection of all necrotic skin, fat, fascia, and muscle to include apparently normal soft tissue at the margins of the advancing cellulitis, since viable organisms can be isolated at the periphery.

Meleney originally described necrotizing fasciitis as "hemolytic streptococcal gangrene," but it is now clear that a mixed flora is present in 50 to 75 per cent of cases (Feingold, 1982). In 29 patients with upper extremity fasciitis, one-half had cultures growing only a single organism—most often hemolytic *Streptococcus*. In the remaining patients, the multiple organisms included gram-negative aerobes and a variety of anaerobes as well as *Eikenella corrodens* (Schecter and associates, 1982). In this study, the survival rate of patients with upper extremity necrotizing fasciitis was only 91 per cent despite broad-spectrum antibiotics and radical debridement. Delay in seeking medical attention was critical, since all the patients who died had presented initially in shock.

TENOSYNOVITIS

Infection of the tenosynovium most often is due to penetrating injury, particularly over the volar joint creases where the skin is separated from the flexor tendon sheath by only a thin layer of subcutaneous tissue. Surgical procedures involving the sheaths and hematogenous spread are less common causes of infection. In the drug addict population, tenosynovitis of the extensor tendon sheaths has been reported in the aftermath of inadvertent intrathecal injection of unsterile drugs (Fig. 135–18) (Dhaliwal and Garnes, 1982). The tendon sheath is poorly vascularized, is rich in synovial fluid, and offers a hospitable environment for infection, which spreads without obstruction from the proximal to the distal limits of the sheath. In this confined space, sufficient pressure can develop to cause tendon necrosis; even if the tendon is preserved, the attendant inflammation and fibrosis can produce adhesions that limit tendon excursion and finger motion.

Diagnosis

Flexor tenosynovitis presents most commonly in the index, long, and ring fingers and is characterized by the four cardinal signs of Kanavel (1912): flexed posture of the digit, uniform swelling of the digit, tenderness over the length of the involved tendon sheath, and severe pain on attempted hyperextension of the digit. These symptoms may extend into the palm and forearm with involvement of the little finger–ulnar bursa, or the thumb–radial bursa.

Once the diagnosis of tenosynovitis is entertained, prompt treatment should include appropriate parenteral antibiotics; in cases in which the infection is very early and symptoms are still limited primarily to pain on extension, the extremity may be immobilized, elevated, and closely observed. An early infection may resolve following these measures, but failure to respond within about 24 hours should mandate a drainage procedure. In cases in which the diagnosis is in doubt or difficult to differentiate from another process such as septic arthritis, the flexor tendon sheath may be aspirated with a 20 or 22 gauge needle introduced tangentially at a point distant from any superficial infection, to minimize the risk of introducing organisms into a previously uninfected sheath. If the sheath cannot be aspirated safely, exploration of the digit to examine the sheath for distention or turbid contents can be diagnostic without violating intact tenosynovium (Linscheid and Dobyns, 1975).

Treatment

Techniques for treating pyogenic flexor tenosynovitis have included open drainage procedures in which the tendon sheath is opened throughout its length though a midaxial incision. This is now reserved for cases of phlegmonous tenosynovitis where the tendon is necrotic and is excised, plans being made for delayed two-stage reconstruction. Closed tendon sheath irrigation is preferred for other cases, since the tendon and adjacent soft tissue structures of the digit can be preserved. Tendon sheath irrigation was introduced by Carter, Burman, and Mersheimer in 1966, with a report of nine cases successfully treated with hydrogen peroxide and oxytetracycline solution irrigations through

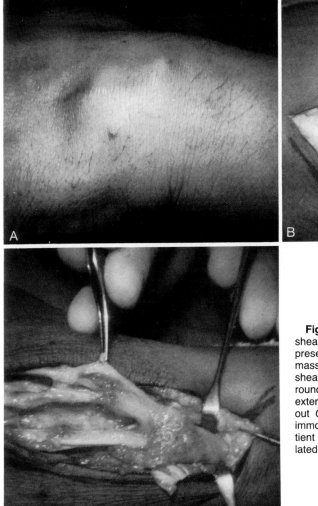

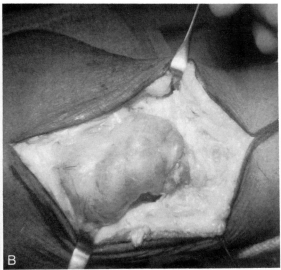

Figure 135–18. Tenosynovitis of the extensor tendon sheaths in a 37 year old male drug abuser. The patient presented with a tense, nontender, movable, dorsal wrist mass (*A*), which proved to be thickened, fibrotic synovial sheath (*B*). Mucoid synovial fluid and rice bodies surrounded and were adherent to degenerated and frayed extensor tendons (*C*). Cultures of the synovial fluid grew out *Candida* species. Synovectomy and two weeks of immobilization were therapeutic temporarily, but the patient returned in 14 months with recurrence of the lobulated dorsal hand swelling.

transverse incisions in the sheath at the palmar crease and distal digital crease over a 24 to 48 hour period. Subsequent reports have confirmed the efficacy of this technique, which produced complete restoration of active and passive motion of the involved digit in 82 and 95 per cent, respectively, of treated patients (Pollen, 1974; Neviaser, 1978). The incision in the distal palm is at the level of the proximal margin of the A1 pulley and can be transverse or zigzag. A 16 gauge catheter is introduced for a distance of 1 to 2 cm and secured in place as the palmar incision is closed. A second incision over the distal joint crease of the digit to allow egress of the irrigating fluid is left open with a small drain in place. Antibiotic irrigating solutions have been proposed (Besser, 1976), but it appears that either isotonic saline or an antibiotic solution is equally useful as a continuous drip or intermittent flush every one to two hours. Irrigation is continued for two or three days with the extremity continuously elevated, and motion is begun as soon as the catheter and drain are removed (Fig. 135–19).

SEPTIC ARTHRITIS

Trauma is the etiologic factor in most cases of septic arthritis from violation of the joint

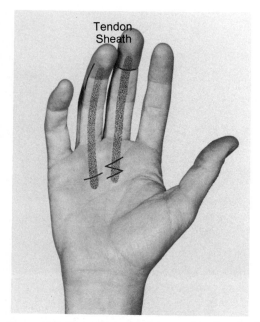

Tendon
Sheath

Figure 135–19. Incisions for drainage of tendon sheath infections include proximal and distal incisions for closed tendon sheath irrigation.

capsule by puncture, burn injury to the joint, or extension from an adjacent bone or soft tissue infection (Lowden, 1975). Seeding of the joint from bacteremia is a less common cause. Several cases of infection of the distal interphalangeal joint of a finger secondary to an infected mucous cyst have been reported (Rangarathnam and Linscheid, 1984) and idiopathic septic wrist is seen in the rheumatoid population (Hart and associates, 1982; Rashkoff, Burkhalter, and Mann, 1983). The involved joint is swollen, warm, erythematous, and tender, and motion is both restricted and painful.

If a septic joint is suspected, diagnosis and treatment should be prompt, since further destruction of the articular surface or adjacent osteomyelitis may lead to a stiff digit. Radiographs show thinning of the joint from cartilaginous loss, resorption of the subchondral bone, and in later cases osteomyelitis and disintegration of the adjacent phalangeal diaphyses (Fig. 135–20). Aspiration of the joint or biopsy of the sequestered bone and cartilage for culture will guide antibiotic selection, but surgery should not be delayed. Treatment requires access to the joint through a dorsal incision, surgical debridement of the involved joint surface and bone, and either packing to keep the wound open

or closure over a catheter for postoperative irrigation. Following resolution of the infection and the resumption of motion, a later arthrodesis or arthroplasty may be required if there is pain, instability, or limited joint mobility.

OSTEOMYELITIS

The critical issue in osteomyelitis is bone necrosis. Microorganisms residing in dead bone, if not removed along with sequestra, can cause flare-ups as late as 50 years after the initial attack. Therefore, the therapeutic plan is determined by the specific clinical situation. Acute hematogenous osteomyelitis can be cured with antibiotics alone if effective therapy is given before extensive bone necrosis occurs. Chronic osteomyelitis requires that all dead bone be surgically removed (Waldvogel and Vasey, 1980).

Etiology

Osteomyelitis in the hand can occur along three routes: hematogenous spread, extension from a contiguous joint or soft tissue infection, and direct inoculation of organisms into the bone. Hematogenous osteomyelitis in the hand is uncommon. The classic case occurs in a prepubertal child, especially one with sickle cell disease or an immunologic disorder, and is due to *Staphylococcus aureus*. The long bones of the lower extremity are most frequently involved, but symmetric hand involvement has been reported (Waldvogel and Vasey, 1980). Acute hematogenous osteomyelitis in the adult differs from that in children. It usually develops during episodes of clinically obvious sepsis and affects the small bones of the wrist or ankle. A wide range of pathogens are reported, including fungi and mycobacteria, particularly in drug addicts and in patients with intravenous lines (Knutson and associates, 1982).

By far the most common cause of bone infection in the hand is by extension from a contiguous soft tissue infection. The phalanges are involved four times more frequently than the metacarpals or carpals. The neglected or inadequately drained felon is a common offender, and the osteitis that frequently accompanies it can progress to sequestration of the tuft and diaphysis of the

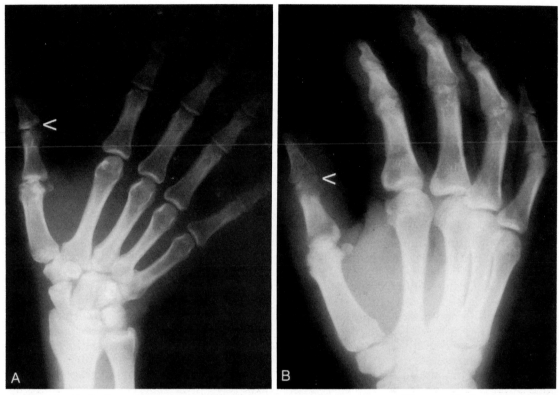

Figure 135–20. Radiographs taken two weeks (*A*) and six weeks (*B*) after a human bite wound to the interphalangeal joint area of a 30 year old woman's thumb. Septic arthritis has resulted in destruction of the articular surface, resorption of subchondral bone, and osteomyelitis of both phalanges (*arrows*).

terminal phalanx and pyarthrosis of the distal interphalangeal joint. Untreated paronychia or any soft tissue infection with a retained foreign body or devitalized tissue predisposes to osteomyelitis of the phalanges. Metacarpal involvement is reported following inadequate drainage of midpalmar or thenar space infections (Resnick, 1976; Michaeli, 1978).

Diagnosis

Early diagnosis of osteomyelitis in the hand is a particular problem, since most cases are secondary to a contiguous soft tissue infection that masks its presence. Pain, fever, leukocytosis, and an elevated sedimentation rate used to diagnose hematogenous osteomyelitis are not helpful. Early radiographs may be normal, since it takes at least ten days for the matrix to be mineralized and for areas of increased density to be detected radiographically. Sclerosis usually indicates that infection has been present for more than one month; lytic lesions occur more rapidly, but

only 3 per cent show this sign in less than one week (Septimus and Musher, 1979). The technetium-99m bone scan is very useful in hematogenous osteomyelitis, since it is positive as early as 24 hours after the onset of disease. However, it has two limitations that become important in the diagnosis of hand infections. First, the scan performed after fracture or surgery cannot differentiate bone repair from bone infection. Second, a single scan cannot differentiate cellulitis from osteomyelitis, and repeated studies at six to 12 hour intervals are necessary as the soft tissue uptake decreases while the uptake in bone remains stable or increases. The gallium scan defines soft tissue infection more clearly and it may have special utility when performed in conjunction with a technetium-99m study (Handmaker, 1980).

Treatment

Prompt surgical exploration is indicated in virtually all cases of contiguous osteomyelitis. It may be the only way to establish the diagnosis and identify the responsible organism in early cases. Debridement and drainage are essential and resection of devitalized soft tissue is recommended without regard for bone cover. Biopsy of the infected bone is the most effective way of identifying the responsible organism.

There is a place for prolonged intravenous antibiotic coverage in cases of acute osteomyelitis, and some of the more cost-effective regimens, with oral antibiotics given for a month on an outpatient basis after one week of parenteral therapy, may be desirable. However, for most cases of acute osteomyelitis, four to six weeks of parenteral therapy is still recommended; an antibiotic should be selected after minimal inhibitory and bactericidal concentrations are determined (Waldvogel and Vasey, 1980).

The role of antibiotics in chronic osteomyelitis is much less clear-cut. The constant feature that is the hallmark of this infection is the presence of necrotic bone. Treatment requires debridement of all sequestra, devitalized tissue, and sinus tracts; this excision may require an amputation or may jeopardize bone stability. There is general agreement that antibiotic therapy is indicated during the healing period, but no consensus on dose and duration. This is not surprising since variables to consider include the area involved, the extent of involvement, the organism, the mode of infection, the duration, and the ability to carry in skin or muscle flap cover. It seems justifiable to tailor the antibiotic regimen to the clinical situation, since there is no good evidence that long-term intravenous therapy is necessary in most cases of contiguous osteomyelitis.

BACTERIAL INFECTIONS

Gangrenous and Crepitant Infections

The gangrenous and crepitant cellulitides are characterized by rapid progress, extensive necrosis, and the need for aggressive surgery to cure them. The classification of these infections is somewhat confusing, since they traditionally are clinical entities rather than specific bacterial infections. They include among others Meleney's progressive synergistic gangrene, clostridial myonecrosis (or gas gangrene), and nonclostridial myositis (or synergistic anaerobic myositis). These infec-

tions are caused by endogenous anaerobic bacteria invading tissue where local conditions have produced low tissue oxygen tension. Thus, these infections are seen in areas of trauma, surgery, burns, ischemia, malignancy, or other forms of tissue damage. Diabetes appears to be a predisposing factor, owing perhaps to small vessel disease and leukocyte dysfunction. Gas in infected areas is an anaerobic metabolite, usually hydrogen, and signifies areas of rapid bacterial multiplication in low oxygen tension. Tissue necrosis and gangrene extend to the skin, subcutaneous tissue, fascia, and muscle on the basis of vascular thrombosis, extracellular bacterial toxins, and ischemic pressure necrosis (Feingold, 1982).

Clostridium, an anaerobic, gram-positive, spore-forming bacillus distributed in the gastrointestinal tract and soil, is the best known of the organisms causing gangrene. Recoverable from many wounds on routine culture, it is pathogenic only under ideal anaerobic conditions, and thus clostridial infection is a clinical rather than a laboratory diagnosis. Rare cases of nontraumatic clostridial infections have been reported (Neimkin and Jupiter, 1985). A variety of anaerobic and facultative bacteria, including coliforms, anaerobic streptococcus, *Bacteroides,* and others, are responsible for nonclostridial crepitant cellulitis.

Seen in the hand after penetrating injury, gangrene presents as swelling, pain, ecchymosis, bullae, and palpable subcutaneous gas developing rapidly and accompanied by signs of systemic toxicity. Radiographs may confirm the presence of gas in the soft tissue, and this demands immediate incision for culture and surgical debridement of necrotic tissue. If gas is absent but there is progressive necrosis or rapidly spreading cellulitis, the same course should be followed. Surgery is almost always essential to treat these infections; necrotic tissue must be debrided since it is inaccessible to antibiotics and the hypoxia must be remedied. There may be a greater role for hyperbaric oxygen in this area in the future.

Mycobacterial Infections

Even before antituberculous chemotherapy was introduced, mycobacterial infections of the hand and wrist were uncommon. From the series reported in the literature, it would appear that tuberculosis of the hand has remained at about the same low incidence over the past 30 to 40 years, but that the newer culturing techniques have permitted the identification of sporadic cases of infections with mycobacteria other than *M. tuberculosis*. The "atypical" mycobacteria were classified by Runyon in 1959 into four major groups on the basis of colonial morphology and pigmentation, but this now appears to be an oversimplification. These ubiquitous environmental bacteria have widely variable pathogenic capabilities and highly variable drug sensitivities. Aside from *M. tuberculosis*, specific chemotherapy must await sensitivity studies, although the general recommendation is the use of at least three drugs. Rifampin and ethambutol are generally combined with isonicotinic acid hydrazide (INH) and others. Minocycline has been found useful in some *M. marinum* cases (Stein, 1982).

The atypical mycobacteria associated with hand infections (Table 135–3) include *M. marinum* (Williams and Riordan, 1973; Cortez and Pankey, 1973; Gunther and associates, 1977; Chow and associates, 1983); *M. kansasii* (Dixon, 1981); *M. gordonae* (Shelley and Folkens, 1984); *M. avium* and *M. intracellulare* (Ellis, 1974); *M. terrae* (Halla, Gould, and Hardin, 1979; Mehta and Hovis, 1983; May and associates, 1983); *M. chelonei* (Stern and Gula, 1986); and *M. fortuitum* (Ariel and associates, 1983).

DIAGNOSIS

The most common symptoms of tuberculosis of the hand and wrist are progressive and painless swelling and stiffness. Pain, paresthesias, and numbness are not uncommon in the later disease stages but are not presenting complaints. In most cases, the hand is the only site of involvement. Pulmonary symptoms or a history of tuberculosis are not customary, and systemic symptoms such as fever or night sweats also are lacking. A striking feature in many series is a major delay between the onset of symptoms and the correct diagnosis (Leung, 1978; Bush and Schneider, 1984). There may be a history of a previous puncture wound as in primary inoculation tuberculosis, described as "prosector's wart" (Hooker, Eberts, and Strickland, 1979), or with *M. marinum*, which appears to be introduced always by direct inoculation. A hematogenous route of spread also may be characteristic of atypical mycobacteria as well as *M. tuberculosis*.

Cutaneous infection with *M. marinum* is the most common mycobacteriosis in the hand and presents as localized, self-limited skin ulceration following skin abrasion in contaminated water, often in swimming pools or tropical fish tanks (Gunther and associates, 1977). The deeper infections were classified originally as dactylitis or tenosynovitis (Robins, 1967), but it has been proposed to abandon this regional classification for a description based on the natural history of the disease (Leung, 1978). The infections are synovial in origin and present as tenosynovitis of the flexor tendons at the wrist, the radial and ulnar bursae, the digital flexor sheaths, and the dorsal wrist compartment. As the disease progresses, the tendon sheaths become increasingly fibrotic and stiff, and tendon rupture may be a late complication. Carpal tunnel syndrome is a common presentation (Lee, 1985), and bone and joint involvement may be secondary to the synovial infection or may arise primarily as tuberculous arthritis or bone lesions of the metacarpals and phalanges (Benkeddache and Gottesman, 1982).

Diagnosis of a mycobacterial hand infection is made from the clinical picture, granulomata on histologic examination of a biopsied portion of synovium, and the presence of acid-fast bacilli on smear. Cultures take six or more weeks to grow and are necessary to differentiate the species of mycobacterium, but the decision to begin therapy is made on a histologic rather than a bacteriologic basis. It is critical to obtain separate cultures for growth of the atypical mycobacteria at 30° to 32° C as well as standard cultures at 37° C. Radiographs show subperiosteal bony prolif-

Table 135–3. Mycobacteria in Hand Infections

Human tuberculosis	*M. tuberculosis*
Group I	
Photochromogens	*M. kansasii*
	M. marinum
Group II	
Scotochromogens	*M. gordonae* ("tap water")
Group III	
Nonphotochromogens	*M. avium*
	M. intracellulare (Battey bacillus)
	M. terrae (radish bacillus)
Group IV	
Rapid growers	*M. chelonei*
	M. fortuitum

eration, diffuse infiltration (honeycombing), and localized destruction, or spina ventosa, in cases with bony involvement (Benkeddache and Gottesman, 1982).

TREATMENT

Exploration and complete surgical synovectomy must be combined with long-term antituberculous medication for curative treatment. Wide exposure and thorough resection of the relatively avascular tuberculous synovium is necessary to prevent recurrence, and bony debridement should be equally vigorous where there is skeletal involvement. Supplementary drug therapy should be continued for 18 to 24 months.

LEPROSY

Leprosy, or Hansen's disease, is caused by *Mycobacterium leprae,* an organism that cannot be cultivated on artificial media but grows only in man and the mouse footpad. A chronic, infectious, granulomatous disease, leprosy occurs only in the colder tissues of the body, i.e., the skin, the peripheral nerves, and the mucous membranes of the mouth and nose. In the peripheral nerves, the target is the Schwann cell, and destruction is caused by an immunologic response rather than the infection itself. The immunologic response is minimal in lepromatous leprosy and maximal in tuberculoid leprosy; this factor, as well as the site, duration, and pathology of nerve involvement, determine the pattern of neurologic injury. In the upper extremity, this may be a motor deficit of the high or low ulnar, median, or radial nerves in any combination. Sensory deficits cause the insensitive, injury-prone hand and may be in a glove pattern, in the distribution of a cutaneous nerve, due to skin involvement, or due to nerve trunk involvement. Other primary symptoms and deformities are due to acute inflammation on an immunologic basis, and include ulnar nerve compression at the elbow, carpal tunnel syndrome, claw hand, intrinsic-plus deformity, pathologic fractures, osteitis, and neurotrophic arthrosis (Brown and Getty, 1979; Pulvertaft, 1983).

The severe secondary deformities of the leprous hand, up to digital loss and mitten-hand, are the result of repeated trauma and ordinary bacterial infections in the denervated hand. Fingers become shortened as recurrent bouts of osteomyelitis and acro-osteolysis lead to progressive bone absorption and soft tissue loss in insensitive digits painlessly injured, infected, or ulcerated with pressure sores.

The drug of choice for the treatment of leprosy is dapsone. It is effective and inexpensive, and is given daily in a 50 to 100 mg dose for at least two years after the disease has been arrested. Surgical management in the hand is limited to draining abscesses and removing necrotic bone in an effort to preserve as much of the remaining tissue as possible. Patient education regarding how to protect the denervated hand is critical, and procedures such as tendon transfer or arthrodesis may improve function (Enna, 1979).

Uncommon Bacterial Infections

Anthrax. Anthrax is an infectious disease of domestic livestock that can be transmitted to man by open wound contact or inhalation. Caused by a gram-positive, aerobic, spore-forming rod, *Bacillus anthracis,* it presents most commonly in a cutaneous form with painless vesicles surrounding an eschar that evolves over 12 to 14 days, sloughs, and slowly heals. Systemic signs include fever, headache, and nausea, and septicemia occasionally develops. Anthrax is treated with penicillin, surgery is not indicated, and disseminated disease is very rare (Wylock, Jaeken, and Deraemaecker, 1983).

Brucellosis. Also known as undulant fever, brucellosis is a systemic febrile illness caused by a gram-negative rod acquired by ingestion, inhalation, or contact of an open abrasion with an infected domestic pig, cow, or goat. Weakness and fever may be accompanied by lymphadenopathy, hepatosplenomegaly, and an acute suppurative monarthritis. Synovial swelling and subarticular erosions characterize the early stages and osteomyelitis can develop. Diagnosis is made by culturing a biopsy specimen and a combination of tetracycline and streptomycin, 2 grams daily for 14 to 21 days, is recommended for treatment (Seal, Oswestry, and Morris, 1974).

Erysipeloid. Erysipeloid of Rosenbach is a disease of fishermen and poultry handlers caused by *Erysipelothrix rhusiopathiae,* a gram-positive, nonmotile bacillus. It presents as localized cutaneous lesions involving the hand, especially the dorsal web spaces, but sparing the fingers distally. A purple-red area of cellulitis, often in a diamond shape with a smooth or vesicular surface, is associated with pruritus, local burning, or pain. This localized form of the disease is usually self-limited and subsides spontaneously; with penicillin treatment, the lesions clear within a week. A diffuse cutaneous form has been described, as has systemic disease with septic arthritis, osteonecrosis, septicemia, and endocarditis. Diagnosed by culture of the infected lesions, penicillin is the drug of choice while culture results are awaited (Barnett and associates, 1983).

Gonorrhea. Gonorrhea is an infectious disease of the human caused by *Neisseria gonorrhoeae,* a gram-negative intracellular diplococcus transmitted by sexual exposure. Extragenital manifestations of the infection can appear during a bacteremic phase with fever, dermatitis, arthritis, and tenosynovitis. In a smaller group of patients, the disseminated form presents as isolated tenosynovitis or septic arthritis. Gonococcal synovitis is a disease of young, sexually active women; 75 per cent of documented cases occur in women and 0.1 to 1.0 per cent of the infected female population become symptomatic.

As in most infectious arthritides, the larger weight-bearing joints are affected most commonly; the wrist and small joints of the hand are not involved as frequently as the knee, shoulder, and ankle. In contrast, tenosynovitis is located in the upper extremity much more often and an antecedent history of blunt trauma or heavy usage has been implicated (Bayer, 1980; Ogiela and Peimer, 1981; Balcomb, 1982; Barrick, 1983). Exploration of the flexor tendon sheath shows a purulent process, which should be treated in the same way as other suppurative processes of the tenosynovium. High dose, intravenous penicillin for seven to ten days remains the chemotherapy of choice. Despite the emergence of resistant genital gonococcal isolates, most organisms isolated from patients with gonococcal arthritis remain penicillin sensitive, and spectinomycin is the current recommendation for resistant organisms (Bayer, 1980).

Pasteurellosis. Many animals can be healthy carriers of *Pasteurella multocida (P. septica),* a small, gram-negative, aerobic, facultatively anaerobic rod found in the mouth and nasal passages. Human infection generally results from the bite or scratch of a household pet: up to 70 per cent of cats and 66 per cent of dogs harbor *P. multocida* in their oral flora. The high incidence of infections following cat scratches is believed to be a reflection of their habitual grooming and transfer of organisms from mouth to paw (Arons, Fernando, and Polayes, 1982). Cellulitis, lymphangitis, tenosynovitis, and osteomyelitis can develop from neglected wounds, and the desirability of prophylactic antibiotic therapy for serious dog and cat bites has been stressed (Lee and Buhr, 1960; Hawkins, 1969). Chemotherapy and surgical management have been discussed earlier under Human and Animal Bites.

Tularemia. An infectious disease of wild animals caused by the gram-negative bacillus *Bacterium tularense,* tularemia is acquired by handling an infected animal or via an arthropod vector, such as a tick bite. It presents as a primary ulceration, commonly on the hand, with regional lymphadenopathy and lymphangitis, fever, chills, and headache. The most useful laboratory test to establish the diagnosis of tularemia is a serial rise in agglutinin titer. Treatment is with streptomycin or gentamicin, continued for about one week after the patient has become afebrile. Surgery is not indicated unless drainage of lymphadenitis is necessary.

Vibrio Hand Infections. Vibrios are gram-negative, facultatively anaerobic rods. One of their subdivisions is the group of noncholera, halophilic organisms found in the marine environment and marine animals and associated with soft tissue infections in man. Minor hand injuries with fish bones or shells can rapidly progress to cellulitis, thrombophlebitis, and vasculitis that lead to intense swelling and necrosis, and rapid onset of septic shock. *Vibrio vulnificus* has been identified in infections causing systemic toxicity within 24 to 48 hours, and vigorous early surgical debridement of areas of cellulitis and fasciotomy to relieve vascular compression is recommended. The relevant *Vibrio* species have been found to be consistently sensitive to cephalothin, chloramphenicol, tetracycline, and the aminoglycosides (Zielinski and Bora, 1984).

FUNGAL INFECTIONS

There are a variety of superficial fungal infections of the hand termed dermatomycoses, or fungal infections of the skin. *Tricho-phyton rubrum* is the most common infecting organism, producing tinea of the skin and onychomycosis of the fingernails. Deep mycoses may involve any tissues of the hand, and although they are relatively uncommon, they present to the hand surgeon sufficiently often to require inclusion in the differential diagnosis of indolent or intractable hand infections.

Deep Fungal Infections

Actinomycosis. Although clinical actinomycosis is usually the result of endogenous infection, most often involving the head and neck, primary infections of the hand do occur after bite injuries, since the organism is part of the normal flora of the mouth (Southwick and Lister, 1979; Rushforth and Eykyn, 1982; Fayman, Schein, and Braun, 1985). *Actinomyces israelii* is an intermediary between bacteria and fungi, existing both as a gram-positive, facultatively anaerobic bacillus and growing in spidery mycelia that cement together to form the characteristic sulfur granules. Trauma, anaerobic conditions, and lowered host resistance predispose to actinomycosis, which presents as a chronic suppurative infection producing abscesses and multiple draining sinuses, and may result in destruction of all local tissues, including bone. The presentation may be delayed for months or a year after the trauma. Treatment involves surgical debridement of the affected area and penicillin continued for at least three months after the infection has cleared.

Candidiasis. *Candida albicans* is a yeast-like fungus causing cutaneous and mucosal infections with erythematous, pruritic, macerated lesions surrounded by white patches. The diagnosis is made by smears demonstrating the budding yeast-mycelial phases, and treatment is with nystatin, clotrimazole, or miconazole topical creams. Chronic paronychia appear to require *C. albicans* in symbiotic balance with lower bowel organisms for their development, and are treated with nystatin cream applied for six to eight weeks, while the hands are protected from water.

Chromomycoses. Dematiacious fungi are pigmented molds that appear yellowish-brown in the infected tissue. All diseases caused by these fungi are classified as chromomycoses and grouped by clinical presen-

tation. Thus, superficial chromomycosis occurs in the keratin layer of the skin; chromoblastomycosis as verrucous, cutaneous lesions; chromomycetoma as suppurative granulomata; and chromohyphomycosis as subcutaneous encapsulated cysts. The last-named entity is of interest to the hand surgeon because the cysts generally appear on the extremities at the site of contact with affected plants, and the cysts may be mistaken for a ganglia, lipomas, or other hand tumors. The clinical behavior is relatively benign compared with that of other fungal diseases, and the lesions are usually solitary, well encapsulated, and slow growing. The disease is more common in immunosuppressed patients. The cysts are treated by complete surgical excision (Monroe and Floyd, 1981).

Coccidioidomycosis. Coccidioidomycosis is caused by *Coccidioides immitis,* a fungus found in the soil of the southwestern United States. It is a systemic mycosis presenting as a respiratory infection with dissemination of the pulmonary infection in fewer than 0.1 per cent of cases, more frequently in the host with compromised defenses. Several cases of extensor or flexor tenosynovitis of the hand have been reported, and surgical synovectomy combined with amphotericin B is the recommended therapy (Iverson and Vistnes, 1973; Gropper, Pisesky and associates, 1983).

Sporotrichosis. Sporotrichosis is a chronic granulomatous fungus infection caused by *Sporothrix schenckii* and usually confined to the cutaneous and subcutaneous tissues of the upper extremity. Found in gardeners, farmers, and fruit pickers exposed to fungus-bearing plants, the infection gains entrance through a minor skin wound, infecting the proximal lymphatics. It presents as a primary, painless, chancre-like hand ulceration with a chain of nodules or ulcers ascending the arm along the lymphatic vessels (Duran and associates, 1957; Becker and Young, 1970). Extracutaneous lesions are less common and include osteomyelitis and tenosynovitis. The bony lesions are multiple, lytic, and destructive and resemble the lesions of tuberculosis (Altner and Turner, 1970). Tenosynovitis with carpal tunnel syndrome and ulnar nerve entrapment has been described, but only one case of tendon sheath involvement in the absence of arthritis has been reported (Atdjian and associates, 1980). Treatment of sporotrichosis is with amphotericin B combined with surgical debridement of the synovium, joints, or bone as needed. The primary cutaneous lesions are not treated surgically.

VIRAL INFECTIONS

Warts

A wart is a hypertrophy of the epidermis caused by the DNA human papillomavirus (HPV), which can be transmitted by direct or indirect contact or by autoinoculation. At present, 22 HPV subtypes have been characterized and the human wart viruses cannot be transmitted to other species. Warts appear at all ages, with the highest incidence at puberty, and common warts usually occur on the hands and fingers. There is a 50 per cent chance that any given wart will involute spontaneously within one year.

Treatment is undertaken both to prevent further transmission of the virus and to effect cosmetic improvement. Warts can be treated successfully with salicylic acid, liquid nitrogen, curettage, or freezing. For multiple recalcitrant common or hand warts, dinitrochlorobenzene (DNCB) or bleomycin has been effective (Rees, 1984). Common warts in the periungual and subungual areas may deform the nail and are tender and painful. They are also difficult to treat, as the nail matrix must be preserved.

Herpes Simplex

This disease is caused by *Herpesvirus hominis,* which is introduced into the skin or mucous membrane with a resultant vesiculopustular eruption that heals spontaneously in a period lasting from a few days to four weeks. In the hand, the herpetic whitlow commonly presents over the distal phalanx where the severe throbbing pain, erythema, and swelling may resemble a pyogenic infection of the pulp space. However, the vesicle formation, absence of pus in the blebs, and a history of exposure to herpes simplex help to distinguish this lesion from a felon or paronychia. The diagnosis can be confirmed by histologic detection of multinucleated giant cells, culture of the virus, or a rise in complement-fixing antibodies after three weeks.

Herpes simplex infections involving the hand have a high incidence in medical or dental personnel in contact with patients' oral secretions, and in children following a primary oral herpes infection (Feder and Long, 1983). Recurrence is not uncommon and treatment has been limited to medical relief and control of symptoms until the self-limited course is completed. The risk of disseminating herpesvirus with an incision and drainage procedure of the finger pulp has been stressed (Louis and Silva, 1979), but unroofing the vesicles or removing the overlying nail to decompress the nail bed has been recommended for pain relief (Fig. 135–21) (Polayes and Arons, 1980).

Other Viral Infections

Orf (ecthyma contagiosum) is a viral infection that most often appears on the hands of persons handling infected sheep. Although the disease is fairly common in man, it is rarely reported in the medical literature since animal handlers recognize the disease and normally do not seek medical advice for it. Vesicular lesions become pustular, drain, and crust—often resembling a smallpox vaccination. Systemic symptoms are rare; the lesions usually heal within five weeks, leaving a residual scar, and one infection confers lifelong immunity.

Milkers' nodule is a pruritic, firm, elevated, red nodule greater than 1 cm in diameter with a central depressed vesicle that occurs on the hands of cattle handlers infected with a paravaccinia virus. The lesions heal spontaneously in five weeks to ten months with persistent hyperpigmentation, and one infection confers lifelong immunity.

ALGAL, PROTOZOAN, AND PARASITIC INFECTIONS

Protothecosis is a rare infection due to algae, and *Prototheca wickerhamii* and *P. zopfii* cause human infections in the extremities. Approximately 20 cases of chronic dermatitis or bursitis of the hand and arm are reported in the literature, and patients with altered host resistance are at greater risk. Treatment involves surgical excision of involved structures. Chemotherapy has not been uniformly successful, although amphotericin B is used in patients with widespread infection (Holcomb and associates, 1981).

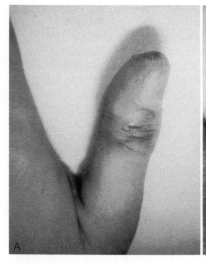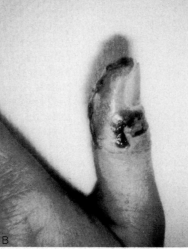

Figure 135–21. An extremely painful vesicular eruption on the thumb of this 27 year old registered nurse was diagnosed as herpesvirus infection (*A*). To provide pain relief, the blebs and vesicles were unroofed without invading the deeper tissues (*B*). The lesions healed spontaneously within three weeks and viral cultures confirmed the diagnosis of herpes simplex infection.

American leishmaniasis is a tropical, protozoan, mucocutaneous infection presenting as a cutaneous ulcer of slow evolution on an exposed area such as the hand or arm. The usual mode of transmission is the sandfly, and the ulcer may clear spontaneously after three to 15 years or recur in the nasopharyngeal region after a latent period, producing destructive lesions known as "espundia." Diagnosed by stain and culture of *Leishmania braziliensis,* the infection is treated with pentavalent antimony (White and Hendricks, 1982).

Parasitic infestation of the upper extremity with cutaneous larva migrans has been described (Belsole and Fenske, 1980). It is caused by nematodal (roundworm) larvae migrating in the epidermis, and is treated with topical thiabendazole. *Onchocerca volvulus* is a filarial nematode residing in the dermis and occasionally migrating via the bloodstream or lymphatics. Tenosynovitis due to this parasite has been reported (Simmons, Van Peteghem, and Trammell, 1980).

REFERENCES

Altner, P. C., and Turner, R. R.: Sporotrichosis of bones and joints: review of the literature and report of six cases. Clin. Orthop., *68*:138, 1970.

Ariel, I., Haas, H., Weinberg, H., Rousso, M., and Rosenmann, E.: *Mycobacterium fortuitum* granulomatous synovitis caused by a dog bite. J. Hand Surg., *8*:342, 1983.

Arons, M. S., Fernando, L., and Polayes, I. M.: *Pasteurella multocida*—the major cause of hand infections following domestic animal bites. J. Hand Surg., *7*:47, 1982.

Atdjian, M., Granda, J. L., Ingberg, H. O., and Kaplan, B. L.: Systemic sporotrichosis polytenosynovitis with median and ulnar nerve entrapment. J.A.M.A., *243*:1841, 1980.

Balcomb, T. V.: Acute gonococcal flexor tenosynovitis in a woman with asymptomatic gonorrhea—case report and literature review. J. Hand Surg., *7*:521, 1982.

Barlow, A. J. E., Chattaway, F. W., Holgate, M. C., and Aldersley, T.: Chronic paronychia. Br. J. Dermatol., *82*:448, 1970.

Barnett, J. H., Estes, S. A., Wirman, J. A., Morris, R. E., and Staneck, J. L.: Erysipeloid. J. Am. Acad. Dermatol., *9*:116, 1983.

Barrick, E. F.: Letter to the editor. J. Hand Surg., *8*:224, 1983.

Bayer, A. S.: Gonococcal arthritis syndromes: an update on diagnosis and management. Postgrad. Med., *67*:200, 1980.

Becker, F. T., and Young, H. R.: Sporotrichosis: a report of 21 cases. Minn. Med., *53*:851, 1970.

Bell, M. S.: The changing pattern of pyogenic infections of the hand. Hand, *8*:298, 1976.

Belsole, R., and Fenske, N.: Cutaneous larva migrans in the upper extremity. J. Hand Surg., *5*:178, 1980.

Benkeddache, Y., and Gottesman, H.: Skeletal tuberculosis of the wrist and hand: a study of 27 cases. J. Hand Surg., *7*:593, 1982.

Besser, M. I. B.: Digital flexor tendon irrigation. Hand, *8*:72, 1976.

Bilos, Z. J., Kucharchuk, A., and Metzger, W.: *Eikenella corrodens* in human bites. Clin. Orthop., *134*:320, 1978.

Bolton, H., Fowler, P. J., and Jepson, R. P.: Natural history and treatment of pulp space infection and osteomyelitis of the terminal phalanx. J. Bone Joint Surg., *31B*:499, 1949.

Boyce, F. F.: Human bites: an analysis of 90 (chiefly delayed and late) cases from Charity Hospital of Louisiana at New Orleans. South. Med. J., *35*:631, 1942.

Brook, I.: Bacteriologic study of paronychia in children. Am. J. Surg., *141*:703, 1981.

Brown, H., and Getty, P.: Leprosy and thumb reconstruction by opponensplasty or phalangizing the first metacarpal. J. Hand Surg., *4*:432, 1979.

Bunnell, S.: *Bunnell's Surgery of the Hand.* 5th Ed. Philadelphia, J. B. Lippincott Company, 1970, pp. 613–642.

Bush, D. C., and Schneider, L. H.: Tuberculosis of the hand and wrist. J. Hand Surg., 9A:391, 1984.

Carter, S. J., Burman, S. O., and Mersheimer, W. L.: Treatment of digital tenosynovitis by irrigation with peroxide and oxytetracycline. Ann. Surg., 163:645, 1966.

Carter, S. J., and Mersheimer, W. L.: Infections of the hand. Orthop. Clin. North Am., 1:455, 1970.

Chow, S. P., Stroebel, A. B., Lau, J. H. K., and Collins, R. J.: Mycobacterium marinum infection of the hand involving deep structures. J. Hand Surg., 8:568, 1983.

Chuinard, R. G., and D'Ambrosia, R. D.: Human bite infections of the hand. J. Bone Joint Surg., 59A:416, 1977.

Cortez, L. M., and Pankey, G. A.: Mycobacterium marinum infections of the hand. J. Bone Joint Surg., 55A:363, 1973.

Dhaliwal, A. S., and Garnes, A. L.: Tenosynovitis in drug addicts. J. Hand Surg., 7:626, 1982.

Dixon, J. H.: Non-tuberculous mycobacterial infection of the tendon sheaths in the hand. J. Bone Joint Surg., 63B:542, 1981.

Duran, R. J., Coventry, M. B., Weed, L. A., and Kierland, R. R.: Sporotrichosis: a report of twenty-three cases in the upper extremity. J. Bone Joint Surg., 39A:1330, 1957.

Eaton, R. G., and Butsch, D. P.: Antibiotic guidelines for hand infections. Surg. Gynecol. Obstet., 130:119, 1970.

Ellis, W.: Multiple bone lesions caused by Avian-Battey mycobacteria. J. Bone Joint Surg., 56B:323, 1974.

Enna, C. D.: Skeletal deformities of the denervated hand in Hansen's disease. J. Hand Surg., 4:227, 1979.

Fayman, M., Schein, M., and Braun, S.: A foreign body related actinomycosis of a finger. J. Hand Surg., 10A:411, 1985.

Feder, H. M., and Long, S. S.: Herpetic whitlow: epidemiology, clinical characteristics, diagnosis, and treatment. Am. J. Dis. Child., 137:861, 1983.

Feingold, D. S.: Gangrenous and crepitant cellulitis. J. Am. Acad. Dermatol., 6:289, 1982.

Fitzgerald, R. H., Cooney, W. P., Washington, J. A., VanScoy, R. E., Linscheid, R. L., and Dobyns, J. H.: Bacterial colonization of mutilating hand injuries and its treatment. J. Hand Surg., 2:85, 1977.

Flynn, J. E.: The grave infections of the hand. In Flynn, J. E. (Ed.): Hand Surgery. Vol. 2. Baltimore, Williams & Wilkins Company, 1982, pp. 688–706.

Glass, K. D.: Factors related to the resolution of treated hand infections. J. Hand Surg., 7:388, 1982.

Goldstein, E. J. C., Barones, M. F., and Miller, T. A.: Eikenella corrodens in hand infections. J. Hand Surg., 8:563, 1983.

Goldstein, E. J. C., Citron, D. M., and Finegold, S. M.: Dog bite wounds and infection: a prospective clinical study. Ann. Emerg. Med., 9:508, 1980.

Goldstein, E. J. C., Citron, D. M., Wield, B., Blachman, U., Sutter, V. L., et al.: Bacteriology of human and animal bite wounds. J. Clin. Microbiol., 8:667, 1978a.

Goldstein, E. J. C., Miller, T. A., Citron, D. M., and Finegold, S. M.: Infections following clenched-fist injury: a new perspective. J. Hand Surg., 3:455, 1978b.

Gropper, P. T., Pisesky, W. A., Bowen, V., and Clement, P. B.: Flexor tenosynovitis caused by Coccidioides immitis. J. Hand Surg., 8:344, 1983.

Grossman, J. A. I., Adams, J. P., and Kunec, J.: Prophylactic antibiotics in simple hand lacerations. J.A.M.A., 245:1055, 1981.

Guba, A. M., Mulliken, J. B., and Hoopes, J. E.: The selection of antibiotics for human bites of the hand. Plast. Reconstr. Surg., 56:538, 1975.

Gunther, S. F., Elliott, R. C., Brand, R. L., and Adams, J. P.: Experience with atypical mycobacterial infection in the deep structures of the hand. J. Hand Surg., 2:90, 1977.

Halla, J. T., Gould, J. S., and Hardin, J. G.: Chronic tenosynovial hand infection from Mycobacterium terrae. Arthritis Rheum., 22:1386, 1979.

Handmaker, H.: Acute hematogenous osteomyelitis: has the bone scan betrayed us? Radiology, 135:787, 1980.

Hart, C. A., Godfrey, V. M., Woodrow, J. C., and Percival, A.: Septic arthritis due to Bacteroides fragilis in a wrist affected by rheumatoid arthritis. Ann. Rheum. Dis., 41:623, 1982.

Hawkins, L. G.: Local Pasteurella multocida infections. J. Bone Joint Surg., 51A:801, 1969.

Holcomb, H. S., Behrens, F., Winn, W. C., Hughes, J. M., and McCue, F. C.: Prototheca wickerhamii—an alga infecting the hand. J. Hand Surg., 6:595, 1981.

Hooker, R. P., Eberts, T. J., and Strickland, J. A.: Primary inoculation tuberculosis. J. Hand Surg., 4:270, 1979.

Iverson, R. E., and Vistnes, L. M.: Coccidioidomycosis tenosynovitis in the hand. J. Bone Joint Surg., 55A:413, 1973.

Johnson, S. M., and Pankey, G. A.: Eikenella corrodens osteomyelitis, arthritis, and cellulitis of the hand. South. Med. J., 69:535, 1976.

Kanavel, A. B.: An anatomical, experimental, and clinical study of acute phlegmons of the hand. Surg. Gynecol. Obstet., 1:221, 1905.

Kanavel, A. B.: Infections of the Hand—A Guide to the Surgical Treatment of Acute and Chronic Suppurative Processes in the Fingers, Hand and Forearm. Philadelphia, Lea & Febiger, 1912.

Kilgore, E. S.: Hand infections. J. Hand Surg., 8:723, 1983.

Kilgore, E. S., Brown, L. G., Newmeyer, W. L., Graham, W. P., III, and Davis, T. S.: Treatment of felons. Am. J. Surg., 130:194, 1975.

Knutson, E. L., Levy, C. S., Curtin, J. A., Allen, H., and Gunther, S. F.: Hematogenous Serratia marcescens osteomyelitis of the carpal scaphoid from an indwelling radial artery catheter. J. Hand Surg., 7:395, 1982.

Koch, S. L.: Felons, acute lymphangitis and tendon sheath infections. J.A.M.A., 92:1171, 1929.

Koch, S. L.: Acute rapidly spreading infections following trivial injuries of the hand. Surg. Gynecol. Obstet., 59:277, 1934.

Koch, S. L.: Osteomyelitis of the bones of the hand. Surg. Gynecol. Obstet., 64:1, 1937.

Lee, K. E.: Tuberculosis presenting as carpal tunnel syndrome. J. Hand Surg., 10A:242, 1985.

Lee, M. L. H., and Buhr, A. J.: Dog-bites and local infection with Pasteurella septica. Br. Med. J., 1:169, 1960.

Leung, P. C.: Tuberculosis of the hand. Hand, 10:285, 1978.

Linscheid, R. L., and Dobyns, J. H.: Common and uncommon infections of the hand. Orthop. Clin. North Am., 6:1063, 1975.

Louis, D. S., and Silva, J.: Herpetic whitlow: herpetic infections of the digits. J. Hand Surg., 4:90, 1979.

Lowden, T. G.: Infection of the digital pulp space. Lancet, 1:196, 1951.

Lowden, T. G.: Acute infections of interphalangeal joints. In Stack, H. G., and Bolton, H. (Eds.): The British

Society for Surgery of the Hand. Brentwood, Essex, England, Westbury Press, 1975, pp. 305–306.

Mandel, M. A.: Immune competence and diabetes mellitus: pyogenic human hand infections. J. Hand Surg., 3:458, 1978.

Mann, R. J., Hoffeld, T. A., and Farmer, B.: Human bites of the hand: twenty years of experience. J. Hand Surg., 2:97, 1977.

Mann, R. J., and Peacock, J. M.: Hand infections in patients with diabetes mellitus. J. Trauma, 17:376, 1977.

Mason, M. L., and Koch, S. L.: Human bite infections of the hand. Surg. Gynecol. Obstet., 51:591, 1930.

Mass, D. P., Newmeyer, W. L., and Kilgore, E. S.: "Seal finger." J. Hand Surg., 6:610, 1981.

May, D. C., Kutz, J. E., Howell, R. S., Raff, M. J., and Melo, J. C.: Mycobacterium terrae tenosynovitis: chronic infection in a previously healthy individual. South. Med. J., 76:1445, 1983.

McConnell, C. M., and Neale, H. W.: Two-year review of hand infections at a municipal hospital. Am. Surg., 45:643, 1979.

McDonald, I.: Eikenella corrodens infection of the hand. Hand, 11:224, 1979.

McKay, D., Pascarelli, E. F., and Eaton, R. G.: Infections and sloughs in the hands in drug addicts. J. Bone Joint Surg., 55A:741, 1973.

Mehta, J. B., and Hovis, W. M.: Tenosynovitis of the forearm due to Mycobacterium terrae (radish bacillus). South. Med. J., 76:1433, 1983.

Michaeli, D.: Osteomyelitis with special reference to the hand. Prog. Surg., 16:38, 1978.

Mock, H. E.: Treatment of hand infections from an economic viewpoint. Surg. Gynecol. Obstet., 21:481, 1915.

Monroe, P. W., and Floyd, W. E., Jr.: Chromohyphomycosis of the hand due to Exophiala jeanselmei (Phialophora jeanselmei, Phialophora gougerotii)—case report and review. J. Hand Surg., 6:370, 1981.

Neimkin, R. J., and Jupiter, J. B.: Metastatic nontraumatic Clostridium septicum osteomyelitis. J. Hand Surg., 10A:281–284, 1985.

Neviaser, R. J.: Closed tendon sheath irrigation for pyogenic flexor tenosynovitis. J. Hand Surg., 3:462, 1978.

Neviaser, R. J.: Infections. In Green, D. P. (Ed.): Operative Hand Surgery. New York, Churchill Livingstone, 1982, pp. 771–791.

Nicholls, R. J.: Initial choice of antibiotic treatment for pyogenic hand infections. Lancet, 1:225, 1973.

Ogiela, D. M., and Peimer, C. A.: Acute gonococcal flexor tenosynovitis—case report and literature review. J. Hand Surg., 6:470, 1981.

Palmieri, T. J., and Schwartz, G. B.: The ambulatory treatment of infections of the hand. Orthop. Rev., 14:97, 1985.

Peeples, E., Boswick, J. A., and Scott, F. A.: Wounds of the hand contaminated by human or animal saliva. J. Trauma, 20:383, 1980.

Polayes, I. M., and Arons, M. S.: The treatment of hepetic whitlow—a new surgical concept. Plast. Reconstr. Surg., 65:811, 1980.

Pollen, A. G.: Acute infection of the tendon sheaths. Hand, 6:21, 1974.

Pulvertaft, R. G.: Report of the committee on paralytic diseases including leprosy. J. Hand Surg., 8:745, 1983.

Rangarathnam, C. S., and Linscheid, R. L.: Infected mucous cyst of the finger. J. Hand Surg., 9A:245, 1984.

Rashkoff, E. S., Burkhalter, W. E., and Mann, R. J.: Septic arthritis of the wrist. J. Bone Joint Surg., 65A:824, 1983.

Rees, R. B.: Treatment of warts. Semin. Dermatol., 3:130, 1984.

Resnick, D.: Osteomyelitis and septic arthritis complicating hand injuries and infections: pathogenesis of roentgenographic abnormalities. J. Can. Assoc. Radiol., 27:21, 1976.

Roberts, A. H. N., and Teddy, P. J.: A prospective trial of prophylactic antibiotics in hand lacerations. Br. J. Surg., 64:394, 1977.

Robins, R. H. C.: Infections of the hand: a review based on 1,000 consecutive cases. J. Bone Joint Surg., 34B:567, 1952.

Robins, R. H. C.: Tuberculosis of the wrist and hand. Br. J. Surg., 54:211, 1967.

Robson, M. C., Schmidt, D., and Heggers, J. P.: Cefamandole therapy in hand infections. J. Hand Surg., 8:560, 1983.

Runyon, E. H.: Anonymous mycobacteria in pulmonary disease. Med. Clin. North Am., 43:273, 1959.

Rushforth, G. F., and Eykyn, S. J.: Actinomycosis of the hand. Hand, 14:194, 1982.

Schecter, W., Meyer, A., Schecter, G., Giuliano, A., Newmeyer, W., and Kilgore, E.: Necrotizing fasciitis of the upper extremity. J. Hand Surg., 7:15, 1982.

Seal, P. V., and Morris, C. A.: Brucellosis of the carpus: report of a case. J. Bone Joint Surg., 56B:327, 1974.

Septimus, E. J., and Musher, D. M.: Osteomyelitis: recent clinical and laboratory aspects. Orthop. Clin. North Am., 10:347, 1979.

Shelley, W. B., and Folkens, A. T.: Mycobacterium gordonae infection of the hand. Arch. Dermatol., 120:1064, 1984.

Shields, C., Patzakis, M. J., Meyers, M. H., and Harvey, J. P.: Hand infections secondary to human bites. J. Trauma, 15:235, 1975.

Simmons, E. H., Van Peteghem, K., and Trammell, T. R.: Onchocerciasis of the flexor compartment of the forearm: a case report. J. Hand Surg., 5:502, 1980.

Smith, R. M., and Manges, W. F.: Roentgen treatment of infection from human bite. Am. J. Roentgenol., 38:720, 1937.

Southwick, G. J., and Lister, G. D.: Actinomycosis of the hand: a case report. J. Hand Surg., 4:360, 1979.

Stein, S. C.: Mycobacteria and the skin. Int. J. Dermatol., 21:82, 1982.

Stern, P. J., and Gula, D. C.: Mycobacterium chelonei tenosynovitis of the hand: a case report. J. Hand Surg., 11A:596, 1986.

Stern, P. J., Staneck, J. L., McDonough, J. J., Neale, H. W., and Tyler, G.: Established hand infections: a controlled prospective study. J. Hand Surg., 8:553, 1983.

Waldvogel, F. A., and Vasey, H.: Osteomyelitis: the past decade. N. Engl. J. Med., 303:360, 1980.

Weckesser, E. C.: Treatment of hand infections. Am. Fam. Physician, 21:145, 1980.

Welch, C. E.: Human bite infections of the hand. N. Engl. J. Med., 215:901, 1936.

White, S. W., and Hendricks, L. D.: American cutaneous leishmaniasis. Int. J. Dermatol., 21:86, 1982.

Williams, C. S., and Riordan, D. C.: Mycobacterium marinum (atypical acid-fast bacillus) infections of the hand. J. Bone Joint Surg., 55A:1042, 1973.

Wylock, P., Jaeken, R., and Deraemaecker, R.: Anthrax of the hand: case report. J. Hand Surg., 8:576, 1983.

Zielinski, C. J., and Bora, F. W.: Vibrio hand infections: a case report and review of the literature. J. Hand Surg., 9A:754, 1984.

Index

Index

Periorbital fat, compartmentalization of, 2323, *2325*
Periosteoplasty, 2756
Periosteum, blood vessels of, 600–602, *601, 602*
Peripheral nerve end organs, sensory receptors of, 646–655
Peripheral nerve grafting, historical background of, 630–632
Peripheral nerves
  central plasticity of, 669
  classification of fibers of, 634, 634*t*
  composition of, *632*, 632–634, *633*
    axoplasmic transport in, 637–638, *639*
    cellular morphology in, 634–637, *635*
    connective tissue elements in, 642–644, *643*
    intraneural architecture patterns in, *643*, 644
    Schwann cell in, 640–642
  conduction in, 638–640
  electrodiagnosis of, 670–675
  injury of, 655–657, *656*
    cause of, 664
    classification of, *656*, 656–657
    level of, 663–664
    timing of repair and, 676–680
  motor end organs and, 655
  neuroma formation and, 669–670
  of hand, physiology of, 4762–4764
  reconstruction of, 675–685, *680, 682*
    by nerve grafting, *682*, 682–683
    epineurium, *680*, 680–681
    nerve bed and, 683
    perineurium or fascicular repair as, *680*, 681
    postoperative care for, 684–685
    tension and, 681–682, *682*
    timing of, 676
    vascularized nerve grafts for, 683–684
  regeneration of
    in distal axon, 660
    in neuron, 657–660, *658, 659*
    in proximal axon, 657–660, *658, 659*
    influencing factors for, 661–666
    relationship to degree of injury in, 660–661
  reinnervation of, 666–669
  repair of
    delay in, 662
    techniques for, *4764–4768*
  structure of, 4314–4315
  vascular supply of, 644–646, *645*
Peripheral nervous system, embryologic development of, in head, 2473–2475, *2474, 2476–2477, 2477*
Persantine, platelet function and, 458
Pes anserinus, 2240
PET (polyethylene terephthalate)
  for alloplastic implants, 708*t*, 712, *713*
  in suture materials, for alloplastic implants, 719*t*, 721
Petit's triangle, 3771
Petrosectomy
  partial, 3401, *3402*
  total, 3401, *3403–3404*, 3404
Peyronie's disease
  Dupuytren's disease and, 5055
  etiology of, 4183–4184
  evaluation of, 4184
  general considerations for, 4185–4187
  penile curvatures in, 4175–4176
  surgical procedure for, 4185, *4185, 4186*
  treatment options for, 4184

Pfeiffer's syndrome, clinical and radiographic findings in, 3023, *3023, 3024*
PGA (polyglycolic acid), in suture materials, for alloplastic implants, 719*t*, 720–721
pH, tissue, as index of flap perfusion, 319*t*, 320
Phalanx
  distal, fractures of, *4604*, 4604–4605
  middle, fractures of, 4602, *4603*, 4604
  proximal, fractures of, 4601–4602, *4602*
  transverse absence of, 5255, 5257
Phalloplasty, 4242–4243
Phallus, reconstruction of, 4237–4239, *4238*
Phantom limbs, 127, 133, 4331
Pharyngeal abscesses, lateral, in pediatric patients, 3178
Pharyngeal constrictor muscles, superior, 2727–2729
Pharyngeal flap
  for velopharyngeal incompetence, operative technique for, 2915, 2917, *2917*
  for velopharyngeal incompetence correction, 2908
  postoperative velopharyngeal incompetence and, 2905–2906
Pharyngeal glands, embryologic development of, 2478, *2479*
Pharyngoplasty
  Hynes procedure for, 2910, *2911, 2912*
  postoperative velopharyngeal incompetence and, 2905–2906
Pharynx
  anatomy of, 3416, *3416*
  cancers of, management of, 3455–3462, *3456, 3458, 3461, 3462*
  walls of
    cancers of, 3457–3458, *3458*
    posterior, augmentation of, for correction of velopharyngeal incompetence, 2908, 2910, *2910–2912*
PHEMA (polyhydroxyethylmethacrylate), 723, *723*
Phenol
  application to skin. *See* Chemical peeling.
  for chemical peeling, 756–757
  full face technique for, 761–764, *762–766*
Phenoxybenzamine (Dibenzyline), 315, 4910, 5021
Phentolamine (Regitine), 315, 5019–5020, 5442
Phenytoin (Dilantin), 2533
Philtrum
  abnormalities of, from bilateral cleft lip repair, correction of, 2851, *2852*, 2853
  reconstruction of, 2185–2186, *2186*, 2789–2790, *2789, 2790*
Phocomelia, intercalated, 5242–5243, *5243, 5244*, 5245
Phosphorus burns, 5439
Photoelectric tests, for flap perfusion assessment, 319*t*, 320–321
Photographer, medical, role of, 37–38
Photographic records, mock surgery on, 1209, *1210*
Photography
  camera for, 38
  color transparencies, vs. black and white print, 38
  lighting for, 38
  of soft tissue wounds in face, 901
  patient positioning for, 38
  preoperative
    for corrective rhinoplasty, 1809–1810, *1810, 1811*
    for facialplasty, 2367
  standards for comparison of, 36–37
  studio for, 38

Trauma *(Continued)*
   malignant melanoma and, 3637
Traumatic segmental arterial spasm (TSAS), 5016–5017
Treacher Collins syndrome
   auricular deformities in, 3120
   bilateral microtia, 2108
   causation of, heredity and, 2931
   classification of, 3105–3106
   clinical features of, 3105t, 3105–3106
   congenital aural atresia and, 2148
   craniofacial skeletal features of, 3111, *3111*
   description of, *2956*, 2956–2957
   differential diagnosis of, 3054
   ear deformities and, 2098
   embryologic development of, 2475, *2476–2477*, 2491–2492
   embryology of, 2455
   genetic considerations in, 3106, 3109
   historical aspects of, 3101, *3104*, 3104–3105
   incomplete form of, 2952, *2953*
   pathogenesis of, 2547, 3109–3110, *3110*
   phenotypic expression of, variations in, 3101, *3102, 3103*
   racial groups and, 3106, *3109*
   radiographic features of, 3105–3106, 3106t, *3107*
   sideburns, anterior placed in, 3119, 3123
   treatment of, 3110–3111
      for eyelid deformities, 3113, 3116–3117, *3116, 3117*
      for mandibular hypoplasia, *3118*, 3119
      for maxillary and orbital deficiencies, 3111–3113, *3111, 3112, 3314–3315*
      using multiple operations, *3120–3122*, 3123
Trefoil flap technique, for columella lengthening, 2856–2857, *2858*
Trench foot (immersion foot), 852
Triamcinolone, intralesional injection of
   for abnormal scars, 738
   for keloids, 739, *739*
Triangular fibrocartilage complex (TFCC), rupture of, in rheumatoid arthritis, 4713, *4713*
Triazene, craniofacial cleft formation and, 2929
Triazolam (Halcion), 140
Tricalcium phosphate, for alloplastic implants, 716–717
Trichiasis, 1737, 1742
Trichion, 28, *28*, 1190
Trichloroacetic acid, for chemical peeling, 754–756
Trichoepitheliomas
   clinical presentation of, 3577–3578, *3578*
   dermabrasion of, 777
   laser therapy for, 3671
Trigeminal nerve, injury of, 906
Trigger points, in myofascial dysfunction, 4894–4896
Trigger thumb, congenital, 5116, *5116*
Trigonocephaly
   description of, 1546
   orbital hypotelorism and, 3005
   visual abnormalities in, 3025–3026
Trigonocephaly-metopic synostosis, clinical and radiographic findings in, 3015, *3016*
Triiodothyronine, 798
Tripier flap, 1703, *1704*, 1707
   modified, 2217
Triquetrum, fractures of, 4597
Trismus
   from maxillary surgery, 3333
   intramuscular pathology of, 1479

Trisomy 13 syndrome, 84, *87*
Trisomy 13–15 syndrome, 3234
Trisomy 18 syndrome, 79
Trisomy 21 syndrome, 79
Trochanter, pressure sores of, 3826–3827, *3826, 3828,* 3827t
Trocinate (thiphenamil hydrochloride), 168
Trophic influences, in peripheral nerve regeneration, 664–666
Tropocollagen, 171
Trunk
   cutaneous arteries of, 362–363, 367–368, *364–366*
   tissue expansion for, *502*, 502–503
TSAS (traumatic segmental arterial spasm), 5016–5017
Tube flap, 277, *277*
   development of, 20
   for neck resurfacing, 2200
Tularemia, 5551
Turban tumor, 3577, *3577*
Turbinates, 1798, 1809
Turner's syndrome, 79
   congenital neck webbing in, 2076–2077
   surgical correction of, 2077–2078, *2079–2084*
Turnover flaps, for cheek reconstruction, 2049
Turricephaly–multiple suture synostosis, clinical and radiographic findings in, 3018, *3018*
Twin-screw Morris biphase appliance, for mandibular fixation, 3500, *3503–3507*, 3504–3505, 3507
Two-point discrimination test, 4818, *4818*, 4859, *4860*, 4862, 4978–4979, *4979*

UHMWPE (ultra high molecular weight polyethylene), 711–712
Ulcers
   in hemangiomas, 3206, *3206*
   in lower extremity, 4076–4077, *4078, 4079*
   radiation injury, 844–846, *845, 846*
Ullrich-Noonan syndrome. *See* Turner's syndrome.
Ulna
   distal
      dislocations of, 4639–4640, *4640*
      fractures of, 4638–4639, *4639*
      subluxations of, 4639–4640
   duplication of, 5133
   longitudinal absence deformities of, 5271, 5273
      classification of, 5273–5274, *5274*
      clinical presentations of, 5274–5276, *5276*
      treatment of, 5276–5277, 5279, *5276–5278*
      vs. radial longitudinal absence deformities, 5273t
Ulnar artery, thrombosis of, 452, 5006
Ulnar bursae, infection of, 5543, *5543*
Ulnar carpal tunnel, 4281, *4281*
Ulnar dimelia, 5133, 5356, 5358, 5361–5362, *5357, 5359–5361*
Ulnar nerve
   anatomy of, 4278, 4280, *4279*, 4759
   dorsal branch of, 4280, *4280*
   entrapment of, 679
   entrapment syndrome of, in rheumatoid arthritis, 4704–4705
   injuries of, with brachial plexus injuries, 4802
   regional block of, *4322*, 4323
Ulnar nerve palsy
   distal effects of, 4949, *4949*
   high, tendon transfer for, 4961–4963, *4962*